New Perspectives in Prostate Cancer

New Perspectives in Prostate Cancer

Edited by

Arie Belldegrun MD FACS

Professor of Urology;
Chief, Division of Urologic Oncology;
Director, Urologic Research, Department of Urology,
UCLA School of Medicine,
Los Angeles, USA

Roger S. Kirby MA MD FRCS (Urol) FEBU

Consultant Urologist, St George's Hospital,
London, UK

R. T. D. Oliver MD FRCP

Sir Maxwell Joseph Professor of Medical Oncology,
St. Bartholomew's Hospital,
London, UK

I S I S
MEDICAL
MEDIA

Oxford

British Library Cataloguing in Publication Data.
A catalogue record for this title is available from
the British Library

ISBN 1899066 89 6

Belldegrun, A (Arie)
New Perspectives in Prostate Cancer
Arie Belldegrun, Roger Kirby, Tim Oliver (eds)

Always refer to the manufacturer's Prescribing
Information before prescribing drugs cited in this book.

Additional technical writing and editorial services provided by
Robert Reford (Oxford) and Heather Russell (Newcastle-upon-Tyne)

Typeset by
Creative Associates Ltd., Oxford, UK

Printed by
Dah Hua Printing Press Co. Ltd, Hong Kong

Distributed in the USA by
Mosby-Year Book, Inc, 11830 Westline Industrial Drive
St Louis MO63145, USA

Distributed in the rest of the world by
Oxford University Press, Saxon Way West, Corby
Northamptonshire NN18 9ES, UK

Contents

List of contributors

Jan Adolfsson MD PhD
Associate Professor of Urology, Karolinska Institute, Department of Urology, Huddinge University Hospital, S-141 86 Huddinge, Sweden

Lee F. Allen MD PhD
Departments of Medicine (Division of Hematology/Oncology) and Oncological Sciences (Division of Developmental Therapeutics), Huntsman Cancer Institute, University of Utah Health Sciences Center, Bldg.# 570, Room 410-B, Salt Lake City, Utah 84112, USA

Arie S. Belldegrun MD
Professor, Room 66-118, Department of Urology, UCLA Medical Centre Box 951738, 10833 Le Cont Ave, Los Angeles, CA 90095-1738, USA

George R. P. Blackledge MB BChir MD PhD FRCP
Medical Research and Communications Group, Zeneca Pharmaceuticals, Mereside, Alderley Park, Macclesfield, Cheshire, SK10 4TG, UK

Rosemary A. Blades MD FRCS
Senior Registrar in Urology, Hope Hospital, Stott Lane, Salford, Manchester, UK

Walter Bodmer
Hertford College, Oxford, OX1 3BW, UK

Markella Boudioni
Research Officer, BACUP, 3 Bath Place, Rivington Street, London, EC2A 3JR, UK

Stephen G. Bown MD FRCP
Director, National Medical Laser Centre, Department of Surgery, University College London Medical School, Charles Bell House, 67–73, Riding House Street, London, W1N 7LD, UK

Michael K. Brawer MD
VA Puget Sound Health Care System, Section of Urology (112UR), 1660 South Columbian Way, Seattle, Washington 98108, USA

Albert O. Brinkmann PhD
Associate Professor, Department of Endocrinology and Reproduction, Erasmus University Rotterdam, P.O. Box 1738, Rotterdam 3000 DR, The Netherlands

Nicholas Bruchovsky MD PhD FRCPC
Professor of Medicine, University of British Columbia; Clinical Professor of Medicine, University of Washington; Head, Department of Cancer Endocrinology, BC Cancer Agency, Vancouver Cancer Center, 600 West 10th Avenue, Vancouver, British Columbia V5Z 4E6, Canada

Lisa Cannon-Albright
Division of Genetic Epidemiology, Department of Medical Informatics,University of Utah School of Medicine, University of Utah, 391 Chipeta Way–Suite D2, Salt Lake City, Utah 84108, USA

Stanley S.-C. Chang MD PhD
Consultant Urologist and Chairman, Faculty of Medicine, Tzu-Chi College of Medicine, Taiwan

Timothy J. Christmas MD FRCS (Urol) FEBU
Consultant Urologist, Department of Urology, Charing Cross Hospital, Fulham Palace Road, London, W6 8RF, UK

A. Collins
Research Associate, Department of Surgery, The Medical School, University of Newcastle-upon-Tyne, Framlington Place, Newcastle-upon-Tyne, NE2 4HH, UK

E. David Crawford
Professor and Chairman, Colorado University, Health Sciences Center, Campus Box C319, Denver, CO 80262, USA

Angus G. Dalgleish MD FRCAPath FRCAP FRCP
Foundation Chair of Oncology and Visiting Professor at the Institute of Cancer Research, Division of Oncology, St. George's Hospital Medical School, Cranmer Terrace, London, SW17 0RE, London, UK

David P. Dearnaley MA MD MRCP FRCR
Bob Champion Senior Lecturer and Head of Urology Unit, Academic Radiotherapy & Oncology, The Royal Marsden NHS Trust and Institute of Cancer Research, Downs Road, Sutton, Surrey, SM2 5PT, UK

Jean B. deKernion MD
Chairman, Department of Urology, The Fran and Ray Stark Professor of Urology, UCLA School of Medicine, 10833 Le Conte Avenue, Los Angeles, CA 90095-1738, USA

Alan H. Drummond
British Biotech Pharmaceuticals Ltd., Watlington Road, Cowley, Oxford, OX4 5LY, UK

Nicholas J. R. George MD FRCS
Senior Lecturer in Urology, Department of Urology, University Hospital of South Manchester, Nell Lane, West Didsbury, Manchester, M20 8LR, UK

Mitchell H. Gold MD
Resident, Department of Urology, University of Washington, 1660 So. Columbia Street, MS: 112UR, Seattle, WA 98108, USA

S. Larry Goldenberg MD
Consultant Urologist, Associate Professor, University of British Columbia, Vancouver, British Columbia

Martin Gleave MD
Consultant Urologist, Assistant Professor, University of British Columbia; Assistant Clinical Professor, University of Washington, Seattle, Washington, USA

Richard Hanover MD JD FCLM
Boro Medical, P.C., 147 East 26th Street, New York, NY 10010, USA

David Hrouda FRCS
Urology Research Fellow, Department of Urology, St. George's Hospital, Blackshaw Road, London, SW17 0QT, UK

Elijah O. Kehinde MBBS FRCS(Eng) FMCS (Nig) Dip Urol (Lond)
Assistant Professor of Urological Surgery, Consultant Urological Surgeon, Department of Urological Surgery, College of Medicine, Sultan Quaboos University P.O. Box 35, Al Khod, Muscat 123,Oman

W. Kevin Kelly DO
Genitourinary Oncology Service, Division of Solid Tumor Oncology, Department of Medicine, Memorial Sloan Kettering, 1275 York Avenue, New York City, NY 10021, USA

Michael G. Kirby MB BS LRCP MRCS MRCP
The Surgery, Nevells Road, Letchworth, Hertfordshire, SG6 4TS, UK

Roger S. Kirby
Consultant Urologist, 95 Harley Street, London W1N 1DF and St. George's Hospital, Blackshaw Road, London, SW17 0QT, UK

David Kirk DM FRCS
Consultant Urologist, Honorary Professor, Department of Urology, Gartnavel General Hospital, 1053 Great Western Road, Glasgow, G12 OYN, UK

Fernand Labrie MD PhD FRCP(c)
Director of Research, CHUL Research Center, Laval University Medical Center, 2705 Laurier Boulevard, Sainte-Foy, Québec, G1V 4G2, Canada

Mark S. Litwin MD MPH FACS
Departments of Urology and Health Services, UCLA Schools of Medicine and Public Health, Box 951738, Los Angeles, CA 90095-1738, USA

Philip O. Livingston MD
Immunology Service, Department of Medicine, Memorial Sloan-Kettering Cancer Center, 1275 York Avenue, New York City, NY 10021, USA

L. J. McWilliam FRCPath
Lecturer/Consultant Histopathologist, University Hospital of South Manchester, Nell Lane, West Didsbury, Manchester, M20 8LR, UK

John Mendelsohn MD
Genitourinary Oncology Service, Division of Solid Tumor Oncology, M.D. Anderson Cancer Center, Holcombe Boulevard, Box 91, Houston, Texas 77030, USA

Kiarash Michel MD
Department of Urology, UCLA School of Medicine, Clark Urological Centre, Box 951738, Los Angeles, CA 90095-1738, USA

Michael S. Morton PhD
Clinical Biochemist, Tenovus Cancer Research Centre, University of Wales College of Medicine, Tenovus Cancer Research Centre, Tenovus Building, Heath Park, Cardiff, CF4 4XX, UK

Jean Mossman
Chief Executive, BACUP, 3 Bath Place, Rivington Street, London, EC2A 3JR, UK

Judd W. Moul MD FACS
Attending Urologic Oncologist, Urology Service, Department of Surgery, Walter Reed Army Medical Center, Washington DC; Associate Professor of Surgery, Department of Surgery, Uniformed Services University of the Health Sciences, 4301 Jones Bridge Road, Bethesda, MD 20814-4799, USA

John Naitoh MD
Urologic Oncology Fellow, Department of Urology, UCLA School of Medicine, 10833 Le Conte Avenue, Los Angeles, CA 90095-1738, USA

David E. Neal MS FRCS BSc MB
Professor of Surgery, Head of School of Surgical Sciences, Department of Surgery, The Medical School, University of Newcastle-upon-Tyne, Framlington Place, Newcastle-upon-Tyne, NE2 4HH, UK

Susan L. Neuhausen
Division of Genetic Epidemiology, Department of Medical Informatics, University of Utah School of Medicine, University of Utah, 391 Chipeta Way–Suite D2, Salt Lake City, Utah 84108, USA

Don W. W. Newling
Department of Urology, Academic Hospital Vrije Universiteit, P.O. Box 7057, Amsterdam 1007 MB, The Netherlands

R. T. D. Oliver MD FRCP
Sir Maxwell Joseph Professor of Medical Oncology, Medical Oncology Department, Colston Ward, 1st Floor King George V Building, St. Bartholomew's Hospital, West Smithfield, London, EC1A 7BE, UK

C. Parkes
Wolfson Institute of Preventative Medicine, Charterhouse Square, London, EC1, UK

David F. Penson MD
Robert Wood Johnson Clinical Scholar, Yale University School of Medicine, 333 Cedar Street, P.O. Box 208025, New Haven, CT 06520-8025, USA

E. Robinson
PhD Student, Department of Surgery, The Medical School, University of Newcastle-upon-Tyne, Framlington Place, Newcastle-upon-Tyne, NE2 4HH, UK

Neal Rosen MD PhD
Laboratory of Molecular Oncogenesis, Department of Cell Biology, Sloan-Kettering Institute and Department of Medicine, Cornell University Medical College, New York, NY, USA

Jack A. Schalken PhD
Research Director in Urology, Professor of Veterinarian Oncology, Department of Urology, University Hospital Nijmegen, Geert Grooteplein 10, P.O. Box 9101, 6500 HB Nijmegen, The Netherlands

Howard I. Scher
Genitourinary Oncology Service, Division of Solid Tumor Oncology, Department of Medicine, Memorial Sloan Kettering Cancer Center, 1275 York Avenue, New York, NY 10021, USA

Laura Sepp-Lorenzino PhD
Laboratory of Molecular Oncogenesis, Department of Cell Biology, Sloan-Kettering Institute, NY, USA

Mark H. Skolnick
Division of Genetic Epidemiology, Department of Medical Informatics, University of Utah School of Medicine, University of Utah, 391 Chipeta Way–Suite D2, Salt Lake City, Utah 84108 and Myriad Genetics, Inc., 390 Wakara Way, Salt Lake City, Utah 84108, USA

Susan F. Slovin MD PhD
Clinical Assistant Attending, Genitourinary Oncology Service, Division of Solid Tumor Oncology, Department of Medicine, Memorial Sloan Kettering, 1275 York Avenue, New York City, NY 10021, USA

M. H. Sokoloff MD
Department of Urology, UCLA School of Medicine, Clark Urological Centre, Box 951738, Los Angeles, CA 90095-1738, USA

Mark S. Soloway MD
Department of Urology, University of Miami School of Medicine, P.O. Box 016960 (M814), Miami, Florida 33101, USA

P. L. Stern PhD
CRC Department of Immunology, Paterson Institute for Cancer Research, Christie Hospital NHS Trust, Wilmslow Road, Manchester, UK

Clive Turner
Merebridge House, Old Hall Drive, Pinner, Middlesex, HA5 4SW, UK

Tapio Visakorpi MD PhD
Senior Scientist, Laboratory of Cancer Genetics, Institute of Medical Technology, University of Tampere and Tampere University Hospital, P.O. Box 607, Tampere FIN-33101, Finland

N. J. Wald
Wolfson Institute of Preventative Medicine, Charterhouse Square, London, EC1, UK

Michael J. Zelefsky
Department of Radiation Oncology, Memorial Sloan-Kettering Cancer Center, 1275 York Avenue, New York, NY 10021, USA

Foreword

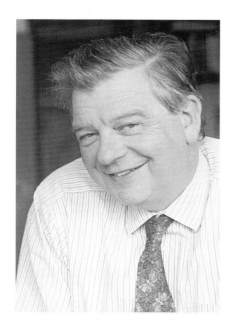

Prostate cancer remains a major problem and very important questions are still to be answered about strategies for screening and treatment, as well as opportunities for new and fundamental understanding of its biology. There have been enormous advances in knowledge, at the genetic level, of many cancers; individual steps have been identified and their significance is beginning to be understood. This meeting and book have shown that prostate cancer is being studied actively at this level and gradually the key steps are being identified. The meeting had a truly international flavour, was enormously stimulating, and was unique in bringing together patients with professionals, clinicians and scientists.

This book is dedicated to the memory of Jacques Roboh who died of prostate cancer in 1981. It was sponsored by the Prostate Cancer Charitable Trust which was formed in 1993, following the success of the Helene Harris Memorial Trust for research into ovarian cancer. Both of these charitable trusts are unique in the way they bring together clinicians, scientists and allied research workers for active discussion at the forefront of research.

Our thanks are due to Dr Monty Brill for the co-ordination of this book, Shirley Claff for her indefatigable energy in the administration of the meeting, ensuring that everyone did what they should and on time, all of the contributors and, of course, particularly Clive Bourne and Jean-Jacques Roboh who are the principal movers of the Prostate Cancer Charitable Trust.

This meeting and its precursors demonstrate the enormous importance of the 'private sector' contribution from dedicated individuals; working together is an enormous stimulus to those of us who are involved professionally in the scientific and medical areas. I believe we have a responsibility to bring a number of groups working on prostate cancer together effectively and to consider jointly the most productive directions for future research. This should be one of the best outcomes from this excellent meeting and book.

Walter Bodmer
July 21, 1997

Preface

Prostate cancer is the leading cancer among men in the USA and the second most common malignancy in males worldwide after lung cancer; it is estimated that 38.7 million men in North America, Europe and Japan have prostate cancer. Incidence varies in different countries ranging from 3.5 per 100 000 in Singapore to 48 per 100 000 in Sweden. Rates in the USA, France and the UK are almost identical at 33 per 100 000.

The cause for the wide variability of prostate cancer in different countries is still unclear although racial/ethnic factors and differences in lifestyle and diet have all been suggested as contributors. International co-operation and the joint efforts of scientists and clinicians worldwide are crucial, therefore, to define the genetic and epidemiological differences that hold the key to early detection, prevention and therapy of this unique men's health hazard.

This volume which summarizes highlights of the *Second International Forum on Prostate Cancer* held at the Royal College of Physicians (London, December 1996), is a testimony for the rapidly growing collaboration and exchange of information fostered by creation of the Prostate Cancer Charitable Trust in association with the Imperial Cancer Research Fund (ICRF). Founded in 1993 by Clive Bourne, a patient and philanthropist with great vision, this young organization is rapidly securing its position as one of the premiere international ambassadors for progress in prostate cancer research and therapy.

Since the inaugural symposium in Cambridge in 1994 and its associated publication *Preventing prostate cancer: screening versus chemoprevention* (Cold Spring Harbor Laboratory Press, 1995), the field of prostate cancer research has expanded dramatically, as evidenced by the wealth of new and exciting information presented in this book. The growing body of knowledge regarding aetiology and pathogenesis (chapters 2,5,7–10,38), epidemiology (12,36), immunology and immunogenetics (4,11,32), screening (15,16), diagnosis (13,14,17), staging and molecular markers (3,6,18), medical and surgical therapy (19–31, 33–35) and quality-of-life assessments (37) is all included in the book so as to give the reader the feel for the enormously stimulating and productive London meeting. The participants truly represented a multidisciplinary team of basic biologists and scientists from top university laboratories and industry, academic clinicians and community physicians and patient advocates.

Undoubtedly the true highlight of this meeting was delivered by 'an interested bystander' (rather than a prostate cancer expert) as he refers to himself in the introductory chapter of this book. Sir Walter Bodmer, Principal of Hertford College, University of Oxford, former Director General of the ICRF and a founding trustee of the Prostate Cancer Charitable Trust, has been the scientific leader of this organization since its inception. With well over 500 publications and seats on numerous advisory boards, Sir Walter Bodmer, with his boundless energy and charisma, is highly devoted to our overall mission. His critical analysis and perspective of all presentations, as the last speaker of this symposium, has clearly signalled the road ahead and the challenges we all face trying to make a major impact by understanding the fundamentals of prostate cancer and design new therapeutic avenues.

In the clinical arena, the treatment of localized and advanced prostate cancer remains a matter of considerable controversy. It is still not clear which patients need treatment, which modality should be used optimally to treat localized or locally advanced disease or what is the role of screening healthy men? Are there significant advantages to early versus delayed or intermittent hormonal therapy? Does chemotherapy have a role in the treatment of metastatic prostate cancer? What is the best approach for hormone refractory patients? At least one-third of the chapters in this book are devoted to these issues and although by no means comprehensive, an attempt has been made to summarize state-of-the-art clinical approaches in 1997. We hope to update the currently ongoing clinical trials after the meeting in Amsterdam in May 1998.

Arie Belldegrun MD FACS
Trustee, UCLA School of Medicine, Los Angeles, California, USA

Roger S. Kirby MD FRCS
Trustee, St. George's Hospital, London, UK

R. T. D. Oliver MD FRCP
Sir Maxwell Joseph Professor of Medical Oncology
St. Bartholomew's Hospital, London, UK

Chapter 1
New perspectives in prostate cancer: an introduction

W. F. Bodmer

Introduction

The aim of this chapter is to summarize highlights of the *Second International Forum on Prostate Cancer* from my point of view. As someone working in colorectal cancer, who is neither a clinician nor a urologist, I have been an interested bystander following the advances in the field, particularly through the Prostate Cancer Meetings. This enormously stimulating meeting covered a mixture of many different areas and included the involvement of patients, together with professionals, clinicians and scientists. I believe it is extremely important and productive to bring all these different groups together.

Treatments, old and new

There still seems to be enormous uncertainty as to when to treat and how to treat. The differences in opinion that were brought out so effectively by the cases that Mark Soloway described, leave me with the very strong impression that there is still a great deal that we need to know about what to do in a given situation. Should treatment be deferred or not? What sort of conservative treatment can be offered? How should one balance treatment with the quality-of-life issues? These difficulties are compounded by the effects of the age of the patient. Mike Kirby pointed out the difficulties general practitioners face in giving advice. The uncertainties leave a great deal of room for opinion and prejudice and an inevitable tendency to prejudge an issue, given the absence of clear-cut answers.

The fact that there is not a significant difference between treatments does not mean that there is *no* difference; it does mean that the difference is not large enough to detect with the numbers of patients that have been analysed. It is standard statistical practice to calculate the magnitude of effect that can be detected with a given number of patients, and this leaves no doubt that, if small percentage effects are to be detected, however important they may be, very large numbers of patients must be studied. This has been shown clearly by the overviews, for example, of breast cancer adjuvant treatment. These questions become even more difficult when the treatments are dramatic, as in the case of prostate cancer, rather than the relatively easy giving of a comparatively benign drug, such as tamoxifen, which can be administered to thousands of patients. I do not see an easy route in the area of prostate cancer for answering questions about whether some of the major differences in treatment do give rise to small significant differences in survival.

I remain unconvinced about the value of intermittent therapy. The obvious parallels with antibiotic treatment of bacterial infections surely suggest that one would not treat such infections with intermittent low levels of antibiotics. That is likely to be the best way to select for antibiotic-resistant variants, and leads me to doubt the *a priori* arguments for intermittent therapy. Can the case really be made for doing such a large-scale trial which may at best have marginal effects, and at worst on *a priori* criteria may not be effective at all?

The meeting started and ended with discussions of a variety of new approaches to treatment. As an outsider, I wonder whether there still might not be some gains to be achieved from better anti-androgen treatments, such as with bicalutamide. Given improved approaches to finding drugs with greater specificity, will it be possible to find more specific and effective anti-androgens? Is there a case for considering prevention trials using the anti-androgens, following the approach of the tamoxifen prevention trials with breast cancer? The latter development followed the demonstration of successful treatment of late-stage disease, then effective adjuvant treatment and from that to subsequent prevention trials. Perhaps a prostate cancer prevention trial could first be considered in identified high-risk groups?

I was impressed by Fernand Labrie's discussion of the extent to which androgens can be produced by non-prostate sources, and the variety of enzymes that are being uncovered by advances in molecular biology. If these can be sorted out with respect to their tissue specificity, then it should be possible to select drugs that differentially inhibit enzymes active in one tissue rather than another. This is just one of many examples where modern technology interfaces with a classical approach to drug discovery. The case is the same for the matrix metalloproteinase inhibitors; these have already given rise to interesting and novel drugs, and one must expect new and more specific versions to be developed in the future.

The way in which photodynamic therapy might be developed as an alternative to radical surgery was described by Stephen Bown. Another aspect of high technology development is in the newer approaches to conformal radiotherapy.

PSA testing, early diagnosis and tumour models

As always, there was much discussion about the prostate-specific antigen (PSA) test — perhaps even too much! It is a marvellous test but still an enormous puzzle. Is it mainly a sign of damage to the prostate, as it seems to give high levels in benign disease? The evidence strikes me as showing that it is tissue specific and not at all tumour specific. The PSA test is a classical example of the dilemma of a screening test for which, despite the small proportion of false positives, the population being tested is so large that the *number* of false positives becomes very large. Then, when the risk of damage in investigation is significant, there is a very complicated balance between the benefits of the screening and the morbidity it induces. I have the impression that we are no better off in dealing with this dilemma now than at the previous meeting 2 years ago. Once again, Mark Soloway's cases were very interesting. If there is no positive biopsy but a persistent low, though raised, level of PSA, what should be done? Is the low persistent level of PSA really an indication that there is still residual tumour present, or not? We do not know enough about tumour biology to answer that question. There is still, therefore, an overwhelming need for a second-level test to answer such questions. This is similar to the problem of evaluating ovarian screening by ultrasound, where most of the lesions detected are benign and a further level of test is needed to decide which really need to be treated. Once such a second-level test is available, then there will be no doubt about the enormous value of PSA screening, even perhaps on a population-wide basis.

There have been enormous advances in the understanding of PSA function. Hans Lilja described an elegant monoclonal antibody-based serological analysis specifically determining bound versus free PSA, which may perhaps be a better indicator than the total PSA level.[1] Some loss of sensitivity may well be tolerated if the number of false positives can indeed be reduced by a factor of two. The more we understand about the PSA test and its biological basis, the more likely we are to be successful in applying it to screening for prostate cancer (Chapter 15).

The discussion on the inadequacies of current diagnostic procedures was very telling. A biopsy may easily miss a tumour because of the problem of sampling, and there is a need for improved imaging beyond the current conventional approaches. The conformal approach to radiotherapy seems an obvious beneficial development, but, once again, there is a delicate balance to be faced between narrowing down the field so much to avoid damage to adjacent tissues, especially the nerves, and then risking not having good local control. From a biological point of view, I find it impossible to imagine that local control is not important; if some cancer cells remain alive, they are surely going to go on to evolve metastases, much as would the initial tumour. The balance of risks is, once again, between over-conservative treatment and, nevertheless, wanting to conserve as much as possible.

There is a real lack of good animal models, and even a lack of a reasonable range of prostate carcinoma-derived cell lines. In the colorectal field we routinely work with 50 or 60 cell lines that are representative of a wide range of tumours, and this number could easily be expanded to 150. I do not believe there is a problem with cell lines changing in culture. If there *is* a problem, it is that they represent a different balance of types of tumours than do fresh samples, because they are most probably selected with respect to which tumours can readily give rise to cell lines in culture. Cell lines, therefore, are useful models, for example, for investigating growth factor effects and adhesion properties, but if the spectrum of cell lines available is too narrow, then results with cell lines may be unrepresentative of the generality of tumours.

Xenografts, whether using cell lines or transplantable tumours only, are undoubtedly useful but are, nevertheless, a very poor model of the human situation. A late-stage tumour is effectively injected into the bloodstream so that the whole process of the early development of a tumour and its metastasis is effectively bypassed. For colorectal cancers, for example, it is now beginning to be possible to manipulate the mouse's genetic constitution to give models that begin to approach a spontaneous tumorigenesis that is more likely to be relevant to the human situation. A good spontaneous tumour model would enable issues connected with the biology of the tumour and the role of PSA, as well as novel approaches to early detection and treatment, to be explored with much greater confidence in their relevance to the human situation.

The discussion of the reverse transcriptase–polymerase chain reaction (RT–PCR) approach to detecting PSA in the blood, by Arie Belldegrun, was very interesting but perhaps a little disappointing. I believe that there is a considerable future in such approaches to early detection of cancers, but that they are much more likely to be effective if the test is based on a search for specific mutations rather than for tissue-specific expression, such as PSA. Nevertheless, such approaches have been used by Peter Selby and others simply for detecting epithelial cells in the blood by looking for an epithelial-specific cytokeratin using the RT–PCR technique.[2] This should, at the very least, provide a useful guide to the load of epithelial cells in the blood. I believe it is quite wrong to assume that, because there are epithelial cells circulating in the blood, metastasis has necessarily occurred. Surely, there could be early escape of epithelial cells into the circulation long before the major series of evolutionary steps that enable metastasis to occur has taken place. Thus, in my view, there is still considerable promise in monitoring for early detection of epithelial cells and their genetic abnormalities as an approach to early detection of tumours. Such an approach has been tried for colorectal cancer in looking for *ras* mutants in the stool.[3] Combining sensitive PCR techniques with epithelial-cell separation from the blood, using appropriate monoclonal antibodies, may considerably increase the resolution of this approach to early detection of cancers. Perhaps high-risk individuals in cancer families can provide a basis for exploring these approaches for monitoring the development of early disease.

Genetics

Genetics lies at the heart of understanding all cancers, and family studies have provided exciting advances in the discovery of genes that are relevant to sporadic cancers, especially in the colorectal field. The use of the Utah Family Resource to substantiate the recent discovery by the Johns Hopkins group of a subset of prostate cancer families that are linked to the 1q24–25 region, was well illustrated by Susan Neuhausen. Hard work will undoubtedly eventually lead to the identification of the relevant gene by positional cloning. However, there is no guarantee that the gene will be relevant to the sporadic disease, as is clear from the fact that so far *BRCA1* mutations have not been found in sporadic breast cancers. It is also important not to exaggerate the contribution of inherited susceptibility, since it is surely unlikely that more than, at most, a few percent of cases will be familial. *BRCA1* and *2* have been particularly frustrating for the analysis of breast and ovarian tumours, in contrast to the considerable contribution to understanding colorectal cancer progression that has come from the identification of the *APC* and mismatch repair gene mutations.

Small families are a problem in many countries, but fortunately not in Utah, and probably not in Oman. If only small families are available for study, it is much harder to detect heterogeneity, and families may only be classified once a gene and its mutations have been identified. Linkage cannot classify a family with respect to which gene is involved, if there are too few analysable individuals in the family. This, for example, makes it very difficult to assess what proportion of cancers are indeed familial.

The study of sibpairs, and its extension to multiple affecteds, is one approach to the search for genes with low penetrance. This can be focused on the extremes of the affecteds — say, those with prostate cancer onset under the age of 55 — which are the ones where a genetic effect is most likely to be present. Selection of cases in this way reduces the probability of studying chance sporadic coincidences, which dilute the power of detecting genetic effects using the multiple-affected approach. Such studies will surely be worthwhile in the search for prostate cancer susceptibility genes with relatively higher frequency but low penetrance.

The studies of prostate cancer in the Middle East by Elijah Kehinde, and in Afro-Caribbeans by Judd Moul, again emphasize the intriguing evidence for major population differences in the incidence of prostate cancer. The impression remains that, notwithstanding a certain regression to the incidence in the population in which migrants are embedded, the acquisition of the incidence rate from the embedded population is much slower for prostate cancer than it is for the classical example of breast cancer. In the latter case, Japanese women who have a very low breast cancer incidence acquire very rapidly, after migration to the United States of America, the relatively high incidence of their American counterparts. The lack of a similarly rapid change in the incidence of prostate cancer still does suggest that there may be a significant genetic component to such differences in population incidence.

This is a major challenge to the population geneticist. Is it likely that there is a single gene variant that influences prostate cancer susceptibility and that is commoner in some populations than in others — and, if so, has it been subject to natural selection, as in the case of the inherited haemoglobinopathies? If there is a genetic contribution to the differences in population incidence, then I believe it is unlikely that this will be due to more than one gene. In that case, understanding the population differences may make a significant contribution to understanding the basis for a relatively common genetic contribution to prostate cancer susceptibility. Of course, this does not exclude, by any means, the importance of environmental — especially dietary — effects. However, as in all dietary studies, it is very, very hard to pin down any particular relevant component of the diet. There are always more hypotheses and ideas than concrete evidence. Even in the colorectal cancer field, where there have been many case–control studies and population differences investigated, there still is no clear-cut definition of what component in the diet is most important in determining differences in colorectal cancer incidence. In that case, animal-model studies have clearly shown that effects of the diet may be strongly correlated with the gut microbial flora.[4]

The incidence of clearly inherited cancer susceptibility is likely to be similar in all populations, as it is largely due to the balance between mutations and the selection against them. If there is a lower overall incidence of a cancer, connected most probably with environmental factors, then the relative proportion that is genetic will be expected to be higher. Thus, Oman with its improved socioeconomic conditions and good opportunities for clinical and scientific investigation, and still with a population with large families, might provide an ideal setting for looking for more prostate cancer families.

The clue to finding the genes involved in genetic susceptibility, whether in clear-cut Mendelian families using positional cloning, or through population association studies, is the testing of candidate genes for mutations that can explain the cancer susceptibility. All positional cloning is, ultimately, testing candidate genes to see whether they fit with the hypothesis — namely, whether they are mutated in the affected individuals of families or whether they are clearly associated with cancer susceptibility in the population at large. In positional cloning, genetic studies of families identify a region within which candidates should lie, and intelligent guesses as to which genes have the appropriate functions that are more likely to explain a cancer susceptibility can speed the process of ultimate identification of the relevant gene. Increasingly in the future, I believe, intelligent guesses as to function will play a more important role. Soon we will know something about all the 50,000–100,000 genes, and perhaps a little about their function. Then it should be possible to scan that information to pick out likely candidates.

There are now straightforward techniques for identifying polymorphisms within, or close to, any chosen candidate gene. Case–control studies can then be done to see whether a given polymorphic variant associates significantly with the disease. This is an approach with wide applicability in the study of disease susceptibility. For prostate cancer, the androgen receptor gene is an obvious candidate. Other possibilities, for example, include missense variant polymorphisms in the *p53* gene for which there is some evidence of variation with latitude and a possible relationship to the effects of sunlight on the incidence of skin cancer.

A very promising hunt for the gene on chromosome 10q24–25, whose position was identified by loss of heterozygosity (LOH) studies, has been described by Nigel Spurr.[5] By no means all studies have identified LOH at this position, showing how variable this approach can be in identifying potentially interesting genetic regions in cancers. This is presumably because of the high background LOH levels resulting from aneuploidy. (Very recently this gene has been identified by three groups independently as a phosphatase with sequences also related to microfilament structures and called PTEN[6,7]. This is an exciting new discovery that may prove relevant to several other cancers in addition to those of the prostate.)

Comparative genome hybridization, as described by Tapio Visakorpi, is another important technique that can identify regions that carry potential genetic changes in cancers. This was the clue that led to the identification of the androgen receptor amplification. A model for such amplification is methotrexate, which selects for high levels of the enzyme dihydrofolate reductase, because the higher the enzyme level the more a cell can manage to cope with high levels of methotrexate. The mechanism for response to this selection is amplification of the gene for the enzyme. Thus, the parallel for the androgen-receptor amplification would be that, as less and less androgen becomes available, the cell is still able to respond by increasing the amount of receptor through gene amplification and enabling it to cope with lower and lower levels of androgen. The cells are still hormone sensitive and that, perhaps, is why androgen-receptor amplification does not necessarily signal a bad prognosis. A further genetic event is presumably needed before cells become truly androgen insensitive, and it is not clear why, when that occurs, there is any selection to mutate to a non-functioning androgen receptor. Perhaps there is some negative selection associated with the anti-androgens. The analogous situation for breast cancers that become tamoxifen insensitive suggests that, at that stage, they become autocrine with respect to one or more polypeptide growth factors. This further stage of the disease then becomes very difficult to treat. The various reviews of growth factors such as IGF1, TGFα and FGF8 perhaps signal the next stages in the progression of prostate cancers after they have become androgen insensitive.

Amongst the many other genetic regions implicated was 5q14–23, which overlaps the position of the *APC* gene. However, to my knowledge, there have been no *APC* mutations found in prostate cancer. The study of *APC* and other mutations in colorectal cancers emphasizes the importance of changes in the attachment of cells to each other and to the basement membrane as early events in epithelial tumorigenesis. Perhaps this should provide some clues for candidate genes involved in the early stages of prostate cancer. Particularly relevant to this are the changes in E-cadherin described by Jack Schalken. E-cadherin molecules are the main factors controlling epithelial cell–cell attachment, which involves catenins, especially β-catenin, inside the cell. Recently, β-catenin mutations have been described by several groups[8], including our own, in colorectal tumours and in melanomas. Changes in integrin levels in colorectal cancers were first described nearly 10 years ago, and are probably also important in indicating disruption of epithelial cell–extracellular matrix attachment, which may be another important element in the escape to growth independence during early stages of tumorigenesis.

Mutations affecting growth factors and their receptors are relatively uncommon, even though such changes are clearly important, at least for the later stages of tumour progression. The mutations that are found are more likely to affect signalling processes, such as that involved in the *ras* pathway, because they may disrupt a wider range of functions relevant to the growth of a tumour, resulting in the geneticist's 'pleiotropy'. Teleologically, one hit at that level in the cell may be able to affect a variety of functions which, jointly, are more likely to give the tumour a selective advantage. The same is likely to be true with respect to attachment, which is not merely a physical association but results in signalling pathways entirely analogous to those mediated by growth factor attachments to their receptors. That is, perhaps, why the *APC* mutations play such a key role in the earlier stage of colorectal tumorigenesis, and the challenge is to find the prostate cancer equivalent.

The general nature of carcinogenesis

The fundamental notion that cancer is essentially a somatic evolutionary process can be traced back to the early years of this century. Somatic cells do not enjoy the sexual process of hybridization; in somatic evolution, therefore, mutations must accumulate successively so that each new mutation giving rise to a selective advantage occurs in the clone of cells that carries all previous mutations. The selective advantages are by no means necessarily with respect to growth rate, but may involve increasing independence and a reduced death rate. The fundamental problem is to identify the individual mutational steps and their functions, and then to use this information to improve prevention, early detection and treatment. Prostate cancer progression is beginning to look like the pathway that is already relatively well defined for colorectal cancer. The difficulty in studying the prostate is that the early stages, corresponding to the colorectal adenoma to carcinoma sequence, are not readily accessible. In colorectal cancers, *ras* mutations follow the *APC* changes and then come the *p53* mutations, which are now widely believed to be selected for because of their effects on reducing the probability of apoptosis. This makes sense, since the early changes leading to looser attachment of cells to each other and to the extracellular matrix probably result in an increased rate of apoptosis. These early changes of tissue architecture may give rise to responses analogous to those in wound healing and non-specific inflammation, which latter results in early angiogenesis that is enough for the initial stages of tumour growth without further specific selection. Changes in growth factors and autocrine tumour growth follow later, with larger tumour mass and perhaps apoptosis. Only at these late stages may there be strong selection for the angiogenesis needed to keep a large tumour growing. Then, following treatment, comes selection for drug resistance and perhaps escape from immune attack.

One of the great puzzles about the growth of carcinomas is their long lag period. Recent work[9] with Ian Tomlinson on models that take into account programmed cell death and differentiation, as well as growth rate, suggest that tumours may not grow following a continuous exponential curve: they may, instead, increase stepwise, each step leading to a finite increase in tumour size. Following such an increase, some time may elapse before the next mutation that is selected for sweeps through the tumour cell population. Only after several such steps may exponential growth be initiated. Until that time, the tumour is benign. A considerable period may elapse before the next advantageous mutation arises and takes a hold, and so a long lag period can easily be accounted for. It must be recalled that the cells of the gut turn over fully every 3–4 days, and this applies as much to an adenoma as to the normal epithelial tissue. Thus, with this huge cell turnover, there is plenty of opportunity for the mutation and selection that is a necessary part of tumour somatic evolution. There must, presumably, be an analogous series of changes in the development of prostate cancer, but these details have still to be filled in.

New therapies

There are two radically new approaches to therapy, which are widely discussed and were represented at this meeting: these are (1) gene therapy involving attempts to kill specifically at least a significant subset of tumour cells, and (2) immunotherapy involving highly targeted, often DNA-based approaches. Gene therapy approaches often make use of tissue-specific promoters to direct expression of a gene product to a cancer, in order to render it specifically susceptible to a particular drug treatment. Thus, promoters from the enzyme tyrosinase have been used to direct production of a viral thymidine kinase, which is susceptible to the drug ganciclovir, to melanoma cells. For the prostate, promoters from PSA, or the prostate-specific membrane antigen, PSM, can be used to direct tissue-specific expression. Since only a relatively small proportion of tumour cells will be reached by the DNA, these approaches to treatment will not work unless there is a significant bystander effect — namely, that killing of a cell somehow induces killing of a large number of surrounding cells. This could, perhaps, be achieved by targeting a substance that is secreted from the cancer cells, such as TNFα, and so kills surrounding cells. To avoid systemic effects of TNFα released into the blood, it might be possible to use antibody to TNF to inhibit its more widespread actions. The work of Richard Vile, Ian Hart and others,[10] however, shows that there may be a considerable bystander effect through the induction of tumour-specific immune responses. It appears that, when cells are killed, for example, by the herpes virus thymidine kinase approach, the killing results in necrosis that seems to create very good targets for antigen presentation by macrophages or dendritic cells. Thus, only in immunocompetent animals do you get a cure. Ironically, therefore, this approach to gene therapy may effectively be a form of immunotherapy. It raises many questions such as whether a tumour ever presents its own antigen and, if not, what triggers effective pick up by professional antigen-presenting cells of tumour cell material.

It was reassuring to hear from Susan Slovin that monoclonal antibody approaches to immune therapy have not been forgotten. They have been tried for a long time, at least since the early 1980s, when monoclonal antibody-based approaches to the diagnosis and treatment of cancer were first being tried. It takes some time to develop such new approaches, and this has led to a general negative attitude about antibody-based therapy. Yet Riethmuller[11] has reported significant positive therapeutic effects of treating colon carcinomas with the antibody raised against antigen 17-1A. Similar results have been obtained by Epenetos[12] using anti-mucin antibodies for the treatment of minimal residual disease in ovarian cancer. I believe there is still much opportunity for the effective use of monoclonal antibodies for therapy. One common difficulty in trying out new therapies is that the case for a trial is often best made for treatment of late-stage disease, when other treatments have failed. But that may be the least appropriate stage for the effectiveness of an antibody treatment, which may work best with small tumour burden almost in an adjuvant setting.

Technetium-labelled monoclonal antibody against PSM has been shown by Keith Britton and his colleagues[13] to be an effective imaging agent for prostate cancer. There may, furthermore, be changes in mucin type 1 in prostate cancer similar to those in ovarian and breast cancer, opening up a variety of possibilities for monoclonal antibody-based imaging and immunotherapy of prostate cancer.

There are a variety of possibilities for trying to generate tumour-specific cytotoxic T cells in order to effect immunotherapy. There have, over the last 10–15 years, been enormous advances in our basic understanding of the mechanisms of

T-cell immune response. Antigen is presented in the form of peptide fragments, and approaches have been developed by Thierry Boone[14] to identify the determinants that a given cytotoxic T cell sees. Through this and other approaches, it is now possible to identify potential target antigens and aim to generate T-cell responses against these. Tissue-specific targets, such as PSA and PSM, may be good candidates. Thus, it seems unlikely that there would normally be a tendency to develop autoimmunity to PSM, since it is expressed in an immunologically privileged site. Furthermore, overexpression of a product, or its expression in an unusual form, can turn it into a target for cytotoxic T cells. The difficulty so far has been that when, for example, T-cell cytotoxic responses are generated to *p53* or *ras* mutations, they do not seem to kill a tumour carrying those mutations. Unless there is effective killing, generating the cytotoxic T-cell response will presumably be ineffective as a form of immunotherapy. Pramod Srivastava, for example, believes that unless one immunizes with a whole range of antigens there will be no cytotoxic effects.[15] His approach is not to use the whole cell as an immunogen, but to use heat-shock proteins, which carry a range of peptides sampled from the cell and which seem to form a remarkably good immunogen.

T-cell attack on a tumour will be ineffective if the tumour does not express HLA class I determinants, unless, as has been claimed for MUC1, T-cell responses may occasionally be HLA independent. Abnormal expression of HLA class I determinants has been described on many tumours, and explained as an escape response to tumour immune attack. The apparent extent of loss of HLA class I expression in the prostate is impressive. This suggests that there are prostate determinants that have developed during the evolution of the tumour, against which it is possible to mount a specific immune T-cell attack. However, if you cannot get to the tumour before it has escaped from the endogenous immune attack by selection for altered HLA expression, immune therapy will be ineffective. This implies that immunotherapy must be started early.

Generalized immune surveillance cannot be effective, otherwise cancers would not develop. It seems likely that tumours are, either directly or indirectly, very poor presenters of antigens, so that natural immune response may develop only relatively late in the evolution of a cancer. If, however, a strong immune response can be induced early, by a better understanding of immunogenicity, then immune therapy may be effective.

Conclusions

It is surely the advances that come from the laboratory that have the greatest promise for new approaches to dealing with prostate cancer. These include understanding the function of PSA, the role of changes in androgen-receptor expression, the role of growth factors, the developing knowledge concerning the genetic changes, and the understanding of the role of molecules involved in adhesion. It is through the understanding of the biology of prostate cancer that those PSA-positive cases that should be treated will, in the end, be identified. The signatures of genetic changes that they carry may then, for example, be the basis for a targeted immune attack, so that the genetic description of a cancer will not so much predict prognosis as determine it. Early detection through looking for mutations in released epithelial cells in the blood offers considerable promise. Will some form of anti-androgen treatment work in prevention, following the lines of the tamoxifen prevention trials for breast cancer?

A most significant feature of the meeting was the way it brought people together from so many different backgrounds. Furthermore, its support demonstrates the enormous importance of the 'private sector' contribution that individuals can make. It is precisely that working together that is such a stimulus to those of us who are involved professionally in the scientific and medical areas. There are a number of groups working in this way to help solve the problems of prostate cancer, and I believe that we have a responsibility to work together effectively and to consider jointly the productive directions that future research should take. That should be the best outcome from this excellent meeting.

References

1. Lilja H, Christensson A, Dahlen U *et al*. Prostate specific antigen in human serum occurs predominantly in complex with alpha-I chymotrypsin. Clin Chem 1991; 37: 1618–1625
2. Burchill SA, Bradbury MF, Pittman K *et al*. Detection of epithelial cancer cells in peripheral blood by reverse transcriptase polymerase chain reaction. Br J Cancer 1995; 71: 278–281
3. Smith-Ravin J, England J, Talbot IC, Bodmer WF. Detection of c-Ki-ras mutations in faecal samples from sporadic colorectal cancer patients. Gut 1995; 36: 81–86
4. Wasan HS, Novelli M, Bee J, Bodmer WF. Dietary fat influences on polyp phenotype in multiple intestinal neoplasia in mice. Proc Natl Acad Sci USA 1997; 94: 3308–3313
5. Gray IC, Phillips SMA, Lee SJ *et al*. Loss of the chromosomal region 10q23-25 in prostate cancer. Cancer Res 1995; 55: 4800–4803
6. Steck PA, Pershouse MA, Jasser SA *et al*. Identification of a candidate tumour suppressor gene, *MMAC1* at chromosome 10q23.3 that is mutated in multiple advanced cancers. Nature Genet 1997; 15: 356–362
7. Li J, Yen C, Liaw D *et al*. *PTEN*, a putative protein tyrosine phosphatase gene mutated in human brain, breast and prostate cancer. Science 1997; 275: 1943–1947
8. Ilyas M, Tomlinson IPM, Rowan A *et al*. β-Catenin mutations in cell lines established from human colorectal cancers. Proc Natl Acad Sci (USA) 1997; 94: 10330–10334
9. Tomlinson IPM, Bodmer WF. Failure of programmed cell death and differentiation as causes of tumors: some simple mathematical models. Proc Natl Acad Sci USA 1995; 92: 11130–11134
10. Hart IR, Vile RG. Targeted gene therapy. Br Med Bull 1995; 51: 647–655
11. Fogler WE, Klinger MR, Abraham KG *et al*. Enhanced cytotoxicity against colon carcinoma by combinations of non-competing monoclonal antibodies to the 17-1A antigen. Cancer Res 1988; 48: 6303–6308
12. Syrigos KN, Epenetos AA. Radioimmunotherapy of ovarian cancer. Hybridoma 1995; 14: 121–124
13. Fenely MR, Chengazi VU, Kirby RS *et al*. Prostatic radioimmunoscintigraphy: preliminary results using technetium-labelled monoclonal antibody, CYT-351. Br J Urol 1996; 77: 373–381
14. Boon T, van der Bruggen P. Human tumour antigens recognized by T lymphocytes. J Exp Med 1996; 183: 725–729
15. Suto R, Srivastava PK. A mechanism for the specific immunogenicity of heat shock protein-chaperoned peptides. Science 1995; 269: 1585–1588

Chapter 2
Genetic susceptibility to prostate cancer

S. L. Neuhausen, M. H. Skolnick and L. Cannon-Albright

Introduction

Prostate cancer is a pervasive disease in the United States, with approximately 244,000 cases diagnosed in 1995.[1] It is the most commonly diagnosed cancer in men and the second most common cause of cancer mortality, with 40,400 deaths per year.[1] Estimates are that one in six men will be diagnosed as having prostate cancer over the course of a lifetime. Risk factors for prostate cancer include age, ethnicity, country of origin and a family history.[2] The risk of prostate cancer is greatly increased after the age of 65 years, with 80% of the cases diagnosed in men over 65. The highest incidence of clinical disease is in African-Americans and the lowest is in Japanese living in Japan.[3–5] With migration to the United States, the rate of prostate cancer increases in Asians.[6] Meikle and Smith[7] hypothesized that, in the pathogenesis of prostate cancer, genetic and hormonal factors are permissive and environmental factors are promotional in genetically susceptible men.

In this chapter, aspects of prostate cancer related to familial prostate cancer are examined. Subjects include relative risks associated with a family history, evidence that familial clustering has a genetic component, testing for prostate cancer in men with a family history, and genetic linkage analysis to localize predisposing prostate cancer genes.

Family history

Increased relative risks of prostate cancer in first-degree relatives of patients have been reported, with risks ranging from 1.9 to 17.0.[8–16] Risk estimates vary, owing to diverse methodologies of collection and analysis, including differences in criteria for selection of probands and in overall study designs. However, these studies provide a body of evidence that prostate cancer is familial. The relative risk rises markedly with increasing closeness of the affected relative,[14] with increasing number of individuals affected within the family,[17] and with decreasing age of the patient.[12,13,17] Familial clustering of cancer may be due to genetic and/or shared environmental risk factors.

In large population-based studies in Utah, familial relative risks were estimated for risks to relatives for the same cancer, as well as for risks of cancers at other sites.[12,18,19] Clustering of cancer sites among relatives of cancer probands was systematically studied utilizing the Utah Population Database (UPDB). The UPDB comprises three Utah sources, including a genealogy of the Utah pioneers and their descendants, the Utah Cancer Registry (a population-based registry of the Surveillance, Epidemiology, and End Results Program of the National Cancer Institute), and Utah death certificates.[20,21] The records of these three sources are linked together into the UPDB database on the basis of unique concordance of name and birth date.

To examine the familial relative risks (FRR) of prostate cancer, 6350 probands were identified.[19] All their first-degree relatives in the UPDB were identified and data on all cancers present in the relatives were examined. The FRR for first-degree relatives for prostate cancer was 2.21 with 95% confidence intervals (CI) of 2.05–2.38. Based only on probands with prostatic cancer diagnosed before 60 years of age (551 probands), the estimate of FRR for prostatic cancer was 4.10 with 95% CI of 2.00–7.10. This is similar to the findings in an earlier report of Cannon et al.,[12] which utilized the same database (although with 10 fewer years of data and a different analysis), and reported a relative risk to brothers of 2.38, with increasing risk of prostate cancer with decreasing age. Examination of FRR for other cancer sites in first-degree relatives of probands with prostate cancer showed statistically significant risks for colon cancer (FRR = 1.27, 95% CI 1.1–1.4), non-Hodgkin's lymphoma (FRR = 1.24, 95% CI 1.1–1.5), rectal cancer (FRR = 1.25, 95% CI 1.1–1.5), and brain/central nervous system (CNS) cancer (FRR = 1.25, 95% CI 1.0–1.5).[19] Isaacs et al.[22] also reported a statistically significant higher risk of CNS cancers among hereditary families, classified as those with a minimum of three first-degree relatives or three successive generations affected with prostate cancer, or two relatives affected with prostate cancers at less than 56 years of age.

In a second study utilizing the UPDB, Cannon-Albright et al.[18] examined familial relationships between all pairs of probands with cancer at a given site compared with sets of matched control subjects. In contrast to the study by Goldgar et al.,[19] even quite distant degrees of relationship between cases were considered, rather than only first-degree relatives. Familial clustering was measured by the Genealogical Index of Familiality (GIF). Of the more common cancers, prostate cancer showed a clear excess of familiality and ranked third for the highest measure of familiality behind melanoma and leukaemia. Prostate cancer showed a stronger familial aggregation than breast or colon cancers, which are known to have genetic components. The GIF values for prostate cancer are shown in Table 2.1. Because excessive familial risk can be due to shared exposure to an environmental risk and/or to a common genetic mutation, examination of familial clustering of a disease by both near and distant genetic relationships is valuable. In the more distant relationships, it is likely that shared familial environment will be less, and the probability of shared genotypes can be measured. When GIF was examined, stratified by path length, there was an excess of familiality at even distant relationships, indicating that a common gene has predisposed to prostate cancer.[18]

Segregation analyses of prostate cancer families provided further evidence that genetic susceptibility is a risk factor for prostate cancer.[17] Carter et al.[17] reported autosomal dominant inheritance of a rare (q = 0.0030), high-risk allele that accounts for a significant proportion of early-onset prostate cancer and 9% of overall prostate

Table 2.1. Familiality of prostate cancer with age-of-onset subgroups

Group	n	Case GIF	Mean control GIF	p value
Total with prostate cancer	8060	3.70	2.76	< 0.001
Youngest 1/3 (less than 69 years)	2688	3.89	2.80	< 0.001
Oldest 2/3	5372	3.76	2.77	< 0.001

cancer by the age of 85. It was estimated that penetrance by the age of 85 is 88% for carriers, whereas only 5% of non-carriers will be affected with prostate cancer. Narod et al.[23] reported a significantly higher relative risk for brothers of men with prostate cancer (RR 2.62, 95% CI 1.69–4.06) than for men with no affected first-degree relatives. The relative risk for fathers (RR 1.2) was not significant, suggesting that familial prostate cancer may be due to a recessive or X-linked gene. Monroe et al.[24] also reported an elevated risk of prostate cancer in brothers compared with sons of prostate cancer cases and proposed an X-linked or recessive mode of inheritance. Accordingly, there appears to be a clear genetic component to prostate cancer susceptibility, although the mode of inheritance is not defined.

In a comparison of cases of hereditary prostate cancer and those with no family history, the only characteristic of hereditary prostate cancer appears to be an early age of onset.[25] There are no differences in clinical state at presentation, preoperative prostate-specific antigen (PSA) level, final pathological state, prostatic weight, nor multifocality of the disease. In contrast to the two early-onset breast cancer genes, BRCA1 and BRCA2, hereditary prostate cancer appears to be a relatively site-specific disease. In the Utah kindreds, there are few other types of cancer observed in excess among relatives of men with prostate cancer, with the most prevalent being breast and colorectal cancer, and non-Hodgkin's lymphoma.

Screening studies of prostate cancer in high-risk families

Screening of males with an increased risk of prostate cancer may be important to identify those with early-stage prostate cancer, which is more treatable than more advanced-stage cancers. One group of high-risk individuals compromises those with a family history of prostate cancer. In one Utah study utilizing the UPDB, a set of 17 sibpairs with prostate cancer was identified.[26] First-degree male relatives of these prostate cancer siblings between the ages of 55 and 80 years with no personal history of prostate cancer were invited to participate in a screening study for prostate cancer. Thirty-four men in 17 families underwent a PSA test, digital rectal examination (DRE), transrectal ultrasound (TRUS), and systematic and clinically directed core needle biopsies. Six had elevated PSA (18%), and three of those were diagnosed as having prostate cancer. Both PSA and DRE were abnormal in four, and TRUS showed a lesion in seven men. Altogether, eight previously unknown, clinically relevant prostate cancers were identified in the 34 siblings (24%), compared with one case in 15 healthy men with no family history (7%). Only needle core biopsies were able to identify all eight prostate cancers. Using a similar screening protocol in the general population, Catalona et al.[27] identified only 36 prostate cancers in 1630 men (2.2%), with a biopsy performed only if warranted.

In a second Utah study (unpublished data), PSA values of 172 first-degree male relatives (over the age of 40) of prostate cancer cases in 18 of the Utah kindreds were compared with Caucasian age-matched population controls with (1136 men) and without a family history (10,278 men). There was a significantly higher incidence of PSA greater than 4 ng/ml in relatives (20/172, or 12%) than in population controls without a family history of prostate cancer (622/10,278, or 6%) ($p = 0.004$). Seven of the 20 relatives with PSA values above 4 ng/ml were diagnosed as having a minimum of histological prostate cancer (five of these cases were also part of the study by McWhorter et al.[26]). The problem with such targeted screening is that it may detect histological prostate cancer which is not clinically relevant, and unnecessary surgery may be performed. However, these limited data suggest that targeted screening in families with a history of prostate cancer is beneficial.

Linkage analysis

Linkage analysis measures the cosegregation of two or more loci and is widely used to localize genetic disease by examining the cosegregation of genetic markers with the disease. When two loci are linked, they are physically located near one another on the same chromosome. Utilization of short tandem repeat (STR) markers allows testing of a minimum number of markers with a maximum amount of information. Genetic linkage analysis is by maximum likelihood estimation and Lod score calculation of the recombination fraction in the pedigrees. Lod scores are summed across the families analysed. Traditionally, a Lod score of 3.0 has been considered strong evidence for linkage and a Lod score of –2.0 as evidence against linkage. A key to successful genetic linkage analysis is to identify large informative kindreds that have a high likelihood of segregating the genetic disease of interest.

Based on the study by Cannon et al.[12] showing familial clustering of prostate cancer, high-risk prostate kindreds in Utah were ascertained through the UPDB. The UPDB provides access to pedigrees spanning seven to eight generations; these include thousands of descendants from a single individual, owing to early polygamy, high fertility and low non-paternity (approximately 1%).[20] The UPDB was shown to be genetically representative of a Northern European population,[28] making this population appropriate for inferences about cancer in Caucasians of Northern European descent. The high degree of cooperation and the large extended families found in the Utah population are especially important for studying prostate cancer, because penetrance of the gene appears to be reduced by age and there is sex specificity, making informative sibships difficult to find. Two examples of pedigrees ascertained through the UPDB are shown in Figure 2.1. In these pedigree drawings, only affected individuals (for whom we have DNA is available or whose haplotype can be inferred) and their ancestors are shown; unaffected siblings and branches have been removed from the pedigree to maintain confidentiality.

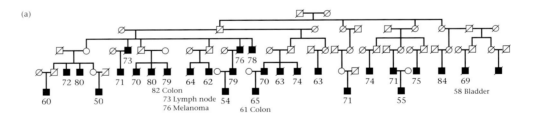

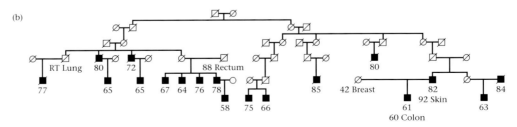

Figure 2.1. Pedigrees of two families with hereditary prostate cancer: (a) Family 4305; (b) Family K4344. Only affected individuals (for whom DNA is available or whose haplotype can be inferred) and their ancestors are drawn. Unaffected children, siblings and branches have been removed from the pedigree to maintain confidentiality. Key: ■ , prostate cancer; ∅ , deceased; numerals indicate age of diagnosis; sites of other cancers are also indicated as ▨ and ■ .

Studies to localize a gene predisposing to prostate cancer utilize this set of high-risk prostate cancer kindreds which now includes 67 kindreds with 3–64 cases of prostate cancer. DNA samples have been gathered for 364 men with prostate cancer and over 2000 relatives, many to infer genotypes of deceased cases. Each of these kindreds descends from a common ancestor and the number of prostate cancer cases observed in the descendants significantly exceeds that expected ($p < 0.05$). The authors are continuing to sample additional family members in these kindreds by extending to branches of the families. In a sample of kindreds containing multiple first-degree relatives with prostate cancer, 10% were diagnosed in men less than 60 years, 4% in men less than 55 years, and 1% in men less than 50 years of age. Carter et al.[25] have defined hereditary prostate cancer as meeting one of the following three criteria: (1) a cluster of three or more affected first-degree relatives; (2) prostate cancer in three successive generations of lineage, or (3) a cluster of two relatives affected at less than 56 years. Forty of the Utah kindreds meet one or more of the criteria; the other kindreds have either more distant relatives or older ages of onset.

For an initial genomic screen, the authors examined polymorphic markers that were either flanking or within candidate genes. Candidate genes are as follows: (1) genes whose functions are relevant to the neoplastic process; (2) previously defined tumour-suppressor genes involved in hereditary cancer syndromes; (3) genes in which mutations in prostate cancer tumours have been observed. Thirteen families were examined for linkage, using Linkage statistical software.[29] Genes included the androgen receptor (AR), TP53, BRCA1, BRCA2, CDKN2 (P16), RB1, LPL, and E-cadherin. Polymorphic markers flanking or within the gene were analysed, and no evidence for linkage was observed at any of the loci (Table 2.2). In addition to candidate genes, several chromosomal regions have been suggested as harbouring tumour-suppressor genes for prostate cancer, based upon cytogenetic analyses and/or allele loss [loss of heterozygosity (LOH)] studies in sporadic prostate tumours. These regions are described in the report by Cannon-Albright and Eeles,[30] and include segments of chromosome arms 3p, 7q, 8p, 9q, 10p, 10q, 11p, 13q, 16q, 17p, 18q and Y. Screening was performed with 34 markers representing 11 chromosome arms (no Y chromosome markers owing to maternal transmission in our kindreds) to test for cosegregation of the marker and prostate cancer. A slightly positive LOD

Table 2.2. Test of candidate genes using an age-specific model

Gene	Marker	LOD score at $r = 0.00$	$r = 0.01$	No. of families
CDKN2	D9S942	−14.5	−12.8	13
BRCA1	D17S855	−7.8	−6.7	13
	D17S1322	−0.5	−0.3	13
BRCA	D13S260	−5.3	−4.2	13
	D13S171	−1.1	−1.0	13
TP53	D17S796	−7.2	−6.2	13
	D17S786	−6.1	−5.4	13
E-cadherin	D16S514	−7.8	−6.7	13
	D16S515	−9.2	−7.6	13
LPL	LPL–2	−9.4	−8.1	13
AR on X	ARX	−9.7	−8.6	6
RB1	D13S119	−9.4	−4.0	9

score in one kindred for D10S212 had previously been reported,[30] but further follow-up disproved linkage. None of the candidate regions appeared to be responsible for the inheritance of common prostate cancer, although not all regions were excluded significantly.

A genome-wide search to localize a prostate cancer predisposition gene was instigated using nine of the same kindreds. Expected Lod scores (ELODs) (Table 2.3) were calculated with an age-dependent model using a recombination fraction of 0.05 analysed by Slink.[31] Initially, the genome was examined with a genetic map density of 20 cM with a variable number of STR markers screened for each kindred (Table 2.3): no significant evidence for linkage was detected using Fastlink.[29,32,33] Because of expectations of genetic heterogeneity, when LOD scores of more than 0.8 are observed in any of the families, additional markers are analysed in that region in order either to confirm and strengthen linkage or to disprove it. The authors are still continuing to follow up on some putative regions. To increase the rate of analysis, they have focused on kindreds K4305 and K4310 and examined only prostate cancer cases within the kindreds for excess allele sharing (Table 2.3). When there was excess allele sharing at a marker, Lod scores were calculated and flanking markers were examined. No putative localization regions have been identified on the basis of this approach; a set of 32 families at high risk of prostate cancer is now being examined.

Many other research groups have been collecting high-risk prostate cancer families and performing genomic searches. Recently, Smith et al.[34] published localization to chromosome 1q24–25. They examined 91 families (79 North American and 12 Swedish), with an average number of 4.9 men affected per family and an average age of 65 years. Accounting for genetic heterogeneity, they were able to obtain a maximum multipoint Lod score of 5.43. They estimated that one-third of their families were linked to the region. Two African American families gave a combined two-point Lod score of 1.4. Other cancer-predisposing genes are thought to be tumour-suppressor genes, based on LOH studies. No LOH has previously been reported in this region and studies are now in progress to examine whether there is LOH within prostate cancer family members.

The authors have now examined this region in a set of 32 prostate cancer kindreds (unpublished work). Initial two-point Lod scores for the 32 kindreds combined were highly negative at the four markers examined. Multipoint analysis provided significant evidence for linkage in the presence of heterogeneity, with a Lod score of

Table 2.3. Kindreds examined in the genomic search

| Kindred | ELODs (θ = 0.05) | | Diagnosis age (years) | | | | | No. of markers examined | |
	Av.	Max.	Total no. of cases	Range	Median	No. of cases with DNA	Total no. with DNA	Kindred	Cases only
K4057*	0.01	0.02	4	69–82	76	3	11	156	—
K4058*	0.00	0.03	14	46–84	69	6	34	156	—
K4305	1.45	2.48	29	50–85	71	15	175	280	120
K4309	0.42	0.95	13	61–82	71	6	56	165	—
K4310	1.10	3.35	39	55–88	72	15	86	225	100
K4325	0.48	1.76	20	52–85	70	9	42	156	—
K4343	0.46	1.30	10	59–83	71	4	30	230	—
K4344	1.17	2.38	43	58–88	73	15	78	230	—
K4347	0.62	1.67	28	54–87	67	18	54	230	—

*These were some of the authors' first families; under a different model they had acceptable LOD scores.

1.49 and an estimated 10% of families linked. The authors are continuing to genotype additional markers in the region in linked families in order to establish haplotypes and to try to narrow the region by identifying genetic recombinants.

In their previous genomic search set, the authors had examined D1S254, a marker in the 1q24–25 region, and had observed no evidence for linkage. However, upon examination of Lod scores in individual kindreds, K4343 was found to have a value of 0.49 under a dominant model. At the time, the authors were examining other more promising Lod scores and therefore did not explore the possibilities of this hint. This example underscores the difficulties in performing genomic searches and possible reasons for lack of localization. First, the authors were examining only a small number of their families and, because of genetic heterogeneity, there was not sufficient power to detect a true linkage. Secondly, the families include distantly related cases of prostate cancer and, because of the high incidence of prostate cancer in the general population, it is likely that there are phenocopies in the families that will reduce Lod scores. For these families, the authors are now following a strategy initially to examine closely related individuals in a family. Thirdly, the inheritance model is not known and must be estimated, so that Lod scores may be underestimates. The authors now analyse using an age-specific model, a dominant model and an unspecified model, and examine Lod scores. Lastly, by utilization of a more dense map of polymorphic markers, a series of positive Lod scores in a region may be observed, thus giving a basis to explore that region more closely. With the identification of the 1q24–25 linkage,[34] the 1q24–25-linked families will be removed from the authors' genomic search set. This will reduce the effects of heterogeneity due to these families on Lod scores in the genomic search, and possibly will enable other loci to be identified.

The authors' 1q24–25 linked families can now be examined in order to refine the region genetically. Currently, paraffin-embedded tumour tissue from cases of familial prostate cancer are being collected and microdissected in order to examine LOH in the region. After the construction of haplotypes within the families, the age-specific penetrance, the risks of other cancers, and the interactions of environmental risks and of modifier genes in these high-risk kindreds can be examined.

Conclusions

A family history of prostate cancer confers an increased risk of prostate cancer, with increasing risks with decreasing age and increasing number of close relatives. Localization of a prostate cancer-predisposing gene on 1q24–25, which may explain a maximum of 33% of families with prostate cancer, provides evidence that the risk factor is due to a genetic predisposition. With this localization, researchers can now isolate this gene and determine actual risk estimates for prostate cancer in linked families. There is, clearly, genetic heterogeneity for inherited prostate cancer and more linkage analysis is necessary in order to identify other genetically predisposing prostate cancer genes.

Acknowledgements

This work was supported by grants CA62154 and CA48711 from the National Institutes of Health, the Utah Cancer Registry (supported by NCI: CN6700 with additional support from the Utah State Department of Health and the University of Utah), and by Myriad Genetics, Inc. The authors would like to thank Thao Tran, Kim Nguyen and Maggie Higbee for technical assistance.

References

References

1. American Cancer Society. Cancer facts and figures, 1995.
2. Pienta K J, Esper P S. Risk factors for prostate cancer. Ann Intern Med 1993; 118:793–803
3. Carter H B, Piantadosi S, Isaacs J T. Clinical evidence for and implications of the multistep development of prostate cancer. J Urol 1990; 143: 742–746
4. Parkin D M, Pisani P, Ferlay J. Estimates of the worldwide incidence of 18 major cancers in 1985. Int J Cancer 1993; 54: 594–606
5. Whittemore A S. Trends in prostate cancer incidence and mortality. In: Doll R, Fraumeni J F, Muir C S (eds) Cancer surveys. Cold Spring Harbor, NY: Cold Spring Harbor Laboratory Press, 1994: 309–322
6. Morgan M S, Griffiths K, Blacklock N. The preventive role of diet in prostatic disease. Br J Urol 1996; 77: 481–493
7. Meikle W A, Smith J A. Epidemiology of prostate cancer. Urol Clin North Am 1990; 17: 709–718
8. Morganti G, Gianferrari L, Cresseri A et al. Recherches clinico-statistiques et genetiques sur les neoplasies de la prostate. Acta Genet Med Gemellol (Roma) 1956; 6: 304–305
9. Woolf C M. An investigation of the familial aspects of carcinoma of the prostate. Cancer 1960; 13: 739–744
10. Krain L: Some epidemiologic variables in prostatic carcinoma in California. Prev Med 1974; 3: 154–159
11. Schuman L M, Mandel J, Blackard C et al. Epidemiologic study of prostatic cancer: preliminary report. Cancer Treat Rep 1977; 61: 181–186
12. Cannon L, Bishop D T, Skolnick M et al. Genetic epidemiology of prostate cancer in the Utah Mormon genealogy. Cancer Surv 1982; 1: 47–69
13. Meikle A W, Smith J A, West D W. Familial factors affecting prostatic cancer risk and plasma sex-steroid levels. Prostate 1985; 6: 121–128
14. Steinberg G D, Carter B S, Beaty T H et al. Family history and the risk of prostate cancer. Prostate 1990; 17: 337–347
15. Spitz M R, Currier R D, Fueger J J et al. Familial patterns of prostate cancer: a case–control analysis. J Urol 1991; 146: 1305–1307
16. Ghadirian P, Cadotte M, Lacroix A, Perrett C: Family aggregation of cancer of the prostate in Quebec: the tip of the iceberg. Prostate, 1991; 19: 43–52
17. Carter B S, Beaty T H, Steinberg G D et al. Mendelian inheritance of familial prostate cancer. Proc Natl Acad Sci U S A 1992; 89: 3367–3371
18. Cannon-Albright L A, Thomas A, Goldgar D E et al. Familiality of cancer in Utah. Cancer Res 1994; 54: 2378–2385
19. Goldgar D E, Easton D F, Cannon-Albright L A, Skolnick M H. Systematic population-based assessment of cancer risk in first-degree relatives of cancer probands. J Natl Cancer Inst 1994; 86: 1600–1608
20. Skolnick M, Bean L, May D et al. Mormon demographic history. I. Nuptiality and fertility of once married couples. Popul Stud 1978; 32: 5–19
21. Skolnick M, Bean L L, Dintelman S M, Mineau G. A computerized family history data base system. Sociol Soc Res 1979; 63: 506–523
22. Isaacs S D, Kiemeney L A L M, Baffoe-Bonnie A et al. Risk of cancer in relatives of prostate cancer probands. J Natl Cancer Inst 1995; 87: 991–996
23. Narod S, Dupont A, Cusan L et al. The impact of family history on early detection of prostate cancer. Nature Med 1995; 1: 99–101
24. Monroe K R, Yui M C, Kolonel L N et al. Evidence of an X-linked or recessive genetic component to prostate cancer risk. Nature Med 1995; 1: 827–829
25. Carter B S, Bova G S, Beaty T H et al. Hereditary prostate cancer: epidemiologic and clinical features. J Urol 1993; 150: 797–802
26. McWhorter W P, Hernandez A D, Meikle A W et al. A screening study of prostate cancer in high risk families. J Urol 1992; 148: 826–828
27. Catalona W J, Smith D S, Ratliff T L et al. Measurement of prostate-specific antigen in serum as a screening test for prostate cancer. N Engl J Med 1991; 324: 1156–1161
28. McLellan T, Jorde L G, Skolnick M H. Genetic distances between the Utah Mormons and related populations. Am J Hum Genet 1984; 36: 836–837
29. Lathrop G M, Lalouel J M, Julier C, Ott J. Multilocus linkage analysis in humans: detection of linkage and estimation of recombination. Am J Hum Genet 1985; 37: 482–489

30. Cannon-Albright L, Eeles R. Progress in prostate cancer. Nature Genetics 1995; 4: 336–338
31. Weeks D E, Ott, J, Lathrop G M, Slink. A general simulation program for linkage analysis. Am J Hum Genet 1990; 47: A204 (abstr)
32. Cottingham R W, Idury R M, Schaffer A A. Faster sequential genetic linkage computations. Am J Hum Genet 1993; 53: 252–263
33. Schaffer A A, Gupta S K, Shriram K, Cottingham R W. Avoiding recomputation in linkage analysis. Human Hered 1994; 44: 225–237
34. Smith J R, Freije D, Carpten J D *et al*. Major susceptibility locus for prostate cancer on chromosome 1 suggested by a genome-wide search. Science 1996; 274: 1301

Chapter 3
Genetic markers of prostate cancer: progression and androgen resistance
T. Visakorpi

Introduction

An accumulation of genetic changes affecting expression of critical genes is thought to underlie malignant transformation and cancer progression. It has been estimated that 5–10 genetic alterations have to be accumulated into a cell before it becomes fully transformed. Additional changes are then required for acquisition of metastatic potential, for example. This multistep cancer progression hypothesis is best known in colorectal cancer.[1] It is likely that development and progression of prostate cancer is also caused by an accumulation of genetic changes. The genes that are dysregulated in the progression of normal cells to highly aggressive, and metastatic, treatment-refractory cancer are nowadays categorized into three groups: these are (1) dominant oncogenes, (2) recessive tumour-suppressor genes (TSG) and (3) mutator genes. These genes are involved in many critical functions of the cell, including growth-stimulatory pathways, cell proliferation, cell death, differentiation, adhesion, angiogenesis, DNA repair and genetic instability. Identification of genetic alterations and genes associated with the development and progression of prostate cancer would be important in order to gain detailed information on the mechanisms of the disease.[2] This would probably provide new tools for assessment of prognosis and prediction of treatment response. Knowledge of the disease mechanisms could also enable the development of new treatment modalities. In this chapter, an attempt is made to summarize what is known about the genetic basis of the development and progression of prostate cancer. First, however, the natural history of prostate cancer is briefly discussed.

Natural history

Prostate cancer is the most common malignancy among men in many Western industrialized countries. Furthermore, the incidence of prostate cancer has increased rapidly in recent years, partly owing to the increased use of serum prostate-specific antigen (PSA) measurements for early diagnosis and screening of the disease.[3,4] Most prostate cancers arise from the secretory epithelial cells of the peripheral zone of the prostate gland.[5] Prostatic intraepithelial neoplasia (PIN) is often found in close proximity to invasive cancer and is considered to be a premalignant lesion. PIN is characterized by proliferation and anaplasia of cells lining ducts and acini and is associated with basal cell layer disruption.[5–7] It has been estimated that more than 50% of 70–80-year-old men have foci of microscopic adenocarcinoma in their prostate gland.[8] This type of histological prostate cancer is found at an equally high frequency in many populations (e.g. in Japanese and US men), even though the incidence rates of clinical prostate cancer are dramatically different.[9] Thus, the progression of these latent histological cancers to clinically evident tumours represents a major rate-limiting step in prostate tumorigenesis.

Clinically detected primary prostate carcinomas display a wide range of phenotypic features and malignant potential. The tumour stage (TNM classification) and histological grade are routinely used to assess the prognosis of patients. The average 5-year survival of patients with localized disease is 80%, and 30% for patients with distant metastases.[10] However, there is considerable heterogeneity in biological aggressiveness and patient prognosis within a given stage or histological grade.

About one-third of prostate cancers are diagnosed at stages C and D, when surgical cure is no longer possible.[11] Patients with such advanced disease are usually treated with androgen deprivation therapy [orchiectomy or leuteinizing hormone-releasing hormone (LHRH) agonists]. About 70–80% of the patients respond to this treatment and disease palliation is achieved for several months or years. Eventually, however, the disease progresses despite the ongoing therapy. The prognosis after relapse is poor: the average survival of patients is only 6 months, and there is no effective treatment for hormone-refractory prostate cancer. Thus, the failure of endocrine therapy is one of the most important problems in the management of a patient with prostate cancer.[12,13] Prostate cancer metastasizes locally to lymph nodes and haematogenously most commonly to bone. As there is no cure for advanced prostate cancer, the acquisition of metastatic potential is a very important change in the phenotype of the prostate tumour.

Primary prostate cancer

Ploidy

DNA aneuploidy is a characteristic feature of malignant cells and is usually found in about 50–75% of solid tumours.[14,15] On average, 40–50% of prostate carcinomas have been found by DNA flow cytometry to be aneuploid. DNA aneuploidy has been associated with advanced clinical stage of disease, high histological grade and poor prognosis of patients.[16] Thus, it has been suggested that measurements of DNA content should be used to predict prognosis for all patients with newly diagnosed prostate carcinomas in a routine clinical setting.[17,18]

DNA flow cytometry can be used only to detect gross deviation in the total cellular DNA content in the malignant cell, whereas classical cytogenetics reveals both numerical and structural chromosomal aberrations. Cytogenetic studies have found clonal chromosomal abnormalities in only approximately 25% of prostate cancers, suggesting that, in the majority of cases, normal cells have been analysed. Conventional cytogenetic analysis is limited by the low mitotic rate and poor growth of prostate cancer cells, the overgrowth of fibroblasts and the poor morphology of metaphase spreads.[19–24] The most common chromosome copy-number changes found by cytogenetics have been losses of chromosomes 1, 2, 4, 5, and Y and gains of chromosomes 7, 14, 20 and 22. Structural rearrangements involving chromosome arms 2p, 7q and 10q and deletions at 7q, 8p and 10q have also been reported.[21,22] In addition, double minute chromosomes (DMs), which are a cytogenetic hallmark of gene amplification, have occasionally been reported.

The advantage of fluorescence *in situ* hybridization (FISH) is that no metaphase preparations from the tumour are needed to detect numerical and structural chromosomal changes. Even formalin-fixed and paraffin-embedded interphase nuclei can be utilized.[25] Prostate carcinomas have shown chromosome copy-number changes by FISH, using chromosome-specific repeat-sequence probes, in 44–97% of primary prostate carcinomas[26–39] and in virtually all recurrent prostate carcinomas.[32] The detected frequencies of aberrations depend largely on the number and selection of probes used in each study. The most frequently altered chromosomes detected by FISH have been 1, 7, 8, 10, 17, 18 and X. Several studies have suggested that trisomy 7 is associated with progression of prostate cancer[28,29,37] Copy-number aberration of chromosomes 8 has also been associated with short progression-free time after prostatectomy, whereas aneusomy of Y has been associated with poor overall survival.[38]

Loss of heterozygosity and tumour-suppressor genes

Loss of heterozygosity (LOH) has been considered to indicate those chromosomal regions that may harbour TSGs. LOH in primary prostate cancer has often been found at the chromosomal regions 5q, 6q, 8p, 10q, 13q, 16q, 17q and 18q.[40–45] Despite the fact that so many regions of losses have been indicated by LOH studies, the target TSGs are not known. Loss of the entire short arm of chromosome 8, or small regions of it, appears to be the most common genetic defect in primary prostate cancer. LOH at 8p has been found in up to 70% of prostate carcinomas, and also in PIN lesions.[46–48] At least three minimal regions of deletions, one at 8p11–12, the other at 8p21, and the third at 8p22, have been reported, suggesting the presence of several TSGs in this chromosomal region.[46,47,49–51] Homozygous deletion has also been reported in the 8p22 region. In a recently published study, this region was narrowed down to 730–970 kb, which should facilitate positional cloning of the TSG;[52] however, no candidate TSGs are known in chromosome 8p.

Another chromosome that has commonly shown LOH is 10q. Allelic loss at 10q has been seen in up to 40–50% of primary prostate cancers, and also in 25% of PIN.[40,41,53–55] Minimal region of loss has been mapped to 10q23–q24.[56] Recently, a candidate TSG, MXI1, was identified at 10q25.[57] It was found to be mutated in prostate carcinomas, which showed deletions of 10q24–q25. MXI1 codes for a transcription factor that negatively regulates MYC activation.[58,59] Since MXI1 is located outside the minimal commonly deleted region at 10q, it seems that this region also harbours another TSG.

Many of the regions commonly showing LOH (5q, 13q, 16q, 18q, etc.) in prostate cancer, contain known TSGs, such as the retinoblastoma gene *(RB1)*, adenomatous polyposis coli *(APC)*, α-catenin, E-cadherin and deleted in colorectal cancer *(DCC)*. Nevertheless, there is only limited evidence that any of these genes is really involved in the development of prostate cancer. Reduced expression of *RB1*, which is located in 13q14, has been documented in primary prostate tumours, but only a few *RB1* mutations have been detected.[60] Chromosome 5q contains two putative TSGs, α*-catenin* (5q21–q22) and *APC* (5q21). PC-3 prostate cancer cells lack the expression of a-catenin expression as a consequence of a homozygous deletion.[42,61] However, the role of α-catenin in the development of primary prostate cancer is not known and further work is required. LOH at the APC locus has been reported in 20–40% of advanced prostate cancers, but expression data and evidence of gene mutations in the remaining allele are still missing.[62,63] Chromosome 18q also contains two putative TSGs, *DCC* (18q21), and the recently found *DPC4* (18q21).[64] Neither has been shown to contain mutations in prostate cancer, whereas decreased expression of the *DCC* gene has been reported.[65]

With regard to prostate cancer, one of the most thoroughly studied genes is *E-cadherin* (16q22), which is a Ca^{2+}-dependent cell–cell adhesion molecule. Decreased expression of *E-cadherin* has been found in prostate cancers, especially in those with a high grade or aggressive clinical behaviour. However, no mutations in the coding region of the *E-cadherin* gene have yet been found in primary prostate tumours.[66–68] The gene may be downregulated, possibly through mechanisms that do not involve gene mutation. For example, Bussemakers and colleagues[69] have shown that the *E-cadherin* promoter is inactive in the TSU-Pr1 prostate cancer cell line, possibly owing to the binding of a repressor molecule. It has been thought that *E-cadherin* could act as a suppressor of invasiveness of malignant cells, because highly invasive tumour cells have lost their phenotype after being transfected with wild-type *E-cadherin* cDNA.[70] Recent data, however, suggest that the minimal commonly deleted region at 16q is closer to the telomere (16q23–qter) than the *E-cadherin* locus.[71] Thus, there might be another TSG in 16q that could be important in the development of prostate cancer.

Mutations in the *p53* gene, located at 17p13.1, may be the most common genetic change in human cancers.[72] The role of the wild-type p53 protein as a negative regulator of cell growth after DNA damage has occurred is well known. The p53 protein functions at the G1/S checkpoint of the cell cycle and inhibits the progression of genetically damaged cell through the S phase.[73] Furthermore, it may induce apoptosis by interacting with the *MYC* oncogene.[74] The role of *p53* mutations in prostate cancer development appears to be less significant than in many other tumours. Three prostate cancer cell lines (PC-3, DU145, TSUPr-1) and 10–20% of primary prostate cancers contain *p53* mutations.[75–77] Mutations of the *p53* gene often lead to prolonged half-life of the protein, causing accumulation of the protein in the nuclei.[72] Such p53 accumulation seems to be associated with high cell proliferation activity of prostate tumours and poor prognosis.[78]

Gains and losses by comparative genomic hybridization

Comparative genomic hybridization (CGH) is a novel molecular cytogenetic technique that enables screening for DNA sequence copy-number aberrations in the entire tumour genome in a single hybridization. In CGH, differentially labelled tumour and normal DNA are co-hybridized to the normal metaphase chromosomes and the hybridization intensity variations between the two DNAs are quantified.[79–81] Five studies on genetic changes detected by CGH on prostate cancer have been published so far.[82–86] The author and colleagues have found DNA sequence copy-number changes affecting one or more chromosomal regions in 74% of primary prostate carcinomas, by using CGH.[83] A characteristic feature of prostate cancer was the finding of losses and deletions up to five times more often than DNA gains and amplifications. These results suggest that early development of prostate cancer may be, to a large extent, attributable to deletions of specific chromosomal regions that harbour TSGs. The most commonly lost regions in primary tumours involve 6q, 9p, 8p, 13q, 16q and 18q, which have also been implicated by LOH studies.

Progression of prostate cancer

Genetic alterations

The author and colleagues have studied genetic changes in nine hormone-refractory recurrent prostate carcinomas by CGH and compared the number and nature of genetic aberrations with those found in a series of 31 primary prostate tumours.[83] The mean number of genetic aberrations in the recurrent tumours was three times higher than in primary tumours, and the frequency of gains was almost five times greater (Figure 3.1). These results suggest that the recurrent tumours are genetically more advanced and probably more unstable than the primary prostate tumours. This would explain the aggressive nature and the poor

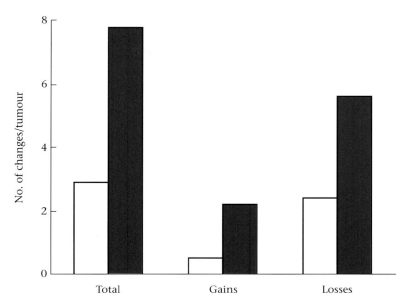

Figure 3.1. Comparison of genetic aberrations in primary (□, n = 31) and recurrent (■, n = 9) prostate carcinomas, showing mean number of genetic changes per tumour.

response to secondary therapy that is characteristic of these recurrent tumours. An LNCaP prostate cancer model system was also studied; in this, serial passages of the androgen-responsive parental LNCaP cell line into nude mice had resulted in establishment of several sublines that are androgen-independent and metastatic.[87,88] Comparison of the CGH findings between the sublines and parental line revealed that the sublines had on average twice as many genetic alterations as the parental line.[85] A recent study by Cher and colleagues[86] also supported the author's finding of a high frequency of genetic changes in the hormone-refractory prostate carcinomas.

In order to explore the possibility that the higher number of genetic changes in recurrent tumours[83] is due to patient-to-patient differences in the genetic composition of tumours, instead of progression-related phenomena, the author and colleagues have analysed primary tumours and local recurrences in 10 prostate cancer patients by FISH and six chromosome-specific repeat-sequence probes.[32] This study showed that the recurrent tumours exhibited systematically more chromosome copy-number changes and cell-to-cell heterogeneity than the corresponding primary tumours, indicating that the genetic progression and genetic instability of the tumour truly underlie the clinical progression of the disease.

The specific chromosomal regions that the author and colleagues[83] found, by CGH, to be particularly often involved in hormone-refractory recurrent prostate carcinomas, included the loss of 5q and the gains of 7p, 8q and Xq (Figure 3.2). Gain of 8q was found in 89% of the recurrent tumours, and it usually involved the entire long arm. Recently, Cher and colleages[86] found 8q gain in 85% of prostate cancer metastases samples taken prior to any treatment. In addition, Van Den Berg and colleagues[89] found that four out of 44 prostatectomy samples showed amplification of 8q24 by FISH and region-specific microdissection probe. Three of the 44 patients in this series presented lymph-node metastases, all of which had the 8q24 amplification. Thus, it seems that 8q gain is strongly associated with the aggressive phenotype of prostate cancer. Although, in most of the tumours, the 8q

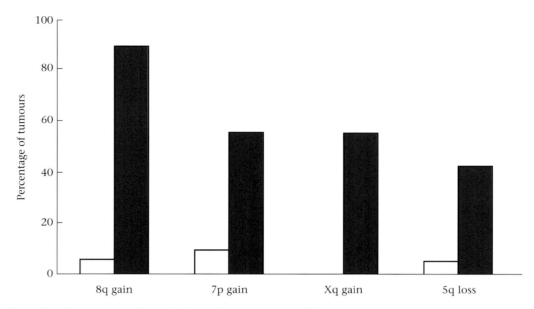

Figure 3.2. Comparison of genetic aberrations in primary (□, n = 31) and recurrent (■, n = 9) prostate carcinomas, showing frequency of gains and losses of the most commonly affected chromosome arms.

gain seems to involve the whole arm, there are two minimal commonly amplified regions, 8q21 and 8q24;[83,86] thus, it is likely that there are several target genes for this alteration. One possible target gene of amplification in 8q24 is the *MYC* oncogene. Elevated expression of *MYC* has been associated with high histological grade in prostate cancer.[90,91] However, amplification of MYC, studied by gene-specific Southern analysis, seems to be rare in primary prostate cancer.[92] Thus, there may be other, currently unknown, target genes even at the distal 8q.

Androgen receptor

The CGH study conducted by the author and colleagues showed that about one-half of the hormone-refractory prostate carcinomas have gain at chromosome Xq. The minimal region of the gain was Xp11–q13, and it has subsequently been shown that the target gene of amplification is likely to be the androgen receptor (*AR*) (AR, localized to Xq12) gene.[93] So far, the author and colleagues have analysed 54 recurrent prostatic tumours (transurethral resection specimens) from patients who had been treated by endocrine monotherapy (orchiectomy, oestrogen, or LHRH analogue) and who had experienced local progression during the treatment.[94] Fifteen (28%) of these samples have shown high level *AR* gene amplification by FISH. The author and colleagues have also analysed primary tumours, taken prior to any therapy from 26 of these sample patients. None of these primary tumours has shown the amplification, suggesting that *AR* gene amplification is selected for during the androgen withdrawal. Interestingly, patients whose tumour developed *AR* gene amplification, initially responded better to the androgen-withdrawal therapy than those whose tumour did not develop the amplification, suggesting that a long period of selection force is required before *AR* amplification emerges. The *AR* gene amplification is associated with overexpression of the gene as measured by mRNA *in situ* hybridization, supporting the idea that the *AR* is the real target gene of the amplification. Those 15 samples that showed *AR* gene amplification were also analysed for gene mutations, using polymerase chain reaction/single-stranded conformation polymorphism

(PCR–SSCP) analysis and sequencing. One of the tumours has shown missense mutation in the hormone-binding domain of the gene. This mutation, however, did not change the properties of the receptor molecule in transfection assay. Thus, it seems that the amplified *AR* gene is usually of the wild type.

The author's findings tend to suggest that *AR* gene amplification improves the cell's ability to survive and grow in the androgen-deficient conditions, when the supply of androgens is rate limiting for cell growth. *AR* amplification may well be the first *in vivo* example, where gene amplification is a common causative mechanism for drug resistance and therapy failure. Many similar mechanisms have previously been described where transformed or tumorigenic cell lines placed in culture in the presence of a specific metabolic inhibitor or cytotoxic drug are able to amplify a specific gene, the increased expression of which then counteracts the effects of the drug.[95]

The finding of *AR* gene amplification may have several clinical implications. It suggests that recurrent hormone-refractory prostate carcinomas are not always truly androgen independent, as usually thought; instead, they may be highly dependent on the residual adrenal androgens remaining in the serum after castration. Studies are now needed to assess whether so-called maximal androgen blockade (MAB) therapy would be particularly effective against tumours that contain *AR* gene amplification. For example, whether *AR* gene amplification could predict the response to the secondary MAB therapy should be studied. So far, the author and colleagues have documented the case of one patient in whom tumour recurred with *AR* amplification during endocrine monotherapy, and the patient was subsequently treated with MAB. An excellent treatment response was obtained initially; unfortunately, however, the disease subsequently progressed once again.[96]

Before the finding of *AR* gene amplification, the role of *AR* gene mutations in the development and progression of prostate cancer had already been studied extensively. Early studies suggested that mutations in the *AR* gene are rare,[97–100] but a more recent investigation, in which the whole coding region of the *AR* gene was analysed, found mutations in 44% of stage C and D prostate carcinomas.[101] In addition, Taplin *et al*.[102] found *AR* gene mutations in five out of 10 metastatic hormone-refractory prostate cancers. Some mutations may lead to altered function of the AR molecule. They may, for example, diminish ligand specificity of the AR molecule in such a way that it can be activated by steroids other than androgens, or even by anti-androgens.[97,102–104] Such mutations may also explain the so called anti-androgen withdrawal syndrome, which refers to the patient's favourable response to withdrawal of anti-androgen treatment.[105] In the light of both the author's finding of *AR* gene amplification and findings by others of *AR* gene mutations, it seems that the aberrations in the AR molecule may play a major role in the failure of endocrine treatment of most of the prostate cancers.

Metastases

The prognosis of cancer patients is largely determined by the development of distant metastases. Cher and colleagues[86] have studied untreated metastatic specimens by CGH. Most commonly they found gains at 8q and losses at 8p, 10q 13q, 16q and 17p. These regions were earlier also implicated by CGH in the primary and hormone-refractory tumours,[82,83] suggesting that there may not be many purely metastasis-associated genes.

However, one putative metastasis-suppressor gene in prostate cancer has already been identified. Microcell-mediated transfer of human chromosomes 11 and 17 to Dunning rat prostate cancer cells was shown to decrease the metastatic potential of the hybrid cells without suppressing the *in vivo* growth rate or tumorigenicity.[106,107] Dong and colleagues[108] later identified a cDNA clone from the 11p11.2 suppressor region that was differentially expressed in the non-metastatic subline but not in the parental metastatic cell line. Following cloning of this *KAI1* gene, it was shown in transfection experiments that this single gene was responsible for the suppression of the metastatic potential in the rat AT6.1 prostate cancer cells. *KAI1* encodes for a membrane glycoprotein, is expressed in a wide variety of normal tissues and is evolutionarily highly conserved. Normal human prostate epithelial cells express the gene, whereas prostate cancer cell lines (PC-3, LNCaP, DU145) derived from metastatic lesions do not. The *KAI1* gene belongs to a family of membrane glycoproteins; it codes for a 2.4 kb mRNA and is assumed to function in cell–cell interactions and possibly in cell migration. Recently, it has also been demonstrated that most of the primary prostate tumours and all metastases show decreased expression of *KAI1*.[109] However, no mutations or LOH in the gene have, so far, been found. Thus, the mechanisms of downregulation of *KAI1* in prostate cancer remain to be determined in subsequent studies.

Conclusions

Recent years have shed light on the molecular mechanisms underlying the development and progression of prostate cancer. Several common chromosomal aberrations have been identified. The next task is to try to find the genes that are affected by these alterations. Some good candidate genes, such as *MXI1*, *AR*, *E-cadherin* and *KAI1*, have been recognized. Many other genes, however, remain to be identified. As more and more genes associated with the development of prostate cancer are found, the critical question — which of them are most important — will arise.

It has been suggested that some of the cancer-related genes could be classified as gatekeeper genes. These genes are normally responsible for maintaining a constant cell number in renewing cell populations. A mutation in such a gene leads to expansion of the mutated cell clone. For example, the *APC* gene has been suggested to be such a gatekeeper gene of colonic epithelial cells.[110] Is there a gatekeeper gene that determines which of the very frequent small prostate carcinoma lesions (latent carcinomas) ever progress to a clinical disease? Finding such a gene would certainly improve understanding of the progression of prostate cancer, and such knowledge would probably be useful in developing targeted therapies for prostate cancer.

In recent years, much attention has been given to the familial clustering of prostate cancer, and it has been suggested that there is a hereditary form of prostate cancer in the same manner as there are hereditary forms of colorectal or breast cancer. Recently, Smith and colleagues[111] reported a genome-wide analysis of families at high risk of prostate cancer: they found significant linkage on chromosome 1 (1q24–q25) in one-third of such families. This is the first clear evidence that there is a hereditary type of prostate cancer. The next step will be to identify the gene (or genes) itself and to determine its function; perhaps it will be a gatekeeper gene.

References

1. Fearon E R, Vogelstein B. A genetic model for colorectal tumorigenesis. Cell 1990; 61: 759–767
2. Kallioniemi O-P, Visakorpi T. Genetic basis and clonal evolution of human prostate cancer. Adv Cancer Res 1996; 68: 225–255
3. Jacobsen S J, Katusic S K, Bergstralh E J et al. Incidence of prostate cancer diagnosis in the eras before and after serum prostate-specific antigen testing. JAMA 1995; 274: 1445–1449
4. Potosky A L, Miller B A, Albertsen P C, Kramer B S. The role of increasing detection in the rising incidence of prostate cancer. JAMA 1995; 273: 548–552
5. Ware J L. Prostate cancer progression: implications of histopathology. Am J Pathol 1994; 145: 983–993
6. Bostwick D G, Brawer M K. Prostatic intra-epithelial neoplasia and early invasion in prostate cancer. Cancer 1987; 59: 788–794
7. Epstein J I. Pathology of prostatic intraepithelial neoplasia and adenocarcinoma of the prostate: prognostic influences of stage, tumor volume, grade, and margins of resection. Semin Oncol 1994; 21: 527–541
8. Sheldon C A, Williams R D, Fraley E E. Incidental carcinoma of the prostate: a review of the literature and critical reappraisal of classification. J Urol 1980; 124: 626–631
9. Yatani R, Chigusa I, Akazaki K et al. Int J Cancer 1984; 29: 611–616
10. Huben R P, Murphy G P. Prostate cancer: an update. CA 1986; 36: 274–292
11. Kosary C L, Ries L A G, Miller B A et al. (eds) SEER Cancer Statistics Review, 1973–1992: Tables and Graphs. NIH Pub. No. 96-2789. Bethesda, Maryland: National Cancer Institute, 1995.
12. Gittes R F. Carcinoma of the prostate. N Engl J Med 1991; 324: 236–245
13. Stearns M E, McGarvey T. Biology of disease. Prostate cancer: therapeutic, diagnostic, and basic studies. Lab Invest 1992; 67: 540–552
14. Hedley D W. Flow cytometry using paraffin-embedded tissue: five years on. Cytometry 1989; 10: 229–241
15. Merkel D E, McGuire W L. Ploidy, proliferative activity and prognosis. DNA flow cytometry of solid tumors. Cancer 1990; 65: 1194–1205
16. Visakorpi T, Kallioniemi O-P, Koivula T, Isola J. New prognostic factors in prostatic carcinoma. Eur Urol 1993; 24: 438–449
17. Shankey T V, Kallioniemi O-P, Koslowski J M et al. Consensus review of the clinical utility of DNA content cytometry in prostate cancer. Cytometry 1993; 14: 497–500
18. Pollack A, Zagars G K, el-Naggar A K et al. Near-diploidy: a new prognostic factor for clinically localized prostate cancer treated with external beam radiation therapy. Cancer 1994; 73: 1895–1903
19. Brothman A R, Peehl D M, Patel A M, McNeal J E. Frequency and pattern of karyotypic abnormalities in human prostate cancer. Cancer Res 1990; 50: 3795–3803
20. Brothman A R, Peehl D M, Patel A M et al. Cytogenetic evaluation of 20 cultured primary prostatic tumors. Cancer Genet Cytogenet 1991; 55: 79–84
21. Lundgren R, Mandahl N, Heil S et al. Cytogenetic analysis of 57 primary prostatic adenocarcinomas. Genes Chromosomes Cancer 1992; 4: 16–24
22. Sandberg A A. Chromosomal abnormalities and related events in prostate cancer. Hum Pathol 1992; 23: 368–380
23. Micale M A, Mohamed A, Sakr W et al. Cytogenetics of primary prostatic adenocarcinoma. Clonality and chromosome instability. Cancer Genet Cytogenet 1992; 61: 165–173
24. Arps S, Rodewald A, Schmalenberger B et al. Cytogenetic survey of 32 cancers of the prostate. Cancer Genet Cytogenet 1993; 66: 93–99
25. Hyytinen E, Visakorpi T, Kallioniemi A et al. Improved technique for analysis of formalin-fixed paraffin-embedded tumors by fluorescence in situ hybridization. Cytometry 1994; 16: 93–99
26. Macoska J A, Micale M A, Sakr W A et al. Extensive genetic alterations in prostate cancer revealed by dual PCR and FISH analysis. Genes Chromosom Cancer 1993; 8: 88–97
27. Micale M A, Sanford J S, Powell I J et al. Defining the extent and nature of cytogenetic events in prostatic adenocarcinoma: paraffin FISH vs. metaphase analysis. Cancer Genet Cytogenet 1993; 69: 7–12
28. Alcaraz A, Takahashi S, Brown J A et al. Aneuploidy and aneusomy of chromosome 7 detected by fluorescence in situ hybridization are markers of poor prognosis in prostate cancer. Cancer Res 1994; 54: 3998–4002

29. Bandyk M G, Zhao L, Troncoso P *et al.* Trisomy 7: a potential cytogenetic marker of human prostate cancer progression. Genes Chromosom Cancer 1994; 9: 19–27

30. Baretton G B, Valina C, Vogt T *et al.* Interphase cytogenetic analysis of prostatic carcinomas by use of nonisotopic in situ hybridization. Cancer Res 1994; 54: 4472–4480

31. Jones E, Zhu X L, Rohr L R *et al.* Aneusomy of chromosomes 7 and 17 detected by FISH in prostate cancer and the effects of selection in vitro. Genes Chromosom Cancer 1994; 11: 163–170

32. Koivisto P, Hyytinen E, Palmberg C *et al.* Analysis of genetic changes underlying local recurrence of prostate carcinoma during androgen deprivation therapy. Am J Pathol 1995; 147: 1608–1614

33. Persons D L, Gibney D J, Katzmann J A *et al.* Use of fluorescent in situ hybridization for deoxyribonucleic acid ploidy analysis of prostatic adenocarcinoma. J Urol 1993; 150: 120–125

34. Persons D L, Takai K, Gibney D J *et al.* Comparison of fluorescence in situ hybridization with flow cytometry and static image analysis in ploidy analysis of paraffin-embedded prostate adenocarcinoma. Hum Pathol 1994; 25: 678–683

35. Qian J, Bostwick D, Takahashi S *et al.* Chromosomal anomalies in prostatic intraepithelial neoplasia and carcinoma detected by fluorescence in situ hybridization. Cancer Res 1995; 55: 5408–5414

36. Steilen H, Ketter R, Romanakis K *et al.* DNA aneuploidy in prostatatic adenocarcinoma: a frequent event, as shown by fluorescence in situ hybridization. Hum Pathol 1994; 25: 1306–1313

37. Takahashi S, Qian J, Brown J A *et al.* Potential markers of prostate cancer aggressiveness detected by fluorescence in situ hybridization in needle biopsies. Cancer Res 1994; 54: 3574–3579

38. Takahashi S, Alcaraz A, Brown J A *et al.* Aneusomies of chromosomes 8 and Y detected by fluorescence in situ hybridization are prognostic markers for pathological stage C ($pT_3N_0M_0$) prostate carcinoma. Clin Cancer Res 1996; 2: 137–145

39. Visakorpi T, Hyytinen E, Kallioniemi A *et al.* Sensitive detection of chromosome copy number aberrations in prostate cancer by fluorescence in situ hybridization. Am J Pathol 1994; 145: 1–7

40. Carter B S, Ewing C M, Ward W S *et al.* Allelic loss of chromosomes 16q and 10q in human prostate cancer. Proc Natl Acad Sci U S A 1990; 87: 8751–8755

41. Bergerheim U S R, Kunimi K, Collins V P, Ekman P. Deletion mapping of chromosomes 8, 10 and 16 in human prostatic carcinoma. Genes Chromosom Cancer 1991; 3: 215–220

42. Isaacs W B, Bova G S, Morton R A *et al.* Molecular biology of prostate cancer. Semin Oncol 1994; 21: 514–521

43. Kunimi K, Bergerheim U S R, Larsson I-L *et al.* Allelotyping of human prostatic adenocarcinoma. Genomics 1991; 11: 530–536

44. Cooney K A, Wetzel J C, Consolino C M, Wojno K J. Identification and characterization of proximal 6q deletions in prostate cancer. Cancer Res 1996; 56: 4150–4153

45. Cunningham J M, Shan A, Wick M J *et al.* Allelic imbalance and microsatellite instability in prostatic adenocarcinoma. Cancer Res 1996; 56: 4475–4482

46. Bova G S, Carter B S, Bussemakers M J G *et al.* Homozygous deletion and frequent allelic loss of chromosome 8p22 loci in human prostate cancer. Cancer Res 1993; 53: 3869–3873

47. Trapman J, Sleddens H F B M, van der Weiden M M *et al.* Loss of heterozygosity of chromosome 8 microsatellite loci implicates a candidate tumor suppressor gene between the loci D8S87 and D8S133 in human prostate cancer. Cancer Res 1994; 54: 6061–6064

48. Emmert-Buck M R, Vocke C D, Pozzatti R O *et al.* Allelic loss on chromosome 8p12-21 in microdissected prostatic intraepithelial neoplasia. Cancer Res 1995; 55: 2959–2962

49. MacGrogan D, Levy A, Bostwick D *et al.* Loss of chromosome arm 8p loci in prostate cancer: mapping by quantitative allelic imbalance. Genes Chromosom Cancer 1994; 10: 151–159

50. Macoska J, Trybus T, Benson P *et al.* Evidence for three tumor suppressor gene loci on chromosome 8p in human prostate cancer. Cancer Res 1995; 55: 5390–5395

51. Matsuyama H, Pan Y, Skoog L *et al.* Deletion mapping of chromosome 8p in prostate cancer by fluorescence in situ hybridization. Oncogene 1994; 9: 3071–3076

52. Bova G S, MacGrogan D, Levy A *et al.* Physical mapping of chromosome 8p22 markers and their homozygous deletion in a metastatic prostate cancer. Genomics 1996; 35: 46–54

53. Macoska J A, Micale M A, Sakr W A *et al.* Extensive genetic alterations in prostate cancer revealed by dual PCR and FISH analysis. Genes Chromosom Cancer 1993; 8: 88–97

54. Sakr W A, Macoska J A, Benson P et al. Allelic loss in locally metastatic, multisampled prostate cancer. Cancer Res 1994; 54: 3273–3277

55. Phillips S M A, Morton D G, Lee S J et al. Loss of heterozygosity of the retinoblastoma and adenomatous polyposis susceptibility gene loci and in chromosomes 10p, 10q and 16q in human prostate cancer. Br J Urol 1994; 173: 390–395

56. Gray I, Phillips S, Lee S et al. Loss of the chromosomal region 10q23-25 in prostate cancer. Cancer Res 1995; 55: 4800–4803

57. Eagle L R, Yin X, Brothman A R et al. Mutation of the MXI1 gene in prostate cancer. Nature Genet 1995; 9: 249–255

58. Edelhoff S, Ayer D E, Zervos A S et al. Mapping of two genes encoding members of a distinct subfamily of MAX interacting proteins: MAD to human chromosome 2 and mouse chromosome 6, and MXI1 to human chromosome 10 and mouse chromosome 19. Oncogene 1994; 9: 665–668

59. Shapiro D N, Valentine V, Eagle L et al. Assignment of the human MAD and MXI1 genes to chromosomes 2p12–p13 and 10q24–q25. Genomics 1994; 23: 282–285

60. Bookstein R, Rio P, Madreperla SA, et al. Promoter deletion and loss of retinoblastoma gene expression in human prostate carcinoma. Proc Natl Acad Sci USA 1990; 87: 7762–7766

61. Morton R A, Ewing C M, Nagafuchi A et al. Reduction of E-cadherin levels and deletion of the α-catenin gene in human prostate cancer cells. Cancer Res 1993; 53: 3585–3590

62. Phillips S M A, Morton D G, Lee S J et al. Loss of heterozygosity of the retinoblastoma and adenomatous polyposis susceptibility gene loci and in chromosomes 10p, 10q and 16q in human prostate cancer. Br J Urol 1994; 73: 390–395

63. Brewster S F, Browne S, Brown K W. Somatic allelic loss at the DCC, APC, nm23-H1 and p53 tumor suppressor gene loci in human prostatic carcinoma. J Urol 1994; 151: 1073–1077

64. Hahn S A, Schutte M, Shamsul Hoque A T M. DPC4, a candidate tumor suppressor gene at human chromosome 18q21.1 Science 1996; 271: 350–353

65. Gao X, Honn K V, Grignon D et al. Frequent loss of expression and loss of heterozygosity of the putative tumor suppressor gene DCC in prostate carcinomas. Cancer Res 1993; 53: 2723–2727

66. Umbas R, Isaacs W B, Brinquier P P et al. Decreased E-cadherin expression is associated with poor prognosis in patients with prostate cancer. Cancer Res 1994; 54: 3929–3933

67. Umbas R, Schalken J A, Aalders T W. Expression of cellular adhesion molecule e-cadherin is reduced or absent in high-grade prostate cancer. Cancer Res 1992; 52: 5104–5109

68. Otto T, Rembrink K, Goepel M et al. E-cadherin: a marker for differentiation and invasiveness in prostatic carcinoma. Urol Res 1993; 21: 359–362

69. Bussemakers M J G, Giroldi L A, van Bokhoven A, Schalken J A. Transcriptional regulation of the human e-cadherin gene in human prostate cancer cells. Biochem Biophys Res Commun 1994; 203: 1284–1290

70. Vleminckx K, Vakaet L Jr, Mareel M et al. Genetic manipulation of e-cadherin expression by epithelial tumor cells reveals an invasion suppressor role. Cell 1991; 66: 107–119

71. Cher M L, Ito T, Weidner N et al. Mapping of regions of physical deletion on chromosome 16q in prostate cancer cells by fluorescence in situ hybridization (FISH). J Urol 1995; 153: 249–254

72. Hollstein M, Sidransky D, Vogelstein B, Harris C C. p53 mutations in human cancers. Science 1991; 253: 49–53

73. Lane D P. p53, guardian of the genome. Nature 1992; 358: 15–16

74. Hermeking H, Eick D. Mediation of c-myc induced apoptosis by p53. Science 1994; 265: 2091–2093

75. Isaacs W B, Carter B S, Ewing C M. Wild-type p53 suppresses growth of human prostate cancer cells containing mutant p53 alleles. Cancer Res 1991; 51: 4716–4720

76. Bookstein R, MacGrogan D, Hilsenbeck S G et al. p53 is mutated in a subset of advanced-stage prostate cancers. Cancer Res 1993; 53: 3369–3373

77. Dahiya R, Deng G, Chen K M-K et al. p53 tumour-suppressor gene mutations are mainly localised on exon 7 in human primary and metastatic prostate cancer. Br J Cancer 1996; 74: 264–268

78. Visakorpi T, Kallioniemi O-P, Heikkinen A et al. Small subgroup of aggressive, highly proliferative prostatic carcinomas defined by p53 accumulation. J Natl Cancer Inst 1992; 84: 883–888

79. Kallioniemi A, Kallioniemi O-P, Sudar D et al. Comparative genomic hybridization for molecular cytogenetic analysis of solid tumors. Science 1992; 258: 818–821

80. Kallioniemi O-P, Kallioniemi A, Piper J *et al.* Optimizing comparative genomic hybridization for analysis of DNA sequence copy number changes in solid tumors. Genes Chromosom Cancer 1994; 10: 231–243

81. du Manoir S, Speicher M R, Joos S *et al.* Detection of complete and partial chromosomal gains and losses by comparative genomic hybridization. Hum Genet 1993; 90: 590–610

82. Cher M L, MacGrogan D, Bookstein R *et al.* Comparative genomic hybridization, allelic imbalance and fluorescence in situ hybridization on chromosome 8 in prostate cancer. Genes Chromosom Cancer 1994; 11: 153–162

83. Visakorpi T, Kallioniemi A, Syvänen A-C *et al.* Genetic changes in primary and recurrent prostate cancer by comparative genomic hybridization. Cancer Res 1995; 55: 342–347

84. Joos S, Bergerheim U, Pan Y *et al.* Mapping of chromosomal gains and losses in prostate cancer by comparative genomic hybridization. Genes Chromosom Cancer 1995; 14: 267–276

85. Hyytinen E R, Thalmann G N, Zhau H E *et al.* Genetic changes associated with the acquisition of androgen-independent growth, tumorigenicity and metastatic potential in a prostate cancer model. Br J Cancer 1997; 75: 190–195

86. Cher M L, Bova G S, Moore D H *et al.* Genetic alterations in untreated metastases and androgen-independent prostate cancer detected by comparative genomic hybridization and allelotyping. Cancer Res 1996; 56: 3091–3102

87. Wu H-C, Hsieh J-T, Gleave M E *et al.* Derivation of androgen-independent human LNCaP prostatic cancer cell sublines: role of bone stromal cells. Int J Cancer 1994; 57: 406–412

88. Thalmann G N, Anezinis P E, Chang S-M *et al.* Androgen-independent cancer progression and bone metastasis in the LNCaP model of human prostate cancer. Cancer Res 1994; 54: 2577–2581

89. Van Den Berg C, Guan X-Y, Von Hoff D. DNA sequence amplification in human prostate cancer identified by chromosome microdissection: potential prognostic implications. Clin Cancer Res 1995; 1: 11–18

90. Fleming W H, Hamel A, MacDonald R *et al.* Expression of the c-myc proto-oncogene in human prostatic carcinoma and benign prostatic hyperplasia. Cancer Res 1986; 46: 1535–1538

91. Buttyan R, Sawczuk I S, Benson M C *et al.* Enhanced expression of the c-myc protooncogene in high-grade human prostate cancers. Prostate 1987; 11: 327–337

92. Latil A, Baron J-C, Cussenot O *et al.* Oncogene amplifications in early-stage human prostate carcinomas. Int J Cancer 1994; 59: 637–638

93. Visakorpi T, Hyytinen E, Koivisto P *et al.* In vivo amplification of the androgen receptor gene and progression of human prostate cancer. Nature Genet 1995; 9: 401–406

94. Koivisto P, Kononen J, Palmberg C *et al.* Androgen receptor gene amplification: a possible molecular mechanism for androgen deprivation therapy failure in prostate cancer. Cancer Res 1997; 57: 314–319

95. Kellens R E. Gene amplification in mammalian cells. A comprehensive guide. New York: Marcel Dekker, 1993

96. Palmberg C, Koivisto P, Hyytinen E *et al.* Androgen receptor gene amplification in a recurrent prostate cancer after monotherapy with nonsteroidal potent anti-androgen "Casodex" (bicalutamide) with a subsequent favorable response to maximal androgen blockade. Eur Urol 1997; 31: 216–219

97. Culig Z, Hobisch A, Cronauer M V *et al.* Mutant androgen receptor detected in an advanced-stage prostatic carcinoma is activated by adrenal androgens and progesterone. Mol Endocrinol 1993; 7: 1541–1550

98. Newmark J R, Hardy D O, Tonb D C *et al.* Androgen receptor gene mutations in human prostate cancer. Proc Natl Acad Sci USA 1992; 89: 6319–6323

99. Ruizeveld de Winter J A, Janssen P J A, Sleddens H M E B *et al.* Androgen receptor status in localized and locally progressive hormone refractory human prostate cancer. Am J Pathol 1994; 144: 735–746

100. Suzuki H, Sato N, Watabe Y *et al.* Androgen receptor gene mutations in human prostate cancer. J Steroid Biochem Mol Biol 1993; 46: 759–765

101. Tilley W D, Buchanan G, Hickey T E, Bentel J M. Mutations in the androgen receptor gene are associated with progression of human prostate cancer to androgen independence. Clin Cancer Res 1996; 2: 277–285

102. Taplin M-E, Bubley G J, Shuster T D *et al.* Mutation of the androgen-receptor gene in metastatic androgen-independent prostate cancer. N Engl J Med 1995; 332: 1393–1398

103. Berrevoets C A, Veldscholte J, Mulder E. Effects of antiandrogens on transformation and transcription activation of wild-type and mutated (LNCaP) androgen receptors. J Steroid Biochem Mol Biol 1993; 46: 731–736

104. Schoenberg M P, Hakimi J M, Wang S *et al*. Microsatellite mutation (CAG24-18) in the androgen receptor gene in human prostate cancer. Biochem Biophys Res Comm 1994; 198: 74–80

105. Moul J W, Srivastava S, McLeod D G. Molecular implications of the antiandrogen withdrawal syndrome. Semin Urol 1995; 13: 157–163

106. Ichikawa T, Ichikawa Y, Dong J *et al*. Localization of metastasis suppressor gene(s) for prostatic cancer to the short arm of human chromosome 11. Cancer Res 1992; 52: 3486–3490

107. Rinker-Schaeffer C W, Hawkins A L, Ru N *et al*. Differential suppression of mammary and prostate cancer metastasis by human chromosomes 17 and 11. Cancer Res 1994; 54: 6249–6256

108. Dong J-T, Lamb P W, Rinker-Schaeffer C W *et al*. KAI1, a metastasis suppressor gene for prostate cancer on human chromosome 11p11.2. Science 1995; 268: 884–886

109. Dong J-T, Suzuki H, Pin S S *et al*. Down-regulation of the KAI1 metastasis suppressor gene during the progression of human prostate cancer infrequently involves gene mutation or allelic loss. Cancer Res 1996; 56: 4387–4390

110. Kinzler K W, Vogelstein B. Lessons from hereditary colorectal cancer. Cell 1996; 87: 159–170

111. Smith J R, Freije D, Carpten J D *et al*. Major susceptibility locus for prostate cancer on chromosome 1 suggested by a genome-wide search. Science 1996; 274: 1371–1374

Chapter 4
Role of growth factors and cytokines in the development and progression of prostate carcinoma

K. Michel and A. Belldegrun

Introduction

The role of oncogenes in the development of human cancers has been well substantiated. Cellular growth factors can become oncogenic through mutation or overexpression. Alternatively, overexpression or overstimulation of their associated receptors or second messengers can lead to oncogenesis. In fact, research suggests that several growth factors and interleukins may be important in the development and/or progression of prostate cancer. With the increasing incidence of prostate adenocarcinoma in our society, and the lack of effective therapy for advanced disease, new therapeutic modalities to treat advanced prostate carcinoma are necessary. In order to develop such therapeutic modalities, exploring and understanding the pathogenesis of prostate cancer and the factors involved in the malignant transformation are imperative. In this chapter, the potential role of several growth factors (epidermal growth factor, transforming growth factor α, insulin-like growth factor, fibroblast growth factor, and transforming growth factor β) and cytokines (interleukins 2 and 6, IL-2 and IL-6) in the development and progression of prostate cancer are discussed.

Epidermal growth factor (EGF)/transforming growth factor α (TGFα)

Epidermal growth factor (EGF) is a potent promoter of cellular growth and mitosis.[1] Transforming growth factor α (TGFα) is, likewise, a peptide growth factor with mitogenic activity, which structurally and functionally resembles EGF.[2–4] In fact, TGFα may more appropriately be classified as a member of the EGF family. Both ligands bind the EGF receptor (EGFR) and not only induce mitosis and confer anchorage-independent cell growth, but also inhibit fibronectin expression and enhance expression of plasminogen activators.[2]

EGFR is a 170 kD transmembrane glycoprotein that possesses tyrosine kinase activity.[1,4–7] Ligand binding of the receptor activates this activity, which in turn phosphorylates a number of cellular proteins, including phospholipase C, γ MAP kinase and the *ras* GTPase-activating protein (GAP).[1,8] These cellular proteins all induce increased cellular metabolism.[1,8] EGFR possesses great homology to the avian viral *erb*B gene. EGFR is considered to be a member of the c-*erb*B family, the overexpression of which has recently been associated with multiple human malignancies.[1] EGFR (c-*erb*B-1) overexpression is most commonly noted in squamous cell carcinomata. Its overexpression is also a prognostic indicator of poor outcome in patients with lung, bladder or breast carcinomata.[8]

Overexpression of the c-erbB-2 (HER-2, or *neu*) receptor is more commonly associated with the development of adenocarcinomata. Furthermore, a number of researchers have demonstrated that activation of the EGFR (c-erbB-1) can result in cross-phosphorylation of the c-erbB-2 protein in cells that express both receptors.[9–11] This might be achieved by heterodimerization of the EGFR and the c-erbB-2 protein, which is induced by EGF or TGFα binding.[12,13] This binding dramatically increases the capacity for self-phosphorylation of the dimerized receptor. The association of c-erbB-3 overexpression with human cancers is currently less well defined.

Cell line studies have demonstrated that addition of the supernatant of prostate cancer cell line PC-3 to other prostate cancer cell lines (LNCaP, and DU-145) enhances their cell growth rate dramatically.[3] Purification of the supernatant has revealed TGFα to be the important mitogen and cell growth promoter. Subsequent studies have shown that most prostate cancer cell lines, as well as fresh BPH and prostate cancer specimens, express TGFα.[2,3] However, EGF expression in prostate cancer cell lines and fresh prostate specimens has been noted in only a few studies.[14,15] Furthermore, studies have demonstrated that EGFR is expressed predominantly in the basal epithelial cell layer of BPH specimens, and relatively little or no EGFR expression is noted in the luminal epithelial cells.[15–17] Expression of TGFα, however, is noted predominantly in the luminal epithelium, with relatively little in the basal epithelial layer.[8] Furthermore, the transition of prostate specimens from benign prostatic hyperplasia (BPH) to prostate intra-epithelial neoplasia (PIN) to prostate adenocarcinoma is associated with decreased basal epithelial EGFR expression and increased EGFR expression in the luminal epithelium.[15,17] Ultimately, prostate adenocarcinomata (where no basal cell layer is noted) express EGFR only in the luminal epithelium and not in any adjacent stromal components. Interestingly, such a relationship has also been noted in breast tissue.[16] Normal breast tissues reveal EGFR expression predominantly in the periacinar muscular layer (analogous to prostatic basal epithelial cells), with little expression in the ductal epithelium. A shift of EGFR expression from muscular to ductal epithelial cells is also noted in the transition from benign to malignant breast tissue.[16]

There is dispute, however, regarding the overall expression of EGFR in BPH versus prostate adenocarcinoma, as to whether *over* or *under*expression of EGFR is associated with development of prostate cancer.[17–19] The same debate and conflicting data also exist regarding total TGFα expression in BPH versus prostate cancer specimens.[15,20,21]

Interestingly, exogenous dihydrotestosterone (DHT) and testosterone also stimulate growth of prostate cancer cell lines *in vitro*, and potentiate the mitogenic effect of exogenous EGF and TGFα. Studies have demonstrated that addition of exogenous androgens to prostate cancer cell lines enhances EGFR and TGFα mRNA and EGFR protein expression.[22,23] Competitive inhibition of EGFR in fact blocked not only the EGF/TGFα effect, but also the mitogenic effect of DHT/testosterone when added alone or in conjunction with EGF/TGFα.[22,24] These results suggest that the mitogenic effect of androgens on prostate cancer cell lines is mediated through an EGFR-dependent mechanism. Loss of androgen-dependent activation of the EGFR may be an important change in the development of hormone-resistant prostate cancer.

Insulin-like growth factor (IGF)

Insulin-like growth factors 1 and 2 (IGF-1 and IGF-2) are ubiquitous growth-hormone-dependent, single-chained polypeptides that share great homology with pro-insulin.[25,26] IGF-1 and IGF-2 induce increased cellular metabolic and mitogenic activity.[25]

Two IGF receptors (IGFR1 and 2) have been identified. IGFR1 is fairly similar to the insulin receptor.[27] Both mediate their actions through a tyrosine kinase moiety and both receptors contain an α and a β subunit.[28] The β subunits are identical and the α subunits differ only in their specificity for IGF and insulin. IGFR2, however, is quite unlike IGFR1 or the insulin receptor.[29] Unlike the other two, IGFR2 is a single polypeptide receptor and its function has not yet been elucidated. IGFR1 is the more important receptor for induction of cellular growth and division. IGFR1 preferentially binds to IGF-1, with an affinity four times higher than that for IGF-2 and 1000-fold higher than for insulin.[27,30]

The presence of six IGF-binding proteins (IGFBPs) has also been noted.[31] IGFBPs can act as a reservoir for IGF. By binding IGF, the IGF half-life is prolonged and a constant supply of IGF is maintained in a given milieu.[32] Furthermore, IGFBPs can be present in a 'free' or 'membrane-bound' form.[33] *Free* IGFBPs impart an inhibitory effect by competitively *blocking* IGF–IGFR binding in a dose-dependent manner, thereby blocking IGF-mediated function.[34–36] However, *membrane-bound* IGFBPs *enhance* IGF-mediated effects by a yet undetermined mechanism.[37] Several possibilities including (a) the suppression of rapid IGF degradation, (b) the facilitation of IGF binding to its receptor by alteration of the receptor orientation, (c) the promotion of receptor aggregation, or (d) the activation of transmembrane signalling independent of IGF binding to the IGF receptor, have been suggested.[37] Therefore, independent of cell type and micromilieu, the production of different IGFBP subtypes can result in enhancement or inhibition of IGF-mediated cellular anabolic and mitogenic activity.

IGF-mediated functions also depend on the presence of other cofactors, highlighting the complexity of the regulation of cell growth and cell division. For example, blocking the *epidermal* growth factor receptor (EGFR) will result in ablation of IGF-mediated functions.[38] Interestingly, EGF has been shown to stimulate IGFBP production;[39] perhaps blocking of EGFR activity results in the altered IGFBP production, ultimately leading to inhibition of IGF-mediated effects.

Studies evaluating the expression of IGF-1, IGF-2, IGFR and IGFBP have failed to demonstrate IGF-1 expression at the protein or mRNA level in prostate epithelial cells.[38,40–42] However, IGF-1 expression is noted in the prostatic stroma, highlighting the importance of stromal–epithelial interactions.[41,43] IGFR1 and 2 are expressed by prostate cancer cell lines and in *ex vivo* prostate adenocarcinoma specimens.[38,44] Furthermore, immunohistochemical studies suggest that although stromal elements are capable of IGFBP production, the majority of IGFBPs are expressed in the luminal epithelial cells of benign and malignant prostatic epithelia.[45] Recent studies have demonstrated increased IGFBP2 and decreased IGFBP3 serum levels in patients with prostate cancer, compared with controls.[46,47]

The importance of IGF in tumour cell growth, invasiveness and metastatic potential is highlighted in a recent study by Burfeind *et al.*[48] IGFR1 expression in prostate cancer cells was blocked using IGFR1 anti-sense. The blocked expression of IGFR1 resulted in dramatically decreased prostate cancer cell growth, as well as loss of invasiveness and metastatic potential.[48]

Under non-malignant conditions, cell growth and cell division are influenced by IGF-dependent mechanisms. The key elements in these highly regulated interactions include IGF-1, IGF-2, the IGFRs, and IGFBPs, as well as other cofunctional regulatory elements such as EGF. Whereas prostatic epithelial cells express IGFR1 and the preponderance of IGFBPs, IGF expression (in particular IGF-1 expression) is mainly localized to the prostatic stroma. Therefore, this normally highly regulated IGF loop can be altered by increased IGF production by the stroma or epithelial cells, altered IGFBP expression, altered IGFR function and normal negative feedback, or by altered concentrations of other peptides, hormones or environmental factors that effect IGF-mediated function. Such changes may ultimately lead to the loss of cell growth and mitotic control, thus imparting the potential for cellular malignant transformation.

Fibroblast growth factor (FGF)

Fibroblast growth factors (FGFs) are ubiquitous polypeptides comprising eight subtypes.[49,50] FGFs are further classified as acidic (aFGF) or basic (bFGF).[51] aFGF is expressed predominantly in the brain and retina, whereas bFGF has a more generalized expression; prostatic cells express bFGF.[52] FGF has several associated functions, namely neo-angiogenesis, promotion of maturation and differentiation of mesenchymal cells, migration of endothelial and mesenchymal cells, and proliferation of the extracellular matrix (ECM).[49,53]

FGF binds specifically to membrane-bound FGF receptors (FGFR).[49,51,54] Two FGFR subtypes, FGFR1 and FGFR2, have been identified. FGFR1 is expressed by cells in the ECM, whereas FGFR2 is expressed by epithelial cells. Furthermore, FGFRs contain a tyrosine kinase moiety that mediates their activity.[55]

The association between FGF and prostatic diseases is currently under evaluation. Whereas the increased expression of FGF in BPH is well substantiated,[56–59] and a potential cause-and-effect relationship between FGF expression and prostatic stromal and epithelial hyperplasia is suggested, the link between FGF and prostate cancer is less well defined.[60,61] Prostate cancer cell lines LNCaP, PC3 and DU145 have all been shown to express FGF and FGFR.[62,63] Furthermore, exogenous FGF stimulates cell growth in the LNCaP and DU145 cell lines, whereas no change in PC3 cell growth is noted.

The expression of FGF in surgical prostate specimens has also been evaluated.[54] FGF expression is high in prepubertal boys, subsequently decreasing post-pubertally, only to increase again (to prepubertal levels) with the development of BPH. The overall expression of FGF in prostate cancer is relatively low. However, although initial studies revealed no correlation between the total FGF expression and prostate cancer,[60] recent reports suggest that FGF8 levels are elevated in prostate cancer specimens compared with 'normal' or BPH specimens. Furthermore, the level of FGF8 expression seems to correlate with the stage of the cancer.[50]

Although it is not clear whether FGF plays a role in the *development* of prostate cancer, it is suggested that altered FGF and FGFR expression may be associated with the transition to more aggressive, less differentiated, more metastatic prostate adenocarcinomas. Gouchan *et al.*[64] demonstrated that, if a combination of well-differentiated rodent prostate cancer epithelial cells (Dunning R3327PAP) and stromal elements are subcutaneously injected into rats, the tumours maintain their differentiated, slow-growing, non-metastatic phenotype. However, when the epithelial cells are injected alone (that is, without any concomitant stromal elements) the cells de-differentiate into an anaplastic, fast-growing, metastasizing subtype, killing the animals in a matter of weeks.

Analysis of the two different (well differentiated, and poorly differentiated) cell subtypes reveals a change in their associated FGF and FGFR expression. In normal prostates, *stromal* cells mainly secrete FGF7 and express FGFR1; the normal prostatic *epithelial* cells predominantly express FGFR2b (which has a specificity for FGF7), and to a much lower extent express FGFR2c (which has a specificity for FGF2). Although, normally, prostatic epithelial cells express FGF receptors, they do *not* produce or express FGFs to any significant extent. This relationship between FGF and FGFR expression is preserved in the well-differentiated rat prostate tumours. However, analysis of the poorly differentiated tumours reveals that, unlike the well-differentiated prostate cancer epithelial cells, the poorly differentiated prostatic epithelial cells express FGF (FGF2, 3 and 5; FGF3 and 5 are embryonic FGF) and exclusively express FGFR2c. As noted previously, FGFR2c has specificity for FGF2, and under 'normal' conditions prostatic epithelial cells predominantly express FGFR2b and only minimally express FGFR2c. This alteration in FGF and FGFR expression highlights the development of autocrine stimulation in the transition from well-differentiated, minimally aggressive, non-metastasizing cancers to poorly differentiated, aggressive, metastasizing cancers. Evaluation of another poorly differentiated, aggressive, readily metastasizing rat prostate cancer cell line (Dunning R3327AT3) reveals exactly the same changes in FGF and FGFR expression that were noted in the de-differentiated Dunning R3327PAP cells, highlighting the possible importance of this altered FGF and FGFR expression in the development of more aggressive prostate cancers.

Transforming growth factor β (TGFβ)

Transforming growth factor β (TGFβ) is a superfamily of five protein subtypes. TGFβ1–3 are expressed in mammals, of which TGFβ1 and 2 are the most important subtypes in human biology.[65] TGFβ has a binding specificity to the TGFβ receptor (TGFβR). TGFβR comprises two subunits, TGFβR1 and TGFβR2 which form a heterodimer.[66] Inactivation or functional mutation of either subunit renders the TGFβR ineffective.[67,68]

TGFβ was initially isolated from the supernatant of a sarcoma cell line.[69] When this was added to a benign fibroblast culture, the fibroblasts developed a transformed phenotype and malignant pattern of growth. Instead of their usual well-organized, density-dependent, monolayer pattern of growth, the fibroblasts developed an erratic, multilayered, density- and anchorage-*independent* cell growth pattern.

Subsequent studies evaluated the effect of TGFβ on different malignant cell lines. Initially, exogenous TGFβ was shown to inhibit cell growth rates in most malignant cell lines.[65,70,71] However, more recent results highlight the fact that the effect of exogenous TGFβ on malignant cell line growth rates is high dependent on the growth conditions used (such as the absence or presence of serum in the growth media, or the use of plastic versus collagen matrix-containing flasks for culture).[71,72] For example, whereas, in the presence of serum-free media, a cell line may exhibit inhibited growth rates when exposed to exogenous TGFβ, the same cell line may develop an increased rate of cell proliferation if serum-containing medium is used instead. This interesting observation suggests the important role of co-growth factors in modulating the effect of TGFβ.

Compilation of studies reveals that TGFβ possesses many tumour-related functions. Thus, TGFβ has the following properties:

1. It enhances malignant cellular growth *in vivo*;[73]
2. It induces angiogenesis;[74]
3. It confers tumour invasiveness by enhancing heparinase and collagenase expression;[75,76] tumour cells expressing high levels of heparinase and collagenase can degrade basement membranes and extracellular matrices more readily;
4. It induces immunosuppression, and decreases B-cell, T-cell, NK and LAK cell proliferation and cytolytic activity through IL-2- (and possibly IL-1) dependent mechanisms.[77–83]

TGFβ, therefore, seems to be an ideal factor for tumorigenesis, as it can stimulate malignant cellular growth, it can impart tumour invasiveness and metastatic potential through increased protease expression, and increased tumour viability through neo-angiogenesis. Furthermore, TGFβ can enable the malignant cells to escape tumour immunosurveillance by inducing immunosuppression of all arms of the immune system.

Given the apparent importance of TGFβ in tumorigenesis, recent research has focused on the potential role of TGFβ in the development of prostate cancer. Immunohistochemical studies reveal that *extra*cellular TGFβ is increased in prostate cancer specimens compared with BPH or normal prostatic tissues. Furthermore, increased *intra*cellular TGFβ expression is associated with de-differentiation of prostate cancers.[84] Interestingly, inducing malignant transformation of normal mouse prostatic epithelial cells with *ras* and *myc* transfections results in increased TGFβ expression.[85]

To elucidate further the potential role of TGFβ in tumour progression, Steiner *et al.* transfected rat prostate cancer cells with the TGFβ gene.[73] These cells produced significantly higher amounts of TGFβ and, when implanted, grew more rapidly and metastasized more readily than those cancer cells that had not been transfected. At the time of tumour harvesting, the tumours producing high levels of TGFβ were also less necrotic and, therefore, more viable.

As previously highlighted, TGFβ seems to impart several important tumorigenic-related effects (Figure 4.1). It therefore follows that inhibiting TGFβ expression may alter the biology of a given tumour. In fact, inhibition of TGFβ expression in different tumour models has resulted in complete eradication of the given tumours in *in vivo* models.[86–88] Similar models evaluating the efficacy of TGFβ blockade for treatment of prostate cancer are currently under way.

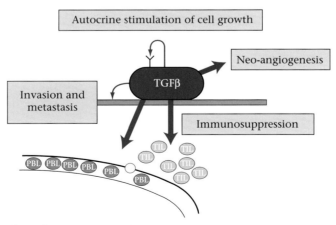

Figure 4.1. Effects of TGFβ on tumorigenesis.

Interleukins (IL-6 and IL-2)

Although there is little information regarding the possible role of cytokines in the development and progression of prostate cancer, some data regarding the possible roles of IL-6 and IL-2 in prostate cancer tumorigenesis are available. IL-6 has been shown to function as an autocrine factor in several human tumours[89–93] and its possible role in the development and progression of prostate cancer has also been suggested. Although IL-6 expression, and expression of its receptor (IL-6R), have been documented in human prostate cancer cell lines LNCaP, DU-145 and PC-3,[89,94] the effect of IL-6 on the cell lines' growth rates and behaviour is unclear. Whereas exogenous IL-6 moderately stimulates the LNCaP growth rate, it has not been shown to impart any change in the growth rates of the more aggressive PC-3 and DU-145 cell lines.[95] Furthermore, no correlation has been noted between the level of IL-6 expression and the presence of prostate cancer versus BPH or normal prostatic tissue.[94,96] Recent data, however, suggest that IL-6 may be an important factor in chemotherapy resistance of prostate cancers. It has been demonstrated that antibody-mediated suppression of IL-6 function renders the chemoresistant prostate cancer cell lines, DU-145 and PC-3, significantly more chemosensitive.[97]

Prostate cancer has classically been considered to be a relatively non-immunogenic human tumour, as judged by the relative absence of tumour-infiltrating lymphocytes (TIL) on histological evaluation of prostate cancer specimens; however, recent research suggests a different viewpoint. Reports reveal that prostate adenocarcinoma can incite a significant immune reaction, and that irradiated prostate cancer cells in conjunction with IL-2 can be used for vaccine therapy. Using this model, regression of primary prostate cancers as well as that of distant metastatic sites has been demonstrated.[98] Furthermore, using this construct, an immune memory can be stimulated, thereby delaying or preventing the development of local recurrences or of distant metastases.[98] These data have spawned new ideas about ways of stimulating host tumour responses against harboured prostate cancers, for eradication of local and distant disease.

Conclusions

Understanding the mechanisms involved in malignant transformation and tumorigenesis may provide insight into potential means of altering, halting or even reversing these processes. The lack of effective therapeutic modalities for the treatment of advanced prostate cancer necessitates further insight into these mechanisms. Likewise, further elucidation of the role of growth factors and cytokines in the development and progression of prostate cancer may provide strategies for treatment of advanced prostate cancer and prostate cancer in general. Review of the role of growth factors in prostate cancer tumorigenesis highlights the importance of stromal–epithelial interactions, the frequent development of unregulated autocrine stimulation, and the importance of co-regulatory elements in dictating the ultimate cellular effect of growth factors. Furthermore, cytokine biology connotes the importance of tumour immunogenicity even in the prostate cancer model. As indicated, utilization of a stimulated immune system may be an effective means of eradicating prostate cancers *in vivo*. Improved understanding of tumorigenesis has already led to the development of new approaches for the treatment of prostate cancer and cancers in general. Although impressive results have been noted *in vitro* and *in vivo*, the efficacy of these therapeutic modalities in treating cancers in humans has yet to be determined.

References

1. Prigent S A, Lemoine N R. The type 1 (EGFR-related) family of growth factor receptors and their ligands. Prog Growth Factor Res 1992; 4: 1–24
2. Wilding G, Valverius E, Knabbe C, Gelmann E P. Role of transforming growth factor-α in human prostate cancer cell growth. Prostate 1989; 15: 1–12
3. Hofer R H, Sherwood E R, Bromberg W D *et al*. Autonomous growth of androgen-independent human prostatic carcinoma cells: role of transforming growth factor-α. Cancer Res 1991; 51: 2780–2785
4. Thompson DM, Gill G N. The EGF receptor: structure, regulation, and potential role in malignancy. Cancer Surv 1985; 4(4): 767–788
5. Stoscheck C M, King L E Jr. Role of epidermal growth factor in carcinogenesis. Cancer Res 1986; 46: 1030–1037
6. Untawale S, Zorbas M A, Hodgson C P *et al*. Tranforming growth factor alpha production and autoinduction in a colorectal carcinoma cell line (DiFi) with an amplified epidermal growth factor receptor gene. Cancer Res 1993; 53: 1630–1636
7. Saitoh T, Masliah E, Jin L W *et al*. Protein kinases and phosphorylation in neurological disorders and cell death. Lab Invest 1991; 64: 596–616
8. Gullick W J. Prevalence of aberrant expression of the epidermal growth factor in human cancers. Br Med Bull 1991; 47(1): 87–98
9. King C R, Borrello I, Bellot F *et al*. EGF binding to its receptor triggers a rapid tyrosine phosphorylation of the erbB-2 protein in the mammary tumour cell line SK-BR-3. EMBO J 1988; 7: 1647–1651
10. Kokai Y, Dobashi K, Weiner D B *et al*. Phosphorylation process induced by epidermal growth factors alters the oncogenic and cellular neu (NGL) gene products. Proc Natl Acad Sci USA 1988; 85: 5389–5393
11. Stern D F, Kamps M P, Cao H. Oncogenic activation of p185neu stimulates tyrosine phosphorylation in vivo. Mol Cell Biol 1988; 8: 3969–3973
12. Wada T, Qian X, Green M I. Intermolecular association of the p185neu protein and EGF receptor modulator EGF receptor function. Cell 1990; 61: 1339–1347
13. Goldman R, Levy R B, Peler E, Yarden Y. Heterodimerization of the c-erbB-1 and c-erbB-2 receptors in human breast carcinoma cells: a mechanism for receptor transregulation. Biochemistry 1990; 29: 11024–11028
14. Connolly J M, Rose D P. Autocrine regulation of DU145 human prostate cancer cell growth by epidermal growth factor-related polypeptides. Prostate 1991; 19: 173–180
15. Glynne-Jones E, Goddard L, Harper M E. Comparative analysis of mRNA and protein expression of epidermal growth factor receptor and ligands relative to the proliferative index in human prostate tissue. Hum Pathol 1996; 27(7): 688–694
16. Maygarden S J, Strom S, Ware J L. Localization of epidermal growth factor receptor by immunohistochemical methods in human prostatic carcinoma, prostatic intraepithelial neoplasia, and benign hyperplasia. Arch Pathol Lab Med 1992; 116: 269–273
17. Ibrahim G K, Kerns B-JM, Macdonald J A *et al*. Differential immunoreactivity of epidermal growth factor receptor in benign, dysplastic, and malignant prostatic tissues. J Urol 1993; 149: 170–173
18. Eaton C L, Davies P, Phillips M. Growth factor involvement and oncogene expression in prostate tumours. J Steroid Biochem 1988; 30(1–6): 341–345
19. Maddy S Q, Chisholm G D, Busuttil A, Habib F K. Epidermal growth factor receptors in human prostate cancer: correlation with histological differentiation of the tumour. Br J Cancer 1989; 60(1): 41–44
20. Tukeri L N, Sakr W A, Wykes S M *et al*. Comparative analysis of epidermal growth factor receptor gene expression and protein product in benign, premalignant, and malignant prostate tissue. Prostate 1994; 25: 199–205
21. Myers R B, Kudlow J E, Grizzle W E. Expression of TGF-α, epidermal growth factor and the epidermal growth factor receptor in adenocarcinoma of the prostate and benign prostatic hyperplasia. Mod Pathol 1993; 6(6): 733–737
22. Liu X, Wiley H S, Meikel W. Androgens regulate proliferation of human prostate cancer cells in culture by increasing transforming growth factor-α (TFG-α) and epidermal growth factor (EGF)/TGF-α receptor. J Clin Endocrinol Metab 1993; 77(6): 1472–1478
23. Limonta P, Dondi D, Marelli M M *et al*. Growth of the androgen-dependent tumor of the prostate: role of androgens and of locally expressed growth modulatory factors. J Steroid Biochem Mol Biol 1995; 53(1–6): 401–405

24. Fiorelli G, De Bellis A, Longo A *et al*. Growth factors in the human prostate. J Steroid Biochem Mol Biol 1991; 40(1–3): 199–205
25. Rosenfeld R G, Lamson G, Pham H *et al*. Insulin-like growth factor-binding proteins. Recent Prog Horm Res 1990; 46: 99–163
26. Daughaday W, Rotwein P. Insulin-like growth factors I and II. Peptides messenger ribonucleic acid and gene structures, serum and tissue concentrations. Endocr Rev 1989; 10: 68–91
27. Rosenfeld R G, Hintz R L. Somatomedin receptors: structure, function, and regulation. In: Conn P M (ed) The receptors, Vol 3. Orlando: Academic Press, 1986; 281–329
28. Ullrich A, Gray A W, Tam A W *et al*. Insulin-like growth factor 1 receptor primary structure: comparison with insulin receptor suggests determinants that define functional specificity. EMBO J 1986; 5: 2503–2512
29. Morgan D O, Edman J C, Standring D N *et al*. Insulin-like growth factor II receptor as a multifunctional binding protein. Nature 1987; 329: 301–307
30. Rosenfeld R G. Somatomedin action and tissue growth-factor receptors. In: Robbins R J, Melmed S (eds) Acromegaly. New York: Plenum Press, 1987; 45–53
31. Shimasaki S, Ling N. Identification and molecular characterization of insulin-like growth factor binding proteins (IGFBP-1,-2,-3,-4,-5,-6). Prog Growth Factor Res 1991; 3: 243–266
32. Nissley S P, Rechler M M. Insulin-like growth factors: biosynthesis, receptors, and carrier proteins. In: Li C H (ed) Hormonal proteins and peptides, Vol 12. New York: Academic Press, 1984: 127–203
33. Conover C A, Ronk M, Lombana F, Powel D. Structural and biological characterization of bovine insulin-like growth factor binding protein-3. Endocrinology 1990; 127(6): 2795–2803
34. Cohen P, Lamson G, Toshihiro O, Rosenfeld R G. Transfection of the human insulin-like growth factor binding protein-3 gene into Balb/c fibroblasts inhibits cellular growth. Mol Endocrinol 1993; 7: 380–386
35. Bicsak T A, Simonaka M, Malkowski M, Ling N. Insulin-like growth factor protein (IGF-BP) inhibition of granulosa cell function: effect on cyclic adenosine 3, 5-monophosphate, deoxyribonucleic acid synthesis, and comparison with the effect of an IGF-I antibody. Endocrinology 1990; 126(4): 2184–2189
36. Ritvos O, Ranta T, Jalkanen J *et al*. Insulin-like growth factor (IGF) binding protein from human decidua inhibits the binding and biological action of IGF-I in cultured choriocarcinoma cells. Endocrinology 1988; 122(5): 2150–2157
37. Andress D L, Birnbaum R S. Human osteoblast-derived insulin-like growth factor (IGF) binding protein-5 stimulates osteoblast mitogenesis and potentiates IGF action. J Biol Chem 1992; 267(31): 22467–22472
38. Connolly J, Rose D P. Regulation of DU145 human prostate cancer cell proliferation by insulin-like growth factors and its interaction with the epidermal growth factor autocrine loop. Prostate 1994; 24: 167–175
39. Martin J L, Baxter R C. Insulin-like growth factor-binding proteins (GF-bps) produced by human skin fibroblasts: immunological relationships to other human IGF-BPs. Endocrinology 1988; 123: 1907–1915
40. Reiter E, Bonnet P, Sente B *et al*. Growth hormone and protein stimulate androgen receptor, insulin-like growth factor-I (IGF-I) and IGF-I receptor levels in the prostate of immature rats. Mol Cell Endocrinol 1992; 88: 77–87
41. Barni T, Vannelli B, Sadri R *et al*. Insulin-like growth factor-I and its binding protein IGFBP-4 in human prostatic hyperplastic tissue: gene expression and its cellular localization. J Clin Endocrinol Metab 1994; 78: 778–783
42. Yee D, Paik S, Lebovic G S *et al*. Analysis of insulin-like growth factor I gene expression in malignancy: evidence for a paracrine role in human breast cancer. Mol Endocrinol 1989; 3: 509–517
43. Bonnet P, Reiter E, Bruyninx M *et al*. Benign prostatic hyperplasia and normal prostate aging: differences in type I and II 5α-reductase and steroid hormone receptors messenger ribonucleic acid (mRNA) levels, but not in insulin-like growth factor mRNA levels. J Clin Endocrinol Metab 1993; 77: 1203–1208
44. Cohen P, Peehl D, Lamson G, Rosenfeld R G. Insulin-like growth factors (IGFs), IGF receptors, and IGF-binding proteins in primary cultures of prostate epithelial cells. J Clin Endocrinol Metab 1991; 73(2): 401–407
45. Tennant M K, Thrasher J B, Twomey P A *et al*. Insulin-like growth factor-binding protein-2 and -3 expression in benign human prostate epithelium, prostate intraepithelial neoplasia, and adenocarcinoma of the prostate. J Clin Endocrinol Metab 1996; 81(1): 411–420

46. Cohen P, Peehl D M, Stamey T *et al.* Elevated levels of insulin-like growth factor-binding protein-2 in the serum of prostate cancer patients. J Clin Endocrinol Metab 1993; 76: 1031–1035

47. Kanety H, Madjar Y, Dagan Y *et al.* Serum insulin-like growth factor-binding protein-2 (IGFBP-2) is increased and IGFBP-3 is decreased in patients with prostate cancer; correlation with serum prostate-specific antigen. J Clin Endocrinol Metab 1993; 77: 229–233

48. Burfeind P, Chernicky C L, Rininsland F *et al.* Antisense RNA to the type I insulin-like growth factor receptor suppresses tumor growth and prevents invasion by rat prostate cancer cells in vivo. Proc Natl Acad Sci USA 1996; 93: 7263–7268

49. Gospodarowicz D, Ferrara N, Schweigerer L, Neufeld G. Structural characterization and biological functions of fibroblast growth factor. Endocr Rev 1987; 8(2): 95–114

50. Leung H Y, Dickson C, Robson C N, Neal D E. Over-expression of fibroblast growth factor-8 in human prostate cancer. Oncogene 1996; 12: 1883–1835

51. Culig B, Hobisch A, Conauer M V *et al.* Regulation of prostatic growth and function by peptide growth factors. Prostate 1996; 28: 392–405

52. Luo D, Lin Y, Liu X *et al.* Effect of prostatic growth factor, basic fibroblast growth factor, epidermal growth factor, and steroids on the proliferation of human fetal prostatic fibroblasts. Prostate 1996; 28: 352–358

53. Pienta K, Isaccs W, Vindivich D, Coffey D. The effects of basic fibroblast growth factor and suramin on cell motility and growth of rat prostate cancer cells. J Urol 1991; 145: 199–202

54. Yan G, Fukabori Y, McBride G *et al.* Exon switching and activation of stromal and embryonic fibroblast growth factor (FGF)-FGF receptor genes in prostate epithelial cells accompany stromal independence and malignancy. Mol Cell Biol 1993; 13: 4513–4522

55. Xu J, Nakahara M, Crabb J W *et al.* Expression and immunochemical analysis of rat and human fibroblast growth factor receptor (flg) isoforms. J Biol Chem 1992; 267: 17792–17803

56. Hamaguchi A, Tooyama I, Yoshiki T, Kimura H. Demonstration of fibroblast growth factor receptor-1 in human prostate by polymerase chain reaction and immunohistochemistry. Prostate 1995; 27: 141–147

57. Begun F, Story M, Hopp K *et al.* Regional concentration of basic fibroblast growth factor in normal and benign hyperplastic human prostates. J Urol 1995; 153: 839–843

58. Geller J, Soinit L, Baird A *et al.* In vivo and in vitro effects of androgen on fibroblast growth factor-2 concentration in the human prostate. Prostate 1994; 25: 206–209

59. Nishi N, Matho Y, Kunimoto K *et al.* Comparative analysis of growth factors in normal and pathologic human prostates. Prostate 1988; 13: 39–48

60. Meyer G, Yu E, Siegel J *et al.* Serum basic fibroblast growth factor in men with and without prostate carcinoma. Cancer 1995; 70: 2304–2311

61. Gleave M E, Hsieh J T, Von Eschenbach A C, Chung L W. Prostate and bone fibroblasts induce human prostate cancer growth in vivo; implications for bidirectional tumor–stromal interaction in prostate carcinoma growth and metastasis. J Urol 1992; 147: 1151–1159

62. Nakamoto T, Chang C, Li A, Chodak G. Basic fibroblast growth factor in human prostate cancer cells. Cancer Res 1992; 52: 571–577

63. Culig Z, Hobisch A, Cronauer M *et al.* Androgen receptor activation in prostatic tumor cell lines by human insulin-like growth factor-1, keratinocyte growth factor, and epidermal growth factor. Cancer Res 1994; 54: 5474–5478

64. Yan G, Fukabori Y, McBride G *et al.* Exon switching and activation of stromal and embryonic fibroblast growth factor (FGF)-FGF receptor genes in prostate epithelial cells accompany stromal independence and malignancy. Mol Cell Biol 1993; 13(8): 4513–4522

65. Massague J. The transforming growth factor-β family. Annu Rev Cell Biol 1990; 6: 597–641

66. Kim I Y, Ahn H, Zelner D *et al.* Loss of expression of transforming growth factor β type I and type II receptors correlates with tumor grade in human prostate cancer tissues. Clin Cancer Res 1996; 2: 1255–1261

67. Chen F, Weinber R A. Biochemical evidence for the auto-phosphorylation and transphosphorylation of transforming growth factor β receptor kinases. Proc Natl Acad Sci USA 1995; 92: 1565–1569

68. Wrana J L, Attisano L, Wieser R *et al.* Mechanism of the activation of the TGFβ receptor. Nature 1994; 370: 341–347

69. De Larco J E, Todaro G J. Growth factors from murine sarcoma virus-transformed cells. Proc Natl Acad Sci USA 1978; 75(8): 4001–4005

70. Ware J L. Growth factors and their receptors as determinants in the proliferation and metastasis of human prostate cancer. Cancer Metastasis Rev 1993; 12: 287–301

71. Roberts A B, Anzano M A, Wakefield L M et al. Type β transforming growth factor: a bifunctional regulator of cellular growth. Proc Natl Acad Sci USA 1985; 82: 119–123.

72. Moses H L, Tucker R F, Leof E B et al. Type β transforming growth factor is a growth stimulator and a growth inhibitor. In: Feramisco J, Ozanna B, Stiles C (eds) Cancer cells, Vol 3. New York: Cold Springs Harbor Press, 1985: 65–75

73. Steiner M S, Barrack E R. Transforming growth factor β-1 overproduction in prostate cancer; effects on growth in vivo and in vitro. Mol Endocrinol 1992; 6: 15–25

74. Roberts A B, Spron M B, Assoian R K et al. TFG type β: rapid induction of fibrosis and antiogenesis in vivo and stimulation of collagen formation in vitro. Proc Natl Acad Sci USA 1986; 83: 4167–4171

75. Welch D R, Fabra A, Nakajima M. Transforming growth factor β stimulates mammary adenocarcinoma cell invasion and metastatic potential. Proc Natl Acad Sci USA 1990; 87: 7678–7682

76. Sehgal I, Baley P A, Thompson T C. Transforming growth factor β1 stimulates contrasting responses in metastatic versus primary mouse prostate cancer-derived cell lines in vivo. Cancer Res 1996; 56: 3359–3365

77. Espevik T, Figari I S, Ranges G E, Palladino M A Jr. Transforming growth factor β1 (TGFβ1) and recombinant human tumor necrosis factor-α reciprocally regulate the generation of lymphokine-activated killer cell activity. J Immunol 1988; 140(7): 2312–2316

78. Wahl S M, Hunt D A, Wong H L et al. Transforming growth factor β is a potent immunosuppressive agent that inhibits IL-1 dependent lymphocyte proliferation. J Immunol 1988; 140(9): 3026–3032

79. Kehrl J H, Roberts A B, Wakefield L M et al. Transforming growth factor β is an important immunomodulatory protein for human B lymphocytes. J Immunol 1986; 137(12): 3855–3860

80. Ristow H. BSC-1 growth inhibitor/type β transforming growth factor is a strong inhibitor of thymocyte proliferation. Proc Natl Acad Sci USA 1986; 83: 5531–5533

81. Kehrl J H, Wakefield L M, Roberts A B et al. Production of transforming growth factor β by human T lymphocytes and its potential role in the regulation of T cell growth. J Exp Med 1986; 164: 1037–1050

82. Rook A H, Kehrl J H, Wakefield L M et al. Effects of transforming growth factor β on the functions of natural killer cells: depressed cytolytic activity and blunting of interferon responsiveness. J Immunol 1986; 136(10): 3916–3920

83. Torre-Amione G, Beauchamp R D, Koeppen H et al. A highly immunogenic tumor transfected with a murine transforming growth factor β1 cDNA escapes immune surveillance. Proc Natl Acad Sci USA 1990; 87: 1486–1490

84. Eastham J A, Truong L D, Rogers E et al. Transforming growth factor β1: comparative immunohistochemical localization in human primary and metastatic prostate cancer. Lab Invest 1995; 73(5): 628–635

85. Thompson T C, Truong L D, Timme T L et al. Transforming growth factor β1 as a biomarker for prostate cancer. J Cell Biochem 1992; Suppl 16H: 54–61

86. Fakhrai H, Dorigo O, Shawler D L et al. Eradication of established intracranial rat gliomas by transforming growth factor β antisense gene therapy. Proc Natl Acad Sci U S A 1996; 93: 2909–2914

87. Jachimczak P, Bogdahn U, Schneider J et al. The effect of transforming growth factor β2 specific phosphorothioate antisense oligodeoxynucleotides in reversing cellular immunosuppression in malignant glioma. J Neurosurg 1993; 78: 944–951

88. Spearman M, Taylor W R, Greenberg A H, Wright J A. Antisense oligonucleotide inhibition of TGFβ1 gene expression and alteration in the growth and malignant properties of mouse fibrosarcoma cells. Gene 1994; 149: 25–29

89. Siegall C B, Schwab G, Nordan R P et al. Expression of the interleukin 6 receptor and interleukin 6 in prostate carcinoma. Cancer Res 1990; 50: 7786–7788

90. Kawano M, Hirano T, Matsuda T et al. Autocrine generation and requirement of BSF-2 IL-6 for human multiple myeloma. Nature 1988; 332: 83–85

91. Taga T, Kawanashi K, Hardy R R et al. Receptors for B cell stimulatory factor 2: quantitation specificity, distribution and regulation of their expression. J Exp Med 1987; 166: 967–981

92. Yamasaki K, Taga T, Hirata Y *et al.* Cloning and expression of the human interleukin-6 (BSF-2/IFNβ2) receptor. Science 1988; 241: 825–828

93. Siedall C B, Nordan R P, Fitzgerald D J, Pastan I. Cell specific cytotoxicity of a chimeric protein composed of interleukin-6 and pseudomonas exotoxin (IL6-PE40) on tumor cells. Mol Cell Biol 1990; 10: 2443–2447

94. Twillie D A, Eisenberger M A, Carducci M A *et al.* Interleukin-6; a candidate mediator of human prostate cancer morbidity. Urology 1995; 45(3): 542–549

95. Okamoto M, Lee C, Oyasu R. Interleukin-6 as a paracrine and autocrine growth factor in human prostatic carcinoma cells in vitro. Cancer Res 1997; 57: 141–146

96. Siegsmund M J, Hitoshi Y, Pastan I. Interleukin 6 receptor mRNA in prostatic carcinomas and benign prostate hyperplasia. J Urol 1994; 151: 1396–1399

97. Borsellino N, Belldegrun A, Bonavida B. Endogenous interleukin 6 is a resistance factor for cis-diamminedichloroplatinum and etoposide-mediated cytotoxicity of human prostate carcinoma cell lines. Cancer Res 1995; 55: 4633–4639

98. Vieweg J, Rosenthal F M, Bannerji R *et al.* Immunotherapy of prostate cancer in the Dunning rat model: use of cytokine gene modified tumor vaccines. Cancer Res 1994; 54(7): 1760–1765

Chapter 5
Epidermal growth factor and its receptor in prostatic growth

D. E. Neal, A. Collins and E. Robinson

Introduction

Each year, 11,000 men in England and Wales develop clinically apparent prostate cancer and 8000 of them die. Most of the tumours are advanced, and initial treatment in the majority is by androgen ablation, which results in subjective improvement in 70%. However, this approach offers only temporary control and eventually proliferation of hormone-unresponsive phenotypes occurs. Upregulation of peptide growth factors or their receptors may be the underlying explanation for androgen resistance. In addition, disturbance of control of the pattern of growth factor secretion in the prostate may be the cause of benign prostatic hyperplasia (BPH).

There are five principal families of peptide growth factors that are currently known to be involved in normal and abnormal prostatic growth. They include transforming growth factors α and β (TGFα and TGFβ), epidermal growth factor(EGF), insulin like growth factors (IGF-I and IGF-II) and some members of the fibroblast growth factor family (FGF).

Epidermal growth factor and transforming growth factor α (Table 5.1)

EGF is a 53-amino-acid peptide with mitogenic activity, the action of which is mediated by binding to a membrane-bound receptor. EGF was originally isolated from murine submaxillary gland extracts and its distribution is widespread, with high levels in milk, prostatic fluid and urine. EGF is mitogenic for prostatic epithelial cells *in vitro*.[1] Castration in adult mice results in extreme prostatic

Table 5.1. Epidermal growth factor (EGF), transforming growth factor α (TGFα) and the epidermal growth factor receptor (EGFr) in the prostate

Cell type	Properties						
	Produce EGF	EGF mRNA	Produce TGFα	TGFα mRNA	Response to EGF	EGF receptor	EGFr mRNA
Normal epithelial	+				+	+	+22
Benign epithelial	+	+30* −	+38		Stimulate	+	+
Prostate cancer	+29	+22	+38				+
DU145	+33	+	+32,42	++	+	++	++30
PC-3	+	+	+32,42	++	+	++	++30
LNCaP	+34	++			+	++	+

*Superscript numbers are those of listed references.

involution, accompanied by a marked reduction in the amount of EGF in the prostate. Conversely, replacement of testosterone in these animals stimulates prostatic growth and restores the tissue levels of EGF.[2] This is in contrast to the role of TGFβ1, which is upregulated by castration and may play the principal role in castration-induced prostatic cell death.[3] This relationship between EGF and TGFβ1 has been supported by experiments using human prostatic epithelial cells.[4]

EGF and TGFα share a common amino-acid sequence containing six characteristically spaced cysteine residues, and have a sequence homology of about 35%. This structural conservation accounts for their ability to interact with the same receptor.[5] Other members of this family include amphiregulin, heregulin-1 and cripto-1.

The epidermal growth factor receptor (EGFr)

EGF and TGFα exert their effects through the epidermal growth factor receptor (EGFr or c-*erb*B1). The differences in the action of these two ligands, on cell growth and function, may be due to different conformational changes induced within the receptor by binding of each ligand.[6] Amphiregulin also acts through the EGFr whereas heregulin binds to c-*erb*B3. Many of the EGFr analogues (c-*erb*B2 and c-*erb*B3) form homodimers or heterodimers in response to ligand activation or to marked over-expression. The EGFr is a 175 kD transmembrane protein with an extracellular EGF binding domain, a small hydrophobic region that spans the plasma membrane and an intracellular domain that has tyrosine kinase activity as well as target tyrosine residues for autophosphorylation. The EGFr (c-*erb*B1 gene) has considerable sequence homology with the gp65[erbB] protein from the avian erythroblastosis virus. Dimerization is a necessary prelude to activation of receptor tyrosine kinase in the non-mutated receptor. The downstream events following receptor activation include binding via intermediate proteins with homology to src (SH2) proteins including shc and grb2; to phospholipase C and phosphoinositidase-3-kinase. Activation of SH2 proteins results in linkage to and activation of *ras* and thereby to activation of MAP-kinase.

The EGFr is distributed throughout the body and is present on normal fibroblasts, corneal cells, kidney cells, prostate epithelium and basal urothelium. Increased expression of EGFr protein is directly transforming in some cell lines, and some human solid tumours, including bladder cancer, have increased levels of EGFr protein. This appears to be achieved by a variety of mechanisms, including gene amplification, upregulation of mRNA, and increased translation or post-translational modification of the protein.

Elevated levels of EGFr have been demonstrated in a variety of human tumours and cell lines.[7] The EGFr mRNA and protein has been demonstrated in human prostatic carcinomas, BPH and normal prostate.[7–9] Increased levels of EGFr mRNA, measured by Northern blotting, are associated with greater tumour extent and with loss of differentiation.[8] However, this conflicts with findings utilizing immunohistochemical techniques, where significant decreases in EGFr expression were found in prostate cancer compared with normal prostate or BPH.[10,11] Ware[12] suggested that this discrepancy may be due to modification of the EGFr in prostate cancer that prevents its detection by standard immunohistochemical techniques, or that TGFα secretion by tumours may downregulate the receptor. Measurement of EGF binding sites in prostatic cancer tissue has also produced conflicting results. Maddy and colleagues[13] demonstrated that tumours with a higher Gleason score had a lower number of EGF binding sites, whereas Davies and Eaton[14] reported that poorly differentiated tumours have higher numbers of EGF binding sites. These conflicting results may be due to different assay techniques or tissue sources. One other possibility relates to the fact that EGFr levels are relatively high in the basal cells of prostatic glands but are lower in the transitional or luminal cells of glands and ducts; on immunocytochemistry, comparison of tumour cells is more likely to be made with these basal cells, whereas it may be that comparison should be made with the transitional or luminal cells from benign glands. A recent careful analysis by Maureen Harper's group,[15] using immunocytochemistry, *in situ* hybridization and Northern blotting, showed that TGFα could be found at mRNA level in BPH. Similarly, no correlation was found between the results of *in situ* hybridization and immunocytochemistry, which suggests that post-translational processing is important in determining final EGFr levels. These authors commented on the high levels of EGFr found in the basal epithelium of BPH with lower levels in secretory luminal epithelium. It is known that, as the epithelial cells migrate from the basal area into the lumen, there is upregulation of androgen receptor levels. The EGFr in normal prostate cells is thought to be downregulated by androgens. It might be expected, therefore, that transitional and luminal cells would be more likely to have lower EGFr levels, as the levels of androgen receptor are high in these cells. The authors therefore suggest that comparison of tumour cells should be made with secretory luminal epithelium rather than with basal cells. This would mean that poorly differentiated tumours would have increased expression of EGFr levels compared with BPH,[15] assuming that luminal cells are relevant to the development of cancer.

The highest levels of expression of EGFr mRNA have been found in the human androgen-independent prostate cancer cell lines DU-145 and PC-3.[8] However, these cell lines show no significant proliferative response when treated with EGFr ligands.[16,17] Both these cells lines produce TGFα.[17,18] The autologous production of growth factors may be linked to the loss of steroid responsiveness in these two cell lines, and reduced response to exogenous growth factors.[16] In contrast, the androgen-sensitive cell line LNCaP expresses lower levels of EGFr mRNA and responds to exogenous EGF and TGFα.[8,18,19] These findings have also led to the suggestion that part of the progression to hormone independence may involve a switch in the predominant ligand from EGF to TGFα.[8] In LNCaP cell lines, androgens upregulate EGFr expression; this is in marked contrast to the normal rat prostate, in which androgens downregulate EGFr expression.[18] This abnormal response may be due to the point mutation found in the androgen receptor of the LNCaP cell line. In recent experiments, the PC3 prostate cancer cell line, which normally lacks the androgen receptor, was stably transfected with the androgen receptor. EGF was positively mitogenic, as were androgens. Cells with the transfected androgen receptor demonstrated a twofold upregulation of EGFr in response to androgens, but in this particular cell line androgen did not induce the secretion of EGF or TGFα into conditioned medium.[20]

c-*erb*B2

The proto-oncogene c-*erb*B2 (also known as *neu* or HER-2) encodes a transmembrane glycoprotein that is related to the EGFr. To date, the ligand(s) for c-*erb*B2 is unknown, although several groups have reported a candidate ligand for the c-*erb*B2 receptor [*neu* differentiation factor (NDF), or heregulin-, (HRG-)] and elucidation of its structure has revealed it as an additional member of the EGF family. Two further members of the *erb*B receptor family are HER-3/p160[erbB3] and HER-4/p180[erbB4]. Recent evidence suggests that heregulin is the physiological ligand for c-[erbB3] (or HER-3). It is possible, however, that the two newly discovered EGF-family members [epiregulin and/or SMDF (sensory and motor neuron-derived factor)] may turn out to be HER-2 activators. The c-erbB2 protein has partial homology with the intracellular domain of the EGFr.[21] Amplification of the c-*erb*B2 gene has been found in human breast cancer[22] and gastric cancer.[23] However, the definitive ligand for c-*erb*B2 has not yet been identified.

In an immunohistochemical study[10] of the expression of c-*erb*B2, the epithelium in benign glands stained strongly for c-*erb*B2 in five of 34 patients (15%). Five of 29 (17%) malignant glands also showed strong positive staining; an additional eight patients with prostate cancer (28%) had weak positive staining of glandular structures and an additional 16 patients with BPH had weak positive staining, mainly in the basal layers of glands. No stromal staining was identified. There was no evidence that high-grade or high-stage tumours contained high levels of c-*erb*B2.

EGF and related peptides

Both EGF and TGFα are secreted from larger precursors cleaved by proteolytic enzymes. Pre-pro-EGF is 1217 amino acids long and the TGFα precursor is 160 amino acids long. The EGFr ligand TGFα has been identified in several tumour cell lines.[24–26] In general, studies have indicated that the normal prostate expresses higher levels of EGF than TGFα, and high levels of EGF are found in seminal plasma. It has been shown that seminal EGF originates from the prostate. EGF is secreted in response to androgens in a simple positively regulated manner in the rat.[27] However, secretion of TGFα does not decrease in response to castration, but does show a slight increase in response to androgens.

Several studies have shown that EGF and TGFα are potent mitogens of cultured prostatic epithelial cells (Figures 5.1 and 5.2). Recent immunocytochemical work has shown that TGFα is undetectable in BPH, but is detected in the epithelium of prostate cancers.[28] EGF has been identified in extracts of prostatic tissue from BPH and prostate cancer[29] (Table 5.2). In addition, both EGF and TGFα have been detected in the human prostate cancer cell lines DU145, PC-3 and LNCaP.[7,18,30,31] Immunocytochemistry for TGFα has shown low amounts in the epithelium of BPH and an increase in intensity of staining in prostatic carcinoma.[32] The least-

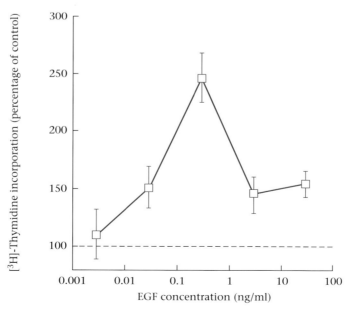

Figure 5.1. Effect of EGF on proliferation of primary cultured epithelial cells.

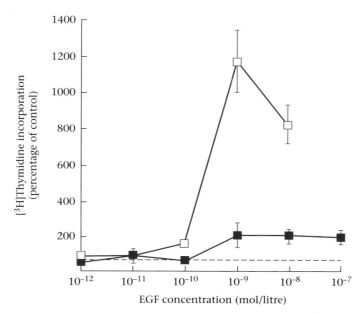

Figure 5.2. Effect of EGF (■) on proliferation of primary cultured stromal cells from the prostate, showing that the combination (□) of EGF plus androgen (mibolerone) induced more marked proliferation than either added alone (mibolerone would normally induce a 200% increase in proliferation); (----) baseline level of proliferation.

Table 5.2. Secretion of TGFα and EGF by prostatic stromal and epithelial cells.

Sample	EGF (ng/ml)	TGFα (ng/ml)
Stroma (S)	ND	0.45
S + androgen	ND	0.61
Epithelium	ND	ND
DU145	10	1.03
Basal medium	ND	ND

ND, not detected.

differentiated tumours expressed the greatest amounts of immunoreactive TGFα. Recent work from the authors' department has failed to detect immunoreactive EGF in conditioned media from prostatic stromal cells grown from human prostatectomy specimens, whereas TGFα was detected and showed a slight increase in response to androgens (Table 5.2). In these experiments, addition of mibolerone with EGF had a synergistic effect on stromal cell growth (Figure 5.2). EGF also had a mitogenic effect on epithelial cells (Figure 5.1).

High levels of EGF are found in the stroma of lymph nodes and bone marrow, and recent studies of the TSU-prl tumour cell line have shown that EGF is strongly chemotactic for prostate cancer cell lines.[33] Stromal conditioned media from LNCaP and DU145 cell lines both contain EGF, but the androgen-independent cell line DU145 contained much more EGF.

Interestingly, it has been shown that EGF can increase transcription of oestrogen-responsive reporter genes, which can be blocked by means of neutralizing antibodies to EGF.[34] Recent work on the androgen receptor has found similar activation of androgen-responsive reporter genes by IGF-I and EGF.[35]

Conclusions

EGF is androgen regulated, decreasing following castration and increasing in response to external androgens. TGFα is not found at high levels in benign epithelium, but is upregulated in cancer — particularly in tumours of high grade. EGF in cell culture studies has been shown to activate androgen-responsive elements, suggesting that high levels of expression or activation of the EGFr may be able to circumvent androgen-regulated growth. The EGFr is not tightly androgen regulated, but levels tend to decrease in response to androgens. It is found in benign basal cells at high levels, but is downregulated in transitional and luminal secretory cells in BPH. Compared with these secretory luminal cells EGFr may be upregulated in prostate cancer — a finding supported by studies using Northern blotting and *in situ* methods. The EGF/TGFα pathway is just one of the biochemical paths that may circumvent androgen control: others, including IGF-I and the FGF family, are also important.

References

1. McKeenan W L, Adams P, Rosser M P. Direct mitogenic effects of insulin, epidermal growth factor, glucocorticoid, cholera toxin, unknown pituitary factors and possibly prolactin, but not androgen, on normal rat prostate epithelial cells in serum-free primary culture. Cancer Res 1984; 44: 1998–2010
2. Hiaramatsu M, Kashimata M, Minami N *et al.* Androgenic regulation of epidermal growth factor in the mouse ventral prostate. Biochem Int 1988; 17: 311–317
3. Kyprianou N, Isaacs J. Identification of a cellular receptor for transforming growth factor beta in rat ventral prostate and its negative regulation by androgens. Endocrinology 1988; 123: 2124–2131
4. Sutkowski D M, Chan-Jye F, Sensibar J *et al.* Interaction of epidermal growth factor and TGFα in human prostatic epithelial cells in culture. Prostate 1992; 21: 133–143
5. Derynck R. The physiology of transforming growth factor-alpha. Adv Cancer Res 1992; 58: 27–52
6. Winkler M E, O'Conner L, Winget M, Fendly B. Epidermal growth factor and transforming growth factor alpha bind differently to the epidermal growth factor receptor. Biochemistry 1989; 28: 6373–6378
7. Derynck R, Goeddel D, Ullrich A *et al.* Synthesis of messenger RNAs for transforming growth factors alpha and beta and the epidermal growth factor receptor by human tumours. Cancer Res 1987; 47: 707–712
8. Morris G L, Dodd J G. Epidermal growth factor receptor mRNA levels in human prostatic tumours and cell lines. J Urol 1990; 143: 1272–1274
9. Ching K Z, Ramsey E, Pettigrew N *et al.* Expression of mRNA for epidermal growth factor, transforming growth factor-alpha and their receptor in human prostate tissue and cell lines. Mol Cell Biochem 1993; 126: 151–158
10. Mellon K, Thompson S, Charlton R G et a. p-53, c-erbB-2 and the epidermal growth factor receptor in the benign and malignant prostate. J Urol 1992; 147: 496–499
11. Ibrahim G K, Kerns B, MacDonald J A *et al.* Differential immunoreactivity of epidermal growth factor receptor in benign, dysplastic and malignant prostatic tissues. J Urol 1993; 149: 170–173
12. Ware J L. Growth factors and their receptors as determinants in the proliferation and metastasis of human prostate cancer. Cancer Metastasis Rev 1993; 12: 287–301
13. Maddy S Q, Chisholm G, Busuttil A, Habib F K. Epidermal growth factor receptors in human prostate cancer: correlation with histological differentiation of the tumour. Br J Cancer 1989; 60: 41–44
14. Davies P, Eaton C. Binding of epidermal growth factor by human normal, hypertrophic and carcinomatous prostate. Prostate 1989; 14: 123–132
15. Glynn-Jones E, Goddard L, Harper M E. Comparative analysis of mRNA and protein expression for epidermal growth factor receptor and ligands relative to the proliferative index in human prostate tissue. Hum Pathol 1996; 27: 688–694
16. MacDonald A, Habib F. Divergent responses to epidermal growth factor in hormone sensitive and insensitive human prostate cancer cell lines. Br J Cancer 1992; 65: 177–182

17. Hofer D R, Sherwood E, Bromberg W D *et al*. Autonomous growth of androgen-independent human prostatic carcinoma cells. Role of transforming growth factor-A. Cancer Res 1991; 51: 2780–2785

18. MacDonald A, Chisholm G, Habib F K. Production and response of a human prostate cancer line to transforming growth factor-like molecules. Br J Cancer 1990; 62: 579–584

19. Schuurmans A L G, Bolt J, Veldscholte J, Mulder E. Regulation of growth of LNCaP human prostate tumour cells by growth factors and steroid hormones. J Steroid Biochem Mol Biol 1991; 40: 193–197

20. Brass A L, Barnard J, Patai B L *et al*. Androgen up-regulates epidermal growth factor receptor expression and binding affinity in PC3 cell lines expressing the human androgen receptor. Cancer Res 1995; 55: 3197–3203

21. Downward J, Yarden Y, Mayes E *et al*. Close similarity of epidermal growth factor receptor and v-erbB oncogene protein sequences. Nature 1984; 307: 521–527

22. King C R, Draus M H, Aaronson S A. Amplification of a novel v-*erb*B related gene in a human mammary carcinoma. Science 1985; 229: 974–976

23. Fukushige S I, Matsubara K I, Yoshida M *et al*. Localisation of a novel v-*erb*B related gene c-*erb*B2 on human chromosome 17 and its amplification in a gastric cancer cell line. Mol Cell Biol 1986; 6: 955–958

24. Todaro G J, Fryling C, DeLarco J E. Transforming growth factors produced by certain human tumour cells: polypeptides that interact with epidermal growth factor receptors. Proc Natl Acad Sci USA 1980; 77: 5258–5262

25. Mydlo J H, Michaeli J, Cordon Cardo C *et al*. Expression of transforming growth factor alpha and epidermal growth factor receptor messenger RNA in neoplastic and non-neoplastic human kidney tissue. Cancer Res 1989; 49: 3407–3411

26. Bennett C, Paterson I, Corishley C M, Luqmani Y A. Expression of growth factor and epidermal growth factor receptor encoded transcripts in human gastric tissues. Cancer Res 1989; 49: 2104–2111

27. Nish N, Oya H, Matsumoto K *et al*. Changes in gene expression of growth factors and their receptors during castration-induced involution and androgen induced regrowth of rat prostates. Prostate 1996; 28: 139–152

28. Myers R B, Kudlow J E, Grizzle W E. Expression of transforming growth factor-alpha, epidermal growth factor and the epidermal growth factor receptor in adenocarcinoma of the prostate and benign prostatic hyperplasia. Mod Pathol 1993; 6: 733–737

29. Shaikh N, Lai L, McLoughlin J *et al*. Quantative analysis of epidermal growth factor in human benign prostatic hyperplasia and prostatic carcinoma and its prognostic significance. Anticancer Res 1990; 10: 873–874

30. Connolly J M, Rose D. Secretion of epidermal growth factor and related polypeptides by human prostate cancer cell line. Prostate 1989; 15: 177–186

31. Connolly J M, Rose D. Production of epidermal growth factor and transforming growth factor-alpha by the androgen-responsive LNCaP human prostate cancer cell line. Prostate 1990; 16: 209–218

32. Harper M E, Goddard L, Glynne-Jones E *et al*. An immunocytochemical analysis of TGF-α expression in benign and malignant prostatic tumors. Prostate 1993; 23: 9–23

33. Rajan R, Venderslice R, Kapur S *et al*. Epidermal growth factor (EGF) promotes chemomigration of a human prostate tumour cell line and EGF immunoreactive proteins are present at sites of metastasis in the stroma of lymph nodes and medullary bone. Prostate 1996; 28: 1–9

34. Ignar-Trowbridge D M, Teng C T, Ross K A *et al*. Peptide growth factors elicit estrogen-receptor-dependent transcriptional activation of an estrogen-responsive element. Mol Endocrinol 1993; 7: 992–998

35. Culig Z, Hobisch A, Cronauer M V *et al*. Androgen receptor activation in prostatic tumour cell lines by insulin like growth factor I, keratinocyte growth factor and epidermal growth factor. Cancer Res 1994; 54: 5474–5478

Chapter 6

E-cadherin expression in prostate cancer: prognostic and therapeutic implications

J. A. Schalken

Introduction

Prostate cancer is one of the most prevalent malignant diseases among men and, despite tremendous efforts, the prognosis for patients with metastatic prostate cancer has not changed significantly during the past five decades. Clearly, a better insight into the molecular basis of the development of prostate cancer may provide a rationale for more accurate prognostic algorithms and for new therapeutic strategies. As an example, E-cadherin is discussed in this chapter.

Combined results from many investigators indicate that prostate carcinogenesis results from two mechanisms that work in concert, i.e. the accumulation of genetic changes and changes in stromal–epithelial interaction. Thus, a prostate epithelial cell, as a target cell, is subjected to several critical genetic hits and the resulting population is permissive to malignant outgrowth, owing to changes in the paracrine and cell–matrix interaction with the surrounding stroma.

Genetic changes in prostate cancer

As the accumulation of genetic changes is associated with the development of cancer, researchers have focused in the past decade on identification of the relevant 'cancer genes'. Early attempts to characterize specific genetic changes in prostate cancer were greatly hampered by the fact that classical cytogenetics did not appear to be altogether appropriate for the analysis of primary prostate cancer. Only with the development of molecular genetic methods (restriction fragment length polymorphism (RFLP), microsatellite polymerase chain reaction (PCR)) and advanced cytogenetics (fluorescence *in situ* hybridization (FISH), comparative genomic hybridization (CGH)), were the genetic changes associated with the development of prostate cancer characterized in some detail. The results have been reviewed by Bova and Isaacs,[1] and are summarized in Table 6.1. This information provides an initial step towards a better understanding of the molecular basis of prostate cancer development. The number of candidate genes that are implicated by these genetic alterations, however, has grown steadily. Whereas, in the early 1980s, only oncogenes would be considered in molecular oncology, nowadays a plethora of genes are to be considered, ranging from those encoding detoxifying enzymes (e.g. GST-pi;[2]) to invasion-suppressor proteins such as E-cadherin. In an attempt to gain insight into the role of a specific molecular change in the entire cascade associated with the development of cancer, Figure 6.1 has been made to discriminate various pathways and examples of genes that are part of such a pathway.

Table 6.1. *Genetic changes in prostate cancer: molecular genetic and comparative genomic hybridization studies.*

Loss		Gain	
Candidate gene	Frequency (%)	Candidate gene	Frequency (%)
8p21-12	80*		
8p22	32–100*	8q24(myc)	6–89[†]
13q (Rb)	60–70	1q	25–50
2qcen-q31	42	2p	20–50
5cen-q 23.3 (α-catenin)	39	3p	30–45
6q14-23.2	39	3q	30–45
		7	30–56
7q31.1	30–70		
9p21 (INK4a)	20–43*	11p	25–50
10p11.2	30–44	17q	25–50
10q23-24	44–62	Xq	40–60
16q22-ter (E-cadherin)	30–56		
17p13-ter 17q21	20–50		
18 cen-q22.1	20–40		

*Metastases; [†]androgen-independent tumours.
Adapted from ref. 1 with permission.

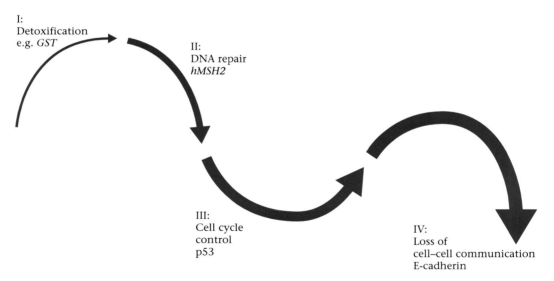

Figure 6.1. *Genetic pathways in cancer development.*

The first molecular pathway that can be discriminated is that involving *detoxifying enzymes*. When these are inactivated or less efficient, the chance of acquiring a mutation is higher, simply because the cells are exposed longer to the aetiological agent, whereby the relative risk to develop cancer increases. The evidence for the importance of this specific molecular pathway in the development of cancer is increasing, and for prostate cancer it is suggested that the *GST-pi* gene has a role.[2]

Conceptually, the relative risk of developing cancer owing to an increased mutation frequency caused by failure in detoxification pathways is increased, albeit to a lower extent than one would anticipate. This is likely to be explained by the fact that the mutations cause a mismatch in the DNA and a complex molecular machinery repairs these. Therefore, the second important pathway is that of *inactivation of DNA repair enzymes*. The role of DNA mismatch repair genes has so far not been substantiated, whereas it is for HNPCC (Human Non Polyposis Colorectal Carcinoma). The relative risk of developing cancers is very high in patients carrying a germ-line mutation in, for instance, *hMSH2* (Human Mut S Homolog 2). In addition, in sporadic tumours replication errors are common and are easily measured by microsatellite instability. However, there is no clear association with gross genetic instability. This is due to the fact that the cell cycle is a highly controlled series of events, in which genetic integrity is a prerequisite for completion of the cell cycle.

The third genetic pathway that can, conceptually, be corrupted and that is critical for maintenance of genetic stability is that of *cell cycle control*. Cancer research has focused a great deal on p53, a protein that later appeared to be involved in cell cycle control. This protein can be considered as the molecular switch to make the cell cycle proceed. The decision is based on the accuracy of DNA replication. Hence, inactivation of p53 is associated with an increase in genetic instability. The accumulation of genetic changes is probably accelerated by at least two orders and likewise the chance of developing an aggressive malignancy is high when p53 is inactivated, often by a mutation. Clearly, loss of cell cycle control leads to an increase in the total number of tumour cells only when this is not balanced by cell death. Thus, interactions with pathways associated with programmed cell death play a pivotal role in the entire cell cycle control machinery.

In order to become truly life threatening, the malignancy has to acquire metastatic properties. Therefore, the fourth molecular pathway is that associated with *invasion and metastasis*. Loss of local control is probably one of the rate-limiting steps that leads to cellular anarchy. For carcinoma, loss of the cell–cell adhesion molecule E-cadherin seems to play a particularly important role. Interference with E-cadherin-mediated interactions is directly related to a loss in intercellular communication.

The four pathways are interrelated and cannot be considered independent as they have to occur sequentially. However, as Figure 6.1 symbolizes, the likelihood of developing a metastatic tumour increases exponentially from left to right.

Prognostic significance of E-cadherin

Combining genetic studies with the above considerations, with respect to the relative importance of specific molecules in the cascade that leads to the development of metastatic cancer, has led the author and colleagues to investigate E-cadherin. The E-cadherin gene, mapped to chromosome 16q22.1 is of particular interest because the product of this gene (also known as uvomorulin, Cell-CAM 120/80 or Arc-1), is a cell–cell adhesion molecule that plays a critical role in embryogenesis and organogenesis by mediating epithelial cell–cell recognition and adhesion processes (for a review see Birchmeier and Behrens[3]). Moreover, it has been demonstrated that experimental inactivation of E-cadherin, using either antibodies or antisense RNA, can result in the acquisition of invasive potential, and that transfection of invasive adenocarcinoma cells with E-cadherin cDNA can render the expressing cells non-invasive.[4] Therefore, E-cadherin can be considered as an invasion-suppressor gene. The first studies to examine E-cadherin in prostate cancer were carried out in the Dunning rat model and showed a strong correlation between the lack of E-cadherin and invasive and/or metastatic potential.[5]

When primary human prostate cancer specimens were stained with E-cadherin, it appeared that aberrant E-cadherin staining was associated with increased Gleason score and thus the correlation with differentiation was confirmed. More importantly, if was subsequently shown that this aberrant immunoreactivity was associated with a poor prognosis.[6] Now that procedures have been developed for the reliable staining of paraffin-embedded specimens,[7] prospective studies are under way to evaluate prospectively the prognostic value of E-cadherin immunohistochemistry.

Therapeutic implications

The knowledge that prostate cancer metastasis is associated with a progressive loss of E-cadherin may even open new therapeutic avenues. The consideration that dedifferentiation is a hallmark of aggressive cancer, and that E-cadherin is critical for maintaining the differentiated state, makes it tempting to speculate that E-cadherin upregulation can, in fact, be a target for pharmacological treatment of prostate cancer. 'Differentiation therapy' is a relatively longstanding concept in the treatment of cancer. Classical mediators are, for instance, retinoids and vitamin D analogues. More recently, it has been shown that drugs inhibiting certain enzymes in the cytochrome *P*-450-dependent catabolism of retinoic acid (4-hydroxylase) can result in increased levels of tissue retinoic acid. Thus, this might be a more effective way to induce differentiation. Indeed, initial studies with an imidazole (R75251) have indicated that the effect is associated with changes in differentiation, as studied by keratin immunohistochemistry.[8] Thus, a better understanding of the differentiation process has now led to the definition of a new target for the therapy of prostate cancer.

Conclusions

Cancer development is a complex process in which genetic and epigenetic factors act in concert. A better understanding of both is likely to lead to better options for diagnosis, prognosis and treatment. E-cadherin is one of the first genes to be identified by molecular genetics as being implicated in prostate cancer development and it seems to play a pivotal role in progression to metastatic disease. Even though the exact mechanism of defective cadherin function has not been fully elucidated,[9] transcriptional downregulation seems to be fairly common. Since this is theoretically reversible, it can also be hypothesized that treatment resulting in upregulation of E-cadherin would prevent progression of the disease. Considering the unique natural history of prostate cancer, this seems a useful approach. Since several other molecular changes and pathways associated with the development of prostate cancer are currently being resolved, it is likely that, with increasing pace, diagnostic and prognostic algorithms will become available and new therapeutic strategies can be defined.[2,10]

References

1. Bova G S, Isaacs W B. Review of allelic loss and gain in prostate cancer. World J Urol 1996; 14: 338–346
2. Nelson W G, Simons J W. New approaches to adjuvant therapy for patients with adverse histopathologic findings following radical prostatectomy. Urol Clin North Am 1996; 23: 685–696

3. Birchmeier W, Behrens J. Cadherin expression in carcinomas: role in the formation of cell junctions and the prevention of invasiveness. Biochim Biophys Acta 1994; 1198: 11–26

4. Vleminckx K, Vakaet L Jr, Mareel M *et al.* Genetic manipulation of E-cadherin expression by epithelial tumor cells reveals an invasion suppressor role. Cell 1991; 66: 107–119

5. Bussemakers M J, van Moorselaar R J, Giroldi L A *et al.* Decreased expression of E-cadherin in the progression of rat prostatic cancer. Cancer Res 1992; 52: 2916–2922

6. Umbas R, Isaacs W B, Bringuier P P *et al.* Decreased E-cadherin expression is associated with poor prognosis in patients with prostate cancer. Cancer Res 1994; 54: 3929–3933

7. Ruijter E T, Miller G J, Aalders T W *et al.* Rapid microwave stimulated fixation of entire prostatectomy specimens. J Pathol 1997; in press

8. Smets G, Van Ginckel R, Daneels G *et al.* Liarozole, an antitumor drug, modulates cytokeratin expression in the Dunning AT-6sq prostatic carcinoma through in situ accumulation of all-trans-retinoic acid. Prostate 1995; 27: 129–140

9. Giroldi L A, Bringuier P P, Schalken J A. Defective E-cadherin function in urological cancers: clinical implications and molecular mechanisms. Invasion Metastasis 1994; 14: 71–81

10. Schalken J A. New perspectives in the treatment of prostate cancer. Eur Urol 1997; 31(suppl): 20–23

Chapter 7
Mechanisms of local invasion and metastasis in prostate cancer

D. Hrouda and R. S. Kirby

Introduction

The last few years have seen major advances in the understanding of the cellular and molecular events involved in the acquisition of invasive and metastatic ability by cancer cells. Figure 7.1 illustrates some of the steps in the metastatic cascade that must occur in order for a cancer cell to metastasize successfully.[1]

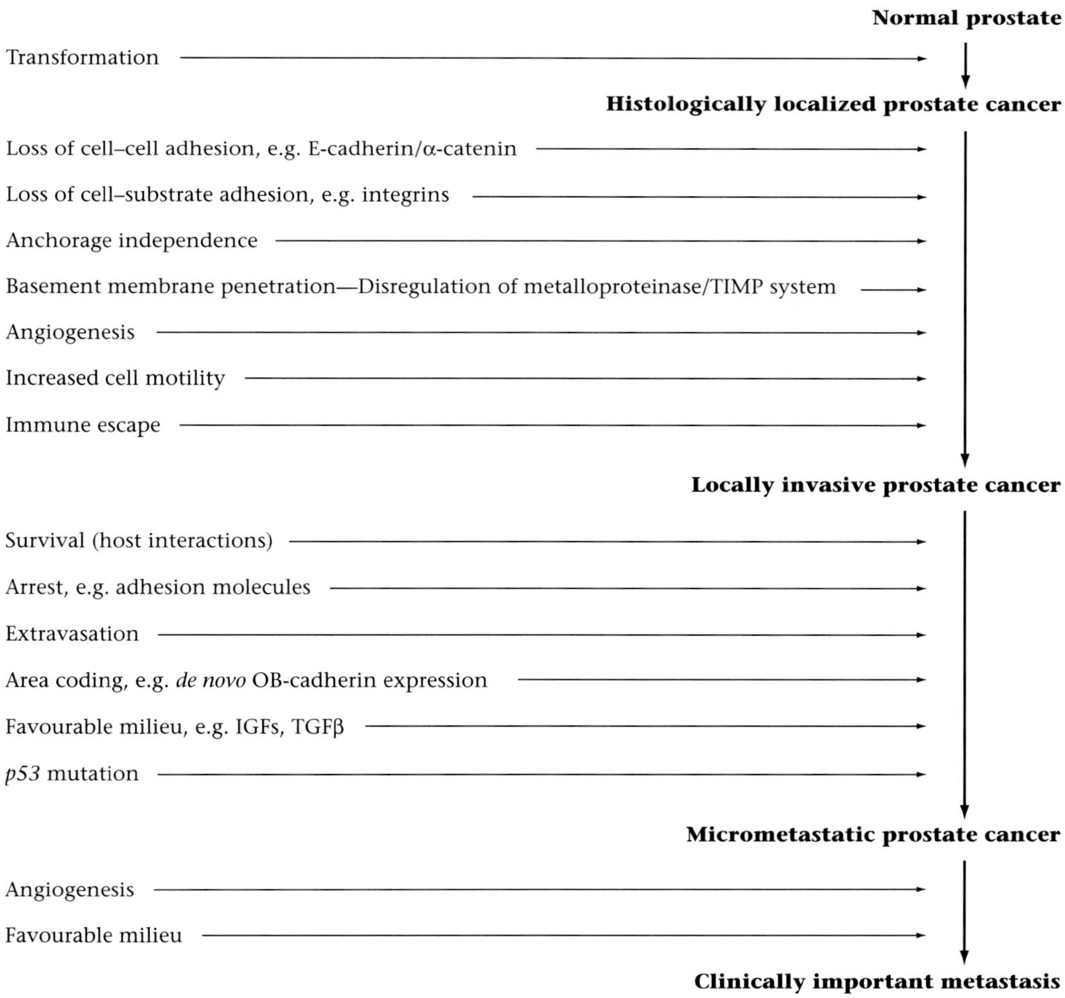

Normal prostate

Transformation

Histologically localized prostate cancer

Loss of cell–cell adhesion, e.g. E-cadherin/α-catenin

Loss of cell–substrate adhesion, e.g. integrins

Anchorage independence

Basement membrane penetration—Disregulation of metalloproteinase/TIMP system

Angiogenesis

Increased cell motility

Immune escape

Locally invasive prostate cancer

Survival (host interactions)

Arrest, e.g. adhesion molecules

Extravasation

Area coding, e.g. *de novo* OB-cadherin expression

Favourable milieu, e.g. IGFs, TGFβ

p53 mutation

Micrometastatic prostate cancer

Angiogenesis

Favourable milieu

Clinically important metastasis

Figure 7.1. Steps involved in the 'metastatic cascade'.

Cellular adhesion

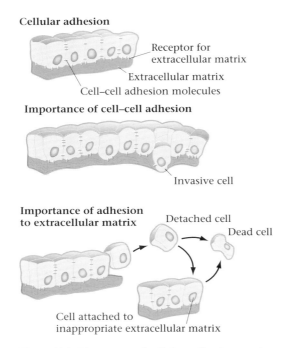

Receptor for
extracellular matrix

Extracellular matrix

Cell–cell adhesion molecules

Importance of cell–cell adhesion

Invasive cell

**Importance of adhesion
to extracellular matrix**

Detached cell

Dead cell

Cell attached to
inappropriate extracellular matrix

*Figure 7.2. Two types of cellular adhesion need
to be disrupted in order for cells to migrate:
adhesion between individual cells and adhesion
between cells and the extracellular matrix.
Cancer cells are anchorage-independent.*

In normal tissues, cells remain attached because of cell–cell adhesion and cell–extracellular matrix adhesion. Each mechanism of adhesion has a different role during local invasion and metastasis (Figure 7.2).

Cell–cell adhesion

Cadherins, a group of calcium-dependent transmembrane glycoproteins that interact homotypically, appear to be the molecules most involved in cell–cell adhesion. The glycoprotein E–cadherin, in the new nomenclature cadherin 1, has been most extensively studied. The intracytoplasmic *C*-terminus of E-cadherin binds to another protein, α-catenin, that mediates binding to microfilaments of the cytoskeleton.[2]

There is good experimental evidence that E-cadherin downregulation plays a role in invasiveness. Lack of E-cadherin expression was found to be strongly correlated with metastatic potential in the Dunning rat model.[3] Restoration of defective cadherin–catenin function in the PC-3 human prostate cancer cell line negated the ability of that cell line to form tumours when injected into nude mice.[4] Conversely, blocking the function of E-cadherin using binding disrupting antibody or viral transformation increased the invasiveness of MDCK cells.[5]

There is also clinical evidence that cadherins and catenins are involved with prostate cancer invasion and metastasis. Aberrant expression of the cadherin–catenin complex is a frequent occurrence in prostate cancer and appears to be strongly correlated with Gleason grade, stage, metastasis and progression after radical prostatectomy.[6,7]

Decreased cell–substrate attachment

Cellular adhesion to the extracellular matrix is an additional interaction that has to be disrupted in order for invasion and metastasis to occur. This interaction does not simply keep cells from 'floating away': cell–substrate adhesion is essential for survival and proliferation. Unattached cells stop growing and apoptose, a phenomenon known as anchorage independence.[8]

Cell–substrate adhesion is largely mediated by integrins, which are heterodimeric glycoproteins composed of α and β chains. The existence of numerous α chains and three β chains enables cells to form multiple specific receptors. The integrins bind specifically to one or two extracellular matrix proteins such as collagen, laminin, fibrinogen and fibronectin, apart from αIIbβ3 and αvβ3 integrins, which bind to multiple ligands.[9]

Alterations in the composition of integrins on the tumour cell, and in the affinity of the integrin receptors, have been reported in cancer progression. Integrins α2, α4, α5, αv and β4 are all expressed in normal prostatic basal cells but

Prostate cancer cell

Receptor

Adhesion molecule

Stromal cell
of bone

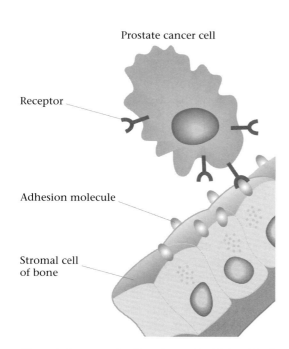

Figure 7.3. Normal cells only survive if they bind to extracellular matrix with the right 'area code'.

lost in prostate cancer, whereas α3β1 and α6β1 integrins remain expressed in invasive cancer.[10] High expression of α6 integrin correlates with more invasive tumour cells when tested in SCID mice.[11] It has been postulated that production of α6β1 integrin may explain the pattern of prostate cancer spread along laminin-coated surfaces such as nerves and blood vessels.[10]

Overexpression of β3 integrins has been found to correlate directly with metastatic potential in melanoma.[12] Recently, αIIbβ3 integrin, previously thought to be expressed only in cells from megakaryocyte lineage, has been described in the human prostate cancer cell lines DU-145 and PC-3 in addition to prostate cancer tissue from three patients.[13] These investigators showed that antibodies to αIIbβ3 were able to inhibit invasion of DU-145 cells through a reconstituted basement membrane, thus suggesting a role for αIIbβ3 integrin in invasion.

Normal cells denied anchorage stop proliferating and undergo apoptosis because one of the nuclear proteins, known as cyclin E-CDK2 complex, which regulates the growth and division of cells, becomes less active. Tumour cells display anchorage independence, possibly because the cyclin E-CDK2 complex stays active even when the cells are unattached.[14] It has been suggested that proteins made by oncogenes convey a false message to the nucleus that the cell is properly attached, when it is not. Another important concept is that of 'area coding', whereby cells survive only if the extracellular matrix to which they adhere bears the right 'area code' which is specific for one tissue by virtue of expression of the appropriate integrin (Figure 7.3). This is made possible by the existence of multiple specific integrin receptors. The binding of integrins to extracellular matrix proteins often occurs at a structure made up of just three amino acids — arginine–glycine–aspartic acid (RGD). RGD peptides injected into mice with subcutaneous melanomas are capable of preventing metastasis, presumably by occupying receptor sites and thus preventing the cancer cells from adhering at distant sites.[15]

Overcoming the basement membrane barrier

Epithelial cells are separated from the rest of the body by a basement membrane. There is progressive loss of basement membrane with increasing grade of prostate cancer.[16] This barrier cannot be breached by normal cells, but white cells and cancer cells are able to penetrate the basement membrane by releasing enzymes termed matrix metalloproteinases (MMPs). Metalloproteinases are categorized on the basis of substrate specificity and include collagenases, stromelysins and gelatinases. These enzymes are involved in the normal turnover of connective tissue matrix. There are tissue inhibitors of metalloproteinases, known as TIMPs, produced by both normal and neoplastic cells and tissues, that may inactivate latent or active enzymes and thus regulate their proteolytic activity. It is thought that, in cancer, there is disregulation of this system due to inappropriate expression of metalloproteinases or downregulation of TIMPs.[17] This facilitates invasion and metastasis, by enabling the cancer cell to pass through its own basement membrane, to penetrate the basement membrane of an endothelial cell to gain access to the bloodstream and, following arrest in a distant capillary bed, to reinvade through the vascular endothelium. It has been shown that DU-145 prostate cancer cells transfected to express MMP-7 (matrilysin) are rendered more invasive.[18]

Angiogenesis

For a three-dimensional tumour to expand beyond approximately 2 mm in diameter, new capillary blood vessels are required;[19] the acquisition of angiogenic capability is, therefore, an important step in the progression of tumours from prostatic intraepithelial neoplasia or small non-progressive prostate cancer to expanding invasive tumours. Failure to acquire angiogenic potential may explain why many histologically detectable prostate cancers remain clinically latent during the lifetime of the host. Autopsy-diagnosed latent prostate cancers have been found to have very low blood capillary density ratios compared with clinically significant tumours that have metastasized.[20,21] Increased frequency of vessel formation has been found to predict metastatic disease in prostate cancer.[22,23]

Ingrowth of new capillaries also facilitates the entrance of neoplastic cells into the circulation and, once they have seeded at a distant site, angiogenesis is required for metastases to flourish. The presence of metastases consisting of non-angiogenic clones might explain why, in some tumours, micrometastases can sometimes remain dormant for years.

There are several ways in which tumours can initiate angiogenesis, including the production of angiogenic factors by the tumour cells, mobilization of angiogenic factors from adjacent tissues or stimulation of the release of angiogenic factors from macrophages. Many angiogenic factors have now been described, including vascular endothelial growth factor, basic fibroblast growth factor and thymidine phosphorylase.[24] Angiogenesis inhibitors regulated by suppressor oncogenes or produced by tumours also appear to be important. Naturally occurring inhibitors of angiogenesis include thrombospondin and angiostatin.[25] Angiostatin, a proteolytic fragment derived from plasminogen, was initially described by Judah Folkman's group, who reported that an angiogenic inhibitor produced by a primary tumour inhibited vascularization of seeded secondaries in the Lewis lung carcinoma model.[26] It has now been demonstrated that the human prostate cancer cell lines PC-3, DU-145 and LNCaP express enzymatic activity that can generate bioactive angiostatin from human plasminogen.[27] It has been postulated that this activity could offer an explanation for the relatively indolent course of many prostate cancers, but the importance of angiostatin in humans is yet to be defined.

Increased cell motility

Motogenic cytokines that may induce random movement of tumour cells, including autocrine motility factor (AMF), migration stimulating factor and scatter factor (SF),[28] have been identified in several tumour types, including prostate cancer. There is some evidence to support a role for these cytokines in prostate cancer metastasis Only the metastatic variant of PC-3 cells is capable of responding to tumour-secreted AMF with increased motility, and the AMF receptor gp78 was found to be aberrantly distributed and regulated in the metastatic variant.[29] SF is expressed by bone stromal cells and it has been shown that the majority of bone and lymph node metastases express the SF receptor, which is the c-MET proto-oncogene product.[30] The mode of action of motility factors, in particular their interaction with the cell adhesion molecules, has not been defined.

Immune escape

Interactions between tumour cells and cells of the immune system, principally T lymphocytes, is mediated by cell-surface molecules. Tumour antigen is presented on the surface of the tumour cell by class I major histocompatibility complex (MHC). Adhesion molecules are an important part of this interaction, in particular intercellular adhesion molecule I (ICAM-1). It has been shown that MHC class I expression is often impaired in prostate cancer, particularly in metastatic disease,[31] and ICAM-1 is downregulated in the metastatic prostate cancer cell line LNCaP.[32] The ability to escape immune surveillance may be an important step in allowing tumour progression.

Adhesive interactions of tumour cells and capillary endothelial cells

Cancer cells are vulnerable in the blood and it is thought that they probably need to attach fairly promptly to the endothelium of a small vessel. Cancer cells often get trapped in the first vascular bed downstream of their origin, usually the lungs; however, in the case of tumours drained by the portal system, spread is usually first to the liver. Some cancer cells may enhance their ability to adhere in the distant capillary bed by producing factors that cause platelets to aggregate around them and effectively make them larger and stickier. Platelets produce a rich supply of growth factors that may help the cancer cells they bind to survive.[33] This may explain why some drugs that interfere with platelets appear to have antitumour activity.

Cellular interactions required in the arrest of tumour cells in distant capillary beds are reminiscent of the trafficking of leucocytes and their extravasation at inflammation sites. Many of the leucocyte adhesion molecules are expressed by tumour cells and may mediate the binding of transformed cells to activated endothelial cells. For example, ELAM-1, one of the calcium-dependent selectins, recognizes a carbohydrate domain expressed on cancer cells.[34] Another illustration of the role of lymphocyte adhesion molecules in malignant spread was the finding that the metastatic behaviour of a rodent pancreatic carcinoma cell line depended on the expression of a variant form of the lymphocyte homing molecule and hyaluronate receptor, CD44.[35] Subsequently, human prostate cancer cells were shown to express CD44 variant isoforms.[36]

'Seed and soil'

The concept of seed and soil, described by Paget 100 years ago, is still relevant today.[37] It was thought for a long time that the predominance of prostate cancer metastases in the spine was due to retrograde flow from the vesical venous plexus into the pelvic emissary veins during a Valsalva manoeuvre. However, mere physical trapping of tumour cells at the first vascular bed encountered clearly cannot be the whole story.

The reason for the predilection of prostate cancer for bone has long fascinated clinicians. The concept of area coding may form at least part of the explanation (Figure 7.3). Osteoblast (OB)-cadherin, in the new nomenclature cadherin 11, is a cell adhesion molecule most commonly expressed in osteoblasts. High levels of cadherin 11 appear to be expressed *de novo* in prostate cancer cell lines, thus providing a possible molecular mechanism for specific affinity between adhesion molecules on prostate cancer cells and the endothelium in bone.[38] Others have demonstrated that the adhesion of PC-3 human prostate cancer cells to an osteoblast-like matrix is mediated by $\alpha2\beta1$ integrin, and this interaction is stimulated by transforming growth factor β (TGF), a major bone-derived growth factor.[39] Although TGFβ is normally a growth-inhibitory cytokine, there is evidence that metastatic prostate cancer cell lines lose TGFβ growth inhibition but respond to TGFβ by induction of matrix metalloproteinase 9 activity.[40]

Another possible explanation is that the bone marrow milieu is favourable for prostate cancer cells in terms of the concentrations of growth factors and hormones. A variety of growth factors are implicated as autocrine/paracrine factors, including fibroblast growth factor, which stimulates growth of LNCaP and stimulates angiogenesis, insulin-like growth factors (IGFs)[41] and cytokines, e.g. interleukin (IL)-6.[42]

Insulin-like growth factor I receptor (IGFR1), a tyrosine kinase receptor, is known to be expressed by prostate cancer cells and is known to be an absolute requirement both for transformation and the maintenance of the transformed phenotype.[43] Bone marrow is an environment rich in IGFs.[44] There is also evidence to suggest a paracrine interaction between prostate-specific antigen (PSA) produced by the tumour cells and IGFs produced by bone stromal cells. PSA is an IGF-binding protein-3 protease, thus causing release of IGF from its latent complex.[45] Thus, PSA produced by prostate cancer cells may make more IGF-1 bioavailable and thus enhance tumour growth. The potential importance of the IGF/IGFR1 pathway was recently demonstrated using Lobund–Wistar rat prostate cancer PA-III cells transfected with an antisense IGFR1 construct to block IGFR1. When injected into nude mice, the antisense IGFR1 transfected cells either developed tumours 90% smaller than controls or remained tumour free.[46]

Genes controlling metastatic phenotype

An increasing number of genetic alterations have been associated with the progression of prostate cancer.[47] Loss-of-heterozygosity (LOH) studies have been used to search for the loss of tumour-suppressor genes throughout the human genome. LOH has been observed on an increasing list of chromosomes but most frequently on chromosomes 8, 16 and 10.

Progression to a metastatic phenotype is thought to be associated with loss of function of invasion/metastasis-suppressor genes. The *E-cadherin* gene located on 16q22.1 has the characteristics of a tumour invasion suppressor gene and the function of its protein product has been described above. The *KAI1* gene is a metastasis-suppressor gene that is located on chromosome 11p11.2. Immunohistochemical staining for KAI1 protein in a small number of patients suggests that downregulation is more frequent in the primary tumours of patients with hormone-refractory metastatic disease than in patients with no known metastases who are undergoing radical prostatectomy.[48] The function of the KAI1 protein is unknown but its position suggests that it may be involved in signalling between cells and their environment.

Inactivation of the *p53* gene has been implicated in prostate cancer progression on the basis of immunohistochemical staining. It is rarely found in primary prostatic tumours,[49] whereas a large proportion of metastases stain positively.[50,51] However, the role of *p53* mutations in prostate cancer progression is still controversial. A recent small study suggested that *p53* gene inactivation is not essential to the development of metastases, because neither the presence nor degree of expression of *p53* correlated with time to progression or time to death. Allelic loss on chromosome 17 did, however, appear to be highly correlated with risk of recurrence, the implication being that another gene or genes on chromosome 17 may be involved in prostate cancer progression.[52] The role of metastasis-suppressor genes such as *NM23* has yet to be established in prostate cancer.

Conclusions

It is anticipated that the elucidation of the mechanisms by which tumours invade and metastasize will provide new cellular and molecular markers of metastatic potential that will enable prediction of which localized, potentially curable, tumours are destined to be life-threatening. There is also hope that these insights into the metastatic cascade may eventually result in effective new therapies being developed for patients with advanced disease. Several new therapeutic strategies are already being assessed: they include metalloproteinase inhibitors such as marimastat, vaccine strategies to 'awaken' the immune response, corrective gene therapy such as *in vivo* transfection of wild-type *p53* into prostate cancer cells, or inhibition of mutated oncogenes using antisense oligonucleotides.[53] Inhibition of angiogenesis with resultant hypoxia-induced cell death is an attractive approach, and several compounds (including cisplatin, suramin, marimastat, linomide, thalidomide and many others) are being evaluated.[25] Other possible strategies might involve restoring normal E-cadherin/α-catenin expression in the tumour cells or blocking expression of $\alpha6\beta1$ integrin. The use of molecules analogous to the RGD peptides might be used to block attachment of cancer cells at distant sites. The IGF-I receptor could be targeted, perhaps by using antisense constructs. Preliminary results using some of these therapies will be available in the next few years.

References

1. Hart I R, Saini A. Biology of tumour metastasis. Lancet 1992; 339(8807): 1453–1457
2. Ozawa M, Kemler R. Molecular organization of the uvomorulin–catenin complex. J Cell Biol 1992; 116(4): 989–996
3. Bussemakers M J, van Moorselaar R J, Giroldi L A *et al*. Decreased expression of E-cadherin in the progression of rat prostatic cancer. Cancer Res 1992; 52(10): 2916–2922
4. Ewing C M, Ru N, Morton R A *et al*. Chromosome 5 suppresses tumorigenicity of PC3 prostate cancer cells: correlation with re-expression of alpha-catenin and restoration of E-cadherin function. Cancer Res 1995; 55(21): 4813–4817
5. Behrens J, Mareel M M, Van Roy F M *et al*. Dissecting tumor cell invasion: epithelial cells acquire invasive properties after the loss of uvomorulin-mediated cell–cell adhesion. J Cell Biol 1989; 108(6): 2435–2447
6. Umbas R, Schalken J A, Aalders T W *et al*. Expression of the cellular adhesion molecule E-cadherin is reduced or absent in high-grade prostate cancer. Cancer Res 1992; 52(18): 5104–5109
7. Morton R A, Ewing C M, Nagafuchi A *et al*. Reduction of E-cadherin levels and deletion of the alpha-catenin gene in human prostate cancer cells. Cancer Res 1993; 53(15): 3585–3590
8. Ruoslahti E, Reed J C. Anchorage dependence, integrins, and apoptosis. Cell 1994; 77(4): 477–478
9. Hynes R O. Integrins: versatility, modulation, and signaling in cell adhesion. Cell 1992; 69(1): 11–25

10. Cress A E, Rabinovitz I, Zhu W *et al*. The alpha 6 beta 1 and alpha 6 beta 4 integrins in human prostate cancer progression. Cancer Metastasis Rev 1995; 14(3): 219–228

11. Rabinovitz I, Nagle R B, Cress A E. Integrin alpha 6 expression in human prostate carcinoma cells is associated with a migratory and invasive phenotype in vitro and in vivo. Clin Exp Metastasis 1995; 13(6): 481–491

12. Honn K V, Tang D G. Adhesion molecules and tumor cell interaction with endothelium and subendothelial matrix. Cancer Metastasis Rev 1992; 11(3–4): 353–375

13. Trikha M, Timar J, Lundy S K *et al*. Human prostate carcinoma cells express functional alphaIIb(beta)3 integrin. Cancer Res 1996; 56: 5071–5078

14. Fang F, Orend G, Watanabe N *et al*. Dependence of cyclin E-CDK2 kinase activity on cell anchorage. Science 1996; 271(5248): 499–502

15. Humphries M J, Olden K, Yamada K M. A synthetic peptide from fibronectin inhibits experimental metastasis of murine melanoma cells. Science 1986; 233(4762): 467–470

16. Fuchs M E, Brawer M K, Rennels M A *et al*. The relationship of basement membrane to histologic grade of human prostatic carcinoma. Mod Pathol 1989; 2(2): 105–111

17. Lokeshwar B L, Selzer M G, Block N L *et al*. Secretion of matrix metalloproteinases and their inhibitors (tissue inhibitor of metalloproteinases) by human prostate in explant cultures: reduced tissue inhibitor of metalloproteinase secretion by malignant tissues. Cancer Res 1993; 53(19): 4493–4498

18. Powell W C, Knox J D, Navre M *et al*. Expression of the metalloproteinase matrilysin in DU-145 cells increases their invasive potential in severe combined immunodeficient mice. Cancer Res 1993; 53(2): 417–422

19. Folkman J. Angiogenesis in cancer, vascular, rheumatoid and other disease. Nature Med 1995; 1(1): 27–31

20. Wakui S, Furusato M, Itoh T *et al*. Tumour angiogenesis in prostatic carcinoma with and without bone marrow metastasis: a morphometric study. J Pathol 1992; 168(3): 257–262

21. Furusato M, Wakui S, Sasaki H *et al*. Tumour angiogenesis in latent prostatic carcinoma. Br J Cancer 1994; 70(6): 1244–1246

22. Weidner N, Carroll P R, Flax J *et al*. Tumor angiogenesis correlates with metastasis in invasive prostate carcinoma. Am J Pathol 1993; 143(2): 401–409

23. Bigler S A, Deering R E, Brawer M K. Comparison of microscopic vascularity in benign and malignant prostate tissue. Hum Pathol 1993; 24(2): 220–226

24. Hanahan D, Folkman J. Patterns and emerging mechanisms of the angiogenic switch during tumorigenesis. Cell 1996; 86(3): 353–364

25. Bicknell R, Harris A L. Mechanisms and therapeutic implications of angiogenesis. Curr Opin Oncol 1996; 8: 60–65

26. O' Reilly M, Holmgren L, Shing Y *et al*. Angiostatin: a novel angiogenesis inhibitor that mediates the suppression of metastases by a Lewis lung carcinoma. Cell 1994; 79(2): 315–328

27. Gately S, Twardowski P, Stack M S *et al*. Human prostate carcinoma cells express enzymatic activity that converts human plasminogen to the angiogenesis inhibitor, angiostatin. Cancer Res 1996; 56: 4887–4890

28. Stoker M, Gherardi E. Regulation of cell movement: the motogenic cytokines. Biochim Biophys Acta 1991; 1072(1): 81–102

29. Silletti S, Yao J P, Pienta K J *et al*. Loss of cell-contact regulation and altered responses to autocrine motility factor correlate with increased malignancy in prostate cancer cells. Int J Cancer 1995; 63(1): 100–105

30. Pisters L L, Troncoso P, Zhau H E *et al*. c-met proto-oncogene expression in benign and malignant human prostate tissues. J Urol 1995; 154(1): 293–298

31. Blades R A, Keating P J, McWilliam L J *et al*. Loss of HLA class I expression in prostate cancer: implications for immunotherapy. Urology 1995; 46(5): 681–686; discussion 686–687

32. Rokhlin O W, Cohen M B. Expression of cellular adhesion molecules on human prostate tumor cell lines. Prostate 1995; 26(4): 205–212

33. Honn K V, Tang D G, Chen Y Q. Platelets and cancer metastasis: more than an epiphenomenon. Sem Thromb Hemost 1992; 18(4): 392–415

34. Matsushita Y, Hoff S D, Nudelman E D *et al*. Metastatic behavior and cell surface properties of HT-29 human colon carcinoma variant cells selected for their differential expression of sialyl-dimeric Le(x)-antigen. Clin Exp Metastasis 1991; 9(3): 283–299

35. Gunthert U, Hofmann M, Rudy W *et al*. A new variant of glycoprotein CD44 confers metastatic potential to rat carcinoma cells. Cell 1991; 65(1): 13–24

36. Bourrguignon L Y, Iida N, Welsh C F *et al.* Involvement of CD44 and its variant isoforms in membrane–cytoskeleton interaction, cell adhesion and tumor metastasis. J Neuro-Oncol 1995; 26(3): 201–208

37. Paget S. Distribution of secondary growths in cancer of the breast. Lancet 1889; i: 571–573

38. Bussemakers M J G, Dikhoff X, van Bokhoven A *et al.* De novo expression of osteoblast (OB)-cadherin 11 in prostate cancer. J Urol 1996; 155: 351A (abstr. 162)

39. Kostenuik P J, Sanchez-Sweatman O, Orr F W *et al.* Bone cell matrix promotes the adhesion of human prostatic carcinoma cells via the alpha 2 beta 1 integrin. Clin Exp Metastasis 1996; 14(1): 19–26

40. Sehgal I, Baley P A, Thompson T C. Transforming growth factor beta1 stimulates contrasting responses in metastatic versus primary mouse prostate cancer-derived cell lines in vitro. Cancer Res 1996; 56(14): 3359–3365

41. Culig Z, Hobisch A, Cronauer M V *et al.* Regulation of prostatic growth and function by peptide growth factors. Prostate 1996; 28(6): 392–405

42. Borsellino N, Belldegrun A, Bonavida B. Endogenous interleukin 6 is a resistance factor for cis-diamminedichloroplatinum and etoposide-mediated cytotoxicity of human prostate carcinoma cell lines. Cancer Res 1995; 55(20): 4633–4639

43. Baserga R. The insulin-like growth factor I receptor: a key to tumor growth? Cancer Res 1995; 55(2): 249–252

44. Yoneda T, Sasaki A, Mundy G R. Osteolytic bone metastasis in breast cancer. Breast Cancer Res Treat 1994; 32(1): 73–84

45. Cohen P, Peehl D M, Graves H C *et al.* Biological effects of prostate specific antigen as an insulin-like growth factor binding protein-3 protease. J Endocrinol 1994; 142(3): 407–415

46. Burfeind P, Chernicky C L, Rininsland F *et al.* Antisense RNA to the type I insulin-like growth factor receptor suppresses tumor growth and prevents invasion by rat prostate cancer cells in vivo. Proc Natl Acad Sci USA 1996; 93(14): 7263–7268

47. Isaacs W B, Bova G S, Morton R A *et al.* Molecular biology of prostate cancer. Semin Oncol 1994; 21(5): 514–521

48. Dong J T, Suzuki H, Pin S S *et al.* Down-regulation of the KAI1 metastasis suppressor gene during the progression of human prostatic cancer infrequently involves gene mutation or allelic loss. Cancer Res 1996; 56: 4387–4390

49. Voeller H J, Sugars L Y, Pretlow T *et al.* p53 oncogene mutations in human prostate cancer specimens. J Urol 1994; 151(2): 492–495

50. Chi S G, deVere White R W, Meyers F J *et al.* p53 in prostate cancer: frequent expressed transition mutations. J Natl Cancer Inst 1994; 86(12): 926–933

51. Dinjens W N, van der Weiden M M, Schroeder F H *et al.* Frequency and characterization of p53 mutations in primary and metastatic human prostate cancer. Int J Cancer 1994; 56(5): 630–633

52. Brooks J D, Bova G S, Ewing C M *et al.* An uncertain role for p53 gene alterations in human prostate cancers. Cancer Res 1996; 56: 3814–3822

53. Hrouda D, Dalgleish A G. Gene therapy for prostate cancer. Gene Ther 1996; 3(10): 845–852

Chapter 8
Neovascularity in human prostate carcinoma

M. K. Brawer

Introduction

Prostate cancer remains the most common malignancy diagnosed in men in the United States. Improved screening and detection have resulted in a dramatic increase in diagnoses from 244,000 new cases in 1995 to 317,000 projected new cases in 1996, a 40% increase, according to the American Cancer Society. A total of 40,000 deaths from prostate cancer in 1995 made it second only to lung cancer as a cause of fatalities from cancer in American men.

At the same time, a variety of treatment options have become available, including variations in surgical procedures as well as radiation, hormonal therapies and other novel methods of treating the disease. The clinician's recommendation of potential courses of therapy and the informed patient's selection among those alternatives have depended heavily on clinical staging information, among other qualitative factors. Both physicians and patients urgently seek more reliable information about the threat posed by this cancer. Estimates of tumour extent, and potentiality of extraprostatic extension, are significant considerations in the treatment decision process.[1-9]

The Gleason score assigned to tissue biopsy samples and serum prostate-specific antigen (PSA) value provide significant predictive power for organ confinement.[1,6,10-12] In addition to Gleason score and PSA levels, other markers — such as DNA ploidy, the number of cancer-positive biopsy cores, the length of each positive core and the percentage of cancer involved in each core — have been shown to provide additional staging information. However, for an individual patient, the ability of this combination to predict extraprostatic extension has been less than ideal. Clinical accuracy of predicting pathological stage has been in the range of 40–60%.[13] The Gleason score/PSA combination is more likely to be accurate at the low and the high end of the respective ranges than for patients who have intermediate Gleason scores[5-7] and moderately elevated PSA (4–10 ng/ml). Inaccuracy is strongly weighted toward understaging. Other potential markers, such as DNA ploidy or relative nuclear roundness, appear promising in research studies but have not been widely accepted in clinical practice. In addition, 'molecular staging' assays for PSA-producing cells are not yet sufficiently accurate or reproducible for clinical application.

Optimized microvessel density

A promising new technique for predicting prostate cancer tumour extent relies on the quantification of tumour angiogenesis or microvessel density (MVD). Numerous clinical studies, including the works of Wakui,[14] Brawer,[15] Weidner[16] and others,[17-23] have been conducted that show the value of MVD analysis as a predictor of tumour aggressiveness and probability of extraprostatic extension (Table 8.1).

Table 8.1. Microvessel density (MVD) in prostate tissue

Tissue	MVD (no. of vessels/mm^2)	
	Mean	Range
Normal prostate	8.6	2.5–14.6
PIN	11.6	6.0–17.8
BPH	70.2	10.0–253.0
Organ-confined cancer	81.2	45.7–116.9
Metastatic cancer	154.6	122.3–240.9

PIN, prostate intra-epithelial neoplasia.
BPH, benign prostatic hyperplasia.

MVD is a quantitative measurement of the number of small blood vessels within a given area of tissue on a histological slide. It is well known that, in order to grow larger than 1 mm^2 in area, cancers must recruit new blood vessels from the host, and this neovascularity can be readily identified by immunohistochemistry in formalin-fixed paraffin-embedded tissue using an antibody to human von Willebrand factor (factor VIII-related antigen) (Figure 8.1). An association between a high degree of neovascularization, measures of tumour extent and aggressiveness and lowered patient survival, has been observed in studies of patients with cancers of the bladder, brain, breast, cervix, endometrium, stomach, head and neck, lung, melanocytes, oral cavity, ovary, rectum, testis and prostate. The following factors, probably acting in concert, are the likely reasons for this association:

1. High vascular density increases the area of vascular surface, which may facilitate the escape of tumour cells into the circulation.
2. Newly formed blood vessels in tumours often are 'leaky', which allows malignant cells to cross their walls with relative ease.

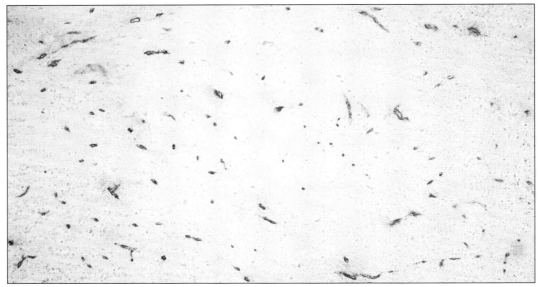

Figure 8.1. Neovascularization demonstrated immunohistochemically in a section of human prostate using an antibody to human von Willebrand factor (factor VIII-related antigen).

3. An angiogenic cell leaving a primary tumour probably is more likely than a non-angiogenic cell to develop into a detectable secondary tumour because secondary tumour growth also depends on neovascularization.
4. Solid tumours comprise both malignant cells and stroma. Tumour MVD may be a measure of the success of a tumour in forming essential stromal support.
5. Enzymes secreted by cells at the tips of growing capillaries may help tumour cells to enter the circulation by digesting the various protein barriers (e.g. connective tissue matrix and basement membrane) that stand between them and the lumina of the tumour vasculature.

MVD satisfies many criteria for being a useful biomarker in prostate cancer. In combination with Gleason score and serum PSA, it significantly increases the predictive accuracy for pathological stage and potential outcome.[14–23] Brawer *et al.*[15] found that the addition of MVD to a Gleason score/PSA model increased the model's ability to identify extraprostatic extension correctly, from 53 to 85%.

Most recently, optimized microvessel density (OMVD) as a predictor of extraprostatic extension was the subject of a multicentre study of 186 patients by Bostwick *et al.*,[23] utilizing computer-enhanced image analysis. The study concluded that the prediction of extraprostatic extension was significantly improved when OMVD was incorporated in a logistic regression model with the Gleason score from the diagnostic needle biopsy and the pre-biopsy serum PSA value.[23] For example, a patient with a Gleason score of 7 and a PSA value of 8 had a 53% probability of extraprostatic extension. Adding OMVD to the model distinguished between probabilities of 37 and 89% for the same patient (see Table 8.2). With a given Gleason score and PSA value, the study indicated that the odds of extraprostatic extension increased 5.97 times with every unit change of log OMVD.

The authors of the study conclude that '...the addition of the OMVD significantly enhanced the power of the Gleason score and serum PSA concentration to predict stage. The predictive accuracy of this combination of biomarkers was sufficiently high to be useful in determining treatment for individual patients.'[23] The authors observed that the probability values produced by the OMVD model '...appear to be useful guides for patient management and may be of greatest value in planning treatment for patients under consideration for radiation therapy, nerve sparing radical prostatectomy, expectant management and androgen deprivation therapy. Accurate pre-operative prediction of extraprostatic extension may also avoid surgery that otherwise might be cancelled intraoperatively.'[23]

Table 8.2. *Percentage probability of extraprostatic extension of cancer, given prostate-specific antigen (PSA), Gleason score and optimized microvessel density (OMVD)*

PSA	Gleason score	OMVD		
		50	100	250
6	6	23	34	51
8	7	50	63	78
4	6	16	24	39
12	5	23	33	50
6	8	70	80	90

Conclusions

MVD assays have been reported from many laboratories but, in prostate cancer, precise quantification appears to require a rigorous image analysis technique. Although a few university medical centres routinely perform the assay, commercial assays are now being developed that allow unstained sections of biopsy cores to be sent by mail to a reference laboratory, with results reported back in a week or less. One such assay, the BioStage™ Tumor Assessment Service developed by Bard Diagnostic Sciences, Redmond, WA, USA, which relies on patented computer algorithms to optimize the identification of microvessels, was used to predict the pathological stage in the study reported by Bostwick et al.[23] Commercial tests for OMVD are expected to cost between US$350 and US$400 and are expected to be reimbursable.

Although few tests in oncology are absolutely definitive, OMVD, along with PSA and Gleason score, may add to the level of confidence for the physician when planning treatment options for managing the patient with prostate cancer.

References

1. Ravery V, Delams V, Boccon-Gibod L A et al. Systematic biopsies accurately predict extracapsular extension of prostate cancer and persistent/recurrent detectable PSA after radical prostatectomy. Urology 1994; 44: 371–377
2. McNeal J E, Bostwick D G, Kindrachut R A et al. Patterns of progression in prostate cancer. Lancet 1986; 1: 60–64
3. McNeal J E, Vilers A A, Redwine E A et al. Capsular penetration in prostate cancer: significance for natural history and treatment. Am J Surg Pathol 1990; 14: 240–247
4. Hering F, Rist M, Roth J et al. Does microinvasion of the capsule and/or micrometastases in regional lymph nodes influence disease-free survival of radical prostatectomy? Br J Urol 990; 66: 177–180
5. Stamey T A, Kabalin J N, McNeal J E et al. Prostate-specific antigen in the diagnosis and treatment of adenocarcinoma of the prostate. II. Radical prostatectomy treated patients. J Urol 1989; 141: 1076–1082
6. Kleer E, Larson-Keller J J, Zincke H, Ostering J E. Ability of preoperative serum prostate-specific antigen value to predict pathologic stage and DNA ploidy. Influence of clinical stage and tumor grade. Urology 1993; 41: 207–212
7. Mukamel E, deKernion J B, Dorey F, Hannah J. Significance of histological prognostic indicators in patients with carcinoma of the prostate. Br J Urol 1990; 65: 46–51
8. Partin A W, Yoo J, Carter H B et al. The use of prostate-specific antigen, clinical stage, and Gleason score to predict pathologic stage in men with localized prostate cancer. J Urol 1993; 150: 110–116
9. Epstein J I, Pizov G, Walsh P C. Correlation of pathologic findings with progression following radical retropubic prostatectomy. Cancer 1993; 71: 3582–3593
10. Bostwick D G, Myers R P, Oesterling J E. Staging of prostate cancer. Semin Surg Oncol 1994; 10: 60–69
11. Ackerman D A, Barry J M, Wicklund R A et al. Analysis of risk factors associated with prostate cancer extension to the surgical margin and pelvic node metastasis at radical prostatectomy. J Urol 1993; 150: 1845–1851
12. Cupp M R, Bostwick D G, Myers R P, Oesterling J E. The volume of prostate cancer in the biopsy specimen cannot reliably predict the quantity of cancer in the radical prostatectomy specimen on an individual basis. J Urol 1995; 153: 1543–1548
13. Brawer M K, Deering R E, Brown M et al. Predictors of pathologic stage in prostatic carcinoma. The role of neovascularity. Cancer 1994; 73: 678–687
14. Wakui S, Furusato M, Itoh T et al. Tumor angiogenesis in prostatic carcinoma with and without bone marrow metastasis: a morphometric study. J Pathol 1992; 168: 257–262
15. Brawer M K, Bigler S A, Deering R E. Quantitative morphometric analysis of the microcirculation in prostate carcinoma. J Cell Biochem 1992; 161: 62–64
16. Weidner N, Carroll P, Flax J et al. Tumor angiogenesis correlates with metastasis in invasive prostate carcinoma. Am J Pathol 1993; 143: 401–409

17. Fregene T, Khanuja P, Noto A C *et al*. Tumor associated angiogenesis in prostate cancer. Anticancer Res 1993; 13: 2377–2382
18. Biegler S A, Deering R E, Brawer M K. Comparison of microscopic vascularity in benign and malignant prostate tissue. Hum Pathol 1993; 24: 220–226
19. Monoroni R, Magi Galluzzi C M, Damand L *et al*. Prostatic intra-epithelial neoplasia. Qualitative and quantitative analyses of the blood capillary architecture on thin tissue sections. Pathol Res Pract 1993; 189: 542–548
20. Hall M C, Tronocoso P, Pollack A *et al*. Significance of tumor angiogenesis in clinically localized prostate carcinoma treated with external beam radiotherapy. Urology 1994; 44: 869–875
21. Vesalainen S, Lipponen P, Talja M *et al*. Tumor vascularity and basement membrane structure as prognostic factors in T1–2M0 prostatic adenocarcinoma. Anticancer Res 1994; 14: 709–714
22. Siegal J A, Yu E, Brawer M K. Topography of neovascularity in human prostate carcinoma. Cancer 1995; 75: 2545–2551
23. Bostwick D G, Wheeler T M, Blute M *et al*. Optimized microvessel density analysis improves prediction of cancer stage from prostate needle biopsies. Urology 1996; 48: 47–57

Chapter 9
Mechanisms of developing androgen independence
A. O. Brinkmann

Introduction

The development and differentiation of the human prostate is an androgen-mediated process.[1] The main androgen in this respect is 5α-dihydrotestosterone, the 5α-reduced metabolite of testosterone. For maintenance of function and structure of the mature prostate also, androgens are indispensable. 5α-dihydrotestosterone acts in the prostate via an interaction with the androgen receptor, resulting in direct regulation of gene expression. The androgen receptor is a member of the superfamily of nuclear receptors, which also includes the other steroid hormone receptors, the thyroid hormone receptors, the retinoid receptors and several orphan receptors.[2]

Adenoma of the prostate is characterized by malignant growth and is a major cause of cancer deaths among men, becoming the greatest cause in men after the age of 75 years in Europe and the USA. Initially, the growth of the majority of prostate cancers is androgen dependent. Consequently, prostate cancer patients benefit temporarily from androgen-suppressing therapies, either by surgical or chemical castration or by anti-androgens, or by a combination. After an initial androgen-dependent growth phase, most prostate tumours enter an androgen-independent stage. The molecular basis for this switch from androgen-dependent to androgen-independent growth is largely unknown. It is not known whether androgen-independent tumours originate from the formation of androgen-independent cells in a population of androgen-dependent cells, or whether androgen-independent cells are selected from an originally heterogeneous tumour.

Despite their androgen independency, most prostate tumours express high levels of androgen receptor in the nuclei of the tumour cells. It has long been speculated, therefore, that the androgen receptor gene could play a role in the initiation or progressive growth of androgen-independent prostate tumours.

Several lines of evidence indicate that the androgen receptor can probably play a role in hormone-refractory prostate cancer. This overview is focused on a possible role of the androgen receptor in the development of androgen independency in prostate cancer. The following aspects are discussed:

1. Ligand-independent activation of the androgen receptor in prostate cancer;
2. Overexpression of the androgen receptor gene by gene amplification in prostate tumours;
3. Activating mutations in the androgen receptor gene in prostate cancer.

Ligand-independent activation of the androgen receptor in prostate cancer

Role of androgen receptor co-activators

It has been known for quite some time that interaction of nuclear receptors with basal transcription factors is necessary for control of hormone-dependent transcription activation. However, more recently it has become clear not only that components of the basal transcription machinery are necessary but also that additional protein factors differing from the basal factors are involved. These additional factors are called 'co-activators'.[3] A co-activator should fulfil the following criteria: binding to activation functional domains (AF-domains) of nuclear receptors; relieving autosquelching of nuclear receptors; increasing transcription activation of nuclear receptors; containing an autonomous activation function; gene knock-outs should have a phenotype of altered hormone action. For almost all nuclear receptors co-activators have been cloned, most of them with a broad specificity. One exception is a very interesting co-activator ARA70, which specifically interacts with the androgen receptor (AR) and enhances AR activity tenfold in the presence of 0.1 nM 5α-dihydrotestosterone or 1 nM testosterone, but not in the presence of the anti-androgen hydroxyflutamide.[4] The action of ARA70 is rather specific, because this co-activator only slightly induces the transcriptional activity of other steroid receptors. It appears that ARA70 is expressed in several cancer cell lines, including the LNCaP cell line, and also in prostate tissue. ARA70 was absent in the AR-negative human prostate cancer cell line DU145. Modulation of expression of ARA70 therefore can also modulate AR activity and it is possible that high levels of ARA70 in prostate tumours might render the tissue still responsive at extremely low levels of activating ligand as well as AR.

Androgen receptor activation by growth factors

It has been shown in a model system (DU 145 cells, co-transfected with AR and androgen-regulated reporter genes) that the growth factors insulin-like growth factor 1 (IGF-1), keratinocyte growth factor (KGF) and epidermal growth factor (EGF) can activate the androgen receptor.[5] Androgen receptor activation by IGF-1, KGF and EGF was completely inhibited by the pure antagonist bicalutamide (Casodex), showing that the growth factor effects are AR mediated. These results provide evidence that the AR signalling pathway may be activated additionally by growth factors in an androgen-depleted environment.

Cross-talk with protein kinase A and protein kinase C activators

There is increasing evidence now that gene expression is regulated by phosphorylation and/or dephosphorylation of transcription factors. DNA binding, transcriptional activity and subcellular trafficking of particular transcription factors have been shown to be directly dependent on the phosphorylation status of the transcription factor.[6] Recently it has been reported that modulators of protein phosphorylation can influence the transcriptional activity of several steroid receptors. In MCF-7 human breast cancer cells, oestrogen-induced transcription activation was increased upon co-treatment with protein kinase activators.[7] Treatment of rat uterine cells with oestradiol or agents which alter intracellular cAMP levels resulted in an increased activity of the oestrogen receptor. This was accompanied by an increase of oestradiol receptor phosphorylation. For the rat AR, transiently transfected in CV-1 cells, and for the human AR stably transfected in Chinese hamster ovary cells, it was found that AR-mediated transactivation was enhanced two- to fourfold by activators of protein kinase A and protein kinase C respectively, in the presence of androgens.[8,9] In a recent study, the effect of modulators of protein kinase A on androgen-independent AR activation was demonstrated.[10] The protein kinase A activator forskolin is able to activate the AR in the absence of androgens several fold after expression in human prostate PC-3 cells. The activation appears to be AR dependent and can be blocked by anti-androgens and protein kinase A inhibitors. This might be a mechanism operating in the progression of prostate cancer and demonstrates that androgen activation can occur even after androgen withdrawal during therapy in prostate cancer patients.

Overexpression of the AR gene by gene amplification in prostate cancer

In a recent study by Visakorpi et al.[11] it was shown by comparative genomic hybridization that amplification of the Xq11–q13 region can be observed in recurring prostate tumours (30%) obtained from patients undergoing androgen deprivation therapy. The mean AR copy number ranges from 3.8 to 21.5 per cell, with the highest number of 40 AR copies per individual tumour cell. In addition, in over 80% of the tumours, strong nuclear AR immunostaining with an anti-AR-antibody was also detectable. This finding might have important implications with respect to growth of the tumour cells under extreme low androgen levels. It is noteworthy that AR amplification occurred only during regrowth of the tumours during endocrine therapy, suggesting a selective mechanism under a very limited supply of androgens.[11] To date, no other upregulating mechanisms of AR expression are known in prostate cancer.

Activating mutations in the AR gene in prostate cancer

Previous studies have established that the human prostate carcinoma cell line LNCaP can be stimulated with respect to growth, not only by androgens but also by progesterone, oestradiol and several anti-androgens.[12] Characterization of the AR in these cells revealed an altered steroid-binding specificity, with an increased preference for progestagens and oestradiol as compared with the steroid-binding specificity of the AR in normal cells.[13] These data strongly suggested a modification of the AR and particularly in the steroid-binding domain. Sequence analysis revealed one point mutation in codon 868 in exon eight coding for the C-terminal end of the steroid-binding domain.[14] The mutation (A → G) resulted in a threonine → alanine substitution. In transfection studies with the mutant receptor, increased binding affinities for progestagens and oestradiol were observed. In addition, these ligands activate transcription at concentrations that are not sufficient for activation of the wild-type AR. These results confirm that the observed point mutation in the LNCaP cell AR is the cause of the broad steroid-binding specificity. Further studies on the importance of the role of threonine 868 in the human AR have indicated that threonine limits the ligand specificity to androgens.[15] Recently, the mutation Thr868Ala was also found in prostatic tumour tissue from patients with metastatic prostate cancer in several different independent studies.[16–19] It can be speculated that this specific mutant AR provides a selective growth advantage in a subset of advanced prostate cancers.

In a recent study, a relatively high number of somatic mutations in the ligand-binding domain were detected in bone marrow biopsies from patients with metastatic prostate cancer.[18] Two mutations were found to change the binding specificity of the AR (Thr868Ser and His865Tyr). Both mutant receptors could be stimulated by progesterone, oestradiol and androstenedione in addition to the normal androgenic stimulation. The His865Tyr mutation has also been reported in another study in an androgen-dependent prostatic carcinoma.[20] The mutant receptor displayed an abnormal specificity of steroid responsiveness, because nanomolar concentrations of oestradiol, hydroxyflutamide, androstenedione and dehydroepiandrosterone (DHEA) had an increased response compared with the wild-type AR. An interesting germ-line mutation was reported in a prostate cancer patient that activated the AR also by oestradiol.[21] The mutation (Arg717Leu) located in exon 5, which is part of the ligand-binding domain, did not alter the ligand binding specificity.

A study in prostate tumour specimens obtained from 26 untreated patients with organ-confined stage B prostate cancer has revealed in one patient a mutation in the AR gene at codon position 721.[22] This mutation resulted in a valine to methionine substitution and appeared to be somatic because the tumour tissue sample contained also wild-type AR sequences and the mutation was not detected in peripheral blood lymphocyte DNA. In the original publication this mutation has not been characterized functionally, but in a later report by the same investigators it was mentioned that the Val721Met mutation did not ablate androgen binding or androgen dependent transcriptional activity.[22] Recently, the Val721Met mutation was also investigated by others.[23] In contrast to the report by Newmark et al.,[22] a difference was observed between the Val721Met mutant and the wild-type androgen receptor. Functional studies with androsterone and androstanediol, two prostatic metabolites of testosterone, indicated a more efficient induction of androgen-responsive genes by this mutant receptor than by the wild-type receptor. Furthermore, high concentrations of the anti-androgen hydroxyflutamide, but not Casodex, enhanced the transactivating function of the mutant receptor.

In a report on the analysis of tumour specimens from seven men with metastatic prostate cancer (stage D2) and under androgen-ablation therapy, a point mutation was detected in one tumour sample from a patient with a poorly differentiated carcinoma of the prostate.[24] The mutation resulted in a valine to methionine substitution at position 706 in exon 4 of the AR. Adrenal androgens such as DHEA and androstenedione, but also progesterone, induced a higher transcription activation via the Val706Met mutant receptor than through the wild-type receptor. The finding that not only testicular androgens but also adrenal androgens can promote transactivation of this mutant receptor may have significance in the process controlling the progression of prostate cancer.

In a recent study, a relatively high number of mutations (44%) were reported in primary prostate tumours sampled prior to initiation of hormonal therapy.[25] Remarkable in this study is the finding of a large number of mutations in exon 1; however, the functional consequences of the mutant receptors were not studied.

Conclusions

Several different mechanisms for developing androgen independency in prostate cancer can be identified that still involve, to some extent, the AR (gene amplification, alternative activation, point mutations). Interesting developments can be expected in the field of associating proteins (e.g. co-activators and co-integrators) with respect to androgen action. Molecular analysis of AR specific co-activators in tumour specimens should yield new insights into progressive tumour growth. Furthermore, conformational consequences induced by specific mutations in the AR can explain, in a relatively small number of cases, the observed changes in ligand specificity and changes in ligand-induced transcription activation. It appears that position 868 (also mutated in the LNCaP cell AR) can be considered as a hot spot. Hardly any mutations in the AR gene have been reported to occur in primary sites. Knowledge of these mutations might have implications for therapy.

References

1. Griffin J E, McPhaul M J, Russell D W, Wilson J D. The androgen resistance syndromes: steroid 5α-reductase 2 deficiency, testicular feminization and related disorders. In: Scriver C R, Baudet A L, Sly W L, Valle D (eds) The metabolic and molecular basis of inherited disease, 7th edn. New York: McGraw-Hill, 1995: II: 2967–2998
2. Evans R M. The steroid and thyroid hormone receptor superfamily. Science 1988; 240: 889–895
3. Horwitz K B, Jackson T A, Bain D L et al. Nuclear receptor coactivators and corepressors. Mol Endocrinol 1996; 10: 1167–1177
4. Yeh S, Chang C. Cloning and characterization of a specific coactivator, ARA70, for the androgen receptor in human prostate cells. Proc Natl Acad Sci USA 1996; 93: 5517–5521
5. Culig Z, Hobisch A, Cronauer M V et al. Androgen receptor activation in prostate tumor cell lines by insulin-like growth factor-1, keratinocyte growth factor, and epidermal growth factor. Cancer Res 1994; 54: 5474–5478
6. Hunter T, Karin M. The regulation of transcription by phosphorylation. Cell 1992; 70: 375–387
7. Cho H, Katzenellenbogen B S. Synergistic activation of estrogen receptor-mediated transcription by estradiol and protein kinase activators. Mol Endocrinol 1993; 7: 441–452
8. Ikonen T, Palvimo J J, Kallio P J et al. Stimulation of androgen-regulated transactivation by modulators of protein phosphorylation. Endocrinology 1994; 135: 1359–1399
9. De Ruiter P E, Teuwen R, Trapman J et al. Synergism between androgens and protein kinase-C on androgen-regulated gene expression. Mol Cell Endocrinol 1995; 110: R1–R6
10. Nazareth L V, Weigel N L. Activation of the human androgen receptor through a protein kinase A signaling pathway. J Biol Chem 1996; 271: 19900–19907
11. Visakorpi T, Hyytinen E, Koivisto P et al. In vivo amplification of the androgen receptor gene and progression of human prostate cancer. Nature Genet 1995; 9: 401–406
12. Schuurmans A L G, Bolt J, Voorhorst M et al. Regulation of growth and epidermal growth factor receptor levels of LNCaP prostate tumor cells by different steroids. Int J Cancer 1988; 42: 917–922
13. Veldscholte J, Voorhorst-Ogink M M, Bolt-de Vries J et al. Unusual specificity of the androgen receptor in the human prostate tumor cell line LNCaP: high affinity for progestagenic and estrogenic steroids. Biochim Biophys Acta 1990; 1052: 187–194
14. Veldscholte J, Ris-Stalpers C, Kuiper G G J M et al. A mutation in the ligand binding domain of the androgen receptor of human LNCaP cells affects steroid binding characteristics and response to anti-androgens. Biochem Biophys Res Commun 1990; 173: 534–540
15. Ris-Stalpers C, Verleun-Mooijman M C T, Trapman J, Brinkmann A O. Threonine on amino acid position 868 in the human androgen receptor is essential for androgen binding specificity and functional activity. Biochem Biophys Res Commun 1993; 196: 173–180
16. Suzuki H, Sato N, Watabe Y et al. Androgen receptor gene mutations in human prostate cancer. J Steroid Biochem Mol Biol 1993; 46: 759–765
17. Gaddipati J P, McLeod D G, Heidenberg H B et al. Frequent detection of codon 877 mutation in the androgen receptor gene in advanced prostate cancers. Cancer Res 1994; 54: 2861–2864
18. Taplin M-E, Bubley G J, Shuster T D et al. Mutation of the androgen receptor gene in metastatic androgen-independent prostate cancer. N Engl J Med 1995; 332: 1393–1398
19. Kleinerman D I, Troncoso P, Pisters L L et al. Expression and structure of the androgen receptor in bone metastases of hormone refractory prostate cancer. J Urol 1996; 155(Suppl): 624A (abstr 1254)
20. Sharief Y, Wilson E M, Hall S H et al. Androgen Receptor gene mutations associated with prostatic carcinoma. Proc 86th AACR Meeting, Toronto, Ontario, Canada, 1995; 36: (abstr 1605)

21. Elo J P, Kvist L, Leinonen K *et al.* Mutated human androgen receptor gene detected in a prostatic cancer patient is also activated by estradiol. J Clin Endocrinol Metab 1995; 80: 3494–3500

22. Newmark J R, Haldy D O, Tonb D C *et al.* Androgen receptor gene mutations in human prostate cancer. Proc Natl Acad of Sci USA 1992; 89: 6319–6323

23. Peterziel H, Culig Z, Stober J *et al.* Mutant androgen receptors in prostatic tumours distinguish between amino-acid sequence requirements for transactivation and ligand binding. Int J Cancer 1995; 63: 544–550

24. Culig Z, Hobisch A, Cronauer M V *et al.* Mutant androgen receptor detected in an advanced-stage prostatic carcinoma is activated by adrenal androgens and progesterone. Mol Endocrinol 1993; 7: 1541–1550

25. Tilley W D, Buchanan G, Hickey T E, Bentel J M. Mutations in the androgen receptor gene are associated with progression of human prostate cancer to androgen independence. Clin Cancer Res 1996; 2: 227–285

Chapter 10
Growth regulation in the prostate: role of the sympathetic nervous system
L. Allen

Autonomic nervous system in the prostate

The prostate is a tubuloalveolar exocrine gland that arises from outgrowths of the urethral epithelium during foetal development. Its development is intimately dependent on androgens,[1–3] although the pathways regulating prostatic growth remain incompletely understood. It has become clear that normal prostate growth and development involves the complex interaction of multiple factors that, in addition to androgens, probably include several other growth factors, stromal/epithelial and cell/extracellular matrix interactions, and the sympathetic nervous system.[3–10] Abnormalities in any of these regulatory pathways may be important in the control of prostate growth and contribute to the pathogenesis and progression of benign and malignant prostate disease.

The prostate gland has a rich autonomic innervation from the hypogastric and pelvic nerves (Figure 10.1).[11–15] Cell bodies located in the upper lumbar spinal cord give rise to sympathetic preganglionic fibres, which provide sympathetic innervation to the prostate through the hypogastric nerve. In the sacral spinal cord, preganglionic parasympathetic fibres arise, which innervate the prostate through the pelvic nerve. Histochemical studies have demonstrated that anatomically cholinergic fibres supply stromal smooth muscle cells and glandular epithelial cells, whereas adrenergic fibres primarily supply stromal cells.[16]

The structural and functional integrity of the prostate both appear to be dependent on its autonomic nervous system innervation. Animal studies have

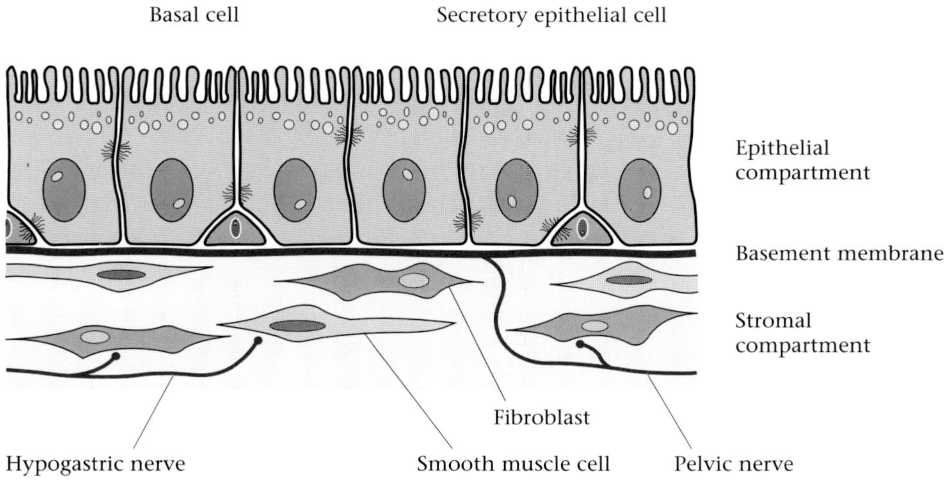

Figure 10.1. Autonomic nervous system innervation to the prostate gland. Functional unit of the prostate gland demonstrating sympathetic (hypogastric nerve) and parasympathetic (pelvic nerve) innervation to the stromal and epithelial cell compartments of the gland.

demonstrated that complete bilateral autonomic denervation results in decreases in weight, total protein content, prostatic binding protein and acid phosphatase levels in the ventral prostate.[17,18] In addition, the denervated glands showed abnormal ultrastructural features consistent with impaired functional activity, including a reduction in microvilli and secretory vesicles.

Sympathomimetic drugs have also been used to demonstrate the importance of the sympathetic nervous system in maintaining functional prostate differentiation. Such drugs have been shown to increase prostatic acid phosphatase[19] and prostatic binding protein concentrations.[18,20,21] Decreased concentrations of neural mediators, particularly noradrenaline, in ventral prostate renal grafts were associated with a significant decrease in prostatic binding protein concentration,[9] and protein levels were found to increase in response to treatment with adrenoceptor agonists.[18] In addition, parasympathomimetic drugs have been shown to induce prostatic fluid secretion, possibly through the direct stimulation of epithelial cells.

Additional animal studies have further characterized the role of sympathetic and parasympathetic innervation in regulating prostate growth. Unilateral sympathectomy was found to result in approximately a 23% decrease in ventral prostate weight and in DNA and protein content on the denervated side, consistent with glandular atrophy.[10] In contrast, unilateral parasympathectomy led to increases in ventral prostate weight and in DNA and protein content on the intact side, consistent with (contralateral) hyperplasia. These data suggest that autonomic innervation to the prostate plays an important role in differentially affecting prostate growth and function.

The effects of autonomic innervation on growth and differentiation have also been demonstrated in several other glandular tissues, e.g. mammary, thyroid, adrenal, ovarian and salivary glands.[22–27] In addition, the sympathetic nervous system has been shown to exert a direct regulatory effect on malignant cell proliferation, for example, mouse neuroblastoma growth both *in vitro* and *in vivo*. Chemical sympathectomy, using 6-hydroxydopamine (an adrenoceptor toxin), was found to suppress neuroblastoma growth *in vivo*.[28–30] In contrast, induction of sympathetic nervous system hypertrophy, by the treatment of newborn mice with nerve growth factor (NGF), was shown to enhance neuroblastoma tumour growth *in vivo*.[29] Co-culture experiments using superior cervical ganglion cells and mouse neuroblastoma cultures suggested that this effect was mediated by the secretion of a mitogenic factor.[30] The sympathetic nervous system, therefore, can play a direct role in stimulating abnormal cell growth and, thereby, could also be an important component in the interplay of regulatory factors controlling normal and abnormal prostate growth.

Epidemiological studies have suggested a strong positive relationship between sympathetic nervous system activity (as manifest by resting heart rate) and the risk of developing cancer and cancer mortality — an effect independent from other risk factors.[31–33] One such study, which utilized a large cohort of men (over 22,000) followed for an average of 19 years, demonstrated that there was a strong association between resting heart rate and prostate cancer mortality:[34] each increment in heart rate of 10 beats/min was associated with a 26% higher risk of prostate cancer death. Prospective studies on risk factors for benign prostatic hyperplasia (BPH) were also consistent with a positive relationship between sympathetic nervous system activity and prostate growth.[35,36] In addition, circulating catecholamine levels were found to increase with increasing age as a result of increased sympathetic nervous system activation and their release into the circulation,[37,38] which parallels the increasing incidence of both benign and malignant prostate disease with age. These data suggest that local neurotropic factors associated with sympathetic activity may have an important influence on the initiation and/or progression of prostate neoplasms.

Adrenoceptors in the prostate

Stimulation of presacral sympathetic nerves controls postganglionic sympathetic activity and results in the release of catecholamines, such as noradrenaline. This neuromediator in turn binds to α_1-adrenoceptors present on the cell membrane, leading to the activation of signal-transduction pathways and results in a cellular response (Figure 10.2). *In vitro* studies of the rat ventral prostate have directly demonstrated the presence of α_1-adrenoceptors,[39] and ligand-binding experiments have confirmed the presence of α_1-adrenoceptors in the human prostate gland.[40–42]

Multiple subtypes of α_1-adrenoceptors, identified pharmacologically and by molecular cloning, may serve to mediate different physiological functions in target tissues.[43–46] These subtypes differ in primary nucleotide sequence and chromosomal localization, and further demonstrate differences in tissue distribution, pharmacology and efficacy of coupling to signal transduction pathways. Several groups have now demonstrated the presence of α_1-adrenoceptors in the human prostate using radioligand binding and functional assays.[47–51] The author and others have further characterized and quantified α_1-adrenoceptor subtypes in the human prostate by RNase protection assays,[52,53] and have demonstrated the presence of mRNAs for each of the three cloned α_1-adrenoceptor subtypes. The level of expression of each receptor subtype mRNA in the human prostate gland was found to differ, with the α_{1a}-adrenoceptor subtype being predominant (69%) followed by the α_{1d}- (27%) and the α_{1b}- (3%) adrenoceptors.[52] This predominance of α_{1a}-adrenoceptor expression in the prostate suggests that this subtype may play a more central role in mediating the physiological effects of adrenoceptor activation in this target tissue.[52,54] *In situ*

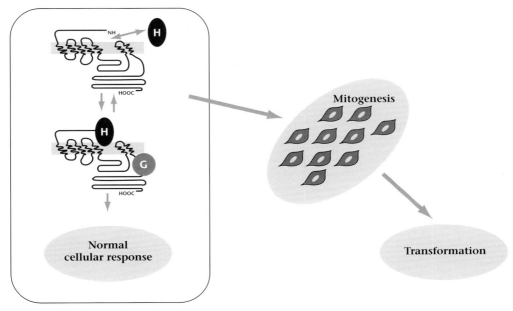

Figure 10.2. Subversion of α_1-adrenoceptor signal-transduction pathways. Subversion of normal cellular signalling pathways of α_1-adrenoceptors resulting in uncontrolled cell proliferation and benign or malignant neoplastic transformation.

hybridization studies employing α_1-adrenoceptor subtype-specific hybridization probes have also been used to localize receptor distribution in the human prostate.[52,53] Autoradiographs confirmed the α_{1a}-adrenoceptor as the predominant receptor subtype mRNA expressed, and localized α_{1a}-adrenoceptor expression predominately to the stromal compartment of the gland; prostate epithelial cells also appeared to express some α_1-adrenoceptor mRNAs.

Functional studies have demonstrated the role of these receptors in mediating prostate smooth muscle contraction,[55–57] an effect blocked by α_1-adrenoceptor antagonists. This regulation of prostatic smooth muscle tone by α_1-adrenoceptors has led to the use of α_1-adrenoceptor antagonists in the treatment of the obstructive symptoms of BPH.[58–60] The outflow obstruction that accompanies BPH consists of static and dynamic components; the static component is related to physical obstruction, resulting from prostate enlargement whereas the dynamic component is related to elevated smooth muscle tone in the prostate.[61] Therapeutic trials of α_1-adrenoceptor antagonists have focused on the dynamic component, attempting to reduce outflow obstruction by modulating sympathetic activity in the prostate; these drugs have proved effective in the management of the obstructive symptoms of BPH.[62–66]

Demonstration of the predominance of the α_{1a}-adrenoceptor subtype in the human prostate has stimulated the development of pharmacological agents that selectively block prostatic α_1-adrenoceptors, rather than vascular α_1-adrenoceptors, in order to minimize adverse cardiovascular side effects. However, it remains to be determined whether other potential effects of adrenoceptor activation, such as the stimulation of cell proliferation[67–70] (see below), will also be mediated through this receptor subtype in the prostate. These findings may have a major effect on our perspective on the therapeutic efficacy of current α_1-adrenoceptor blockers in the treatment of prostate disease, and the utility of the future development of more α_{1a}-adrenoceptor-specific antagonists.

Adrenoceptors as proto-oncogenes

The adrenoceptor family is a member of the larger superfamily of G-protein coupled receptors. Several G-protein-coupled receptors have now been shown to be capable of transforming cells to a malignant phenotype, thereby acting as proto-oncogenes,[71,72] and some have been found to be involved in the development of human disease including thyroid neoplasms.[73,74] The author's laboratory has reported the ability of α_1-adrenoceptors to function as proto-oncogenes, when overexpressed and agonist stimulated.[68] Transfection of these receptors into Rat-1 or NIH-3T3 fibroblasts resulted in a loss of normal growth control mechanisms, leading to abnormal cell proliferation and focus formation *in vitro*; foci were not observed in untransfected cells or cells transfected with expression vector alone. Receptor-expressing cells showed an increased rate of cell proliferation in the presence of adrenoceptor agonists — an effect that could be blocked by concurrent α_1-adrenoceptor antagonist treatment. These cells exhibited a neoplastic phenotype and induced tumours when injected into nude mice; tumour tissue was found to express significant levels of α_1-adrenoceptors. These data suggest that α_1-adrenoceptors can be subverted from their normal signal-transduction pathways and function as proto-oncogenes, inducing agonist-dependent focus formation *in vitro* and tumorigenesis *in vivo* (Figure 10.2).

Additional studies on untransformed fibroblasts expressing α_1-adrenoceptors have suggested that adrenoceptor activation results in the induction and secretion of a mitogenic factor that, in turn, can act in an autocrine or paracrine manner to stimulate cell proliferation. Addition of catecholamines alone (noradrenaline) to serum-free media was found to induce a marked stimulation of cell proliferation; this effect was agonist specific and was blocked by concurrent treatment with an α_1-adrenoceptor antagonist.[69] Collection of medium from receptor-expressing fibroblasts after treatment with noradrenaline demonstrated the ability of this conditioned medium to induce a two- to fivefold increase in [³H]thymidine incorporation in wild-type (non-receptor-expressing) fibroblasts.[69] In contrast, conditioned medium from non-receptor-expressing fibroblasts or from α_1-adrenoceptor-expressing fibroblasts grown in the absence of agonist was found to have no effect on DNA synthetic activity. These data suggest the receptor-mediated induction of a mitogenic factor that can be importantly involved in autocrine/paracrine regulatory pathways controlling cell proliferation of non α_1-adrenoceptor-expressing cells.

Other investigators have also demonstrated the mitogenic activity of catecholamines for bovine aortic endothelial cells, fibroblasts and vascular smooth muscle cells.[75–77] Norepinephrine has also been shown to function as a mitogenic growth factor for epithelial cells in other organs, such as the liver. Catecholamines were found to stimulate DNA synthesis in cultured hepatocytes through α_1-adrenoceptors.[78–81] In addition, the effects of growth inhibitors (such as transforming growth factor-β) on hepatocyte growth could be reduced by the concurrent administration of sympathomimetic agents.[82] During hepatic regeneration, treatment with α_1-adrenoceptor antagonists resulted in an inhibition of DNA synthesis.[70]

Sympathomimetic agents, such as noradrenaline, have also been shown to exert a concentration-dependent, direct mitogenic effect on rat prostate stromal cells *in vitro*, suggesting a potential role for them in the pathogenesis of BPH.[9,67] Their ability to stimulate prostate epithelial cell proliferation, directly or indirectly (i.e. through stromal/epithelial interactions), is currently under investigation. However, on the basis of the available *in vitro* data, it is possible that, in addition to their effects on smooth muscle tone in the prostate, α_1-adrenoceptors may also have a direct effect on prostate growth and thereby ultimately affect the pathogenesis and/or progression of prostate disease.

Effects of α_1-adrenoceptor antagonists on prostate cancer cell growth

The author and colleagues have begun to evaluate the role of α_1-adrenoceptors in regulating prostate cancer cell growth using an *in vitro* co-culture human prostate cancer model.[83] The human prostate cancer cell line, DU-145, was used in conjunction with primary cultures of human prostate stromal cells. Epithelial cell cultures were plated on microporous collagen-coated membrane inserts and then co-cultured in the presence of prostate stromal cells; this permitted the establishment of an *in vitro* model system of the human prostate that was analogous to the *in vivo* microenvironment. Co-cultures were left untreated or treated with various concentrations (5–50 μM) of doxazosin, a quinazoline derivative that is a selective, competitive antagonist of α_1-adrenoceptors.[84] This cell line was shown to exhibit a dose-dependent inhibition of cellular proliferation with complete inhibition of prostate cancer cell growth at doses of doxazosin above 15 μM (Figure 10.3). Similar inhibitory effects of this α_1-adrenoceptor antagonist were also noted on prostate stromal cell growth.

Using a cellular reconstitution model system, therefore, it has been demonstrated that the α_1-adrenoceptor antagonist, doxazosin, can potently

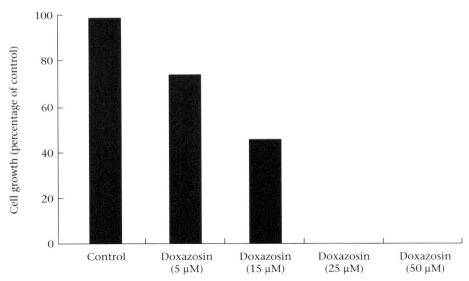

Figure 10.3. Inhibition of human prostate cancer cell growth by a specific α_1-adrenoceptor antagonist. Human prostate cancer cell proliferation (DU-145) in the presence of various concentrations of the α_1-adrenoceptor antagonist, doxazosin. Growth curves performed with epithelial cells grown on permeable collagen-coated membranes in co-culture with human prostate stromal cells.

inhibit the proliferation of human prostate cancer cells, as well as prostate stromal cells *in vitro*. However, because of the equal affinity of this α_1-adrenoceptor antagonist at each of the three α_1-adrenoceptor subtypes, it remains unclear whether this inhibitory effect is mediated preferentially through one of the α_1-adrenoceptor subtypes. In addition, the inhibitory effect of doxazosin on prostate cancer cell proliferation may actually be mediated through other pathways, such as through the direct induction of programmed cell death, i.e. apoptosis;[85] further studies should define the mechanism of growth inhibition by α_1-adrenoceptor antagonists.

High doses of chlorpromazine have been associated with a 33% reduction in the risk of prostate cancer.[86] Chlorpromazine is an antipsychotic drug that has pronounced α_1-adrenoceptor-blocking properties. This finding provides further support for the concept that α_1-adrenoceptor antagonists may have an important clinical role in controlling prostate growth and the development of prostate cancer.

Future directions in the treatment of prostate disease

The sympathetic nervous system appears to play an important role in maintaining prostate structure and function and may also be directly involved in the pathways regulating prostate growth. Abnormal activation of α_1-adrenoceptors, as the result of higher levels of sympathetic nervous system activity or abnormalities in the receptors themselves, could induce abnormal stromal and/or epithelial cell proliferation, resulting in the initiation and progression of benign and/or malignant prostate disease. The presence of adrenoceptors on human prostate stromal cells coupled with the demonstrated ability of adrenoceptor-expressing cells to secrete mitogenic factors in response to agonist stimulation, supports the concept that these receptors could be important physiological mediators of stromal/epithelial cell interactions controlling prostate cell function and growth (Figure 10.4) — a paradigm that parallels that of the mitogenic action of androgen on the prostate.[87–90]

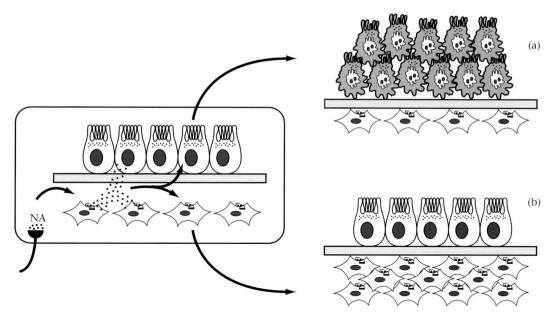

Figure 10.4. Proposed role of adrenoceptors in mediating prostate growth. Activation of α_1-adrenoceptors located on stromal cells by catecholamines released from the sympathetic nervous system (NA, noradrenaline) results in the secretion of a mitogenic peptide. This tropic factor can in turn modulate autocrine and paracrine growth regulatory loops resulting in: (a) malignant transformation of the prostate epithelium leading to the initiation/progression of prostate cancer; and/or (b) stromal hyperplasia, i.e. BPH.

Current investigations focused on defining such adrenoceptor-mediated growth-regulatory pathways in the prostate would provide the rationale for a targeted approach to the treatment of prostate neoplasms, directed at disrupting these autocrine/paracrine feedback loops. Pharmacological agents directed at these receptors, or at specific targets in their second-messenger pathways, could provide a specific and effective therapeutic modality for human prostate disease. Potentially, there would be an important role for such a therapeutic strategy in the treatment of both benign and malignant prostate neoplasms; the profound effects of α_1-adrenoceptor antagonists on prostate cancer cell growth and prostate stromal cell growth *in vitro* support the potential efficacy of such an approach. Ongoing clinical trials using α_1-adrenoceptor antagonists for the symptomatic treatment of BPH should provide important insights, when the incidence of prostate cancer or prostate cancer mortality is correlated with treatment in the study population. Future directions in the management of prostate neoplasms, therefore, may involve a novel treatment modality — the interruption of adrenoceptor-mediated autocrine/paracrine growth regulatory loops in the prostate — and lead to disease stabilization or the regression of established disease. It is hoped that such an approach may prove to have a significant impact on prostate cancer mortality.

References

1. Cunha G R, Alarid E T, Turner T *et al*. Normal and abnormal development of the male urogenital tract. Role of androgens, mesenchymal-epithelial interactions, and growth factors. J Androl 1992; 13(6): 465–475
2. Bruchovsky N, Lesser B, Van Doorn E, Craven S. Hormonal effects on cell proliferation in the rat prostate. Vitam Horm 1975; 33: 61–102
3. Coffey D S, Isaacs J T. Control of prostate growth. Urology 1981; 17(3): 17–24

4. Chung L W. The role of stromal–epithelial interaction in normal and malignant growth. Cancer Surv 1995; 23: 33–42

5. Wilding G. Endocrine control of prostate cancer. Cancer Surv 1995; 23: 43–62

6. Steiner M S. Role of peptide growth factors in the prostate: a review. Urology 1993; 42(1): 99–110

7. Lee C. Role of androgen in prostate growth and regression: stromal–epithelial interaction. Prostate 1996 (Suppl 6): 52–56

8. Cunha G R. Role of mesenchymal–epithelial interactions in normal and abnormal development of the mammary gland and prostate. Cancer 1994; 74(Suppl 3): 1030–1044

9. Thompson T C, Zhau H Y, Chung L W. Catecholamines are involved in the growth and expression of prostatic binding protein by rat ventral prostatic tissues. Prog Clin Biol Res 1987; 239: 239–248

10. McVary K, Razzaq A, Lee C et al. Growth of the rat prostate gland is facilitated by the autonomic nervous system. Biology Reprod 1994; 51(1): 99–107

11. Purinton F T, Fletcher T F, Bradley W F. Gross and light microscopic features of the pelvic plexus in the rat. Anat Rec 1972; 175: 697–706

12. Langworthy O R. Innervation of the pelvic organs of the rat. Invest Urol 1965; 2: 491–511

13. Vaalasti A, Hervonen A. Innervation of the ventral prostate of the rat. Am J Anat 1979; 154: 231–244

14. Nadelhaft I, McKenna K E. Sexual dimorphism in sympathetic preganglionic neurons of the rat hypogastric nerve. J Comp Neurol 1987; 256(2): 308–315

15. Nadelhaft I, Booth A M. The location and morphology of preganglionic neurons and the distribution of visceral afferents from the rat pelvic nerve: a horseradish peroxidase study. J Comp Neurol 1984; 226(2): 238–245

16. Gosling J A. Autonomic innervation of the prostate. In: Hinman F (ed) Benign prostatic hypertrophy. New York: Springer-Verlag, 1983: 349–360

17. Wang J M, McKenna K E, McVary K T, Lee C. Requirement of innervation for maintenance of structural and functional integrity in the rat prostate. Biol of Reprod 1991; 44: 1171–1176

18. Guthrie P D, Freeman M R, Liao S T, Chung L W. Regulation of gene expression in rat prostate by androgen and β-adrenergic receptor pathways. Mol Endocrinol 1990; 4(9): 1343–1353

19. Jacobs S C, Story M T. Autonomic control of acid phosphatase exocrine secretion by the rat prostate. Urol Res 1989; 17(5): 311–315

20. Wang J M, McKenna K E, Lee C. Determination of prostatic secretion in rats: effect of neurotransmitters and testosterone. Prostate 1991; 18(4): 289–301

21. Bruschini H, Schmidt R A, Tanagho E A. Neurologic control of prostatic secretion in the dog. Invest Urol 1978; 15: 288–290

22. Silberstein G B, Strickland P, Trumpbour V et al. In vivo, cAMP stimulates growth and morphogenesis of mouse mammary ducts. Proc Natl Acad Sci USA 1984; 81: 4950–4954

23. Melander A, Ericson L E, Sundler F, Westgren U. Intrathyroidal amines in regulation of thyroid activity. Rev Physiol Biochem Pharmacol 1975; 73: 39–71

24. Burden H W. Ovarian innervation. In: Jones R E (ed) The vertebrate ovary: comparative biology and evolution. New York: Plenum Press, 1978: 615–638

25. Brenner G M, Wulf R G. Adrenergic ß receptors mediating submandibular salivary gland hypertrophy in the rat. J Pharmacol Exp Ther 1981; 218(3): 608–612

26. Walker P. The mouse submaxillary gland: a model for the study of hormonally dependent growth factors. J Endocrinol Invest 1982; 5(3): 183–196

27. Kilpatrick D L, Howells R D, Fleminger G, Udenfriend S. Denervation of rat adrenal glands markedly increases preproenkephalin mRNA. Proc Natl Acad Sci USA 1984; 81(22): 7221–7223

28. Chelmicka-Schorr E, Arnason B G W. Effect of 6-hydroxydopamine on tumor growth. Cancer Res 1976; 36: 2382–2384

29. Chelmicka-Schorr E, Arnason B G W. Modulatory effect of the sympathetic nervous system on neuroblastoma tumor growth. Cancer Res 1978; 38: 1374–1375

30. Chelmicka Schorr E, Jones K H, Checinski M E et al. Influence of the sympathetic nervous system on the growth of neuroblastoma in vivo and in vitro. Cancer Res 1985; 45(12 Pt 1): 6213–6215

31. Severson R K, Nomura A M, Grove J S, Stemmermann G N. A prospective study of demographics, diet, and prostate cancer among men of Japanese ancestry in Hawaii. Cancer Res 1989; 49(7): 1857–1860

32. Wannamethee G, Shaper A G, Macfarlane P W. Heart rate, physical activity, and mortality from cancer and other noncardiovascular diseases. Am J Epidemiol 1993; 137(7): 735–748

33. Persky V, Dyer A R, Leonas J. Heart rate: a risk factor for cancer? Am J Epidemiol 1981; 114: 477–487

34. Gann P H, Daviglus M L, Dyer A R, Stamler J. Heart rate and prostate cancer mortality: results of a prospective analysis. Cancer Epidemiol Biomark Prev 1995; 4: 611–616

35. Gann P H, Hennekens C H, Longcope C et al. A prospective study of plasma hormone levels, nonhormonal factors, and development of benign prostatic hyperplasia. Prostate 1995; 26(1): 40–49

36. Giovannucci E, Rimm E B, Chute C G et al. Obesity and benign prostatic hyperplasia. Am J Epidemiol 1994; 140(11): 989–1002

37. Stromberg J S, Linares O A, Supiano M A et al. Effect of desipramine on norepinephrine metabolism in humans: interaction with aging. Am J Physiol 1991; 261(6 Pt 2): R1484–R1490

38. Supiano M A, Linares O A, Smith M J, Halter J B. Age-related differences in norepinephrine kinetics: effect of posture and sodium-restricted diet. Am J Physiol 1990; 259(3 Pt 1): E422–E431

39. Raz S, Ziegler M, Caine M. Pharmacological receptors in the prostate. Urology 1973; 45: 663

40. Chapple C R, Aubry M L, James S et al. Characterization of human prostatic adrenoceptors using pharmacology receptor binding and localisation. Br J Urol 1989; 63(5): 487–496

41. Lepor H, Shapiro E. Characterization of α_1-adrenergic receptors in human benign prostatic hyperplasia. J Urol 1984; 132(6): 1226–1229

42. Gup D I, Shapiro E, Baumann M, Lepor H. Autonomic receptors in human prostate adenomas. J Urol 1990; 143(1): 179–185

43. Lomasney J W, Cotecchia S, Lorenz W et al. Molecular cloning and expression of the cDNA for the α_{1A}-adrenergic receptor. J Biol Chem 1991; 266(10): 6365–6369

44. Schwinn D A, Lomasney J W, Lorenz W et al. Molecular cloning and expression of the cDNA for a novel α_1-adrenergic receptor subtype. J Biol Chem 1990; 265(14): 8183–8189

45. Cotecchia S, Schwinn D A, Randall R R et al. Molecular cloning and expression of the cDNA for the α_1-adrenergic receptor. Proc Natl Acad Sci USA 1988; 85(19): 7159–7163

46. Weinberg D H, Trivedi P, Tan C P et al. Cloning, expression and characterization of human α adrenergic receptors α_{1A}, α_{1B} and α_{1C}. Biochem Biophys Res Commun 1994; 201(3): 1296–1304

47. Faure C, Pimoule C, Vallancien G et al. Identification of α_1-adrenoceptor subtypes present in the human prostate. Life Sci 1994; 54(21): 1595–1605

48. Chapple C R, Burt R P, Andersson P O et al. Alpha$_1$-adrenoceptor subtypes in the human prostate. Br J Urol 1994; 74(5): 585–589

49. Goetz A S, Lutz M W, Rimele T J, Saussy D L Jr. Characterization of α_1-adrenoceptor subtypes in human and canine prostate membranes. J Pharmacol Exp Ther 1994; 271(3): 1228–1233

50. Muramatsu I, Oshita M, Ohmura T et al. Pharmacological characterization of α_1-adrenoceptor subtypes in the human prostate: functional and binding studies. Br J Urol 1994; 74(5): 572–578

51. Lepor H, Tang R, Meretyk S, Shapiro E. α_1-Adrenoceptor subtypes in the human prostate. J Urol 1993; 149(3): 640–642

52. Price D T, Schwinn D A, Lomasney J W et al. Identification, quantification, and localization of mRNA for three distinct α_1-adrenergic receptor subtypes in human prostate. J Urol 1993; 150(2 Pt 1): 546–551

53. Tseng-Crank J, Kost T, Goetz A et al. The α_{1C}-adrenoceptor in human prostate: cloning, functional expression, and localization to specific prostatic cell types. Br J Pharmacol 1995; 115(8): 1475–1485

54. Forray C, Bard J A, Wetzel J M et al. The α_1-adrenergic receptor that mediates smooth muscle contraction in human prostate has the pharmacological properties of the cloned human α_{1C}- subtype. Mol Pharmacol 1994; 45(4): 703–708

55. Hieble J P, Caine M, Zalaznik E. In vitro characterization of the alpha-adrenoceptors in human prostate. Eur J Pharmacol 1985; 107(2): 111–117

56. Caine M, Raz M, Ziegler M. Adrenergic and cholinergic receptors in the human prostate, prostatic capsule and bladder neck. Urology 1975; 47: 193

57. Lepor H, Tang R, Shapiro E. The α-adrenoceptor subtype mediating the tension of human prostatic smooth muscle. Prostate 1993; 22(4): 301–307

58. Kane M M, Fields D W, Vaughan E D, Jr. Medical management of benign prostatic hyperplasia. Urology 1990; 36(5 Suppl): 5–12

59. Lepor H. The emerging role of alpha antagonists in the therapy of benign prostatic hyperplasia. J Androl 1991; 12(6): 389–394

60. Chapple C R, Christmas T J, Milroy E J. A twelve-week placebo-controlled study of prazosin in the treatment of prostatic obstruction. Urol Int 1990; 1: 47–55

61. Caine M. The present role of alpha-adrenergic blockers in the treatment of benign prostatic hypertrophy. J Urol 1986; 136(1): 1–4

62. Kirby R S. Alpha-adrenoceptor inhibitors in the treatment of benign prostatic hyperplasia. Am J Med 1989; 87(2a): 26s–30s

63. Lepor H, Williford W O, Barry M J et al. The efficacy of terazosin, finasteride, or both in benign prostatic hyperplasia. Veterans Affairs Cooperative Studies Benign Prostatic Hyperplasia Study Group. N Engl J Med 1996; 335(8): 533–539

64. Kawabe K, Moriyama N, Yamada S, Taniguchi N. Rationale for the use of alpha-blockers in the treatment of benign prostatic hyperplasia (BPH). Int J Urol 1994; 1(3): 203–211

65. Caine M. Alpha-adrenergic blockers for the treatment of benign prostatic hyperplasia. Urol Clin North Am 1990; 17(3): 641–649

66. Lepor H, Auerbach S, Puras Baez A et al. A randomized, placebo-controlled multicenter study of the efficacy and safety of terazosin in the treatment of benign prostatic hyperplasia. J Urol 1992; 148(5): 1467–1474

67. Chung L W K, Thompson T C, Chao H et al. Catecholamines are involved in stromal epithelial interactions in rat ventral prostate gland. In: Rodgers et al., eds. Benign Prostatic Hyperplasia: 2nd NIDDK Symposium. Bethesda, MD: U.S. Department of Health and Human Services, Public Health Science, 1986; 11: 27–33

68. Allen L F, Lefkowitz R J, Caron M G, Cotecchia S. G-protein-coupled receptor genes as protooncogenes: constitutively activating mutation of the α_{1B}–adrenergic receptor enhances mitogenesis and tumorigenicity. Proc Natl Acad Sci USA 1991; 88: 11354–11358

69. Topouzis S, Allen L F, Majesky M W. Mitogenic potential of a cloned α_{1C}-adrenergic receptor expressed in Rat-1 fibroblasts. FASEB J 1993; 7(3 Pt1): A1

70. Cruise J L, Knechtle S J, Bollinger R R et al. α_1-Adrenergic effects and liver regeneration. Hepatology 1987; 7(6): 1189–1194

71. Julius D, Livelli T J, Jessell T M, Axel R. Ectopic expression of the serotonin 1c receptor and the triggering of malignant transformation. Science 1989; 244(4908): 1057–1062

72. Gutkind J S, Novotny E A, Brann M R, Robbins K C. Muscarinic acetylcholine receptor subtypes as agonist-dependent oncogenes. Proc Natl Acad Sci 1991; 88(11): 4703–4707

73. Shenker A, Laue L, Kosugi S et al. A constitutively activating mutation of the luteinizing hormone receptor in familial male precocious puberty. Nature 1993; 365: 652–654

74. Parma J, Duprez L, Van Sande J et al. Somatic mutations in the thyrotropin receptor gene cause hyperfunctioning thyroid adenomas. Nature 1993; 365(6447): 649–651

75. Sherline P, Mascardo R. Catecholamines are mitogenic in 3T3 and bovine aortic endothelial cells. J Clin Invest 1984; 74: 483–487

76. Blaes N, Boissel JP. Growth-stimulating effect of catecholamines on rat aortic smooth muscle cells in culture. J Cell Physiol 1983; 116(2): 167–172

77. Nakaki T, Nakayama M, Yamamoto S, Kato R. α_1-Adrenergic stimulation and ß2-adrenergic inhibition of DNA synthesis in vascular smooth muscle cells. Mol Pharmacol 1990; 37(1): 30–36

78. Cruise J L, Houck K A, Michalopoulos G K. Induction of DNA synthesis in cultured rat hepatocytes through stimulation of α_1 adrenoreceptor by norepinephrine. Science 1985; 227(4688): 749–751

79. Refsnes M, Thoresen GH, Sandnes D et al. Stimulatory and inhibitory effects of catecholamines on DNA synthesis in primary rat hepatocyte cultures: role of alpha 1- and beta-adrenergic mechanisms. J Cell Physiol 1992; 151(1): 164–171

80. Cruise J L, Muga S J, Lee Y S, Michalopoulos G K. Regulation of hepatocyte growth: α_1 adrenergic receptor and ras p21 changes in liver regeneration. J Cell Physiol 1989; 140(2): 195–201

81. Takai S, Nakamura T, Komi N, Ichihara A. Mechanism of stimulation of DNA synthesis induced by epinephrine in primary culture of adult rat hepatocytes. J Biochem (Tokyo) 1988; 103(5): 848–852

82. Houck K A, Cruise J L, Michalopoulos G. Norepinephrine modulates the growth-inhibitory effect of transforming growth factor-beta in primary rat hepatocyte cultures. J Cell Physiol 1988; 135(3): 551–555

83. Allen L F, Ferguson S B, Moore M E. Prostate cancer cell inhibition by doxazosin. Eur Urol 1996; 30(Suppl 2): 35

84. Young R A, Brogden R N. Doxazosin. A review of its pharmacodynamic and pharmacokinetic properties, and therapeutic efficacy in mild or moderate hypertension. Drugs 1988; 35(5): 525–541

85. Yang G, Timme T L, Park S *et al*. Induction of apoptosis by doxazosin in the BPH–mouse prostate reconstitution model. Eur Urol 1996; 30(Suppl 2): 27

86. Mortensen P B. Neuroleptic medication and reduced risk of prostate cancer in schizophrenic patients. Acta Psychiatr Scand 1992; 85(5): 390–393

87. Chang S, Chung L W K. Interaction between prostatic fibroblast and epithelial cells in culture: role of androgen. Endocrinology 1989; 125(5): 2719–2727

88. Chung L W K, Gleave M E, Hsieh J *et al*. Reciprocal mesenchymal-epithelial interaction affecting prostate tumour growth and hormonal responsiveness. Cancer Surv 1991; 11: 91–121

89. Sugimura Y, Cunha G R, Bigsby R M. Androgenic induction of DNA synthesis in prostatic glands induced in the urothelium of testicular feminized (Tfm/Y) mice. Prostate 1986; 9(3): 217–225

90. Verhoeven G, Swinnen K, Cailleau J *et al*. The role of cell–cell interactions in androgen action. J Steroid Biochem Mol Biol 1992; 41(3–8): 487–494

Chapter 11
Major histocompatibility complex abnormalities in benign and malignant prostate disease

R. A. Blades, L. J. McWilliam, P. L. Stern and N. J. R. George

Introduction

In the past, prostate cancer has been considered to be poorly immunogenic and little research has concentrated on this aspect of the host–tumour interaction. The process of carcinogenesis and metastasis undoubtedly involves many steps to permit uncontrolled cell division, angiogenesis, invasion and adhesion at sites of metastasis. It is well established that tumour cells express different antigens that potentially render the malignant cell susceptible to attack by the host immune response. Central to the concept of immune surveillance is the necessity for recognition of some aspect of the tumour cell as abnormal/foreign and presentation of such aberrant antigens to the adaptive immune response. In order for cytotoxic T cells to recognize a cell as abnormal, the peptide antigen must be presented to the T cells in association with a major histocompatibility complex (MHC) class I molecule, this phenomenon being known as MHC restriction.[1]

There is abundant evidence for the role of the MHC in tumour progression from studies of cell lines and animal tumours both *in vivo* and *in vitro*. Clones derived from methylcholanthrene-induced sarcomas were found to be heterogeneous with regard to MHC class I expression and those clones with the lowest expression were most tumorigenic in syngeneic mice.[2] Furthermore, transfection of specific class I genes into cell clones with high metastatic potential and loss of this class I product caused complete abrogation of metastasis formation.

Some adenoviruses are known to cause cellular transformation, but only those such as adenovirus 12 which cause loss of class I expression are tumorigenic.[3] Induction of class I expression by interferon γ (INF-γ) or gene transfection reduced the tumourigenicity of these transformed cells.[4] Other widely studied tumour models include the spontaneously arising leukaemias in AKR mice, some of which show loss of just one class I allele (H2-K^k) and demonstrate resistance to specific cytotoxic T cells *in vitro* and always form tumours in immunocompetent AKR mice. Once again, transfection of the K^k gene prevented tumour formation.[5]

These and other studies demonstrate that re-expression of MHC class I molecules can render tumour cells susceptible to the immune response and thereby prevent tumour growth and metastasis. It is conceivable that the immunogenicity of tumours and the resulting control of tumour growth by the immune system depend not only on the existence of tumour-associated antigens but also on the expression of individual MHC antigens on the tumour cell surface. If this is the case, then quantitative and qualitative changes in MHC expression may influence tumour growth and metastasis in immunocompetent hosts.

This chapter concentrates on human leucocyte antigen (HLA) class I expression in prostate cancer, but to put this in perspective it is important to understand the nature of HLA class I and II expression in normal tissue.

HLA class II expression

Most normal epithelia are constitutively HLA class II negative[6] but may express HLA class II in response to inflammation. The prostate is no exception to this observation, with benign prostatic hyperplasia (BPH) generally being HLA class II negative except in areas adjacent to lymphocytic infiltration.[7-9]

De novo HLA class II expression occurs in some tumours independent of lymphocytic infiltrate, with variable effects on tumour progression, although in most cases this occurs on low-grade tumours with good prognosis.[10] HLA class II expression was not observed in the authors' series of prostate cancers, in keeping with earlier reports.[7,8] However, focal class II expression has been reported in low grade carcinomas[11] and following neuraminidase digestion, which resulted in less than 5% of cells staining in a minority of tumours.[9] There is no evidence of HLA class II expression in the widely available cell lines DU-145, PC-3 and LNCaP,[12] although HLA class II expression can be induced by INF-γ in the DU-145 prostate cancer cell line.[8] The lack of class II expression by malignant cells adjacent to lymphocytic infiltrate would suggest that this does not occur *in vivo*, assuming that the T cells are activated, thereby producing the appropriate cytokines.

HLA class I expression

Daar and colleagues[13] studied a wide range of normal tissues post mortem, including one sample of prostate from a 20-year-old man, and concluded that all normal epithelia expressed the class I antigen.

Benign prostatic hyperplasia

The authors have assessed HLA class I expression using commonly available monomorphic antibodies in frozen tissue from 17 patients with BPH, and observed strong membranous expression by epithelial cells (Figure 11.1), as well as expression in stromal tissue.[14] There have been two reports of HLA expression in formalin-fixed benign tissue using antibodies against β_2-microglobulin, with all 13 cases in one study demonstrating membranous staining,[9] in contrast to only 21% of benign cases in the other study.[15] Since the authors' report of HLA class I expression they have found one case of BPH with loss of expression of the HLA-A2 allele, but with normal expression of HLA-B alleles. This observation is currently unexplained. It seems unlikely that this is simply a field change induced by an occult carcinoma, as specimens containing both BPH and prostate cancer failed to show HLA loss in benign areas adjacent to carcinoma.

Primary prostate cancer

There is abundant evidence that many diverse tumours show altered HLA class I expression, with rates of complete loss of expression of 10% in transitional cell carcinoma of the bladder[16] and of 10–15% in cervical squamous cell carcinoma,[17] in the latter case being associated with poor prognosis. Before the authors' investigation of HLA expression, prostate cancer had not been widely studied.

Snap-frozen prostatic tissue was collected from 69 patients presenting with either outflow obstruction or untreated prostate cancer requiring transurethral resection of the prostate. In 51 cases there was histological evidence of prostate cancer, with 29 of these patients having bone metastases diagnosed on routine

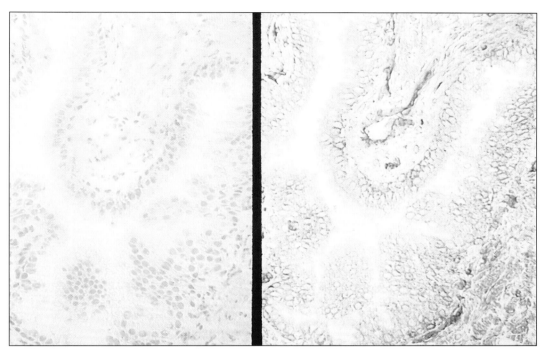

Figure 11.1. Serial sections through a benign prostate gland demonstrating strong membranous HLA class I expression by epithelial cells, as well as expression by stromal tissues which serves as a positive control within each section: (a) stained with H&E, X100 magnification; (b) stained for HLA class I expression using the antibody W6/32. (Reproduced from ref 14, with permission from Elsevier Science Inc.).

isotope bone scans (Table 11.1). HLA expression was assessed by standard immunohistochemical technique using eight different antibodies,[14] in order to assess not merely the presence or absence of the complete class I molecule as defined by the antibody W6/32, but also whether only β_2-microglobulin (β_2m) or HLA-B and -C heavy chains (defined by the antibody HC10) were produced if the complete class I molecule was absent. In addition, isolated allele product loss was examined using five antibodies against the common HLA class I alleles, as the nature of any putative tumour antigen may determine which of these alleles acts as a restriction element for cytotoxic T cells, such that loss of expression of a single HLA allele may prevent presentation of tumour antigen to the immune system. Provided that the remaining class I alleles are expressed normally,

Table 11.1. Clinicopathological parameters for patients with or without metastases

Patient group	Age (years)	PSA ng/ml*	Gleason score	Local tumour stage[†]
Non-metastatic ($n = 22$)	69.4 ± 7.0	54.8 (range 18–207)	7.4	No. ≤ T2 = 13 No. > T2 = 9
Metastatic ($n = 29$)	71.8 ± 6.9	126.7 (range 8–500)	8.4	No. ≤ T2 = 7 No. > T2 = 22

*Normal < 4 ng/ml.
[†]TNM 1992 (ref. 43).

antibodies such as W6/32 will produce positive staining and underestimate potentially significant HLA losses unless allele-specific expression is also assessed.

Sections of prostate labelled by the eight antibodies against the HLA class I antigens were scored by two independent observers. The stromal staining acted as a positive control within each section, and the epithelial staining intensity relative to the latter was scored ++ when equivalent, + when of lesser intensity, and – when absent.

Initial studies using the three antibodies against the HLA heavy chain–β_2m complex (W6/32), free heavy chains (HC10) or β_2m (BM-63) produced similar results, with three main patterns of staining (Table 11.2). Overall, 24% of malignant specimens had complete loss of class I expression (Figure 11.2) and a further 54% had weak staining compared with the stromal staining. Only 22% of cases had normal homogeneous membranous staining of intensity equivalent to

Table 11.2. HLA expression as defined by monomorphic antibodies (W6/32, BM-63 and HC10) in primary prostate cancer from 51 patients, divided according to presence or absence of bone metastases at the time of presentation

	HLA expression		
Patient group	Normal (++)	Reduced (+)	Absent(–)
Non-metastatic ($n = 22$)	7	11	4
Metastatic ($n = 29$)	4	17	8
	11	28	12

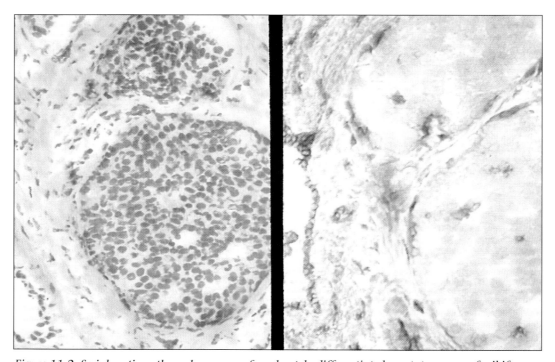

Figure 11.2. Serial sections through an area of moderately differentiated prostate cancer of cribiform type. There is normal HLA class I expression by the epithelium of the benign gland in the bottom left-hand corner, in contrast to the class I-negative prostate cancer highlighted by the blue counterstain: (a) stained with H&E, X100 magnification; (b) stained for HLA class I expression using the antibody W6/32. (Reproduced from ref 14, with permission from Elsevier Science Inc.).

stroma. In view of the large number of cases with abnormal HLA class I expression with these three antibodies, all cases were assessed using the five allele-specific antibodies. For the 51 cases of prostate cancer, only four specimens had normal HLA class I expression when the results of the eight antibodies were combined. In particular, all of the cases with abnormal staining with the three monomorphic antibodies had loss of expression of at least one allele.

There were no significant differences between the cases with or without bone metastases, but the majority of these prospectively collected specimens were from patients with advanced disease, and even those cases with a low clinical stage had an elevated serum prostate-specific antigen in the range known to be associated with extracapsular disease.

Relationship of HLA expression to progression and survival

Correlation of HLA class I downregulation with tumour stage and differentiation has been demonstrated in several tumours, including colorectal cancer,[18] larynx[19] and transitional cell carcinoma of the bladder.[20] In the authors' prospective investigation of HLA class I expression there was no significant association between either global or allele-specific HLA loss and tumour stage or grade. However, the number of cases with clinically localized tumours and negative bone scans was too small to permit separate statistical analysis.

In order to address this dilemma and investigate any relationship to survival, the authors examined HLA expression in 78 cases of untreated prostate cancer presenting between 1980 and 1986 and known to have negative bone scans at presentation. The range of antibodies available for use in formalin-fixed tissue was limited to antibodies against HLA-A heavy chains and HLA-B and -C heavy chains (HC-A2 and HC10, respectively, which were gifts from Dr H. Ploegh, MIT, Massachusetts, USA). Overall, normal or heterogeneous class I expression was found in 36% of cases, and there was an association between HLA class I downregulation and tumour stage but no correlation with Gleason grade (unpublished data). These results are comparable to the two published reports in which fixed archival prostate cancer was evaluated using antibodies against β_2m, with both studies including a larger proportion of low-grade and low-stage cases. The Hammersmith group found heterogeneous expression in 59% of samples and no correlation with Gleason grade,[9] in contrast to the report from Israel in which 43% of cases had heterogeneous class I expression and increased rates of HLA loss in poorly differentiated tumours.[15]

Clinical studies on the relationship of HLA expression to progression and survival in other tumours are scarce and controversial, owing to the small number of cases and short follow-up in many reports.[21-23] The prospective study[14] was hampered by the short follow-up period and it is impossible to draw any meaningful conclusions regarding the influence of HLA expression on survival. Although there was a significant association between survival and HLA expression for the whole group, this was not independent of other factors known to be related to outcome. Despite the prolonged follow-up of the 78 cases from the longitudinal study of the natural history of localized prostate cancer,[24] it was not feasible to confirm or refute the hypothesis that loss of HLA expression permits evasion of immune surveillance and progression of prostate cancer. The major confounding factor in this and other investigations of prostate cancer is that patients tend to be elderly with significant co-morbidity, which frequently results in death from intercurrent disease, thus reducing the number of cases available for follow-up with regard to disease-specific survival.

HLA class I expression in metastatic tissue

If abnormal HLA expression is a significant factor in tumour progression and metastasis, a higher rate of class I downregulation in metastatic deposits would be expected. A dominant role for the adaptive immune response in controlling metastasis is supported by the observation of additional loss of HLA class I expression in lymph node metastases from carcinomas of the breast, colon, bladder and cervix,[25–27] and the reduction of metastatic potential by correction of MHC class I downregulation in animal models.[2] Lymph nodes from seven patients with advanced disease were assessed with all eight antibodies used in the prospective study of frozen prostatic tissue. In six cases there was complete loss of class I expression and one had allele-specific loss. For six of these cases, paired prostate specimens were available, three of which had reduced expression with the monomorphic antibody W6/32 and three complete loss of class I expression. These observations corroborate the report from the Hammersmith Hospital, which reveals increased rates of HLA downregulation in lymph nodes compared with paired radical prostatectomy specimens,[9] thus supporting the hypothesis that loss of HLA expression may be important in tumour progression.

HLA class I expression and lymphocytic infiltration

The relationship of tumour-infiltrating lymphocytes to survival has provoked considerable controversy. The extent of lymphocytic infiltrate does appear to be related to outcome in some tumours[28] and the demonstration of T lymphocytes within tumours is supporting evidence of a regulatory role for the immune system in tumour progression. The nature of lymphocytic infiltrate and its relationship to HLA expression and outcome of prostate cancer has not been widely reported. Qualitative descriptions of lymphocytic infiltrates in prostate cancer generally report a sparse, diffuse pattern with occasional aggregates infiltrating the periphery of the tumour;[7,11] this was also observed in both the frozen and fixed tissue in the authors' present studies. Vesalainen[29] has reported a series of 325 primary prostate cancers, including 141 T1-2M0 tumours, in which lymphocytic infiltrate was semi-quantitatively assessed and found to be independent of tumour differentiation, and with absent or weak infiltrate associated with a higher risk of disease progression.

The authors have scored the degree of lymphocytic infiltration on a four-point scale in haematoxylin- and eosin-stained sections in the 78 archival specimens. Normal HLA expression was found to be associated with a significantly greater degree of lymphocytic infiltration (Table 11.3). Qualitative assessment of the nature of the infiltrating cells using antibodies against leucocyte differentiation antigens is possible only in frozen sections. Using frozen tissue from the original prospective study, both CD4-positive helper T cells and CD8-positive cytotoxic

Table 11.3 Extent of lymphocytic infiltration compared with HLA class I expression in formalin-fixed primary prostate cancer

HLA expression	No or minimal* infiltrate	Mild or moderate* infiltrate
Normal (n = 14)	5 (36%)	9 (64%)
Heterogeneous (n = 14)	7 (50%)	7 (50%)
Absent (n = 50)	35 (70%)	15 (30%)

*Minimal = occasional isolated lymphocyte; mild = occasional small aggregates of lymphocytes; moderate = several aggregates or a heavy diffuse infiltrate.

T cells were identified predominantly at the tumour–stromal interface, but were also present among the malignant cells. There is, however, no evidence in prostate cancer that these T cells are either activated or specific for tumour cells, although both peripheral blood lymphocytes and tumour-infiltrating lymphocytes isolated from a minority of other tumours have been shown to contain tumour-specific cytotoxic lymphocytes.[30]

Mechanisms of HLA class I downregulation

The mechanisms of HLA downregulation are diverse, as shown by investigation of other tumours. Altered HLA class I expression may result from interference at any stage from the initiation of HLA class I gene transcription, through heavy chain assembly with β₂m and peptide in the endoplasmic reticulum, to the stability of cell surface expression.

It seems unlikely that loss of HLA expression by prostate cancer is due to mutations and/or deletions in coding regions of the structural genes for the heavy chain, as this would involve multiple mutations in view of loss of expression of more than one allele product, but this may be the case if loss of expression of several alleles is a staged event occurring successively throughout tumour progression.[31] Loss of heterozygosity has been described on chromosome 6p; however, the relationship to the MHC genes at 6p2 has yet to be defined in detail.[32] Abnormal β₂m expression could be expected to result in global loss of HLA class I expression, as seen in the Daudi cell line.[33] Complete class I loss does not occur in all prostate cancers, however, the association of β₂m with a particular heavy chain occurs with varying affinity, which may explain apparent allele-specific downregulation.[34] The cell line LNCaP was found to be deficient in class I expression, possibly owing to a defect in β₂m transcription.[35,36]

Following translation, heavy chain and β₂m molecules are translocated to the lumen of the endoplasmic reticulum, where they are glycosylated and bind allele-compatible peptides. Sialylation is a common event in prostate cancer and is associated with altered expression of cell surface glycoproteins.[37] However, it does not appear to be the sole cause of impaired HLA class I expression in prostate cancer,[9] as neuraminidase digestion to remove the sialyl residues resulted in 59% of primary carcinomas expressing HLA class I compared with 26% prior to digestion.

Peptides are transported to the lumen of the endoplasmic reticulum via a specific transporter associated with antigen processing (TAP), which is composed of TAP-1 and TAP-2 subunits encoded by genes in the MHC. When peptides bind to specific HLA heavy chains there are conformational changes, which are stabilized by the binding of β₂m molecules. In the absence of the appropriate peptide, heavy chain may associate with β₂m, but the complex is unstable and is unlikely to be expressed at the cell surface. Loss of TAP expression associated with HLA class I downregulation has been found in several tumours.[38,39] One of five prostate cancer cell lines (PPC-1) was found to have loss of HLA class I expression and resistance to cytotoxic T-cell mediated lysis due to underexpression of TAP-2 mRNA, despite abundant class I heavy chain and β₂m mRNA. Induction of TAP-2 by INF-γ led to restoration of functional antigen processing.[35] It seems likely from the preliminary work of Sanda that there are diverse mechanisms of HLA class I downregulation in prostate cancer.

Conclusions

It has been shown that benign prostatic epithelium is HLA class I positive and class II negative, except in areas of lymphocytic infiltration. Downregulation of

HLA class I expression is a common observation in primary prostate cancer and appears to occur more frequently in lymph node metastases. The high levels of HLA class I loss would imply that this phenomenon is likely to have biological significance. Either loss of HLA class I expression is of direct selective advantage to the tumour, or the loss of HLA is an indirect consequence of another factor that confers a selective advantage. The former would appear more plausible, on the basis of animal studies demonstrating abrogation of tumorigenicity by transfection of HLA genes into cell lines deficient in HLA expression.[2]

The finding of apparently normal class I expression by some advanced primary tumours emphasizes the fact that HLA expression must not be viewed in isolation when considering mechanisms of prostate cancer progression. It is possible that the accumulation of oncogene and tumour suppressor gene defects widely documented in prostate cancer may combine to allow tumour escape from any putative immune surveillance even in the presence of HLA class I expression, as loss of accessory molecules such as adhesion factors that are known to occur in prostate cancer may prevent interaction of T lymphocytes with malignant cells. Additionally, production of immunosuppressive growth factors, such as transforming growth factor β, by prostate cancer may contribute to escape from immune regulation.

The high rates of HLA class I downregulation have considerable implications for the development of gene/immunotherapy for prostate cancer. The Dunning rat prostate cancer model has been used to evaluate tumour vaccines involving transfection of cytokine genes into prostate cancer cells. The preliminary results with small tumour burdens were encouraging,[40–42] but successful immunotherapy may need to induce HLA class I expression or use strategies to circumvent HLA-mediated tumour cell recognition.

References

1. Zinkernagel R M, Doherty P C. MHC-restricted cytotoxic T cells: studies on the biological role of polymorphic major transplantation antigens determining T cell restriction — specificity, function and responsiveness. Adv Immunol 1979; 27: 51–177
2. Hämmerling G J, Klar D, Pülm W et al. The influence of major histocompatibility complex class I antigens on tumour growth and metastasis. Biochem Biophys Acta 1987; 907: 245–259
3. Schrier P I, Bernards R, Vaessen R T M J et al. Expression of class I major histocompatibility antigens switched off by highly oncogenic adenovirus 12 in transformed rat cells. Nature 1983: 305; 771–775
4. Hayashi H, Tanaka K, Jay F et al. Modulation of the tumorigenicity of human adenovirus 12 transformed cells by interferon. Cell 1985; 43: 263–267
5. Festenstein H. The biological consequences of altered MHC expression on tumours. Br Med Bull 1987; 43: 217–227
6. Daar A S, Fuggle S V, Fabre J W et al. The detailed distribution of the MHC class II antigens in normal human organs. Transplantation 1984; 38: 293–298
7. Theyer G, Kramer G, Assmann I et al. Phenotypic characterisation of infiltrating leukocytes in benign prostatic hyperplasia. Lab Invest 1992; 66: 96–107
8. Blumenfeld W, Ye J-Q, Dahiya R et al. HLA expression by benign and malignant prostatic epithelium: augmentation by interferon-gamma. J Urol 1993; 150: 1289–1292
9. Sharpe J C, Abel P D, Gilbertson J A et al. Modulated expression of human leucocyte antigen class I and class II determinants in hyperplastic and malignant human prostatic epithelium. Br J Urol 1994; 74: 609–616
10. Garrido F, Cabrera T, Concha A et al. Natural history of HLA expression during tumour development. Immunol Today 1993; 14: 491–499
11. Bigotti G, Coli A, Castagnota D. Distribution of Langerhans cells and HLA class II molecules in prostatic carcinomas of different histopathological grade. Prostate 1991; 19: 73–87

12. Rokhlin O W, Cohen M B. Expression of cellular adhesion molecules on human prostate tumour cell lines. Prostate 1995; 26: 205–212

13. Daar A S, Fuggle S V, Fabre J W et al. The detailed distribution of HLA- A, B, C, antigens in normal human organs. Transplantation 1984; 38: 287–292

14. Blades R A, Keating P J, McWilliam L J et al. Loss of HLA class I expression in prostate cancer: implications for immunotherapy. Urology 1995: 46; 681–687

15. Levin I, Klein T, Kuperman O et al. The expression of HLA class I antigen in prostate cancer in relation to tumour differentiation and patient survival. Cancer Detect Prev 1994; 18: 443–445

16. Nouri A M E, Hussain R F, Oliver R T D. The frequency of major histocompatibility complex antigen abnormalities in urological tumours and their correction by gene transfection or cytokine stimulation. Cancer Gene Ther 1994; 1: 119–123

17. Connor M E, Stern P L. Loss of MHC class-1 expression in cervical carcinomas. Int J Cancer 1990; 46: 1029–1034

18. Momburg F, Degener T, Bacchus E et al. Loss of HLA-A,B,C and de novo expression of HLA-D in colorectal carcinoma. Int J Cancer 1986; 38: 459–464

19. Esteban F, Concha A, Delgado M et al. Lack of MHC class I antigens and tumour aggressiveness of the squamous cell carcinoma of the larynx. Br J Cancer 1990; 62: 1047–1051

20. Tomita Y, Matsumoto Y, Nishiyama T, Fuiwara M. Reduction of major histocompatibility complex class I antigens on invasive and high grade transitional cell carcinoma. J Pathol 1990; 167: 157–164

21. Concha A, Cabrera T, Ruiz-Cabello F, Garrido F. Can the HLA phenotype be used as a prognostic factor in breast carcinoma? Int J Cancer 1991; suppl 6: 146–154

22. Wintzer H-O, Benzing M. von Kleist S. Lacking prognostic significance of ß$_2$microglobulin, MHC class I and class II antigen expression in breast carcinomas. Br J Cancer 1990; 62: 289–295

23. Connor M, Davidson S E, Stern P L et al. Evaluation of multiple biological parameters in cervical carcinoma: high macrophage infiltration in HPV associated tumours. Int J Gynecol Cancer 1993; 32: 103–109

24. George N J R. Natural history of localised prostatic cancer managed by conservative therapy alone. Lancet 1988; 3: 494–497

25. Cordon-Cardo C, Fuks Z, Drobnjak M et al. Expression of HLA-A, B, C antigens on primary and metastatic tumour cell populations of human carcinoma. Cancer Res 1991; 51: 6372–6380

26. Garrido F, Ruiz-Cabello F. MHC expression on human tumours — its relevance for local tumour growth and metastasis. Sem Cancer Biol 1991; 2: 3–10

27. Cromme F V, van Bomme P F J, Walboomers J M M et al. Differences in MHC and TAP-1 expression in cervical lymph node metastases as compared with the primary tumours. Br J Cancer 1994; 69: 1176–1181

28. Oliver R T D, Nouri A M E. T cell immune response to cancer in humans and its relevance for immunodiagnosis and therapy. Cancer Surv 1991; 13: 173–204

29. Vesalainen S, Lipponen P, Talja M, Syrjänen K. Histological grade, perineural infiltration, tumour-infiltrating lymphocytes and apoptosis as determinants of long-term prognosis in prostatic adenocarcinoma. Eur J Cancer 1994; 30A: 1797–1803

30. Knuth A, Wolfel T, Meyer zum Buschenfelde K-H. T cell responses to human malignant tumours. Cancer Surv 1992; 13: 39–52

31. Lehmann F, Marchand M, Hainaut P et al. Differences in the antigens recognized by cytolytic T cells on two successive metastases of a melanoma patient are consistent with immune selection. Eur J Immunol 1995; 25: 340–347

32. Gao X, Wu N, Grignon D et al. High frequency of mutator phenotype in human prostatic adenocarcinoma. Oncogene 1994; 9: 2999–3003

33. Rosa F, Felows M, Dron M et al. Presence of an abnormal β$_2$microglobulin mRNA in Daudi cells: induction by interferon. Immunogenetics 1983; 31: 245–252

34. Neefjes J J, Momburg F. Cell biology of antigen presentation. Curr Opin Immunol 1993; 5: 27–34

35. Sanda M G, Restifo N P, Walsh J C et al. Molecular characterisation of defective antigen processing in human prostate cancer. J Natl Cancer Inst 1995; 87: 280–285

36. Fenton R G, Longo D L. Genetic instability and tumour cell variation: implications for immunotherapy. J Natl Cancer Inst 1995; 87: 241–243

37. Foster C S, Abel P D. Clinical and molecular techniques for diagnosis and monitoring of prostatic cancer. Hum Pathol 1992; 23: 395–401

38. Restifo N P, Esquivel F, Kawakami Y *et al*. Identification of human cancers deficient in antigen processing. J Exp Med 1993; 177: 265–272

39. Cromme F V, Airey J, Heemels M-T *et al*. Loss of transporter protein, encoded by the TAP-1 gene is highly correlated with loss of HLA expression in cervical carcinomas. J Exp Med 1994; 179: 335–340

40. Moody D B, Robinson J C, Ewing C M *et al*. Interleukin-2 transfected prostate cancer cells generate a local antitumour effect in vivo. Prostate 1994; 24: 244–251

41. Vieweg J, Rosenthal F M, Bannerji R *et al*. Immunotherapy of prostate cancer in the Dunning rat model: use of cytokine gene modified tumour vaccines. Cancer Res 1994; 54: 1760–1765

42. Sanda M G, Ayyagari S R, Jaffee E M *et al*. Demonstration of a rational strategy for human prostate cancer gene therapy. J Urol 1994; 151: 622–628

43. Schroder F H, Hermanek P, Denis L, Fair W R, Gospodarowicz M K, Pavone-Macaluso M. The TNM classification of prostate cancer. Prostate Suppl 1992; 4: 129–138

Chapter 12
Increased risk of prostate cancer in men of Afro-Caribbean extraction*

J. W. Moul

Introduction

The age-adjusted incidence of prostate cancer in men of Afro-Caribbean extraction, [hereafter referred to as African-American (Black) males] is 50% higher than in Caucasian (White) men, and Black men have the highest incidence of prostate cancer in the world.[1] Differences in the probability of being diagnosed (9.6 vs 5.2%), lifetime-specific mortality (3 vs 1.4%), and 5-year survival rates (65 vs 78%) between Blacks and Whites are all indicative of a major public health problem in this population.[2] The aetiology for these racial differences in the clinical behaviour of prostate cancer is unknown; hormonal, nutritional, genetic, behavioural and socioeconomic status (SES) factors have all been implicated.[2] Now, in the late 1990s, as more research funding is finally being devoted to prostate cancer, it is critically important to find the cause, or causes, of this racial disparity. The author's research group, the Department of Defense (DoD) Center for Prostate Disease Research (CPDR), is funded to study prostate cancer and disease in the DoD health care system. Because the system is equal access and geographically diverse, and cares for a large number of African-American (AA) men, it is a good setting to study this issue. This chapter reviews the author's ongoing investigations in this area and compares and contrasts it with other recent work in the field.

PSA in Black men

In 1992, Vijayakumar and associates were the first to report that Black American men with newly diagnosed prostate cancer referred for radiotherapy had higher prostate-specific antigen (PSA) levels than their white counterparts.[3] A number of other preliminary reports also suggested that Blacks had higher PSA.[4,5] These early reports lacked proper multivariate adjustment for stage, grade, age and SES. In 1995, the author and colleagues reported on 541 consecutive men with newly diagnosed prostate cancer and showed that, even with adjustment for tumour grade, age and clinical stage, Black men had higher levels of PSA.[6] In this same study, a subsequent consecutive cohort was taken of 91 men (29 Black, 63 White) who underwent a radical prostatectomy and whole-mount processing of the prostate by careful tumour volume assessment.[6] The startling finding was that, even in the military equal-access health care system, the Black men had much higher tumour volumes overall and within each clinical stage (Table 12.1). This

*The opinions and assertions contained herein are the private views of the author and are not to be construed as reflecting the views of the US Army or Department of Defense.

Table 12.1. Tumour volume (TVol) and prostate weight (PWt) for Black and White patients
undergoing radical prostatectomy for prostate cancer, by clinical stage of disease

Clinical stage	Black			White		
	n	TVol*	PWt[†]	n	TVol*	PWt[†]
Total	28	5.42	42.4	63	2.10	39.6
T1a, T1c	11	4.11	40.7	32	1.60	41.0
T2a	3	1.86	40.3	10	1.12	34.7
T2b	10	9.86	42.6	18	4.31	39.9
T2c, T3	4	5.80	47.9	3	4.28	42.0

*Tumour volume (cm^3) geometric mean.
[†]Prostate weight (g) geometric mean.
(From ref. 6 with permission.)

within-stage tumour volume disparity was primarily responsible for the racial
difference in PSA, and PSA was a surrogate for bigger tumours in Black men.

Since this report was published, most,[7–9] but not all,[10] investigators have
confirmed that Black American males in general have higher PSA values than do
White males. Recent work from Vijayakumar and colleagues[7] suggests that the
racial disparity in PSA is primarily due to socioeconomics: they found no racial
differences in PSA in multivariate analysis of Black and of White patients who had
similar insurance; however, for Medicare-only patients, Blacks had significantly
higher PSA. They concluded that Blacks had higher PSA owing to lack of access
and/or lack of health-seeking behaviour. This is not inconsistent with the author's
results; even though the study noted above[6] was performed in the equal-access
military, Blacks may not have availed themselves of early detection opportunities,
and delay in diagnosis may have been responsible for the disparity. Alternatively,
since the Blacks in the author's study were, on average, 3 years younger than the
Whites, potential biological differences that caused the tumours to grow larger
more quickly have not been ruled out.

Use of PSA in Black men: age-adjusted reference ranges for maximal cancer detection

Despite the racial disparity in outcome noted in the Introduction, encouraging
recent data from the Radiation Therapy Oncology Group (RTOG),[11] US Military[12]
and Veterans Administration[12] suggest that, if Black men are afforded the same
access and care, the outcome disparity may be minimized or eliminated. This
information may enable this disease in this population to be combated by
increased public awareness, early detection programmes and proper detection
tools.

The American Urological Association (AUA), American Cancer Society (ACS)
and American College of Radiology have recommended early detection
programmes using digital rectal examination (DRE) and PSA starting at the age of
40 for AA men for a number of years.[14,15] Despite this recommendation, until now
no data existed to document the value of PSA testing for the early and accurate
diagnosis of prostate cancer in this population.

There was an urgent need to examine the proper PSA 'normals' for Black men
and over the last year, a number of groups have examined the clinical utility of
PSA in this population. Smith and associates studied 861 Black men with regard to
the use of PSA and DRE in screening for prostate cancer.[16] A PSA level greater than

4 ng/ml had a sensitivity of 80%, specificity of 39% and positive predictive value of 46% for cancer detection in Black men; this compares with 76, 54 and 34%, respectively, for White men. The DRE had corresponding values of 44, 56 and 40%, respectively, for AA patients. In the opinion of Smith and colleagues, these percentages were suboptimal in this high-risk group and a lower cutoff of PSA was recommended, rather than the traditional 4.0 ng/ml.[16]

A recent study by the author and associates documents the outstanding ability of PSA to detect prostate cancer in both Caucasian and AA men, and develops age-adjusted PSA reference ranges for maximal cancer detection in this high-risk group of men.[17] In this study, between January 1991 and May 1995, serum PSA concentration was determined for 3475 men (1802 Caucasian, 1673 AA) without clinical evidence of prostate cancer (PC) and 1783 men (1,372 Caucasian, 411 AA) with PC. All PSA examinations were performed using Abbott IMx assay (normal 0–4 ng/ml) in a central, single laboratory. PSA concentration was analysed as a function of age and race to determine operating characteristics of PSA for the diagnosis of PC. Serum PSA concentration correlated directly with age for both AA men and Caucasian men ($r = 0.40$, $p = 0.001$ for AA and $r = 0.34$, $p = 0.0001$ for Caucasian). AA men had significantly higher serum PSA concentrations than Caucasian men ($p = 0.0001$) (Figure 12.1). When sensitivity was plotted against 1-specificity, the area under the receiver operator characteristic (ROC) curve was 0.91 for AA men and 0.94 for Caucasian men, indicating that the PSA test is an excellent early detection tool. For comparison, the Papanicolaou smear for cervical cancer, which is an accepted clinical screening test, has a ROC value of only 0.70. When the author and colleagues calculated age-specific reference ranges by methodology identical to that used by Oesterling and colleagues in their 1993 study in Olmstead County, Minnesota,[18] very similar values were found for White

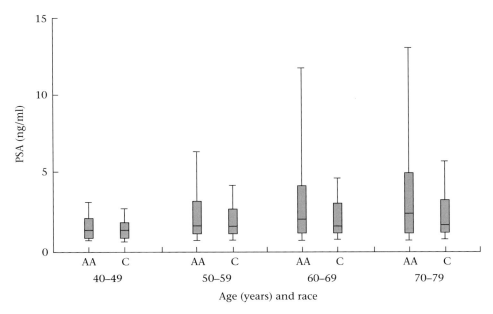

Figure 12.1. Distribution of PSA values for African-American (AA) and Caucasian (C) race by age in decades for 3475 men without clinical evidence of prostate cancer (1802 C and 1673 AA). The vertical line represents the 5th to 95th percentiles with the heavy horizontal bar being the 95th percentile. The boxes represent the 25th to 75th percentile and the mean is a line within the box. Note that AA men have more variability in PSA, which markedly increases the 95th percentiles compared with the C men. (Reproduced from ref. 17 with permission.)

men but higher values for Black men. These ranges were 0–2.4 ng/ml for Black men aged 40–49, 0–6.5 ng/ml for those aged 50–59, 0–11.3 ng/ml for those aged 60–69, and 0–12.5 ng/ml for those aged 70–79. These new ranges were then tested in the group of Black men with prostate cancer to determine how effective the use of these ranges would have been if they had been used to detect the subjects' cancers: unfortunately, these markedly higher ranges would have missed 41% of the cancers (only 59% sensitivity).

The reason why these traditionally derived ranges performed so poorly is because they are simply the 95th percentile of values in the Black controls. Because there is more variability of PSA results in Blacks without evidence of cancer, there is more skewness, which pushes the 95th percentile further to the right (higher); this higher range, however, is not clinically useful. Age-adjusted reference ranges were therefore developed for Black men with prostate cancer, selecting PSA upper limits of normal by decade to maximize cancer detection. In other words, reference ranges by decade in the men with prostate cancer were developed by using the 5th percentile of PSA values. Only the lowest 5% of pre-diagnosis PSA values in the Black men with cancer are 'normal' and the remainder (95%) are above the normal (95% sensitivity).

These ranges have been termed the Walter Reed/Center for Prostate Disease Research (WRAMC/CPDR) age-specific reference ranges for maximal cancer detection (Table 12.2). They maximize sensitivity (cancer detection) without undue loss of specificity [false positives/unnecessary transrectal ultrasonography (TRUS)/biopsy]. These values for maximal cancer detection for Black and White men are compared with the traditional normal (0–4 ng/ml) and the previously developed age-specific reference ranges in Table 12.3.

Table 12.2. Walter Reed/Center for Prostate Disease Research (WR/CPDR) age-adjusted reference ranges of PSA for maximal cancer detection in African-American patients

Age (years)	PSA (ng/ml)	Specificity (%)
40–49	0–2.0	93
50–59	0–4.0	88
60–69	0–4.5	81
70–79	0–5.5	78

(From ref. 17 with permission.)

Table 12.3. Comparison of Walter Reed/Center for Prostate Disease Research (WR/CPDR) PSA reference ranges for maximal prostate cancer detection versus traditional age-adjusted and original normal PSA values

Age (years)	WR/CPDR age-adjusted PSA reference ranges* (ng/ml)		Traditional PSA 'normal' for all men (ng/ml)	Traditional age-adjusted reference ranges[†] (ng/ml)
	African-American	Caucasian		
40–49	0–2.0	0–2.5	0–4.0	0–2.5
50–59	0–4.0	0–3.5	0–4.0	0–3.5
60–69	0–4.5	0–3.5	0–4.0	0–4.5
70–79	0–5.5	0–3.5	0–4.0	0–6.5

*From ref. 17 with permission.
[†]Based on Caucasian men at the Mayo Clinic. (From ref. 18 with permission.)

Clinically localized prostate cancer in AA men

There is an ongoing debate as to whether AA race itself is a prognostic factor for worse outcome in localized (and advanced) prostate cancer. As noted above, data from the RTOG,[11] US military[12] and Veterans Administration,[13] suggest that race alone is not a prognostic factor. In particular, the study by Optenberg and associates deserves further comment.[12] They studied 1606 patients (7.5% Black) who were treated in the US Military health care system between 1973 and 1994. They found that Blacks entered active treatment and exhibited a higher relative risk of cancer in younger age groups, presented with higher stage, and demonstrated increased progression to distant metastatic disease. In multivariate analysis with stage, grade and age, race was not an independent prognostic factor. In fact, for men with metastatic disease there was a clear trend for Blacks to have greater survival. Despite the fact that race itself did not remain as a prognostic factor, what was responsible for Blacks presenting at a younger age with more advanced disease? Along similar lines, a recent Surveillance Epidemiology and End Results (SEER) database study in metropolitan Detroit found that Blacks had a poorer survival than Whites at all stages of disease, which was especially evident in younger men (under 65).[19] Powell *et al.* also found that survival was worse for AA men under the age of 65 but better for men over this age; they used the phrase, 'ethnic survival crossover'.[20] More study is necessary to determine whether younger Black men do have a worse survival and, if so, the cause of this disparity.

The author's group has been studying men who have undergone radical prostatectomy, and comparing outcome and tumour characteristics by race to gain insight. In a consecutive group of 102 radical prostatectomy patients, 32 (31.4%) of whom were Black, Blacks had higher tumour volumes in all clinical stage categories.[21] Overall, the Black men had a mean tumour volume of 4.98 cm^3 versus 3.37 cm^3 in the White patients. This greater tumour volume is associated with more adverse pathological features: capsular involvement (68.8% for Blacks vs 57.1% for Whites), margin positivity (58.1% vs 45.7%) and mean highest Gleason sum (6.38 vs 6.10) were all higher among Black patients.[21] Similarly, Pettaway *et al.* from the M.D. Anderson Cancer Center, found that 61% of AA patients undergoing radical prostatectomy had adverse pathological features.[22] What is now necessary is the collection of more cases with careful pathological assessment and stratification by screening status and age to determine whether young Black men truly have more adverse disease characteristics when afforded similar early detection opportunities.

In a follow-up study, the author and colleagues studied 518 men who had undergone radical prostatectomy at Walter Reed Army Medical Center between 1975 and 1995, comparing Black and White race.[23] Table 12.4 illustrates the pathological variables of the radical prostatectomy specimens between these two groups of men. There were non-significant trends for Blacks to have greater pathological stage and Gleason grade. Most strikingly, the margin positive rate was 50.5% in Blacks compared with 38.4% in Whites ($p = 0.038$). This is very similar to the rate of margin positivity reported by Powell *et al.*[20] and Pettaway *et al.*[22]

The survival analysis for Black and White men was very interesting and points to the need for careful multivariate analysis when trying to determine whether race itself is a prognostic factor. Overall, the AA men had a lower recurrence-free survival. In other words, at a mean follow-up of 23.3 months, Black men were more likely to have had a recurrence, generally defined as a rising PSA, as their first evidence of failure. Even in one multivariate analysis with adjustment for pathological stage, grade, and pretreatment PSA and acid phosphatase, Black race

Table 12.4. Pathological variables of radical prostatectomy specimens in Black and White patients

Variable	Patients		p value
	White n (%) [N]*	Black n (%) [N]*	
Pathological stage			
T1 + T2A	53 (15.3)	9 (8.6)	
T2B + 2C	108 (31.2) [346]	32 (30.5) [105]	NS
T3A + 3B	143 (41.3)	46 (43.8)	
≥ T3C	42 (12.1)	18 (17.1)	
Maximum Gleason sum			
3–4	42 (16.2)	11 (13.1)	
5–6	134 (51.5) [260]	35 (41.7) [84]	NS
7	60 (23.1)	24 (28.6)	
≥ 8	24 (9.2)	14 (16.7)	
Positive margin	133 (38.4) [346]	51 (50.5) [101]	0.038
Seminal vesicles			
Negative	308 (88.3)	90 (85.7)	
Positive unilateral	27 (7.7) [349]	8 (7.6) [105]	NS
Positive bilateral	14 (4.0)	7 (6.7)	
Pelvic lymph nodes			
Negative	336 (97.4) [345]	103 (100) [103]	NS
Positive	9 (2.6)	0 (0)	
Tumour volume (mean cm^3)	4.68 [76]	8.10 [34]	0.040

*[N], Number of White and Black patients available for variable analysis.
NS, Not statistically significant (i.e. $p \geq 0.050$).
(From ref. 23 with permission.)

remained as an independent prognostic factor. However, in another multivariate analysis, when margin positivity was included in the model, race ($p = 0.083$) was no longer an independent prognostic factor.

Because clinical stage and pathological stage categories may not accurately reflect tumour volume and subtle pathological features, such as margin positivity and volume of high-grade cancer, it will be imperative to include these factors in multivariate analysis when deciding whether race itself affects outcome. The author and colleagues are currently conducting a prospective radical prostatectomy (RP) study in which the Armed Forces Institute of Pathology and CPDR are collaborating to compare three-dimensional tumour volumes and careful quantitative histology to outcome of Black and White men. Even if race itself is not found to be an independent prognostic marker when including these comprehensive pathological assessments, what is responsible for the worse pathological findings? Considering that the Black men in the studies by the author and others are 1–3 years younger than the White men, yet have bigger and more adverse pathological tumours, is biology or behaviour and access to blame?

In the author's opinion behaviour and access are largely at fault. AA men have simply not been educated about prostate cancer and the need for early detection. If early detection programmes were more universally available and accepted, starting at the age of 40 years, the majority of prostate tumours would be detected when they were smaller and with fewer adverse pathological features, and this would eliminate the current racial survival disparity. This appears to be borne out by the Detroit Education and Early Detection (DEED) study results.[24] Compared with a non-screening population, the screened AA men undergoing RP had a significantly higher rate of organ-confined disease and lower recurrence rate at early follow-up. By instituting education about prostate cancer and screening PSA in this high-risk population, the DEED project increased the organ-confined rate in these men to 65% — a gratifying result. Furthermore, at a mean follow-up of 18–20 months, of the 15 DEED men screened who underwent RP, only one (7%) has has a recurrence compared with 25% of their non-screened clinic patients. It was also encouraging to see that the DEED screened men had lower mean and median initial PSA values. Considering that pretreatment PSA correlated directly with tumour volume in both Black and White RP patients,[6] the DEED data suggest that screened AA men are being diagnosed when their tumours are smaller. It is tantalizing to speculate that, if the lower WRAMC/CPDR PSA reference range of 2.0 ng/ml in men between the ages of 40 and 49 is used, as discussed earlier,[17] and screening in these younger AA men is encouraged, an even greater impact may be achieved.

Advanced prostate cancer in AA men

Conflicting data have been reported for outcome of Black and White men with metastatic prostate cancer. Whereas SEER data report a worse survival outcome for Black men, stage for stage,[1,25] recent studies have suggested a better survival for Black men with metastatic disease,[12,20,24] or survival equal to that of Caucasian men.[13] Fowler *et al.* have recently studied the PSA response to hormonal therapy in Black and White men, and found no difference.[49] Furthermore, the response to delayed anti-androgen treatment and anti-androgen withdrawal was similar in Black and White patients. Those authors concluded that androgen dependence and androgen independence are similar for Black and White men with prostate cancer. Although this may be true, basing these conclusions simply on PSA response may be naive, and further research is needed.

Are there biological differences in prostate cancer between Black and White patients?

On the basis of the preceding discussion of PSA, PSA-based screening and localized and advanced disease, the question of possible biological differences remains to be answered. Although the author's opinion is that most, if not all, of the racial disparity may be explained by lack of awareness, lack of access and delay in diagnosis, some data suggest true biological differences.

Some of the most compelling evidence for biological difference is the work of Sakr and colleagues from Wayne State University.[26,27] In landmark autopsy studies of young Black or White men who died of other causes, they found that Blacks harboured more high-grade prostatic intraepithelial neoplasia (PIN) than age-matched Whites. Because high-grade PIN is considered to be the precursor of prostate carcinoma, some factor (or factors), presumably biological, is contributing to this PIN disparity. Could this biological factor be genetic, hormonal, a combination of these, or related to environmental factors such as diet?

Hormonal differences between Black and White men have been proposed as constituting a possible biological factor that could explain the racial difference in prostate cancer. Ross and colleagues have found that young Black males have higher testosterone and higher 5α-reductase activity than age-matched Caucasian and Japanese men.[28–30] Furthermore, recent study of the androgen receptor has shown intriguing racial differences.[31–32] AA men, in general, have shorter CAG (glutamine) repeat lengths in their androgen receptor gene sequence; this shorter length reportedly renders the androgen receptor more active. Much more work is necessary to study the androgen signalling pathway to determine whether these differences affect the behaviour of prostate cancer in various racial groups.

Diet has long been postulated to contribute to the behaviour of prostate cancer and to play a role in observed racial differences. Early studies suggested that, as Blacks migrated from Africa and began consuming a Western diet high in fat and meat, this was responsible for the increasing prevalence of prostate cancer.[33] This was based on the assumption that the rate of prostate cancer in Africa was very low. New data from some of the more developed African countries suggest that the rate of prostate cancer in native African Blacks is actually quite high, despite a non-Western diet.[34] Furthermore, recent data from Whittemore *et al.* suggest that a high-fat diet may explain only a minority of the racial difference in prostate cancer.[35] Conversely, Powell and associates feel that a high-fat diet plays a major role in explaining the racial difference in prostate cancer.[36] They feel that a high fat-diet consumed by AAs leads to more bioactive lipids in their biological system that contribute to prostate cancer progression.[37,38] They have studied 12-lipoxygenase (12-LOX), a fatty acid metabolite, in 122 samples of prostate cancer tissue and matched control tissue from patients undergoing RP.[38] Although the results were not statistically significant, the authors did find higher levels of 12-LOX in most subcategories of AAs (T2, poorly differentiated, age 51–60) and used these data to support a dietary link with prostate cancer behaviour by race. Much further work needs to be performed.

It is intriguing to speculate that there may be racial differences in various genes that may contribute to the observed clinical disparity in prostate cancer. Apart from the recent studies of CAG repeats in the androgen receptor, noted above,[31,32] very little focused molecular epidemiology work has been performed. The author's group has not found significant racial differences in the incidence of *ras*,[39] c-*erb*-B2,[40] cathepsin-D,[41] epidermal growth factor receptor (EGFR),[41] p53,[42] bcl-2,[43] p16,[44] and Ki-67 proliferation.[45] Conversely, deVere White and associates recently reported that AAs had a higher rate of p53 protein expression and the racial difference was most striking for diploid tumours.[46] In a separate line of reasoning, Hayes *et al.* studied the family history of prostate cancer in Black and in White patients:[47] they found equal familial prostate cancer by race, and concluded that the ethnic disparity in incidence is influenced by environmental and not genetic factors. Furthermore, the recent discovery of the HPC-1 (hereditary prostate cancer 1) locus on chromosome 1 in both Black and White familial prostate cancer suggests that genetic factors may not be responsible for the racial differences observed.[48]

Conclusions

The incidence of prostate cancer in AA men is higher than that of other racial groups and most studies demonstrate a higher recurrence rate and poorer survival for these men. In studies of localized prostate cancer, Black men generally have higher PSA due to larger tumours. Whether the observed differences are due to environmental or biological factors (or a combination) is open to debate. Known environmental factors that have contributed include lack of access or knowledge and/or unwillingness to seek care, which causes delay in diagnosis and more advanced disease at presentation. Despite this, or in addition, the observation that a subset of Blacks tend to be diagnosed at a younger age, and the findings of autopsy studies that young Blacks harbour more high-grade prostatic intraepithelial neoplasia, suggest that other factors are at play. Whether other environmental promoters, such as a high-fat diet, or genetic differences are responsible, must await further study. Apart from reported genetic differences in the androgen receptor gene, other studies with sporadic and familial prostate cancer have not found significantly different genetic alterations by race. Despite this continuing debate regarding causation, new efforts to educate and screen AA men have a good likelihood of helping to diagnose prostate cancer earlier, so that it can be treated more effectively and the currently observed disparity can be lessened.

References

1. Boring C C, Squires T S, Health C W. Cancer statistics for African Americans. CA 1993; 43: 7–17
2. Morton R A. Racial differences in adenocarcinoma of the prostate in North American men. Urology 1994; 44: 637–645
3. VijayaKumar S, Karrison T, Weichselbaum R R et al. Racial differences in prostate-specific antigen levels in patients with local–regional prostate cancer. Cancer Epidemiol Biomark Prev 1992; 1: 541–545
4. Staggers F M, DeAntoni E P, Crawford E D et al. A profile of African-American participants in Prostate Cancer Awareness Week (PCAW) 1992. J Urol 1994; 151: 291(abstr 255)
5. Bullock A, Smith DS, Basler J et al. Racial differences in prostate cancer detection and staging. J Urol 1994; 151: 291(abstr 257)
6. Moul J W, Sesterhenn I A, Connelly R R et al. Prostate-specific antigen values at the time of prostate cancer diagnosis are higher in African-American men. JAMA 1995; 274: 1277–1281
7. VijayaKumar S, Weichselbaum R, Vaida F et al. Prostate specific antigen levels in African-Americans correlate with insurance status as an indicator of socioeconomic status. Cancer J Sci Am 1996; 2: 225–233
8. Diantoni E P, Crawford E D, Ross C A et al. Age and race specific reference ranges for prostate-specific antigen from a large, community-based study. J Urol 1996; 155: 374(abstr 253)
9. Henderson R J, Eastham J A, Culkin D J et al. Prostate specific antigen (PSA) and PSA density (PSAD) are higher in African Americans without prostate cancer: results of 526 patients. J Urol 1996; 155: 376(abstr 262)
10. McCammon K A, Schellhammer P F, Wright G L, Lunch D F. Age specific PSA levels in African Americans. J Urol 1996; 155: 426(abstr 461)
11. Roach M, Won M, Keller J et al. The prognostic significance of race and survival from prostate cancer based on patients irradiated on Radiation Therapy Oncology Group Protocols (1976–1985) Int J Radiat Oncol Biol Phys 1992; 24: 441–449
12. Optenberg S A, Thompson I M, Friedrichs P et al. Race, treatment, and long-term survival from prostate cancer in an equal-access medical care delivery system. JAMA 1995; 274: 1599
13. Fowler J E, Terrell F. Survival in blacks and whites after treatment for localized prostate cancer. J Urol 1996; 156: 133–136
14. Mettlin C, Jones G, Averett H et al. Defining and updating the American Cancer Society guidelines for the cancer-related checkup: prostate and endometrial cancers. CA 1993; 43: 42–46
15. Early detection of prostate cancer and use of transrectal ultrasound. In: AUA (ed) American Urological Association 1992 Policy Statement Book. AUA: 1992: 4.20
16. Smith D S, Catalona W J, Bullock A D. Operating characteristics of prostate cancer screening tests in African American and white men. J Urol 1996; 155: 376(abstr 264)
17. Morgan T O, Jacobson S J, McCarthy W F et al. Age-specific reference ranges for prostate-specific antigen in black men. N Engl J Med 1996; 335: 304–310
18. Oesterling J E, Jacobson S T, Chute CG et al. Serum prostate-specific antigen in a community-based population of healthy men. JAMA 1993; 270: 860
19. Pienta K T, Demers R, Hoff M et al. Effect of age and race on the survival of men with prostate cancer in the metropolitan Detroit tri-county area, 1937 to 1987. Urology 1995; 45: 93–102

20. Powell I H, Heilbrun L K, Sakr W *et al*. The predictive value of race as a clinical prognostic factor among patients with clinically localized prostate cancer: a multivariate analysis of positive surgical margins. Urology 1997; 49: 726–731

21. Moul J W, Mooneyhan R, Lin T H *et al*. Three dimensional (3D) computerized tumor volume determination in radical prostatectomy specimens from black and white patients. J Urol 1996; 155: 509(abstr 794)

22. Pettaway C A, Troncoso P, Steelhammer L *et al*. Prostate specific antigen and tumor volume in African American and caucasian men. A comparative study based on radical prostatectomy specimens. J Urol 1996; 155: 421(abstr 443)

23. Moul J W, Douglas T H, McCarthy W F, McLeod D G. Black race is an adverse prognostic factor for prostate cancer recurrence following radical prostatectomy in an equal-access health care system. J Urol 1996; 155: 1667–1673

24. Powell I J, Heilbrun L, Littrup P *et al*. Outcome of African American men screened for prostate cancer, the DEED (Detroit Education and Early Detection) study. J Urol 1997; 158: 146–149

25. Parker S L, Tong T, Bolden S, Wingo P A. Cancer statistics. CA 1996; 65: 5–27

26. Sakr W A, Haas G P, Cassin J E *et al*. The frequency of carcinoma and intraepithelial neoplasia of the prostate in young male patients. J Urol 1993; 150: 379–385

27. Sakr W A, Grignon D J, Haas G P *et al*. Epidemiology of high grade intraepithelial neoplasia. Pathol Res Pract 1995; 191: 838–841

28. Ross R, Bernstein L, Judd H *et al*. Serum testosterone levels in healthy young black and white men. J Natl Cancer Inst 1986; 76: 45

29. Ellis L, Nyborg H. Racial/ethnic variations in male testosterone levels: a probable contributor to group differences in health. Steroids 1992; 57: 72

30. Ross R K, Bernstein L, Lobo R A *et al*. 5-Alpha-reductase activity and risk of prostate cancer among Japanese and US white and black males. Lancet 1992; 339: 887

31. Coetzee G A, Ross R K. Re: prostate cancer and the androgen receptor. Letter to the Editor. J Natl Cancer Inst 1994; 86: 872

32. Hakimi J M, Schoenberg M P, Rondinelli R H *et al*. Androgen receptor CAG (glutamine) and GGC (glycine) repeat lengths as potential risk factors for prostate cancer. Am Assoc Cancer Res 1996; 37: 258

33. Jackson M A, Ahluwalia B S, Herson J *et al*. Characterization of prostate carcinoma amongst blacks: a continuation report. Cancer Treat Rep 1977; 61: 167–172

34. Osegbe D N. Prostate cancer in Nigerians: facts and non-facts. J Urol 1997; 157: 1340–1343

35. Whittemore A S, Kolonel L N, Wu A H *et al*. Prostate cancer in relation to diet, physical activity, and body size in blacks, whites, and Asians in the United States and Canada. J Natl Cancer Inst 1995; 87: 652

36. Powell I J. Prostate cancer and African American Men. Oncology 1997; 11: 599–605

37. Wang Y, Corr J G, Thaler H T *et al*. Decreased growth of established human prostate LNCaP tumors in nude mice fed a low fat diet. J Natl Cancer Inst 1995; 87: 1456–1462

38. Gao X, Oringnon D J, Chbihi T *et al*. Elevated 12-lipoxygenase mRNA expression correlates with advanced stage and poor differentiation of human prostate cancer. Urology 1995; 46: 227–237

39. Moul J W, Friedrichs P A, Lance R S *et al*. Infrequent ras oncogene mutations in human prostate cancer. Prostate 1992; 20: 327–338

40. Kuhn E J, Kurnot R A, Sesterhenn I A *et al*. Expression of the c-*erb*-2 oncoprotein in prostate cancer. J Urol 1993; 150: 1427–1433

41. Moul J W, MayGarden S J, Ware J L *et al*. Cathepsin-D and epidermal growth factor receptor (EGFR), immunohistochemistry does not predict recurrence of prostate cancer patients undergoing radical prostatectomy. J Urol 1996; 155: 982–985

42. Bauer J J, Sesterhenn I A, Mostofi F K *et al*. p53 nuclear protein expression is an independent prognostic marker in clinically localized prostate cancer patients undergoing radical prostatectomy. Clin Cancer Res 1995; 1: 1295–1300

43. Bauer J J, Sesterhenn I A, Mostofi F K *et al*. Elevated levels of apoptosis regulator proteins p53 and bcl-2 are independent prognostic biomarkers in surgically treated clinically localized prostate cancer patients. J Urol 1996; 156: 1511–1516

44. Gaddipatti J P, McLeod D G, Sesterhenn I A *et al*. :Mutations of the p16 gene product are rare in prostate cancer. Prostate 1997; 30: 188–194

45. Bettencourt M, Bauer J J, Sesterhenn I A *et al*. Ki-67 expression is a prognostic marker of prostate cancer recurrence after radical prostatectomy. J Urol 1996; 156: 1064–1068

46. deVere White R W, Lunetta J M, Deitch A D *et al.* Racial differences in prostate cancer. J Urol 1996; 155: 529(abstr 875)
47. Hayes R B, Lift J M, Pottern L M *et al.* Prostate cancer risk in US blacks and whites with a family history of prostate cancer. Int J Cancer 1995; 60: 361–364
48. Smith J R, Carpten J, Kallioniemi O *et al.* Major susceptibility locus for prostate cancer on chromosome 1 revealed by a genome-wide search. Science 1996; 274: 1371–1374
49. Fowler J E, Bigler S A, Renfroe D L, Dabagia M D. Prostate specific antigen in black and white men after hormonal therapies for prostate cancer. J Urol 1997; 158: 150–154

Chapter 13
PSA: the most effective serum tumour marker in oncology

M. H. Gold and M. K. Brawer

Introduction

There is no single biological marker that has revolutionized the treatment of malignancy to such an extent as has prostate-specific antigen (PSA). PSA, a 33 kD glycoprotein serine protease, is well known as a clinical marker for prostate adenocarcinoma, which is the most common carcinoma in men, and the second most common cause of cancer-related death.[1] Historically, the majority of cases were diagnosed at a time when the tumour had spread beyond the confines of the prostate gland, making it incurable. The clinical significance of this cancer has given great impetus to the improvement of methods of early detection.

Following the development of serum assays for PSA, there has been increasing enthusiasm for applying this tumour marker to early detection and screening. Of the existing modalities available for early detection of prostate cancer, serum PSA measurement offers several advantages: it is economical, easily performed and readily accepted by the patient, and the results are objective. However, despite widespread clinical use of PSA for early detection of prostate cancer, objective data supporting its use have only recently become available.

Prospective studies have now been published using PSA as the initial test in screening protocols for prostate cancer. Catalona and associates,[2] as well as Brawer and associates,[3] have used a serum PSA level greater than 4.0 ng/ml by the Hybritech Tandem assay and/or an abnormal digital rectal examination (DRE) as the criterion for further cancer work-up.

Despite impressive results of these initial screening studies (detection rates of 2–4%; positive predictive values of approximately one in three), there are significant problems with the use of serum PSA alone as a screening tool. It has been shown that approximately 20% of clinically significant cancers are associated with PSA values within the normal range.[4,5] Furthermore, studies show that many patients with benign prostatic conditions have elevations in serum PSA as well.[6,7] These findings limit the efficacy of PSA alone as a screening tool.

To improve the performance of PSA-based prostate cancer diagnosis, various strategies have been proposed. Many authors have suggested that the quotient of serum PSA/prostate gland volume (PSA index or density) has value as an indicator of malignancy. Data also support serial measurements of serum PSA as a diagnostic test. The rate of increase in PSA (PSA velocity) may be a sensitive indicator of malignancy when followed over a period of years. The most recent development of comparing free versus total PSA in the serum has added additional value and specificity to PSA. A discussion of these strategies and their relevance to the diagnosis and management of prostate cancer follows.

Abnormal vs normal serum PSA levels

Since PSA is an enzyme found in men without disease, the difficulty in using this marker comes in defining the 'normal' range for serum PSA. An increased leakage of PSA into the circulation appears to be the cause of most PSA elevations in prostatic disease. PSA levels in prostatic fluid are approximately a million-fold higher than serum PSA values. An epithelial layer, a basal cell layer and a basement membrane separate the intraductal PSA from the capillary and lymphatic drainage of the prostate. When disease, such as prostatitis or cancer, interferes with this natural barrier, it is believed that the flux of PSA into the serum increases, causing an elevated PSA.[7]

Although prostatic carcinoma may make the most significant contribution to elevating serum PSA, it is not the only contributor. Other factors adding to the flux of PSA into the serum include benign prostatic hyperplasia (BPH), trauma and inflammation. Stamey and associates studied men undergoing simple prostatectomy for BPH with the Pros-check assay.[8] According to their findings, 0.29 ng/ml PSA in the retropubic prostatectomy group and 0.31 ng/ml PSA in the transurethral resection group was contributed by each gram of BPH. In stark comparison, they found that prostate cancer in radical prostatectomy specimens raised serum PSA by 3.5 ng/ml/g cancer. Two additional groups have been unable to link the volume of BPH in radical retropubic prostatectomy specimens with preoperative serum PSA levels.[9,10] Stamey argued that the inconsistency is due to greater serum PSA contribution by prostate cancer present in these patients, which masks the elevation of serum PSA due to BPH.[8] Stamey's insight may have presaged the recognition of the different forms of PSA detected by two different assays. For example, it is well known now that the IMX assay (Abbott Laboratories) selectively measures more free PSA than does the Hybritech Tandem method.[11]

Another lesion found to contribute to serum PSA levels is a premalignant change in the human prostate known as prostatic intraepithelial neoplasia (PIN). PIN is commonly seen in association with invasive carcinoma. In a study of repeat transrectal ultrasound (TRUS)-guided needle biopsies[12] in men with a diagnosis of PIN in the original biopsy, the authors found that all men with a PSA greater than 4.0 prior to the second biopsy had carcinoma in their second biopsy specimen. Only two of 11 (18%) men with PIN grade 1 on the original biopsy had invasive carcinoma on the repeat biopsy. Ten patients with grade 2 or 3 PIN were found to have invasive carcinoma on repeat biopsy, indicating that a large percentage of men with high-grade PIN have undetected carcinoma.

Prostatitis, prostatic massage and prostate needle biopsy have also been identified as causing increased elevations of serum PSA. Acute bacterial prostatitis and urinary retention, which may disrupt the barriers between the lumina and adjacent capillaries, have been associated with increased levels of PSA.[13–15] The authors and others have reported no effect on serum PSA of standard digital rectal examination (DRE).[16,17] Stamey et al.[8] reported serum PSA increased 1.5 to 2 times following prostatic massage, leading to the conclusion that serum PSA should be assessed before or at least several days following prostate massage. Yuan et al.[16] found similar elevations in serum PSA values in 89 of 100 men following prostate needle biopsy, which continued for more than 2 weeks in 27 of the 89 patients. Oesterling and Bergstrahl,[18] in following 19 men after trans-rectal ultrasound (TRUS)-guided prostate needle biopsy, reported that 5 to 21 days (median 14.5 days) were needed for PSA values to return to baseline; PSA levels should, therefore, be monitored prior to prostate needle biopsy. Recent data reported by Tchetgen and associates[19] have suggested an acute elevation in serum PSA levels following ejaculation. The highest relative change occurred 1 h after ejaculation; however, in 8% of subjects such elevation persisted for more than 24 h, with 97% of subjects returning to normal by 48 h. These data stress the importance of asking patients about any recent ejaculation prior to assessing PSA.

In order to define an 'elevated' PSA reading, a 'normal' PSA distribution for men without disease was determined using the Tandem-R assay (Hybritech, San Diego, CA, USA). The manufacturers of the Tandem-R assay suggested a reference range (mean ± 2 standard deviations) of less than 4.0 ng/ml.[20] This was tested by several investigators on men of various ages. In men over 40 years of age who are without disease, Chan et al.[21] described a reference range (mean ± 3 SD) as being up to 2.8 ng/ml; for men up to the age of 40, the reference range was up to 2.0 ng/ml. Ercole et al.[22] further evaluated men over the age of 40 and found the reference range (mean ± 2 SD) to be less than 4.0 ng/ml; for normal males under 40, all tested had PSA values under 4.0 ng/ml, with a reference range of up to 1.8 ng/ml. In the authors' screening study[3] of 1249 men over the age of 50, 1062 (85%) had serum PSA levels less than 4.0 ng/ml, 149 (12%) had levels between 4.1 and 10.0 ng/ml, and 38 (3%) had levels greater than 10.0 ng/ml. Also noted was a trend toward increasing PSA values as men grow older.

The usefulness of serum PSA values in the detection and management of prostatic carcinoma is thus highly dependent upon knowing what is a 'normal' range distribution and on being fully aware of the various contributors to serum PSA levels beyond prostatic carcinoma. When these factors are considered, the usefulness of PSA in prostate cancer screening, treatment and follow-up becomes evident.

PSA as a screening tool

The potential utility of PSA for prostate cancer screening has been demonstrated by numerous studies, including that of Cooner et al.[23] in which a sensitivity and specificity of 0.80 and 0.61, respectively, for a Hybritech PSA value greater than 4.0 ng/ml was described for a population of men undergoing ultrasound-guided prostate biopsy due to hypoechoic peripheral zone lesions. Of those men biopsied, 32% were found to have a carcinoma. Similarly, in the authors' early experience with TRUS, using an abnormal DRE as an indication for biopsy, 32% of those biopsied had a positive biopsy result using the Hybritech Tandem-R assay and a 4.0 ng/ml cutoff.[24] The sensitivity and specificity were 0.68 and 0.60 respectively.

Results from the authors' screening study involving 1249 men and using the Tandem-R PSA assay[3] demonstrated the value of PSA as a predictor of prostate cancer. Patients who were found to have a PSA of 4.0 ng/ml or more were further evaluated with a DRE, TRUS and six systematic transrectal prostate needle biopsies. Prostate cancer was detected in 27% of the group whose PSA values were between 4.1 and 10.0 ng/ml. Of those with PSA values over 10.0 ng/ml, 50% were found to have carcinoma. For eight of 32 patients with proven prostate carcinoma, no abnormality was detected on DRE; four additional carcinomas were found in patients with only asymmetry on their digital rectal examination.

Hudson et al.[5] evaluated 1653 men utilizing the Tandem-R PSA as an initial screening test. Of these patients, 6% had a serum PSA value of between 4 and 9.9 ng/ml. Prostate carcinoma was detected in 22% of these patients by TRUS-guided needle biopsy. Another 2% of patients screened initially using PSA had values of 10 ng/ml or greater. Of these patients, 67% had prostate carcinoma revealed by ultrasound-guided prostate needle biopsy.

Despite these encouraging results, false positives were significant using the Tandem-R PSA as a sole screening device. False positives with resulting reduced specificity are particularly troublesome because of both the financial and psychological costs of undergoing a work-up for presumed prostate cancer. The majority of research during the past 10 years has focused on enhancing the specificity of PSA.

Tools to enhance the specificity of PSA

The test specificity is of particular importance because a higher value would mean that fewer biopsies would be performed in men who have elevated PSA levels yet do not have cancer (Figure 13.1). Four methods — PSA density, PSA velocity, age-specific PSA cutoff values and PSA forms — have been proposed to improve the specificity of PSA testing for prostate cancer detection. The current status and future utility of each of these methods are discussed below.

PSA density

PSA density (PSAD) is defined as the quotient of serum PSA divided by the volume of the prostate gland.[25] The observation that PSA levels are elevated in proportion to the volume of hyperplastic tissue encouraged investigators to correlate the size of the gland, usually measured by TRUS, to levels of PSA in serum.[8,26,27] Given that cancerous cells leak more PSA into the circulation than hyperplastic cells, it seemed intuitive that knowing if a patient had PSA values above those that would be expected for a hyperplastic gland of similar size would help to differentiate between cancer and BPH.

Initial studies demonstrated that men with cancer had a significantly higher PSAD than men with BPH, such that a PSAD value above a given cutoff (initial cutoffs ranged from 0.10 to 0.15) would indicate a likelihood of cancerous findings on biopsy.[25,27–30] Littrup and associates determined that a 16–55% reduction in biopsies could be achieved with a 4–25% loss in the number of cancers detected if

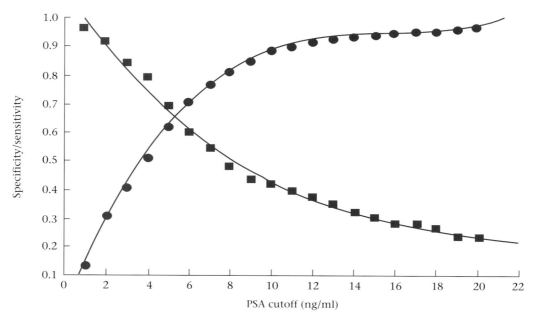

Figure 13.1. Inverse relationship between prostate-specific antigen (PSA) sensitivity (■) and specificity (●) for men undergoing ultrasound-guided needle biopsy. (Modified from ref. 37 with permission.)

a PSAD cutoff of 0.12 or greater was used.[31] Likewise, Bangma and associates, using the same cutoff, calculated a 28% reduction in biopsies with an 11% loss in cancers detected.[32] Subsequent investigations were unable to replicate an improved stratification using PSAD over the use of PSA alone.[33–35] Table 13.1 provides a summary of these investigations.

There are a number of reasons for the conflicting results, some of which are TRUS measurement error, variability of prostatic epithelial/stromal ratios, biopsy sampling error and PSA assay variability.[11,25,36,37] In review of the studies supporting PSA density it is clear that the glands harbouring malignancy were smaller than the benign-appearing ones; with equivalent PSA values, therefore, the smaller gland would have a higher PSAD. If each man has an equal volume of cancer, the clinician is much more likely to obtain a positive biopsy in the smaller gland (Figure 13.2). This rationale suggests that PSAD enhancement in predicting cancer may be spurious. Recent data, however, dispute the sampling error hypothesis. Presti et al.[38] tried to correct for this sampling error by performing sextant biopsies on men with estimated prostatic volumes of 50 cm^3 or less and doubled the number of biopsies to 12 if the gland volume was greater than 50 cm^3. They showed PSAD to be superior to PSA by receiver-operating characteristic analysis for all PSA values between 4 and 20 ng/ml. The significance was lost, however, in the important 4–10 ng/ml grey zone. Despite the larger number of biopsies, the cancer detection rate was significantly lower in the larger prostates (16% vs 33%, $p = 0.02$). Questions of how PSAD changes with age and race are additional concerns.[39–41] Henderson and associates,[39] in a study of men with benign biopsies, confirmed a markedly higher PSA in African-Americans (mean of 7.7 ng/ml, $n = 145$) compared with Caucasians (mean of 4.8 ng/ml, $n = 381$). Among these same patients, they also observed higher PSAD in African-Americans (0.18 vs 0.11). Further prospective analysis is needed to determine the usefulness of PSAD, but at this time many experts believe that the cost of conducting TRUS is not justified by the limited information gained.

Table 13.1. Summary of recent investigations of PSA density

Study	Biopsy	No. of patients	PSA (ng/ml)*		Prostate volume (cm³)*		Prostate-specific antigen density*	
Benson et al.[27]	Positive	98	7.0	(1.7)[†]	28.9	(14.6)[†]	0.30	(0.15)[†]
	Negative	191	6.8	(1.8)	40.1	(20.2)	0.21	(0.11)
Seaman et al.[28]	Positive	115	6.87	1.70)	29.2	(14.2)[†]	0.285	(0.147)[†]
	Negative	311	6.77	(1.71)	42.2	(21.8)	0.199	(0.108)
Brawer et al.[33]	Positive	68	10.7	(11.4)[†]	40.5	(16.6)	0.29	(0.41)[†]
	Negative	159	5.2	(5.0)	42.6	(25.6)	0.14	(0.14)
Bazinet et al.[29]	Positive	217	21.4	(29.6)[†]	37.6	(21.4)[†]	0.63	(0.86)[†]
	Negative	317	9.1	(8.1)	51.6	(27.3)	0.21	(0.25)
Rommel et al.[30]	Positive	612	15.5	(21.6)[†]	42.7	(27.2)[†]	0.47	(0.11)[†]
	Negative	1394	4.9	(4.7)	47.0	(31.6)	0.105	(0.09)
Mettlin et al.[34]	Positive	171	12.0	(16.0)[†]	38.9	(16.4)[†]	0.35	(0.5)[†]
	Negative	650	2.1	(2.3)	33.5	(14.2)	0.08	(0.09)
Ohori et al.[35]	Positive	110	9.3	(0.3–1320)[‡]	28.1	(15.1–228.7)[‡]	0.21	(0.009–39.3)[‡]
	Negative	134	4.8	(0.2–64.1)[‡]	47.3	(13.3–332.6)[‡]	0.09	(0.007–1.82)[‡]

*Values are means, with standard deviations in parentheses.
[†]$p <0.05$.
[‡]Values are medians with ranges in parentheses ($p < 0.05$).
PSAD = prostate-specific antigen density.

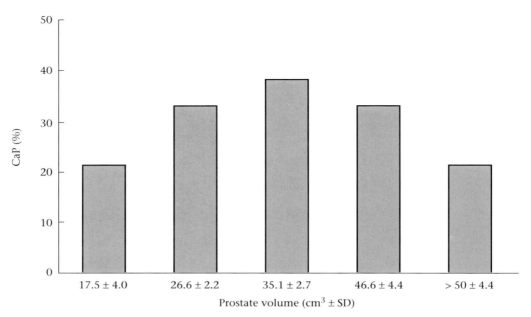

Figure 13.2. Detection of prostate cancer (CaP) from ultrasound-guided biopsies, by prostate volume (population grouped into percentiles).

PSA velocity

Another effort at improving specificity involves measuring the PSA velocity, or the rate of change in PSA values across serial measurements. It was believed that the prostatic growth rate could be monitored by yearly PSA values and, that, it cancer was present, a substantial increase in the PSA determination would be observed. Carter and associates in the Baltimore Longitudinal Aging Study noted that patients with BPH had linear increases in PSA levels over time, whereas patients with cancer had a similar linear increase with a subsequent exponential rise in PSA.[42] These investigators reported that an upward change in serum PSA of 0.75 ng/ml/year helped to identify those men with cancer. Using a velocity of 0.75 ng/ml/year, Carter reported sensitivities of 75% and specificities ranging from 90 to 100%.

It is rational that a patient with prostate cancer would have a greater rise in PSA levels, yet not all reports observed improvement in the specificity of cancer detection using PSA velocity. Brawer and associates, and others, were unable to find significant stratification between patients who did or did not have cancer, measuring PSA velocity in terms of a percentage or absolute change in PSA over 1- to 2-year time intervals.[43,44] Likewise, Catalona and associates revealed that a rate of change of 0.75 ng/ml/year provided no advantage in cancer detection for 224 men who had serum PSA levels measured 1–3 years prior to their first prostate biopsy.[45] The observation that PSA levels fluctuate on a day-to-day basis owing to biological and analytical variation provides a reason for the failure of PSA velocity to enhance the specificity of PSA. Both Nixon and associates and Lanz reported that the biological variation of PSA had a coefficient of variation of 8.94%, which represents a 30% change in serum PSA levels on a day-to-day basis.[46,47] Carter and associates conducted a study showing that measuring PSA velocity is useful if a minimum of three consecutive measurements are taken over a 2-year time period,[48] but this was most significant for men with an initial PSA value greater than 4.0 ng/ml.

The authors have recently demonstrated the value of using a 20% per year increase in PSA as a screening criterion in patients with initial PSA values less than 4.0 ng/ml.[42] The use of a 20% per year increase reflects the 4–5 year doubling time for serum PSA in men with untreated prostate cancer.[49] Using a PSA increase of greater than 20% per year, the authors were able to project a 17.1% positive predictive value for prostate cancer detection. Moreover, tumours amenable to surgical extirpation could be identified. Seven of eight cancers thus identified were pathologically organ confined. However, in contrast to the findings of Carter *et al.*, the present authors were unable to show that an absolute PSA velocity of more than 0.75 ng/ml/year is able to discriminate between carcinoma and BPH when absolute PSA is less than 4.0 ng/ml.

It appears that first-year screening detects the majority of those patients with advanced stage disease, and the subsequent screenings will detect a higher percentage of patients with localized disease (interval cancers). Findings of Catalona *et al.*[50] further support this hypothesis; they found advanced prostate cancer in only 30% of men diagnosed after serial PSA measurements, in comparison to 41% of men diagnosed after screening with a single PSA measurement and 67% of men diagnosed by DRE.

As more patients return for annual serum PSA determination, observations on rate of change or the rate of change of free/total PSA could have added potential. The authors' current recommendations are that all men with a PSA greater than 4.0 ng/ml who previously had a lower level should undergo biopsy.

Age-specific PSA reference ranges

Age-specific PSA reference ranges are based on the concept that PSA levels increase with age and that a PSA cutoff that is more specific for each age group would help to answer the question of when to conduct a biopsy. The upper bounds of PSA levels for each age were established by using 95% confidence intervals of normal[51,52] (Table 13.2). The advantages of age-specific PSA cutoffs are that they ideally would increase cancer detection (greater sensitivity) in men younger than 60 and decrease negative biopsies (greater specificity) in men older than 60 years of age. Oesterling and associates have argued that the greater number of prostate cancers identified in younger men would be more clinically significant and curable.[53] Reissigl and associates found that age-specific cutoffs resulted in an 8% increase in biopsies, with an 8% increase in cancers detected for men aged 45–59 years, whereas 21% fewer biopsies would have been performed in older men with 4% of cancer missed.[54]

Table 13.2. Age-specific PSA reference ranges*

Age (years)	Serum PSA (ng/ml)
40–49	0.0–2.5
50–59	0.0–3.5
60–69	0.0–4.5
70–79	0.0–6.5

*As defined by Oesterling *et al.*[51]

Once again, however, not all studies have demonstrated a particular advantage with age-specific cutoffs across all age groups. Borer and associates analysed the utility of age-specific cutoffs in men aged 60–79 years.[55] They determined that 60% of the cancers missed using age-related cutoffs had the characteristics of life-threatening tumours. Moul and associates demonstrated a significant elevation in the age-specific cutoffs in African-Americans.[56] There is little current rationale to begin screening or early detection at an age younger than 50, unless a patient has significant risk factors and might benefit from early detection.

Etzioni *et al.* compared the expected life years gained using age-specific PSA vs PSA alone for PSA values greater than 4.0 ng/ml[57] (Table 13.3). They found that age-specific PSA appears to add approximately 7 months more than PSA alone per subject; however, the cancer-specific survival was markedly greater in the group using PSA levels of more than 4.0 ng/ml alone. This is due to the increased prevalence of cancer in the older population and therefore a higher detection rate. The authors concluded that the longevity of the population was increased by using PSA greater than 4.0 ng/ml as a criterion, as opposed to age-specific PSA.

PSA remains an essential tumour marker in prostate cancer detection. Although the current data for PSAD, PSA velocity and age-specific PSA cutoffs are not yet conclusive, these refinements represent future directions to avoid costly procedures and to ensure that patients with prostate cancer are correctly identified. At present it is difficult to rationalize the prevention of negative biopsies if a significant proportion of cancers are missed. In this regard, the recognition of PSA isoforms and assays for same may offer the greatest promise.

Table 13.3. Expected survival advantage (years) with two screen-positive criteria — PSA > 4.0 ng/ml and PSA > age-specific cutoff (APSA)

(a) Expected years of life saved per subject screened

Criterion	Percentage local stage	
	65	75
PSA > 4.0	0.114	0.118
PSA > APSA	0.106	0.104
Difference	0.008	0.014

(b) Expected years of life saved per cancer case detected by each screening test

Criterion	Percentage local stage	
	65	75
PSA > 4.0	2.14	2.17
PSA > APSA	2.57	2.52
Difference	–0.43	–0.35

(c) Expected years of life saved per cancer case detected by either PSA > 4.0 ng/ml or PSA > APSA

Criterion	Percentage local stage	
	65	75
PSA > 4.0	2.14	2.17
PSA > APSA	2.00	1.96
Difference	0.14	0.21

Results of decision-analytic model estimating years of life saved attributable to screening for screened subjects and cancer cases detected by each of two screen-positive PSA criteria. In Table 13.3a, the total years of life saved are divided by the number of subjects screened. In Table 13.3b the total years of life saved are divided by the number of cases detected by each screen, on average 72 for PSA > 4.0 ng/ml, and 56 for PSA greater than an age-specific cutoff. In Table 13.3c, the total years of life saved are divided by the number of cases detected by either screen, on average 72, to show that dividing the total years of life saved by the number of cases detected by each screen neglects to account for the different numbers of cases detected by PSA and age-specific PSA.
(Modified from ref. 57 with permission.)

PSA forms

Perhaps the most exciting discovery in the arena of prostate cancer since the discovery of PSA itself is the recognition of two different molecular forms of PSA.[58-60] Complexed PSA is primarily bound to alpha-1-antichymotrypsin and is measured by all commercial assays available. Free or non-complexed PSA is present in much lower amounts in the serum and is measured in varying degrees by all commercial assays. PSA is also bound to alpha-2-macroglobulin; however, this form is not detected by any of the commercial assays available. Stenman and colleagues demonstrated in 1991 a strong correlation between the complexed form of PSA and carcinoma of the prostate.[60] A potential for increasing the sensitivity and, more importantly, the specificity has been reported in a number of studies. Christensson et al. showed that the percentage of free to total was significantly lower in patients with prostate cancer.[61] Using a total PSA of 5 ng/ml, Christennson demonstrated a sensitivity of 95% and a specificity of 55%. However, when he considered the proportion of free PSA to the total PSA in all PSA ranges, he was able to increase the specificity to 73% without affecting the sensitivity. The difficult diagnostic dilemma that plagues most clinicians is the intermediate PSA values in the range 4–10 ng/ml. Luderer et al.[62] examined PSA values in this range for patients with benign and malignant disease and found that the medians of the total PSA did not differ significantly between the two groups, with a p value of 0.13. The differences in the median free to total PSA, however, showed a p value of 0.0004. The median value of free PSA in the cancer group was 14% compared with 21% for the BPH group. They also looked at the enhancement of sensitivity and specificity in patients with a total PSA value greater than 4.0 ng/ml, and found total PSA to have a sensitivity of 92.7% and a specificity of 37.1%.[62] When free PSA was used to investigate the diagnostic grey zone of total PSA values between 4 and 10 ng/ml, it was found that free/total had a higher specificity than total PSA, for almost all sensitivity levels.

Higashihara et al.[63] demonstrated similar findings; they showed a positive predictive value of PSA alone of 24% and a significantly greater positive predictive value of the combination of PSA and free PSA ratio (50%). In using the combination test, they were able to avoid 30 biopsies, at the expense of only two cancers missed. The optimal PSA ratio reported in this study was 12%, compared with the 7% reported by Chen et al.[64] The authors have opted for free/total PSA ratios of less than 10% as being highly indicative of underlying malignancy and those greater than 25% as being highly suggestive of benign disease. Perhaps future studies will look at the diagnostic grey zone within free/total PSA values and stratify patients using PSAD, PSA velocity, age-specific PSA and free/total ratios to arrive at an overall predictive value of cancer.

PSA as a staging tool

For an individual patient, the serum PSA value is not a good indicator of pathological stage. PSA values vary widely among disease stage, and overlapping of stages further confounds the predictive value of PSA to pathological stage. The Johns Hopkins group[9] observed that the elevation in serum PSA for a given volume of tumour is inversely correlated with the grade of the tumour. Given this, a large and potentially higher-stage tumour that is poorly differentiated and a small, relatively well-differentiated tumour may produce similar PSA values. Another explanation is that the stromal and epithelial contributions to total gland volume vary enough between glands to cause spurious variations in serum PSA values. Although this is true, it is known that the mean PSA value generally increases as pathological stage increases.

As mentioned earlier, PSA values can be greatly effected by significant prostatic insult. For this reason, pre-biopsy PSA values are much better correlated to pathological stage than are post-biopsy PSA values. In the authors' study, in which PSA was determined prior to significant prostatic perturbation and then radical prostatectomy was performed, none of the 14 tumours found in men with pre-biopsy values greater than 10.0 ng/ml were organ confined on pathological examination.[65] A recent study by the Washington University group confirms these observations.[22] In this study, 14 of 16 patients with biopsy-proven prostate carcinoma and a serum PSA greater than 10 ng/ml were found to have extracapsular disease. These observations suggest that there is a high degree of correlation between serum PSA values greater than 10 ng/ml by the Hybritech method and the presence of extracapsular tumour extension.

Serum PSA values have also proved useful in the determination of bone metastases in patients with untreated prostate cancer. The Mayo Clinic group[66] found only one of 306 patients with serum PSA values less than 20 ng/ml (Tandem-R) to have a positive bone scan. The probability of a positive bone scan with a serum PSA of 10.0 ng/ml or less was estimated at 1.4%. PSA was found to be a more reliable and accurate indicator of bony metastases than clinical stage, tumour grade, or prostatic acid phosphates (PAP). Of course, any patient with skeletal pain should be fully staged with radionuclide bone scan, but the cost of savings may lead to a more selective approach to ordering bone scans.

One new biological tissue marker is microvessel density (MVD; BioStage, Bard Pharmaceuticals). This is a measurement of the number of blood vessels seen within a specified area of tissue on a needle biopsy specimen expressed in number of vessels per mm^2. Because of the frequency of add mixture within microscopic fields in glands expressing prostatic intraepithelial neoplasia, as well as benign histology, a linear quantification of vessel density is attained and expressed in a number of vessels per mm^2.[67] It is well described that neoplasms must recruit new vessels in order to grow to greater than 1 cubic mm in size.[68] Using computer enhancement techniques Brawer et al.[67] and Deering[69] have reported MVD for benign, PIN, BPH and malignant prostates (Table 13.4). Bostwick et al.[70] assessed the ability of MVD in conjunction with Gleason's score and PSA level in a needle biopsy specimen to predict pathological stage. Using logistic regression analysis he showed that a patient with a Gleason score of 6 and a PSA of 12 had a 43% chance of T3 disease. Adding MVD to the formula gave a range of 29% for the low and 85% for the high density (Table 13.5). MVD, therefore, is seen as a significant adjunct to PSA and Gleason's grade in managing patients with biopsy proven carcinoma.

Table 13.4. Microvessel density in prostate tissue and cancer

Tissue	Microvessel density (no. of vessels/mm²)	
	Mean	Range
Normal prostate	8.6	2.5 – 14.6
PIN	11.6	6.0 – 17.8
BPH	70.2	10.0 – 253.0
Cancer, organ confined	81.2	45.7 – 116.9
Cancer, metastatic	154.6	122.3 – 240.9

(Modified from refs. 67 and 69 with permission.)

Table 13.5. *Probability of extracapsular extension as assessed by Gleason score, PSA and optimized microvessel density (OMVD)*

Gleason score	PSA (ng/ml)	OMVD		
		25	150	750
6	4	0.10	0.30	0.60
6	12	0.29	0.62	0.85
7	4	0.20	0.51	0.78
7	12	0.49	0.79	0.93
8	4	0.38	0.71	0.89
8	12	0.69	0.90	0.97

(Modified from ref. 70 with permission.)

PSA in the management of prostate adenocarcinoma

Within 3 weeks following a radical prostatectomy with negative surgical margins, the serum PSA should theoretically be zero. The half-life of PSA is between 2.2 and 3.2 days; this level should be attained within 3 weeks postoperatively.[71] Unfortunately, none of the currently available assays for PSA can measure levels of zero. The biological sensitivity of the assay (that level of serum PSA that can be distinguished from zero with 95% certainty) varies between commercial assays and must be determined in an individual laboratory by repetitive testing.

Serum PSA is the first indicator of 'recurrent' disease. Carter et al.[72] noted that no patient with undetectable PSA level after radical prostatectomy had clinical evidence of active prostate cancer. Carter further noted that all patients with clinically detectable distant recurrences had elevated PSA postoperatively. Stamey et al.[8] added to these findings, noting that no patient who failed to normalize serum PSA within 3 weeks of radical prostatectomy had a subsequent decrease in PSA levels to undetectable range without adjuvant therapy.

Several studies suggest that the majority of patients with undetectable PSA level following radical prostatectomy will remain without evidence of recurrence, whereas those whose PSA levels remain detectable will experience some type of recurrence. Lange and associates[73] measured PSA level 3–6 months after radical prostatectomy and correlated it with clinical outcome. In men with PSA levels of 0.2 ng/ml or less, only 11% had a recurrence; of those who had PSA levels above 0.4 ng/ml, 100% had a recurrence. In following 86 patients who had undetectable PSA levels after radical prostatectomy, seven (8.1%) had a subsequent rise in PSA levels to a mean of 70.6 ng/ml; 47 followed for less than a year and 32 followed for between 12 and 33 months had persistently undetectable PSA values without evidence of recurrence. Stein et al.[74] report that in all cases in a group of 230 patients with pathological stage T1–2, N0, M0 disease followed for a mean of 48 months after radical retropubic prostatectomy, elevations of serum PSA preceded the clinical recurrence of disease. However, in 41 of 175 patients with current PSA values and no clinical evidence of recurrent prostate cancer, elevated serum PSA levels suggested a recurrence. The 5- and 10-year clinical disease-free survivals were 82% and 72%, respectively. If an elevated serum PSA value was taken to indicate recurrent disease, then the 5- and 10-year disease-free survival decreases to 62% and 41%, respectively. Thus, even 10 years after radical prostatectomy, a significant percentage of patients with apparent recurrent prostate cancer as assessed by biochemical parameters remain without other clinical evidence of the disease.

Detecting low-volume persistent disease can be difficult. DRE is often inconclusive. Bone scan and computerized tomography (CT) scan are generally negative in these patients. Lightner and associates,[75] in evaluating needle biopsy of the anastomosis (NBA) in a group of men with serum PSA value of more than 0.4 ng/ml after radical prostatectomy, found that 42% of the patients had a positive needle biopsy but negative bone scans and CT scans. Notably, no patient with an undetectable PSA value had a positive needle biopsy of the anastomosis. Foster *et al.*[76] confirmed these findings, reporting that positive NBAs occur in about 45% of cases with detectable PSAs. Abi-Aad and associates[77] had similar findings, reporting positive readings among 40% of those patients with elevated PSA following radical prostatectomy.

The development of more sensitive assays for PSA should allow earlier detection of persistent disease. Modifications of the reagents used in the Tandem-R and Tandem-E assays have improved the biological sensitivities of those assays to 0.2 ng/ml. The IMX assay (Abbott Laboratories, Abbott Park, IL, USA) has a biological sensitivity of 0.06 ng/ml. However, repetitive testing of post-cystoprostatectomy sera produced many values between 0.06 and 0.1 ng/ml. Therefore, the present authors have adopted a clinical sensitivity of 0.1 ng/ml for this assay.[78] Takayama *et al.*[79] found a 9- to 12-month lead time in detecting persistent disease using 0.1 rather than 0.4 ng/ml serum PSA to indicate persistent disease.

All patients in this group who reached a serum PSA level of 0.1 ng/ml continued to show a rise in PSA levels. No patient who had a serum PSA value of less than 0.1 ng/ml at 36 months after radical prostatectomy developed recurrent disease. Whether early treatment of patients with biochemical evidence of recurrent disease will result in prolonged survival remains to be determined.

There is evidence that patients in whom PSA levels fail to become normal initially are more likely to have distant metastases, whereas those who develop delayed PSA elevations after radical prostatectomy may be more likely to have a local recurrence. Lange *et al.*[80] treated 29 patients with elevated PSA values, who had negative CT scans and bone scans with pelvic irradiation. PSA values decreased by more than 50% in 82% of the patients; 43% of the patients had an accompanying decrease in PSA serum within 6 months, to an undetectable range. The Stanford group[81] reported similar findings in an evaluation of two groups of patients with adjuvant radiation therapy: they found that only one of 12 (8%) of patients receiving radiation treatment for elevated PSA immediately after prostatectomy versus seven of 15 (47%) of patients receiving radiation treatment for a delayed elevation in PSA after radical prostatectomy had continued suppression of PSA levels at undetectable levels during an average 33-month follow-up. The Southwest Oncology Group and Eastern Cooperative Oncology Group are currently studying the impact of adjuvant radiotherapy on pathological stage T3 disease.

PSA after radiation or hormonal therapy

PSA offers new information on the behaviour of prostate cancer following radiation (XRT) or hormonal therapy. Serum PSA has been found to decrease, with the half-life estimated at 1.4–2.6 months,[82,83] following radiation therapy. The Stanford group[84] followed a group of 183 patients after completion of radiation therapy, most of which had localized disease, for a mean of 61 months: serum PSA was reduced to undetectable levels in 11% of the patients; 25% of patients had a decrease in serum PSA values to the normal range (less than 2.5 ng/ml, Pros-check); elevated PSA levels persisted in 65% of patients. Radiation therapy during the first year caused a reduction in PSA values in 82% of patients, but continued reduction after the first year of therapy occurred in only 8% of patients; PSA values rose in 51% of the patients.

Russell and colleagues[85] reported that pretreatment PSA values are associated with the chance of complete response (normalization of PSA with no tumour detectable by radiographic studies or DRE). In evaluation of 143 men who were treated with external beam irradiation, either photon or fast neutron, for clinically localized prostate cancer, with a median follow-up of 27 months, patients with a pretreatment PSA value less than four times the normal value had an 82% chance of complete response, whereas those with a PSA value greater than four times the normal value had only a 30% chance of complete response. Furthermore, the time to normalization of PSA appears to be important; in the study by Russell and colleagues, 94% of those with normalization of PSA within 6 months remained complete responders during the study, compared with 8% of men with persistently elevated PSA values after 6 months.

The Wisconsin group[83] conducted a similar study of serum PSA and radiotherapy for prostate cancer; they found a post-treatment PSA nadir in the normal range to be the most important prognostic variable. Pretreatment PSA was not predictive of outcome if serum PAP was considered. They also noted that the initial rate of PSA decrease was unrelated to outcome. MVD may help to stratify patients undergoing XRT so that XRT can be compared with RRP on a more accurate stage-for-stage basis.

Kabalin[86] conducted TRUS-guided sextant biopsies on 27 men 18 months after external beam radiation therapy. Persistent prostate carcinoma was detected in 25 of the 27 patients, including 20 or 22 men with normal DRE. All four patients with normal PSA levels (<2.5 ng/ml, Pros-check), including one patient with an undetectable PSA, had positive biopsies. This suggests that rising PSA levels after radiation therapy may indicate persistent disease. Such rises should prompt further evaluation with prostate needle biopsy if the patient is a candidate for salvage radical prostatectomy. Recent data from Zagars and associates[87–89] suggest that any PSA value greater than 0.5 ng/ml after radiation therapy suggests persistent disease.

The PSA nadir appears to be an important indicator of response to hormonal therapy. Stamey et al.[90] followed a cohort of patients with D2 prostate cancer after initiation of hormonal therapy; of these, 22% had a decrease in serum PSA levels to the normal range, whereas 9% had a decrease to undetectable levels. Of 11 patients who were followed with frequent PSA determinations after the induction of hormonal therapy, the PSA nadir was reached within 5 months in nine. In 72% of these 11 patients, increasing PSA values were noted after 6 months.

Miller et al.[91] studied serum PSA levels of 48 patients with D2 prostate cancer who achieved an objective response to hormonal therapy. They found that patients who reached a PSA nadir of less than 4.0 ng/ml had a significantly longer duration of remission than those in whom PSA failed to regain normal levels. No patient gave evidence of progressive disease while the PSA level was decreasing or plateaued at the nadir level. Miller and associates also noted that a rise in serum PSA pre-dated other evidence of disease progression by a mean of 7.3 months. Gillat et al.[92] also reported that PSA levels are significantly related to survival after initiation of hormonal therapy, in their study of 136 men with metastatic prostate cancer whose PSA levels were determined at 3 and 6 months following therapy initiation.

Conclusions

PSA is the most accurate tumour marker in the field of oncology. This analyte can be used successfully to diagnose, stage and monitor prostatic carcinoma. Refinement of PSA assays continues to contribute to their clinical use and allows for earlier detection of persistent disease after radical surgery. Although there have been significant advances in the use of PSA as a tumour marker, shortcomings still exist and the measure continues to be controversial in prostate cancer screening. Further evaluation of new ideas such as free/total PSA, reverse transcriptase–polymerase chain reaction PSA, basic fibroblast growth factor and MVD will contribute to the knowledge of PSA and its clinical applications.

References

1. Silverberg E, Boring C C, Squires T S. Cancer statistics. Cancer 1990; 40: 9–26
2. Catalona W J, Smith D S, Ratliff T L *et al.* Measurement of PSA in serum as a screening test for prostate cancer. N Engl J Med 1991; 324: 1156–1161
3. Brawer M K, Chetner M P, Beatie J *et al.* Screening for prostatic carcinoma with PSA. J Urol 1992; 147: 841–845
4. Stamey T A, Kabalin J N. Prostate specific antigen in the diagnosis and treatment of adenocarcinoma of the prostate: I. Untreated patients. J Urol 1989; 141: 1070–1075
5. Hudson M A, Bahnson R B, Catalona W J. Clinical use of prostate specific antigen in patients with prostate cancer. J Urol 1989; 142: 1011–1017
6. Brawer M K. PSA: a review. Acta Oncol 1991; 30(2): 161–168
7. Brawer M K, Rennels M A, Nagle R B *et al.* Serum PSA and prostate pathology in men having simple prostatectomy. Am J Clin Pathol 1989; 92(6): 760–764
8. Stamey T A, Yang N, Hay A R *et al.* Prostate-specific antigen as a serum marker for adenocarcinoma of the prostate. N Engl J Med 1987; 317: 909–916
9. Partin A W, Carter H B, Chan D W *et al.* Prostate specific antigen in the staging of localized prostate cancer: influence of tumor differentiation, tumor volume and benign hyperplasia. J Urol 1990; 143: 747–752
10. Stamey T A, Kabalin J N, McNeal J E *et al.* Prostate specific antigen in the diagnosis and treatment of adenocarcinoma of the prostate: II. Radical prostatectomy treated patients. J Urol 1989; 141: 1076–1083
11. Wener M H, Daum P R, Brawer M K. Variation in measurement of PSA: the importance of method and lot variability. Clin Chem 1995; 41(12): 1730–1737
12. Brawer M K, Nagle R B, Bigler S A *et al.* Significance of PIN on prostate needle biopsy. Urology 1991; 38(2): 103–107
13. Dalton D L. Elevated serum PSA due to acute bacterial prostatitis. Urology 1989; 33: 465
14. Neal D E, Clejan S, Sarma D, Moon T D *et al.* PSA and prostatitis I. Effect of prostatitis on serum PSA in the human and nonhuman primate. Prostate 1992; 20: 105
15. Armitage T G, Cooper E H, Newling W W *et al.* The value of the measurement of serum PSA in patients with BPH and untreated prostate cancer. Br J Urol 1988; 62: 584
16. Yuan J J J, Coplen D E, Petros J A *et al.* Effects of rectal examination, prostatic massage, ultrasonography, and needle biopsy on serum PSA levels. J Urol 1992; 147: 810–814
17. Brawer M K, Schifman R B, Ahmann F R *et al.* The effect of digital rectal examination on serum levels of PSA. Arch Pathol Lab Med 1988; 112(11): 1110–1112
18. Oesterling J E, Bergstralh E J. PSA following prostate biopsy and TURP: length of time necessary to achieve a stable value. J Urol 1991; 145: 251A
19. Tchetgen M B, Song J T, Strawderman M *et al.* Ejaculation increases the serum prostate-specific antigen concentration. Urology 1996; 47(4): 511–516
20. Myrtle J F, Klimley P G, Ivor L P, Bruni J F *et al.* Clinical utility of prostate specific antigen (PSA) in the management of prostate cancer. In: Advances in Cancer Diagnostics. San Diego: Hybritech Inc., 1986; 1–4
21. Chan D W, Bruzek D J, Oesterling J E *et al.* Prostate-specific antigen as a marker for prostatic cancer: a monoclonal and polyclonal immunoassay compared. Clin Chem 1987; 33: 1916
22. Ercole C J, Lange P H, Mathisen M *et al.* Prostate specific antigen and prostatic acid phosphatase in the monitoring and staging of patients with prostatic cancer. J Urol 1987; 138: 1181–1184

23. Cooner W H, Mosley R B, Rutherford J *et al*. Prostate cancer detection in a clinical urological practice by ultrasonography, digital rectal examination and prostate specific antigen. J Urol 1990; 143: 1146–1152

24. Brawer M K, Lange P H. PSA: its role in early detection, staging and monitoring of prostatic carcinoma. J Endourol 1989; 3(2): 227–236

25. Benson M C, Whang I S, Pantuck A *et al*. Prostate specific antigen density: a means of distinguishing benign prostatic hypertrophy and prostate cancer. J Urol 1992; 147: 815–186

26. Babaian R J, Fritsche H A, Evans R B. PSA and prostate gland volume: correlation and clinical application. J Clin Lab Anal 1990; 4: 135–137

27. Benson M C, Whang I S, Olsson C A *et al*. The use of prostate-specific antigen density to enhance the predictive value of intermediate levels of serum prostate-specific antigen. J Urol 1992; 147: 817–821

28. Seaman E, Whang M, Olsson C A *et al*. PSA density (PSAD): role in patient evaluation and management. Urol Clin North Am 1993; 20: 653

29. Bazinet M, Meshref A W, Trudel C *et al*. Prospective evaluation of prostate-specific antigen density and systematic biopsies for early detection of prostatic carcinoma. Urology 1994; 43: 44–51

30. Rommel F M, Augusta V E, Breslin J A *et al*. The use of PSA and PSAD in the diagnosis of prostate cancer in a community based urology practice. J Urol 1994; 151: 88–93

31. Littrup P J, Kane R A, Mettlin C J *et al*. Cost-effective prostate cancer detection: reduction of low-yield biopsies. Cancer 1994; 74(12): 3146–3158

32. Bangma C H, Kranse R, Blijenberg B G, Schroder F H *et al*. The value of screening tests in the detection of prostate cancer. Part I: results of a retrospective evaluation of 1726 men. Urology 1995; 46(6): 773–778

33. Brawer M K, Aramburu E A G, Chen G L *et al*. The inability of PSA index to enhance the predictive value of PSA in the diagnosis of prostatic carcinoma. J Urol 1993; 150: 369–373

34. Mettlin C, Littrup P J, Kane R A *et al*. Relative sensitivity and specificity of serum PSA level compared with age-referenced PSA, PSA density and PSA change. Cancer 1994; 74: 1615–1620

35. Ohori M, Dunn J K, Scardino P T. Is prostate-specific antigen density more useful than prostate-specific antigen levels in the diagnosis of prostate cancer? Urology 1995; 46: 666

36. Stamey T A. Making the most out of six systematic sextant biopsies. Urology 1995; 45(1): 2–11

37. Brawer M K. How to use PSA in the early detection or screening for prostatic carcinoma. CA 1995; 45(3): 148–164

38. Presti J C Jr, Hovey R, Carroll P R *et al*. Prospective evaluation of prostate-specific antigen and prostate-specific antigen density in the detection of nonpalpable and stage T1C carcinoma of the prostate. J Urol 1996; 156: 1685–1690

39. Henderson R J, Eastham J A, Culkin D J *et al*. Prostate-specific antigen (PSA) and PSA density (PSAD) are higher in African-Americans without prostate cancer: results of 526 patients. J Urol 1996; 155: 262A

40. Hovey R M, Shinohara K, Bhargava V *et al*. Prostate-specific antigen and prostate-specific antigen density in the detection of prostate cancer: ethnic variations. J Urol 1996; 155: 267A

41. McCammon K A, Schellhammer P F, Wright G L *et al*. Age specific PSA levels in African-Americans. J Urol 1996; 155: 461A

42. Carter H, Morrell C H, Pearson J D *et al*. Estimation of prostatic growth using serial PSA measurements in men with and without prostate disease. Cancer Res 1992; 52: 3323–3328

43. Brawer M K, Beattie J, Wener M H *et al*. Screening for prostatic carcinoma with PSA: results of the second year. J Urol 1993; 150(1): 106–109

44. Porter J R, Hayward R, Brawer M K. The significance of short-term PSA change in men undergoing ultrasound guided prostate biopsy. J Urol 1994; 152: 293A

45. Catalona W J, Smith D S, Ratliff T L. Value or measurement of the rate of change of serum PSA levels in prostate cancer screening. J Urol 1993; 150: 300A

46. Lanz K J, Wener M H, Brawer M K *et al*. Biologic variation in serum PSA level. J Urol 1996; 155: 696A(suppl)

47. Nixon R G, Wener M H, Smith K M *et al*. Biological variation of prostate-specific antigen levels in serum: an evaluation of day-to-day physiological fluctuations in a well-defined cohort of 24 patients. J Urol 1997; 157: 2183–2190

48. Carter H B, Pearson J D, Chan D W *et al*. Prostate-specific antigen variability in men without prostate cancer: effect of sampling interval on prostate-specific antigen velocity. Urology 1995; 45: 591

49 Smith D S, Catalona W J. Rate of change in serum prostate specific-antigen levels as a method for prostate cancer detection. J Urol 1994; 152: 1163

50. Catalona W J, Smith D, Ratliff T L. Single and serial measurement of serum prostate antigen as a screening test for early prostate cancer. J Urol 1992; 147(suppl): 450

51. Oesterling J E, Jacobsen S J, Chute C G *et al*. Serum PSA in a community-based population of healthy men: establishment of age-specific reference ranges. JAMA 1993; 270: 860–864

52. Dalkin B L, Ahmann F R, Kopp J B. PSA levels in men older than 50 years without clinical evidence of prostatic carcinoma. J Urol 1993; 150: 1837–1839

53. Oesterling J E, Cooner W H, Jacobsen S J *et al*. Influence of patient age on the serum PSA concentration: an important clinical observation. Urol Clin North Am 1993; 20(4): 671–680

54. Reissigl A, Pointner J, Horninger W *et al*. Comparison of different prostate-specific antigen cutpoints for early detection of prostate cancer: results of a large screening population. Urology 1995; 46: 662

55. Borer J G, Serman J, Solomon M C *et al*. Age-specific reference ranges for prostate-specific antigen and digital rectal examination may not safely eleminate further diagnostic procedures. J Urol 1996; 155: 48A

56. Morgan T O, Jacobsen S J, McCarthy W F *et al*. Age-specific reference ranges for serum prostate-specific antigen in black men. N Engl J Med 1996; 335(5): 304–310

57. Etzioni R, Shen Y, Petteway J C, Brawer M K *et al*. Age-specific PSA: a reassessment. Prostate 1996; 7: 70–77

58. Christensson A, Laurell C B, Lilja H. Enzymatic activity of prostate-specific antigen and its reaction with extracellular serine proteinase inhibitors. Eur J Biochem 1990; 194: 755

59. Lilja H, Christensson A, Dahlen U *et al*. PSA in human serum occurs predominantly in complex with alpha-1 antichymotrypsin. Clin Chem 1991; 37: 1618–1625

60. Stenman U, Leinonen J, Alfthan H *et al*. A complex between PSA and a 1-antichymotrypsin is the major form of PSA in serum of patients with prostatic cancer: assay of the complex improves clinical sensitivity for cancer. Cancer Res 1991; 51: 222

61. Christensson A, Bjork T, Nilsson O *et al*. Serum prostate-specific antigen complexed to alpha 1-antichymotrypsin as an indicator of prostate cancer. J Urol 1993; 150(1): 100–105

62. Luderer A A, Chen Y, Thiel R *et al*. Measurement of the proportion of free to total PSA improves diagnostic performance of PSA in the diagnostic gray zone of total PSA. Urology 1995; 46(2): 187–194

63. Higashihara E, Nutahara K, Kojima M *et al*. Significance of serum free prostate-specific antigen in the screening of prostate cancer. J Urol 1996; 156: 1964–1968

64. Chen Y, Luderer A A, Thiel R P *et al*. Using proportions of free to total prostate-specific antigen, age and total prostate-specific antigen to predict the probability of prostate cancer. Urology 1996; 47(4): 518–524

65. Ellis W J, Brawer M K. The role of tumor markers in the diagnosis and treatment of prostate cancer. In: Lepor H, Lawson R K (eds) Prostate diseases. Philadelphia: Saunders; 1993: 276–291

66. Chybowski F M, Larson Keller J J, Berstralh E J, Oesterling J E *et al*. Predicting radionuclide bone scan findings in patients with newly diagnosed, untreated prostate cancer: PSA is superior to all other clinical parameters. J Urol 1991; 145: 313

67. Brawer M K, Deering R E, Brown M *et al*. Predictors of pathologic stage in prostatic carcinoma: the role of neovascularity. Cancer 1994; 73(3): 678–687

68. Weidner N, Semple J P, Welch W R, Folkman J *et al*. Tumor angiogenesis and metastasis — correlation in invasive breast carcinoma. N Engl J Med 1991; 324: 1–8

69. Deering R E, Bigler S A, Brown M, Brawer M K. Microvascularity in benign prostatic hyperplasia. Prostate 1995; 26(3): 111–15

70. Bostwick D G, Wheeler T M, Blute M *et al*. Optimized microvessel density analysis improves prediction of cancer stage from prostate needle biopsies. Urology 1996; 48: 47–57

71. Oesterling J E, Chan D W, Epstein J I *et al*. Prostate-specific antigen in the pre-operative and post-operative evaluation of localized prostatic cancer treated with radical prostatectomy. J Urol 1988; 139: 766

72. Carter H B, Partin A W, Oesterling J E *et al*. The use of prostate-specific antigen in the management of patients with prostate cancer: the Johns Hopkins experience. In: Catalona W J, Coffey D S, Karr J P (eds) Clinical aspects of prostate cancer. New York: Elsevier Science, 1989; 247–254

73. Lange P H, Ercole C J, Lightner D J *et al*. The value of serum prostate specific antigen determinations before and after radical prostatectomy. J Urol 1989; 141: 873

74. Stein A, deKernion J B, Smith R B *et al*. PSA levels after radical prostatectomy in patients with organ confined and locally extensive prostate cancer. J Urol 1992; 147: 942–946

75. Lightner D J, Lange P H, Reddy P K, Moore L *et al*. Prostate specific antigen and local recurrence after radical prostatectomy. J Urol 1990; 144: 921–926

76. Foster L S, Jajodia P, Fournier G Jr. *et al*. The value of PSA and transrectal ultrasound-guided biopsy in accurately detecting prostatic fossa recurrences following radical prostatectomy. J Urol 1993; 149(5): 1024–1028

77. Abi-Aad A S, Macfarlane M T, Stein A, deKernion J B *et al*. Detection of local recurrence after radical prostatectomy by PSA and TRUS. J Urol 1992; 147: 952–955

78. Vessella R L, Noteboom J, Lange PH. Evaluation of the Abbott IMx (R) automated immunoassay of PSA. Clin Chem 1992; 38: 2044–2054

79. Takayama T K, Vessella R L, Brawer M K *et al*. The enhanced detection of persistent disease after prostatectomy with a new PSA immunoassay. J Urol 1993; 150(2): 374–378

80. Lange P H, Lightner D J, Medini E *et al*. The effects of radiation therapy after radical prostatectomy in patients with elevated PSA levels. J Urol 1990; 144: 927–933

81. Link P, Freiha F S, Stamey T A. Adjuvant radiation therapy in patients with detectable prostate specific antigen following radical prostatectomy. J Urol 1991; 145: 532–534

82. Meek A G, Park T L, Oberman E, Wielopolski L *et al*. A prospective study of PSA levels in patients receiving radiotherapy for localized carcinoma of the prostate. Int J Radiat Oncol Biol Phys 1990; 75: 1982

83. Ritter M A, Messing E M, Shanahan T G *et al*. Prostate-specific antigen as a predictor of radiotherapy response and patterns of failure in localized prostate cancer. J Clin Oncol 1992; 10: 1208–1217

84. Stamey R A, Kabalin J N, Ferrari M. Prostate specific antigen in the diagnosis and treatment of adeonocarcinoma of the prostate. III. Radiation treated patients. J Urol 1989; 141: 1083–1087

85. Russell K J, Dunatov C, Hafermann J T *et al*. Prostate-specific antigen in the management of patients with localized adenocarcinoma of the prostate treated with primary radiation therapy. J Urol 1991; 146: 1046–1052

86. Kabalin J N, Hodge K H, McNeal J E *et al*. Identification of residual cancer in the prostate following radiation therapy: role of transrectal ultrasound guided biopsy and prostate specific antigen. J Urol 1989; 142: 326–331

87. Zagars G K, Pollack A. The fall and rise of serum PSA levels after radiation therapy for prostate cancer. Cancer 1993; 72: 832

88. Zagars G K, von Eschenbach A C, Ayala A G. Prognostic factors in prostate cancer. Cancer 1993; 72: 1709–1725

89. Zagars G K. PSA as an outcome variable for T1 and T2 prostate cancer treated by radiation therapy. J Urol 1994; 152: 1786–1791

90. Stamey T A, Kabalin J N, Ferrari M, Yang N *et al*. Prostate specific antigen in the diagnosis and treatment of adenocarcinoma of the prostate: IV. Anti-androgen treated patients. J Urol 1989; 141: 1088–1090

91. Miller J I, Ahman F R, Drach G W *et al*. The clinical usefulness of serum PSA after hormonal therapy of metastatic prostate cancer. J Urol 1992; 147: 956–961

92. Gillatt D, Gingell C, Smith P J B. Serum PSA for the assessment of response to hormonal therapy. J Urol 1990; 144: 207A

Chapter 14
PSA as routine medicine: the primary care physician's view — an English perspective

M. G. Kirby

Introduction

The two most common diseases of the prostate gland, benign prostatic hyperplasia (BPH) and carcinoma of the prostate, have attracted a remarkable increase in interest in the past few years. This has come about because of the increasing awareness of the prevalence of both benign and malignant disease of this gland.[1]

BPH is one of the most common diseases to affect men beyond middle age — histological disease is present in more than 60% of men in their 60s and 40% of men beyond this age have symptomatic disease, of whom about half have an impaired quality of life.

Cancer of the prostate is also a very common disease, ranking as the fifth most common cancer in the world. In some advanced countries it has become the most common cancer in men, owing mainly to improvement in methods of diagnosis and increased public interest. As a result of this, more patients are presenting to their physician with lower urinary tract symptoms or anxiety about the possibility of prostate cancer.

In England and Wales, the present incidence of prostatic cancer is 0.72 new cases per 1000 men between 55 and 70 years of age, and in 1991, 8500 men died from this disease.[2] In the European Economic Community as a whole, it was estimated that there were 85,000 new cases of prostate cancer diagnosed in 1980 and 35,084 men die annually from prostate cancer.[3] The onset and progression of prostate cancer are insidious and many patients have either locally advanced or metastatic disease at the time of presentation.[4] The incidence of prostatic cancer is strongly correlated with age (Figure 14.1) and coupled with this is demographic changes in our populations with increasing numbers of men living into old age (Figure 14.2).

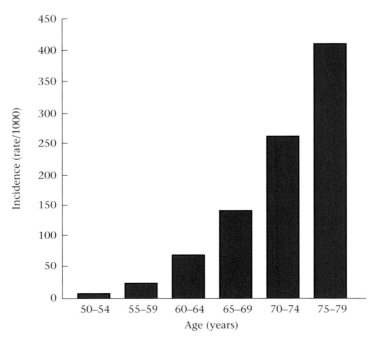

Figure 14.1. Age is the strongest risk factor for prostate cancer. (From ref. 48 with permission.)

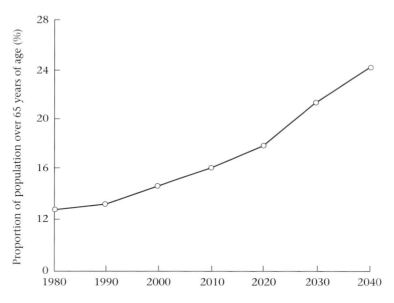

Figure 14.2. There is a worldwide trend towards an ageing population and the incidence of prostate cancer will continue to rise. (From ref. 48 with permission.)

Increasing incidence of carcinoma of the prostate

In recent years, a steady rise in the incidence of clinically significant prostate cancer has been seen in many countries. Figure 14.3 shows figures for the USA but the trend is similar for the UK. There is no doubt that there has been an absolute increase in cancer of the prostate.

The age-adjusted incidence rate for cancer of the prostate in US Afro-Caribbeans is nearly twice that of US Whites, which in turn is twice the reported

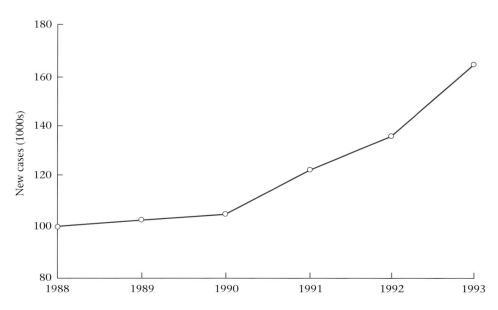

Figure 14.3. There has been a consistent increase in the incidence of clinically significant prostate cancer in recent years. The graph shows the number of new cases diagnosed in the USA, and similar trends have been reported in other countries. (From ref. 48 with permission.)

rate in the UK (20 per 100,000), age adjusted. Age-adjusted mortality rates in the USA and in the UK are very similar.[5,6]

The increasing incidence of carcinoma of the prostate may be the result of any of the following:
1. Improved diagnostic techniques;
2. Improved registration methods;
3. Greater awareness among medical practitioners;
4. Improving life expectancy of men over the age of 70 years;
5. Increase in the incidence of cancer of the prostate;
6. A combination of all these factors.

As a result of these factors there is likely to be a marked increase in prostate cancer deaths during the next two decades[7] (Figure 14.4).

Health care provision

Health care provision varies greatly from country to country in terms of the ratios of urologists to family practitioners and the relationships between them. The number of urologists per capita also varies widely (Figure 14.5). The limited number of urologists in the UK has led to the development of shared care schemes for the management of patients with prostatic diseases.[8] The overall benefit of shared care for prostatic disease is improved patient care and the advantages to all those involved can be significant.

Advantages of a shared-care approach for prostatic diseases
For patients, a shared-care approach has the following advantages:
1. Reduced hospital visits and waiting times;
2. Easier access to local medical advice;
3. Greater continuity of treatment and better follow-up;
4. Greater contact with the family practitioner, who is more aware of their medical/social history.

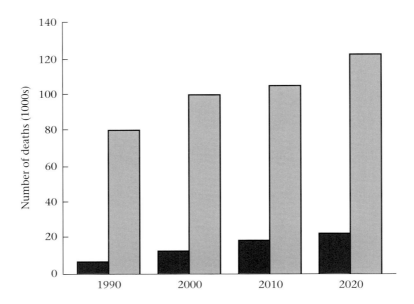

Figure 14.4. A marked increase in prostate cancer deaths is expected to occur during the next two decades. ■ United Kingdom; ■ Europe. (Data from Boyle, 1992). (From ref. 48 with permission.)

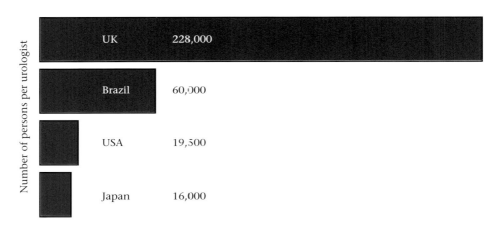

Figure 14.5. Worldwide variations in the number of individuals for whom each urologist is responsible in each country will influence the development of shared care protocols for prostatic disease around the world. (From ref. 8 with permission.)

Family practitioners are aware of the following benefits:
1. Patients may be more open with health care professionals with whom they are familiar;
2. There is an opportunity for family practitioners to broaden their knowledge of prostatic disease and develop new skills;
3. There are the rewards of team working and providing better patient care.
   Urologists find that shared care has the following effects:
1. It reduces hospital admissions and surgical waiting times;
2. It encourages more appropriate referrals;
3. It enables earlier diagnosis of prostate cancer;
4. It makes more time available for patients requiring specialist management;

5. It brings the rewards of stronger relations with community physicians and provision of better patient care.

This concept in the UK has led to an increased awareness of the prevalence, and importance, of both BPH and prostate cancer within the general public and family practitioners, and should lead to an increase in the detection of early and potentially curable tumours.

The PSA test

The investigation of patients with prostatic diseases has been facilitated by the introduction of the prostate specific antigen (PSA) test.[9] PSA is a single-chain glycoprotein of 237 amino acids and four carbohydrate side chains. Functionally, PSA is an organ-specific, kallikrein-like serine protease produced by prostatic epithelial cells lining the acini and ducts of the prostate gland.[10,11] It is organ specific but not disease specific because it is expressed in both benign and malignant processes involving epithelial cells of the prostate.

Under normal physiological conditions, PSA is secreted into the lumina of the prostate ducts; it is present in the seminal plasma in high concentrations and constitutes an important part of the prostatic secretions. Its main function is to liquefy the seminal coagulum[12] (Figure 14.6). Normally, only a small proportion is absorbed into the bloodstream.

Conditions such as prostate cancer will disrupt the basement membrane and result in increased absorption and elevated serum PSA levels.

The test should not be performed under the following circumstances:
1. During an episode of urinary infection;
2. During an episode of retention of urine;
3. Within 72 hours after ejaculation;
4. Shortly after prostatic surgery or biopsy;
5. During an episode of prostatitis;
6. As a routine investigation without adequate counselling.

Used intelligently, PSA is currently the most important, accurate and clinically useful tumour marker for prostate cancer. It has revolutionized the diagnosis, staging, management and follow-up of prostate cancer and it is regarded as the

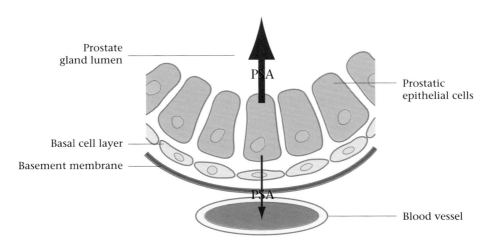

Figure 14.6. PSA is exclusively elaborated from the epithelial cells of the prostate and constitutes an important part of the prostatic secretions. Disruption of the basement membrane results in increased absorption and elevated PSA serum levels. (From ref. 49 with permission.)

most useful tumour marker in oncology today. PSA has been in widespread clinical use since 1987. Since that time it has been used as a marker to measure tumour recurrence after therapy and there have been many studies using it as a marker for early detection of prostate cancer.

Prostate cancer screening

The limited efficacy of current therapy for advanced prostate cancer and the rising death toll from the disease have led to a call for the introduction of prostate cancer screening to facilitate the diagnosis of localized disease.[13] Others have suggested the need for large-scale controlled studies of screening.[14]

This debate has important implications for both individual and public health but, unfortunately, decision-making has been hindered by inadequate data. Screening may reduce morbidity and mortality associated with prostatic carcinoma but as yet this hypothesis is unproven. Opponents to screening suggest that widespread testing may set off a cascade of diagnostic and treatment procedures with potentially serious complications, and the overall balance of benefits and harms is unclear (Table 14.1).

The economic implications of PSA screening are also difficult to quantify but, undoubtedly, testing all men over the age of 50 years would cost the country millions of pounds. Benoit and Naslund[15] have made an interesting comparison between the overall screening cost per prostate cancer detected in men in the USA aged 50–69 years (US$2372) and the overall screening cost per breast cancer detected in women aged 50–69 years (US$10,975). The criteria that need to be fulfilled for screening for a given disease to be acceptable were set out by Wilson and Jungner in 1969;[16] these are not met as yet, in the case of prostate cancer, owing to uncertainties in the natural history of the disease, lack of consensus in the management of some early tumours, and lack of randomized clinical trials.

The current recommendation by the American Cancer Society, the American Urological Association and the American College of Radiology is that men over

Table 14.1. Advantages and disadvantages of screening for prostate cancer

For	Against
• Simple tests available (PSA and DRE) • Detects early, potentially curable lesions • Reassures those who are screened as negative • May reduce prostate cancer morbidity and mortality • Many patients present with metastatic disease • This is an unpleasant disease to die from	• More likely to detect slow-growing tumours • Unproven efficacy in reducing mortality • Some cancers detected may never present clinically • False-positive findings cause anxiety • Expensive and time consuming • TRUS*-guided biopsy carries a 2% risk of serious infection • Active treatments may result in major complications such as incontinence or impotence • The need to wait for results of randomized clinical trials • Cost inefficient

*Transrectal ultrasound scan.

the age of 50 years should undergo an annual digital rectal examination (DRE) and serum PSA determination for the purpose of detecting early prostate cancer.[17,18] Annual screening should begin at the age of 40 years in African-American men or in patients with a known family history of prostate cancer. In the UK there is no enthusiasm for mass screening of the whole population but a case has been made for selective screening for certain high-risk groups in the population, and case finding in patients already in contact with the primary health care service.[19] In practice, more primary care physicians will case find; that is, they will screen patients who consult them because (a) they have symptoms of micturition difficulty (and they may also consult because of other medical problems but then reveal lower urinary tract symptoms), or (b) although asymptomatic, they are seeking advice or wanting to be checked.

Much debate centres on whether to proceed further to mass screening. Despite several pilot studies to assess the place of screening for prostate disease,[20] there is at present no support for mass screening until large-scale trials to establish benefit are conducted and published.[21–23]

The NHS Centre for Reviews and Dissemination has reviewed the evidence for screening[24] and published the following recommendations:

1. Routine testing of men to detect prostate cancer should be discouraged, irrespective of family history;
2. Purchasers should not fund screening services for prostate cancer;
3. Evidence from randomized controlled trials of prostate cancer screening using PSA (or similar tests) and treatment are needed before consideration is given to funding prostate screening;
4. Patients enquiring about prostate screening should be clearly informed about the current state of evidence on the benefits and harms of screening and treatment.

They have also published a document for men considering or asking for PSA tests.[25] This is available from the National Health Information Service, freephone 0800 66 55 44.

Prostatic cancer: risk groups

Those at particular risk for prostatic cancer are (a) those over 50 years of age with a family history of carcinoma of the prostate (those whose father or brother had prostate cancer are twice as likely to have the disease), and (b) those over 50 years of age in Black races (especially in the USA, where the age-adjusted incidence for Blacks is three to four times greater than for a White man in the UK).

Screening procedure

The components of the screening procedure are as follows:

1. Physical examination to include external genitalia and abdomen;
2. DRE;
3. PSA test, after discussion of the implications of the test with the patient.

Interpretation of the results of the PSA test is shown in Table 14.2. A rise of more than 20% per year should lead to an immediate referral for biopsy.

Who should be tested?

1. Available to all men over the age of 50 years;
2. Reduce the age limit to 40 years if family history of prostate cancer or Afro-Caribbean race;
3. All men who request PSA testing (after counselling);

Table 14.2. Interpretation of PSA values

PSA value (ng/ml)	Interpretation
0.5–4.0	Normal
4.0–10.0	20% chance of cancer
10.0	50+% chance of cancer

4. Case finding, not screening;
5. Prostate cancer patients on treatment or watchful waiting;
6. Before prescribing drugs for BPH;
7. Follow-up tests in BPH patients.

Other causes of PSA elevation

PSA may be significantly elevated after prostatic needle biopsy, transurethral resection of the prostate (TURP), urinary tract infection, prostatitis, retention of urine or ejaculation and it is wise to delay measuring serum PSA for at least 1 month after such procedures or events. In the case of ejaculation,[26] a 72 h delay is recommended.

DRE, prostatic massage and TRUS all have minimal effects on serum PSA levels in most patients.[27,28]

Is PSA testing accurate?

The true sensitivity and specificity of PSA screening is unknown as it is unethical for researchers to perform biopsies on men with normal PSA results. The test has a reported sensitivity of up to 80% in detecting prostate cancer in screened men,[29] but the test lacks specificity:[30] 25% of men with BPH have elevated PSA values and PSA values may also fluctuate by as much as 30% for physiological reasons.[31] Screening studies have shown a positive predictive value (PPV), using PSA, of 28–35%.[32–34] This situation has led to a search for techniques to improve the accuracy of PSA screening.

Methods to improve the accuracy of PSA testing

Ways of improving the accuracy of PSA testing include the use of the following:
1. Age-related PSA;
2. PSA velocity;
3. PSA density;
4. Free/complexed PSA ratio;
5. In combination with DRE (the American Cancer Society National Prostate Cancer Detection Project);
6. In combination with TRUS plus biopsy (the American Cancer Society National Prostate Cancer Detection Project).

Age-specific reference ranges of PSA

In Britain the most commonly used test (Hybritech) provides a PSA reference range of 0–4 ng/ml as a normal result. This is not appropriate for all men, since this single range does not account for age difference or the variations that can occur in prostatic volume. The increase in prostate size that occurs with age leads to increased levels of PSA production: 1 g BPH tissue gives rise to 0.2 ng/ml PSA in the serum.[35]

Other factors that increase PSA levels in older men include the following:
1. Chronic subclinical prostatitis;

2. Prostatic intra-epithelial neoplasia (PIN);
3. Ischaemia or infarction;
4. Changes in the normal physiological barrier in the prostatic ducts;
5. Leakage of PSA into capillaries and lymphatics.

In order to clarify the situation, Oesterling and co-workers[36] studied 471 Caucasians aged 40–79 years who had no evidence of prostatic cancer, by DRE, PSA testing or TRUS (Figure 14.7) and produced an age-specific reference range (Table 14.3). Using this method of interpretation increases the sensitivity of PSA in younger men, who can therefore benefit from definitive treatment, and it increases the specificity of PSA in older men, who are less likely to benefit from medical intervention.

PSA velocity

PSA velocity (PSAV) is a measurement of the change in serum PSA over time. This PSA slope is formed by measuring and plotting sequential PSA values (Figure 14.8). Clinically significant prostate cancer is composed of actively dividing cells that elaborate PSA (unless they are very poorly differentiated). Whereas normal prostate tissue and BPH have only very slow cell division rates, patients with prostate cancer might be expected to show sequential PSA rises. This has been confirmed in a small retrospective study,[37] in which a PSAV of at least 0.75 ng/ml per year resulted in the correct identification of 72% of cancer subjects (sensitivity 72%) and the correct

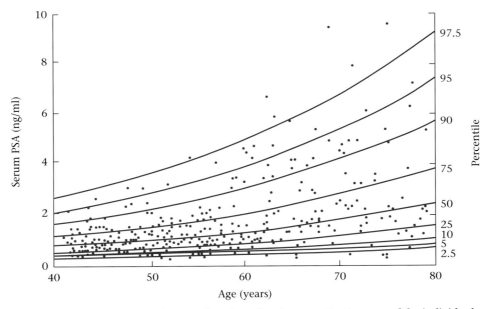

Figure 14.7. Serum PSA concentration as a function of patient age. Scattergram of the individual serum PSA values of 471 men. (From ref. 36 with permission from the American Medical Association.)

Table 14.3. Age-specific reference range for PSA

Age (years)	PSA (ng/ml)
40–49	2.5
50–59	3.5
60–69	4.5
70–79	6.5

(From ref. 8 with permission.)

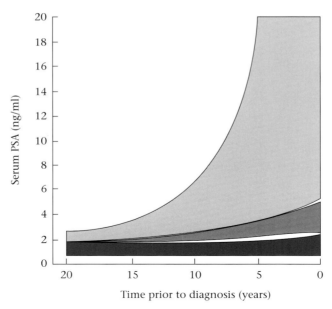

Figure 14.8. Average curves of PSA levels (ng/ml) as a function of years before diagnosis for three diagnostic groups (BPH patients ■, local/regional cancer and metastatic cancer ▨ and a control group ■). (From ref. 8 with permission.)

identification of 92% of BPH subjects (specificity 92%). The authors concluded that PSAV was a potentially useful tool in distinguishing benign and malignant disease and this method of follow-up might be helpful in the early detection of prostate cancer in men with a normal DRE and a normal PSA.

Unfortunately, the interassay estimation of PSA values is subject to a variation of 8–15% in the same patient;[38] at least three determinations should be used to calculate the velocity value and, ideally, these should be made at least a year apart.

Discrepancy in serum PSA levels between different immunoassays can quickly make the evaluation process inaccurate and confusing, and it is important to check that the same methodology has been used on each subject.

Free/complexed PSA ratio
PSA is a powerful protease enzyme that, when present in plasma in a concentration of one million times less than in seminal fluid, is largely bound to one of two inhibitors — α_1-antichymotrypsin (ACT), and α_2-macroglobulin (AMG). AMG completely envelops the PSA molecule and shields all the antigen from the antigen assay, whereas ACT shields only some of the antigenic surface (Figure 14.9), thus enabling the various bound and unbound forms to be distinguished.

The complexed form of PSA and ACT inactivates the protease effects of PSA, and the PSA–AMG complex is also inactivated. Different pathological conditions of the prostate appear to manifest differing patterns of serum-binding of PSA forms. Lilja and co-workers[39] found a median of 18% free PSA in carcinoma and 28% free PSA in BPH, and Christensson *et al.*[40] also confirmed that the complexed/total ratio was significantly higher in patients with prostate cancer than in patients with BPH, free PSA constituting a significantly smaller fraction in cancer patients than in patients with BPH. When this is applied to age-specific reference ranges (Table 14.4),[41] the free/total PSA ratio may increase the ability of PSA to distinguish early prostate cancer accurately from BPH.[40]

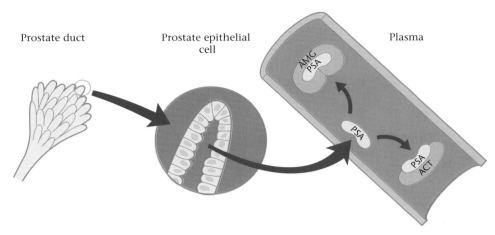

Figure 14.9. PSA is elaborated by epithelial cells within the prostate. In the plasma it may occur as free PSA or conjugated to either ACT or AMG. (From ref. 8 with permission.)

Table 14.4. Age-specific reference ranges (ng/ml) for free (F), complexed (C) and total (T) PSA*

Molecular form of PSA	Age group (years)			
	40–49	50–59	60–69	70–79
F	0.5	0.75	1.0	1.5
C	1.5	2.0	2.5	3.5
T	2.5	3.5	4.5	6.5

(From ref. 41 with permission.)

PSA density

This is not easily measured in primary care because it requires TRUS, which is normally performed by a urologist. The calculation of PSA density (PSAD) depends on the observation that the PSA values in BPH tend to rise proportionately to the volume of the gland. Thus, a correction of the BPH contribution to the PSA value can be made by dividing the PSA value by the gland volume (in cm^3), as calculated by TRUS, to give the PSAD.[42] Values above 0.15 are regarded as suspicious of malignancy.

This concept has been criticized on the grounds that not all BPH tissues elaborate predictable quantities of PSA because the ratio of stroma to glandular tissue is very variable; in addition to this, TRUS measurements of prostate volume are operator dependent and therefore subject to significant variability.

PSAD appears to have some utility in distinguishing BPH from prostate cancer and in identifying those patients with prostate cancer who have mildly elevated or intermediate PSA levels and a normal DRE. However, if age-specific reference ranges are used, PSAD does not provide additional clinical information,[43] and in primary care the use of a specific range is a more practical approach (Figure 14.10)

PSA measurements: management of benign disease

The management of BPH in primary care allows the use of watchful waiting, α-blockers or finasteride. Therapy with α-blockers will not have any impact on the

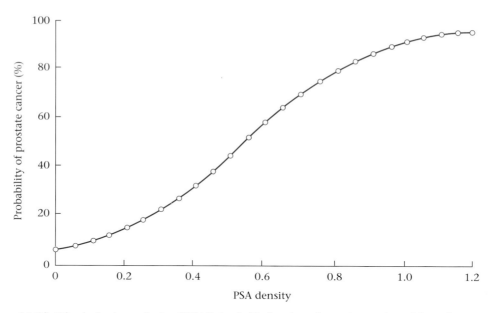

Figure 14.10. Discriminate analysis of PSAD (ng/ml/ml) values for patients whose PSA values are between 4.1 and 10.1 ng/ml. (From ref. 50 with permission from W.B. Saunders Company.)

PSA level but this is not the case with finasteride. This drug is a synthetic 4-azasteroid compound that competitively inhibits 5α-reductase, an enzyme that converts testosterone to dihydrotestosterone (DHT).[44] The drug works by reducing the size of the prostate gland and a decrease of 20% has been recorded after 6 months treatment.[45] The effect on PSA levels was studied by Gormley and co-workers,[46] who noted a 50% decrease in PSA levels at 3 months in patients receiving finasteride (5 mg/day). This caused concern that the use of this drug might mask the presence of prostate cancer. However, a study performed by Guess and co-workers showed that finasteride did not appear to have a greater effect on PSA of malignant origin than on PSA of benign origin.[47]

Clinicians should have an increased suspicion of prostate cancer when a patient on finasteride therapy has not recorded the expected 50% decline from the baseline serum PSA level. It is, therefore, crucial to measure the baseline PSA before starting treatment with finasteride and to check compliance with medication if the PSA fails to fall by 50% after the first 6 months of treatment.[46] Failure to achieve the expected PSA reduction should lead to referral to a urologist.

Summary and conclusions

A Cinderella subject for many years, the prostate has recently become the focus of intense medical and public interest. The exciting advances made in the development of new techniques for investigating patients with prostatic disease, and the advent of effective drug therapy, have led to the involvement of the primary care physician. This progress, together with a heightened awareness of the considerable prevalence of these diseases, has been reflected in the media, which have brought prostatic diseases to the awareness of the public.

As the expectations of our ever-swelling ranks of middle-aged and elderly populations increase, men with prostate problems are presenting to us in greater and greater numbers. Shared care for prostatic disease will enable primary care physicians and urologists to provide these men with the best-quality and most cost-effective care.

The PSA test allows the primary care physician to be reasonably confident that he is managing BPH and not prostate cancer, and allows him to follow the patient up with an awareness that prostate cancer may well develop at a later stage.

The uncertainties of screening for prostate cancer must be acknowledged when physicians counsel patients, and the use of this test should be neither recommended nor discouraged without first ensuring that the patient has complete information about the potential benefits and risks.

Before deciding to be tested, the patient should consider what procedures will follow a positive result and whether he would want to be treated if cancer were diagnosed. In particular, men with a life expectancy of less than 10 years should be advised that screening and treatment are unlikely to be helpful and may well lead to a deterioration in their quality of life.

A prostate assessment in men under the age of 50 is not recommended because the detection rate of abnormalities is extremely low unless there is a family history of the disease.

Interpretation of a PSA test result is not straightforward because values may vary according to the test used and there is debate about the definition of normal values. As a result of this, methods to improve the diagnostic accuracy of the test have been developed.

The primary care physician has an important role to play in monitoring patients with diagnosed prostate cancer. This role will vary according to the facilities offered by the urologist and by the particular interests of the primary care physician. This relationship becomes more important when the patient either fails primary hormone control or develops progressive disease after radical treatment.

When orchiectomy is chosen as the primary treatment, the follow-up may well be carried out in the community or by the urologist. When monthly, or 3-monthly luteinizing hormone-releasing hormone treatments are prescribed, these are usually given in the primary care setting; this requires symptoms and signs to be monitored regularly and the PSA to be repeated at 6-monthly intervals to assess progress.

This test is a valuable monitor of prostate cancer, but problems may arise when the patient becomes focused on the PSA value, particularly when there is a rising PSA in the absence of any clinical or symptomatic change. It is at this stage that a referral back to the urologist will almost certainly be necessary and when a decision on second-line treatment will have to be made.

Shared care is clearly the way forward for managing patients with prostatic disease and, as a result of this, a great deal of responsibility is going to be placed on the primary care physician. Interpretation of the PSA test is a critical factor in the management of these patients and the communication of current knowledge to primary care physicians is critical. The result will be of benefit to primary care physicians and urologists and, most importantly, to patients with prostatic diseases.

References

1. Garraway W M, Collins G N, Lee R J. High prevalence of benign prostatic hypertrophy in the community. Lancet 1991; 338: 469–471
2. OPCS. Mortality data — 1990. In: OPCS Series DH2, 1992
3. Moller-Jensen O, Esteve J, Moller H, Renard H. Cancer in the European Community and its member states. Eur J Cancer 1990; 26: 1167–1256
4. Murphy G P, Natarajan N, Pontes J E *et al.* The national survey of prostate cancer in the United States by the American College of Surgeons. J Urol 1982; 127: 928–934

5. Muir C S, Nectoux J, Staszewski J. The epidemiology of prostatic cancer. Geographic distribution and time-trends. Acta Oncol 1991; 30: 133–140
6. Lytton B. Epidemiology of prostate cancer. Urol Top 1993; 68: 114–116
7. Kirby R S, Oesterling J E, Denis L J. Prostate cancer. Fast Facts. Oxford: Health Press, 1996
8. Kirby R, Kirby M, Fitzpatrick J, Fitzpatrick A. Shared care for prostatic diseases. Oxford: Isis Medical Media, 1994
9. Lundwall A, Lilja H. Molecular cloning of human prostate specific antigen cDNA. FEBS Lett 1987; 214: 317–322
10. Lilja H. A kallikrein-like serine protease in prostatic fluid cleaves the predominant seminal vesicle protein. J Clin Invest 1985; 76: 1899–1903
11. Oesterling J. Prostate specific antigen: a critical assessment of the most useful tumor marker for adenocarcinoma of the prostate. J Urol 1991; 145: 907–923
12. Schellhammer P, Wright G Jr. Biomolecular and clinical characteristics of PSA and other candidate prostate tumor markers. Urol Clin North Am 1993; 20: 597–606
13. Yamanaka H. Incidence and prevention of prostate cancer. Asian Med J 1993; 36: 91–95
14. Schroder F H. Prostate cancer: to screen or not to screen? Br Med J 1993; 306: 407–408
15. Benoit N, Naslund MJ. An economic rationale for prostate cancer screening. Urology 1994; 44: 795–803
16. Wilson J M G, Jungner G. Principles and practice of screening for disease. Geneva: WHO, 1969; 1–34
17. Mettlin C, Jones G, Averette H et al. Defining and updating the American Cancer Society guidelines for the cancer-related checkup: prostate and endometrial cancers. CA 1993; 43: 42–46
18. American Urological Association. Early detection of prostate cancer and use of transrectal ultrasound. In: American Urological Association 1992 Policy Statement Book, Vol 4. Baltimore: American Urological Association, 1992: 20
19. Holland W W, Stewart S. Screening in health care. Nuffield Provincial Hospital Trust, 1990
20. Kirby R S, Kirby M G, Feneley M R et al. Screening for carcinoma of the prostate: a GP based study. Br J Urol 1994; 74: 64–71
21. Brawer M K, Chetner M P, Beattie J et al. Screening for prostatic carcinoma with prostate specific antigen. J Urol 1992; 147: 841–845
22. Benson M C, Whang I S, Panteuck A et al. Prostate specific antigen density; a means of distinguishing between benign prostatic hypertrophy and prostate cancer. J Urol 1992; 147: 815–816
23. Carter B H, Pearson J D, Metter J et al. Longitudinal evaluation of prostate specific antigen levels in men with and without prostate cancer. JAMA 1993; 267: 2215–2220
24. NHS Centre for Reviews and Dissemination. Recommendations. In: Screening for prostate cancer. Effectiveness matters, Vol. 2(2). Heslington, York: University of York, 1997: 3
25. NHS Centre for Reviews and Dissemination. Screening for prostate cancer: the evidence. Information for men considering or asking for PSA tests. Effectiveness matters. Heslington, York: University of York, 1997: 4pp
26. Simbak R, Madersbacher S, Zhang Z F. Impact of ejaculation on serum PSA. J Urol 1996; 150: 895–897
27. Chybowski F, Bergstrahl E, Oesterling J. The effect of digital rectal examination on the serum prostate specific antigen concentration: results of a randomized study. J Urol 1992; 148: 83–86
28. Yuan J, Coplen D, Petros J et al. Effects of rectal examination, prostatic massage, ultrasonography and needle biopsy on serum prostate specific antigen levels. J Urol 1992; 147: 810–814
29. Catalona W J, Richie J P, Ahmann F R et al. Comparison of digital rectal examination and serum prostate specific antigen in the early detection of prostate cancer: results of a multicenter clinical trial of 6,630 men. J Urol 1994; 151: 1283–1290
30. Oesterling J E. Prostate specific antigen: a critical assessment of the most useful tumor marker for adenocarcinoma of the prostate. J Urol 1991; 145: 907-923
31. Stamey T A, Prestigiacomo A, Komatsu K. Physiological variation of serum prostate specific antigen (PSA) from a screening population in the range of 4–10 ng/ml using the Hybritech Tandem-R PSA assay. J Urol 1995; 153(Suppl): 420A (abstr)
32. Cooner W H, Mosley B R, Rutherford C L Jr et al. Prostate cancer detection in a clinical urological practice by ultrasonography, digital rectal examination and prostate specific antigen. J Urol 1990; 143: 1146–1152

33. Catalona W J, Richie J P, Ahmann F R *et al.* Comparison of digital rectal examination and serum prostate specific antigen in the early detection of prostate cancer: results of a multicenter clinical trial of 6,630 men. J Urol 1994; 151: 1283–1290

34. Catalona W J, Smith D S, Ratliff T L, Basler J W. Detection of organ-confined prostate cancer is increased through prostate-specific antigen-based screening. JAMA 1993; 270: 948–954

35. Stamey T, Yang N, Hay A *et al.* Prostate-specific antigen as a serum marker for adenocarcinoma of the prostate. N Engl J Med 1987; 317: 909–916

36. Oesterling J, Jacobsen S, Chute C *et al.* Serum prostate-specific antigen in a community-based population of healthy men: establishment of age-specific reference ranges. JAMA 1993; 270: 860–864

37. Carter H B, Pearson J D, Metter J *et al.* Longitudinal evaluation of prostate specific antigen levels in men with and without prostate cancer. JAMA 1993; 267: 2215–2220

38. Guess H A, Heyse J F, Gormley G J. The effect of finasteride on prostate specific antigen in men with benign prostatic hyperplasia. Prostate 1993; 22: 31–37

39. Lilja H, Christensson A, Dahlen U *et al.* Prostate-specific antigen in serum occurs predominantly in complex with alpha-1 antichymotrypsin. Clin Chem 1991; 37: 1618–1625

40. Christensson A, Bjork T, Nilsson O *et al.* Serum prostate specific antigen complexed to alpha-1-antichymotrypsin as an indicator of prostate cancer. J Urol 1993; 150: 100-105

41. Oesterling J, Jacobsen S, Klee G *et al.* Free, complexed, and total serum PSA: establishment of age-specific reference ranges using newly developed immunofluorometric assays (IFMA). J Urol 1994; 151: 311A

42. Benson M C, Whang I S, Panteuck A *et al.* Prostate specific antigen density; a means of distinguishing between benign prostatic hypertrophy and prostate cancer. J Urol 1992; 147: 815–816

43. Oesterling J, Cooner W, Jacobsen S *et al.* Influence of patient age on the serum PSA concentration: an important clinical observation. Urol Clin North Am 1993; 20: 671-680

44. Rasmusson G. Biochemistry and pharmacology of 5-alpha-reductase inhibitors. In: Furr B, Wakeling A (eds) Pharmacology and clinical uses of inhibitors of hormone secretion and action. London: Baillière Tindall, 1987: 308–325

45. McConnell J. Current medical therapy for benign prostate hyperplasia: the scientific basis and clinical efficacy of finasteride and alpha-blockers. In: Walsh P, Retik A, Stamey T, Vaughn E Jr (eds) Campbell's Urology, 6th edn. Update no.3. Philadelphia: Saunders, 1992: 1–12

46. Gormley G, Stoner E, Bruskewitz R *et al.* The effect of finasteride in men with benign prostatic hyperplasia. N Engl J Med 1992; 327: 1185–1191

47. Guess H, Heyse J, Gormley G *et al.* Effect of finasteride on serum PSA concentration in men with benign prostatic hyperplasia: results from the North American phase III clinical trial. Urol Clin North Am 1993; 20: 627–636

48. Kirby R S, Oesterling J E, Denis L J. Prostate cancer. Fast Facts. Oxford: Health Press, 1996

49. Kirby R S, McConnell J D. Benign prostatic hyperplasia. Fast Facts. Oxford: Health Press, 1996

50. Seaman E, Whang I, Olsson C *et al.* PSA density (PSAD): role in patient evaluation and management. Urol Clin North Am 1993; 20: 653–663

Chapter 15

Prostate-specific antigen as a screening test for prostate cancer: a nested serum sample study

R. S. Kirby, C. Parkes and N. J. Wald

Introduction

In 1993 there were 9530 deaths from prostate cancer in the United Kingdom — the second commonest cause of death from cancer in men. In the USA nearly 400,000 men died from prostate cancer in 1996. Over 90% of deaths occur in men aged over 65 years. Prostate-specific antigen (PSA) (Figure 15.1) is a glycoprotein protease produced only by the prostate gland; its function is to liquefy semen, and low concentrations are normally found in serum (< 4.0 ng/ml) as a result of its absorption across the basement membrane of prostatic acini. As a tumour marker in the diagnosis and management of prostate cancer, concentrations of PSA have been shown to increase with increasing stage of the cancer[1] and increasing tumour volume,[2] but there are insufficient data to evaluate adequately its performance as a screening test for preclinical prostate cancer among apparently healthy men. Studies of men with lower urinary tract symptoms which are mainly the result of benign prostatic hyperplasia (BPH) would be expected to produce

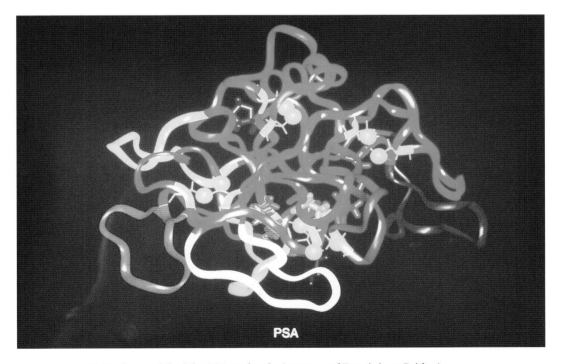

Figure 15.1. Molecular model of the PSA molecule (courtesy of Dominique Bridon).

greater false positive rates. In studies of asymptomatic men in which prostate biopsies were performed only in those with positive results of tests for PSA, the detection rate (sensitivity) of the test cannot be estimated because cancers were not sought in men who screened negative. The results could also be distorted by including so-called incidental prostate cancers that may never have presented clinically. The authors therefore designed a collaborative study to avoid these problems by using stored frozen serum samples collected from four prospective epidemiological studies.

Methods

The project was based on four cohorts totalling 49,261 healthy men: these were the BUPA study[3] (London), the CLUE study[4] (United States), the North Karelia project[5] and the Social Insurance Institution mobile clinic health survey[6] (both in Finland). Serum taken from the men on recruitment was frozen and stored at −70°C. Of men from whom a serum sample was available, 265 (cases) subsequently developed clinical prostate cancer or died of prostate cancer. Of the cases of prostate cancer, 120 were ascertained from national death records and 145 from cancer registries. A nested case–control study was used. Controls were men from the same study who had not developed prostate cancer at the end of follow-up. Five controls were selected per case, except in the CLUE study (two controls selected per case), making a total of 1055. Controls were matched with each case for age at the time of serum collection (within 1 year), duration of storage of the sample (collected within the same year), and the number of freeze–thaw cycles; they were otherwise selected at random. The median age at entry was 57 years (5th–95th percentile 45–68 years). Cases were followed up for a median of 17.5 years and controls for 17.4 years (range 10–20 years).

Samples from each subject were retrieved from storage and assayed in blinded fashion without knowledge of which were from cases or controls by using Tandem R-prostate specific antigen radioimmunoassay kits (Hybritech Tandem-R) at the Wolfson Institute of Preventive Medicine, London. Measurement of serum PSA is not materially affected by freezing and thawing.[7]

In the controls there was no significant change in the concentration of the antigen with duration of storage or number of freeze–thaw cycles, but there were unexplained differences in concentrations between centres. For example, at 50 years of age the median concentrations in the controls were 0.75, 0.75, 0.60 and 0.47 ng/ml in the four centres. The median concentrations in the controls increased with age by 3.7% per year. In the BUPA study the medians at age 50, 60 and 70 years were 0.75, 1.08 and 1.55 ng/ml, respectively. In the analysis the matching was broken and, to allow for variation with centre and age, each PSA concentration was expressed as a multiple of the median for a given centre and age and referred to as the 'level'. The 'normal' medians were derived from the controls by using a weighted linear regression of median concentration on age (in 5-year age groups) for each centre.

Detection rate (sensitivity) was defined as the proportion of cases in the study with a level of PSA above a specified cutoff level. The false positive rate (1-specificity) was defined as the proportion of controls with a value above the same level.

Results

Table 15.1 shows the number of cases from each centre according to the interval between blood collection and diagnosis of prostate cancer. Table 15.2 shows the

Table 15.1. Number of men who developed prostate cancer from each centre according to observation time between blood collection and diagnosis of prostate cancer

Observation time (years)	Centre				All
	BUPA, London	Washington County, Maryland United States	North Karelia, Finland	Social Insurance Institution Finland	
< 3	4	8	0	4	16
3 – <6	12	8	1	8	29
6 – <10	24	10	4	18	56
> 10	35	64	31	34	164
All	75	90	36	64	265

Table 15.2. Level of serum PSA according to observation time between blood collection and diagnosis of prostate cancer

Observation time (years)	PSA (multiples of median*)		
	10th Centile	Median	90th Centile
< 3	8.6	23	58
3 – <6	1.8	4.0	25
6 – <9	1.0	3.6	9.4
≥ 10	0.5	1.8	6.0
All	0.7	2.6	10

*Multiple of median of controls of same age and from same centre.
(Modified from ref. 22, with permission from the BMJ Publishing Group.)

median levels of PSA and the 10th and 90th percentiles for the cases for all centres combined, expressed in multiples of the median. Median levels declined as the interval between blood collection and date of diagnosis increased. With an interval of less than 3 years the median level in cases was 23 multiples of the median. Thereafter it declined rapidly but was raised even as long as 10 years (1.8 multiples of the median, $p < 0.001$, t test) before diagnosis. Figure 15.2 shows the individual results of the 265 cases.

Table 15.3 shows the proportions with levels of PSA greater than or equal to specified values for cancers diagnosed within 3, 6 and 10 years and for controls. By using a cutoff level of 12 multiples of the median, the detection rates for the three observation times were, respectively, 81, 40 and 22%, with a false-positive rate of only 0.5%. Detection was greater in patients who died — 89% (8/9), 65% (13/20) and 33% (17/52), respectively. The results were similar if only cases diagnosed between 1 and 3 years after blood collection were included (that is, excluding the first year). As the median age of cases was similar for those presenting less than 3 years, 3–5, 6–9 and 10 or more years after collection (61, 60, 60 and 57 years, respectively), the early cases were not concentrated in the older men.

The distribution of serum PSA expressed in multiples of the median in cases and controls fitted a log Gaussian distribution well (values were higher than expected only above the 95th percentile in cases and the 99.5th percentile in controls). Figure 15.3 shows the Gaussian distributions in patients who developed prostate cancer within 3 years and in controls; the small overlap between the two

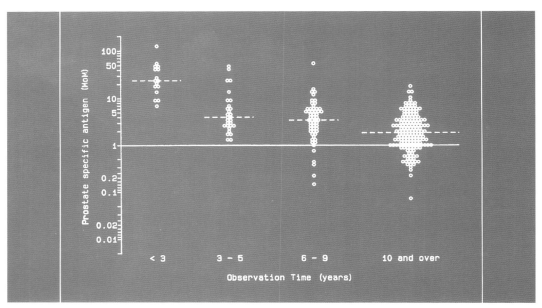

Figure 15.2. Concentration of serum PSA in men who developed clinical prostate cancer according to the interval between blood collection and date of diagnosis (modified from ref. 22, with permission from the BMJ Publishing Group).

Table 15.3. Percentage of cases and controls with levels of PSA above or equal to specified values of multiples of median according to observation time between blood collection and diagnosis of clinical prostate cancer.

PSA (multiples of median*)	Percentage of controls (false positive rate)	Percentages of cases (detection rate)		
		Less than 3 years[†] ($n = 16$)	Less than 6 years ($n = 45$)	Less than 10 years ($n = 101$)
≥ 4	5.4	100 (79–100)	67 (51–80)	54 (45–64)
≥ 6	1.9	100 (79–100)	58 (42–72)	38 (28–47)
≥ 8	1.3	94 (70–100)	49 (34–64)	31 (22–40)
≥ 12	0.5	81 (54–96)	40 (26–56)	22 (14–30)
≥ 16	0.2	75 (48–93)	36 (22–51)	17 (10–24)

*Multiple of median controls of same age and from same centre.
[†]When cases diagnosed within 1 year of sample collection are removed (four cases), detection rates are 100, 100, 92, 83, 75% in the groups.
n = Number of men who developed clinical prostate cancer.
(Modified from ref. 22, with permission from the BMJ Publishing Group.)

curves illustrates the potential value of PSA as a screening test for prostate cancer, in contrast to other serum markers such as cholesterol in coronary heart disease.

To determine if there were any cases of no clinical consequence diagnosed incidentally at necropsy, the records of the 41 cases notified only at necropsy were examined: in 36, prostate cancer was the certified cause of death, not an incidental finding; the five remaining cases occurred over 10 years after blood collection and did not therefore affect the results up to 10 years.

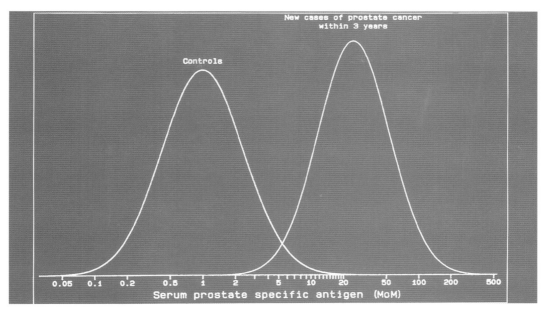

Figure 15.3. Relative frequency distribution of serum PSA in men who developed prostate cancer within 3 years of sample collection and in controls (modified from ref. 22, with permission from the BMJ Publishing Group).

Discussion

The results of this study suggest that a single measurement of the concentration of PSA in healthy men effectively distinguished between men who did and did not develop clinical prostate cancer. By using a cutoff level of 12 multiples of the median, the detection rate over a 3-year period was 81% and the false-positive rate was 0.5%. Although this estimate of detection was based on only 16 cases, the lower limit of the 95% confidence interval was 54%, which represents a reasonable screening performance with a 0.5% false-positive rate.

Our study design, testing asymptomatic men and following up all until either death or clinical presentation with cancer, provides an unbiased evaluation of measurement of PSA as a screening test. It avoided bias from linking levels of PSA with incidental prostate cancer, which is common in elderly men (about one third of prostates examined at routine necropsy have been found to have cancer)[8–10] or from linking levels with prostate cancer in men with prostatic symptoms.

Five other studies similar to that described here have been reported recently.[11–15] Because the studies use different periods of observation, cutoff levels of antigen, ages of men, and assays, direct comparison is complicated. Three of the published reports[11–13] permit a comparison with the results of this study if cutoff levels yielding a 12% false-positive rate are used with an observation time of 5 years to diagnosis. The corresponding detection rates would be 95%[12] (19 cases), 84% (32 cases, this study), 66%[13] (113 cases) and 56%[11] (25 cases). The pooled estimate is 78% (189 cases combined by weighting by inverse of the variance). The results reported here are consistent with the data of others.

Because PSA values are known to increase slowly with age, it is important to adjust for this when interpreting PSA. By using a cutoff of 4 ng/ml (which has been widely cited in the literature), the false-positive rate increased from 0% for men aged under 50 to 26% for men aged 70 years or over (see Table 15.4). Table 15.4 shows how such a cutoff fails to allow for age and yields too high a false-positive rate for use in screening. The effect of age in our study was allowed for by

Table 15.4 Serum PSA and subsequent clinical prostate cancer: detection and false-positive rates with cutoff for PSA of 4 ng/ml (≥ 4 ng/ml) according to age at blood collection and time to diagnosis of cancer

Age (years)	Detection rate			
	No. (%) at < 3 years	No. (%) at < 6 years	No. (%) at < 10 years	No. (%) of false-positive results
< 50	2/2 (100)	3/3 (100)	4/7 (57)	0/130 (0)
50–59	5/5 (100)	12/16 (75)	19/40 (48)	18/250 (3.5)
60–69	7/7 (100)	13/20 (65)	28/45 (62)	31/366 (8.5)
≥ 70	2/2 (100)	4/6 (67)	6/9 (67)	10/39 (26)
All	16/16 (100)	32/45 (71)	57/101 (56)	59/1055 (5.6)

expressing concentration of PSA as a multiple of the normal median for controls of the same age.

The age-specific false-positive rates reported here are consistent with those reported in other studies.[16,17] For a cutoff concentration of 4 ng/ml, Catalona and his colleagues reported a false-positive rate of 2.1% in the age group 50–59 and 6.7% in the age group 60–69[17], close to the results of 3.5 and 8.5% in this study.

Levels of PSA were raised many years before prostate cancer presented clinically. Even more than 10 years (median 14) before clinical presentation, the median level was 1.8 multiples of the median. Since prostate cancer is generally a slow-growing tumour form of cancer, with a cell doubling time that is often as long as 2 years, this observation is not surprising. Clearly this prolonged interval between PSA elevation and clinical presentation may offer an opportunity for early detection and potential cure by radical surgery or radiotherapy.

The authors' data, like those of others,[12] suggested that a test for PSA was more discriminatory for future prostate cancer in younger than in older men. As age increases, the false-positive rate rises and the detection rate falls (see Table 15.4). This effect is best demonstrated by holding the false-positive rate constant; within 3 years the age effect was not discernible, but for cancer developing within 6 years the detection rate (corresponding to a 5% false-positive rate) for men under 58 years was 77% (10/13) compared with 53% (17/32) in older men. At a false-positive rate of 0.5%, the detection rates were 54% (7/13) and 34% (11/32), respectively.

The odds that men with a raised level of PSA will present clinically with prostate cancer depend on the cutoff level and the prevalence of clinical prostate cancer in the age group. The prevalence of prostate cancer in men aged 60–74 years is about 0.8% (estimated from the weighted average product of the incidence and the median survival)[18]. Those with concentrations greater than or equal to12 multiples of the median will have an approximately even (about 50%) chance of presenting with prostate cancer in the next 3 years (derived by comparing the incidence over 3 years multiplied by the detection rate with the false-positive rate from Table 15.3). This estimate will not be materially affected by the fact that the age group 60–74 years is somewhat older than the men in this study. Restriction of measurement of the antigen to men aged 60 or more would not miss all that many cases in the population because prostate cancer is a disease of older men; 98% of deaths in England and Wales occur in men aged 60 or more, although preclinical lesions may of course be present in many younger men.

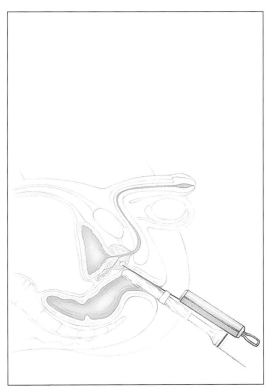

Figure 15.4. Technique of transrectal ultrasound guided prostate biopsy. (Reproduced with permission from Kirby R, Fitzpatrick J, Kirby M and Fitzpatrick A, Shared Care for Prostatic Diseases, Isis Medical Media *1994, p 67.)*

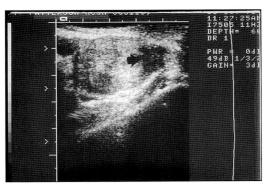

Figure 15.5. Sagittal transrectal ultrasound image of the prostate demonstrating a hypoechoic area (arrowed) characteristic of prostate cancer.

In a screening programme men with positive results would be referred for a diagnostic transrectal biopsy (Figure 15.4) at various sites of the prostate under ultrasound guidance (Figure 15.5). Pathological diagnosis (Figure 15.6) of cancer would be followed by radical prostatectomy (Figure 15.7) radiotherapy or hormonal treatment. The value of different treatments is uncertain since randomised, controlled studies have yet to be completed. It has even been suggested that early prostate cancer should be conservatively managed with active treatment only if there is evidence of spread.[19] The most appropriate treatment and the associated adverse effects, such as incontinence and erectile dysfunction, are currently being evaluated in randomized controlled studies in North America and Scandinavia (see Chapter 31).

Our study[22] shows that the measurements of serum PSA in men aged 60 years or more effectively predict future clinical prostate cancer. Whether this can lead to treatment that could reduce mortality and morbidity from the disease is unknown and can be assessed only in a randomized trial of men invited for screening and in controls not invited for screening. A randomized trial of treatment among those allocated to the screened group may also be needed. With evidence on efficacy and an estimate of the size of any benefit, a judgement could be made on whether screening for prostate cancer is worthwhile. Even a 30% reduction in deaths from prostate cancer among men aged 60–74 would save about 900 lives each year in England and Wales and many more internationally.

Recently the NHS technology review group[20] has called for a UK-based study on PSA-based screening. In fact, two randomized studies of prostate cancer screening are already underway — the prostate, lung and colon (PLC) cancer screening study in the USA[21] and the European randomized study of screening centred at Rotterdam. Data relating to any survival advantage stemming from PSA screening will not be available, however, for many years. There are concerns, moreover, especially in the USA about contamination of the control arm by widespread *ad hoc* PSA testing which may obscure any survival advantage derived from the measurement of this tumour marker.

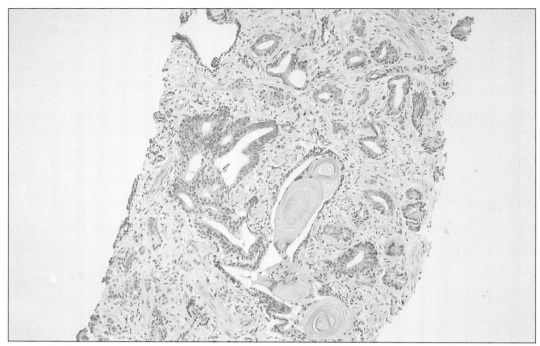

Figure 15.6. A prostate biopsy core containing moderately differentiated prostate cancer.

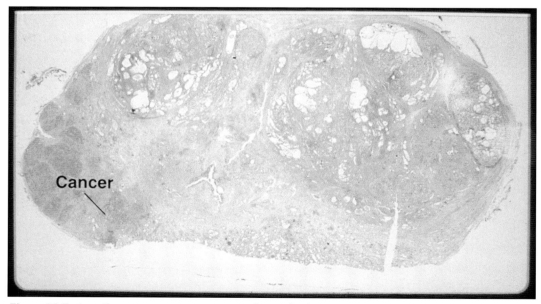

Figure 15.7. A section across a prostate removed at radical prostatectomy revealing a sizeable cancer in the right peripheral zone.

In the meantime what is the concerned clinician to do? Providing full information to the patient and his family is paramount, including an explanation of the implications of testing positive, and the current uncertainty about survival benefit. Studies such as the authors'[22] cannot provide the answers to these important questions, but they do provide some reassurance that PSA testing does appear to detect early cancers which are indeed destined to become clinically manifest, with resultant morbidity, rather than microscopic foci of latent carcinoma. As such it appears to afford the possibility of identifying curable lesions while they are still confined to the prostate and the current suggestion from America is that this technology, now refined by differential assays of free to total PSA, may at last allow us to turn back the steadily rising tide of deaths from this insidious malignancy.

Summary and conclusions

PSA testing can undoubtedly detect considerable numbers of asymptomatic individuals who harbour foci of prostatic adenocarcinoma. However, concerns have been raised that many of the lesions thus identified would never have become clinically manifest within the natural life span of the affected individual and recently PSA testing has been discouraged by the NHS technology group.[20]

In order to address this important question, the nested case–control study described here was conducted with stored serum samples collected from 49,261 men, with follow-up using the national death and cancer registration systems.

The serum from 265 asymptomatic men and 1055 controls matched for age, study centre and duration of storage were analysed for PSA values using the Hybritech monoclonal PSA immunoassay system to determine the distribution of PSA values in those who did and did not develop prostate cancer.

PSA concentrations were significantly higher in men who subsequently developed prostate cancer than in controls. In the first 3 years after blood collection the median concentration was 23 times greater in the cases than in the controls of the same age (that is 23 multiples of the median). A smaller difference persisted thereafter — 4.0 multiples of the median 3–6 years after blood collection, 3.6 between 6 and 10 years and 1.8 after 10 years. In the first 3 years, the proportion of men who developed prostate cancer and had raised levels of PSA (> 12 multiples of the median) (i.e. detection rate or sensitivity) was 81% (95% confidence intervals 54–96%) The proportion of men who did not develop prostate cancer but had levels this high (false-positive rate) was only 0.5%.[22]

These data confirm that PSA measurement is highly discriminatory between men who do and do not develop prostate cancer. Men with a PSA value more than 12 times the multiple of the median appear to have around a 50% chance of developing prostate cancer within the next 3 years. This study confirms that PSA screening does not appear to identify men with clinically insignificant disease, but rather those who harbour disease that is destined to progress. Measurement of this antigen is a good enough screening test to justify randomized studies of screening to determine any reduction of mortality from prostate cancer.

Acknowledgements

The data in this chapter have been previously published in a peer-reviewed Journal.[22] The authors would like to thank Hybritech Ltd for providing the PSA testing kits and Philip Murphy, Lynne George and Hilary Watts for their help with the study. The authors would also like to thank Paul Knekt, K.J. Hetzlsouer and J. Tuomilehto for providing frozen serum samples and information on the outcome of their patient subsets.

References

1. Hudson M A, Bahnson R R, Catalona W J. Clinical use of prostate specific antigen in patients with prostate cancer. J Urol 1989; 142: 1011–1017

2.   Palken M, Cobb O E, Warren B H, Hoak D C. Prostate cancer: correlation of digital rectal examination, transrectal ultrasound and prostate specific antigen levels with tumour volumes in radical prostatectomy specimens. J Urol 1990; 143: 1155–1162

3.   Wald N J, Thompson S G, Densem J W, Boreham J, Bailey A. Serum vitamin E and subsequent risk of cancer. Br J Cancer 1987; 56: 69–72

4.   Helzlsoeur K J, Comstock G W, Morris J S. Selenium, lycopene, alpha-tocopherol, beta-carotene, retinol, and subsequent bladder cancer. Cancer Res 1989; 49: 6144–6148

5.   Puska P, Tuomilehto J, Salonen J T et al. Changes in coronary risk factors during comprehensive five-year community programme to control cardio-vascular diseases (the North Karelia project). Br Med J 1979; ii: 1173–1178

6.   Knekt P, Aromaa A, Maaatela J et al. Serum vitamin E, serum selenium and the risk of gastrointestinal cancer. Int J Cancer 1988; 42: 846–850

7.   Killian C S, Yang N, Emrich L J. Prognostic importance of prostate-specific antigen for monitoring patients with stages B2 to D1 prostate cancer. Cancer Res 1985; 45: 886–891

8.   Franks L. Latent carcinoma of the prostate. J Pathol Bacteriol 1954; 68: 603–616

9.   Breslow N, Chan C, Dhom G et al. Latent carcinoma of the prostate at autopsy in seven areas. Int J Cancer 1977; 20: 680–688

10. Kabalin J N, McNeal J E, Price H M et al. Unsuspected adenocarcinoma of the prostate in patients undergoing cystoprostatectomy for other causes: incidence, histology and morphometric observations. J Urol 1989; 141: 1091–1094

11. Helzlsouer K J, Newby J, Comstock G W. Prostate-specific antigen levels and subsequent prostate cancer: potential for screening. Cancer Epidemiol Biomarkers Prev 1992; 1: 537–540

12. Stenman A H, Hakama M, Knekt P et al. Serum concentrations of prostate specific antigen and its complex with alpha1 antichymotrypsin before diagnosis of prostate cancer. Lancet 1994; 344: 1594–1598

13. Gann P H, Hennekens C H, Stampfer M J. A prospective evaluation of plasma prostate-specific antigen for detection of prostatic cancer. JAMA 1995; 273: 1594–1598

14. Carter B, Pearson J, Metter J et al. Longitudinal evaluation of prostate specific antigen levels in men with and without prostate cancer. JAMA 1993; 267: 2215–2220

15. Whittemore A S, Lele C, Friedman G D et al. Prostate-specific antigen as predictor of prostate cancer in black men and white men. J Natl Cancer Inst 1995; 354–360

16. Oesterling J E, Jacobsen S J, Chute C G et al. Serum Prostate-specific antigen in a community-based population of healthy men. JAMA 1993; 270: 860–864

17. Catalona W, Smith D, Ratliff T et al. Measurement of prostate specific antigen in serum as a screening test for prostate cancer. N Engl J Med 1991; 324 (17): 1156–1161

18. Axtell L M, Asire A J, Myers M H (eds). Cancer patient survival. Report number 5. Bethesda: US Dept Health, Education and Welfare, 1976

19. Johansen J, Adami H, Andersson S et al. High 10-year survival rate in patients with early untreated prostate cancer. JAMA 1992; 267: 2191–2196

20. Chamberlain J, Melia J, Moss S, Brown J. Report prepared for the health technology assessment panel of the NHS executive on the diagnosis, management, treatment and costs of prostate cancer in England and Wales. B J Urol 1997; 79: 1–32

21. Auvinen A, Rietbergen J, Denis L, Schroder F, Prorok P. Prospective evaluation plan for randomised trials of prostate cancer screening. J Med Screening 1996; 3: 97–104

22. Parkes C, Wald N, Murphy P et al. Prospective observational study to assess value of prostate specific antigen as screening test for prostate cancer. Br Med J 1995; 311: 1338–1343

PSA as routine for prostate cancer screening in the United States: an internist's perspective

R. Hanover

Introduction

In this age of promoting cost-effective quality care, should serum prostate-specific antigen (PSA) be used for routine prostate cancer screening and, if so, for whom?

The results of controlled randomized trials assessing the relative merits of prostate cancer screening may not be available for 10–15 years.[1] Meanwhile, there is widespread use of serum PSA to screen asymptomatic men for prostate cancer. The use of this widely available test in an age of promoting quality yet cost-effective health care throughout the United States has fostered much debate as to whether asymptomatic men should be routinely screened by PSA measurement. This controversy gives rise to some far-reaching professional implications that transcend the threshold decision on whether to screen — implications of failing to diagnose or of refraining from diagnosing, and of failing to manage the patient properly if an abnormal PSA is found. Through early intervention with prostatectomy, radiation or other treatment, or through 'watchful waiting', or just by being aware or unaware of his condition, the asymptomatic man with prostate cancer may ultimately suffer physical and emotional pain, deficit, lost chance of survival, loss of consortium, loss of enjoyment of life, loss of earnings, and numerous other forms of harm to himself, third parties and the public at large. Fundamentally, the implications of widespread PSA screening begin with the threshold decision itself.

The current situation in the United States

There is no question that there is extensive use of PSA measurement for prostate cancer screening in the United States. Hicks *et al.*[2] report that 74% of Oklahoma family physicians surveyed believe both a digital rectal examination (DRE) and serum PSA measurement are appropriate for prostate cancer screening. The primary reason reported for ordering PSA for screening was to decrease morbidity and mortality; in addition, 69% of those physicians reporting believed that screening would improve the patient's quality of life. McKnight *et al.*,[3] in a large survey, found that, in the south-eastern United States 98% of urologists and 87% of family physicians reported using serum PSA to screen patients, beginning at a mean age of 49 ± 4 years. None the less, the decision to use PSA as a screening test for prostate cancer remains controversial. Despite evidence that PSA screening increases the early detection of prostate cancers as compared with DRE alone,[4–6] it is not clear whether a change in post-screening patient management will reduce morbidity and mortality or improve quality of life. Indeed, a study by Krahn *et al.*[7] did not support the use of PSA, transrectal ultrasonography (TRUS) or DRE to screen asymptomatic men for prostate cancer — not even those in high-risk populations, such as Black men or men with a father or brother with prostate cancer. Although conceding a marginal reduction in prostate cancer mortality in men between the ages of 50 and 70 years, this study concluded that the morbidity of prostate cancer treatment 'more than offset' the benefits of reduced prostatic cancer mortality. 'Quality-adjusted' life expectancy is diminished by 3–13 days and costs are increased.[7] Concordant views are held by Woolf[8] and by Chodak.[9]

The balance between net benefit and harm helps to define professional standards and guidelines and it is the standard of care that defines one's professional duty to screen or to refrain from screening. Also helping to set the standard of care is the accepted practice of reasonably prudent physicians who practise the same specialty in the same or a similar community. As indicated by the data from Hicks *et al.*[2] and McKnight *et al.*,[3] the majority of American family practitioners and the overwhelming majority of urologists reporting to these studies use PSA to screen for prostate cancer. The American Cancer Society (ACS)[10,11] recommends annual PSA measurement in addition to DRE for men aged 50 and over, or aged 40 and over for African-American men or men with a family history of prostate cancer, until life expectancy is less than 10 years. Also recommended is DRE starting at the age of 40. The American Urological Association (AUA) promotes similar recommendations.[12] However, the American College of Physicians (ACP) now does not recommend routine screening for prostate cancer with DRE or PSA in *average*-risk men of any age, pointing to the lack of direct evidence from controlled trials that the screening and subsequent treatment would provide a net benefit to the average man.[13] The ACP does, however, recommend that patients enrol in studies to help determine whether there may be a place for routine screening.[13] Furthermore, the US Preventive Services Task Force[14] does not recommend routine screening for prostate cancer with DRE, PSA or TRUS. While a diversity of recommendations exist, the current widespread use of PSA to screen for prostate cancer by American generalists and specialists alike is not surprising.

The effectiveness of the PSA test

Serial screening with PSA nearly doubles the percentage of cancers that are confined to the gland when first detected, when compared with DRE alone.[4,5] These cancers are detected at a stage when treatment may offer a cure, or a reduction in mortality or in the morbidities of advanced prostate cancer.[4] However, PSA is not cancer specific and detects benign conditions of the prostate such as benign prostatic hyperplasia (BPH) and prostatitis. Nor is PSA specific to those cancers in which such features as tumour volume or Gleason score suggest that progression is likely; the cancers detected may be relatively indolent, never to cause harm during the patient's lifetime. Moreover, roughly 25% of men with prostatic carcinoma have a 'normal' PSA of below 4.0 ng/ml, and two-thirds of men with a PSA of more than 4.0 ng/ml will have biopsies negative for carcinoma.[6]

It would thus appear to be difficult for a medical professional to be bound to an absolute duty to use PSA to screen every asymptomatic, average-risk patient for prostate cancer. In view of the studies and recommendations discussed above, it would be more plausible to use PSA to screen all patients in *targeted* populations — such as those who are at high or poorly defined risk for prostate cancer and who are also more likely than not to obtain net benefit from treatment. Such patient populations may include the asymptomatic younger patients who could rapidly adapt to treatment complications.

Informed consent

The questions of net harm versus net benefit of PSA screening also raise the issue of whether there is a duty to obtain the patient's informed consent prior to PSA screening. According to the ACP recommendations, it is inappropriate to perform a routine PSA test without a frank discussion of costs, harms, and benefits.[13] The US Preventive Services Task Force[14] suggests that patients requesting treatment should be given objective information about the potential benefits and harms of early detection and treatment, pointing out the availability of patient education materials that review this information.

However, obtaining informed consent is usually required where the *procedure itself* will involve substantial invasion or *disruption* of the body, such as in the case of many surgical or invasive diagnostic procedures. Performing a diagnostic test on a blood sample usually does not require that the patient is given advance information about the test's benefits, alternatives to testing, and foreseeable risks and consequences. General consent to medical treatment usually covers most diagnostic blood tests, including other tumour markers. A noteworthy exception is HIV testing; many jurisdictions require that the patient's informed consent be obtained prior to HIV testing.

Nevertheless, as far as PSA screening is concerned, some have considered obtaining an asymptomatic patient's informed consent prior to screening,[8,10,11] in view of the many possible management options and the consequences of each. After testing, the asymptomatic patient may be found to have an elevated PSA and may ultimately face treatment consequences, including (but not limited to) incontinence, impotence, diminished libido, loss of consortium, mental anguish, labile mood, 'hot flushes', gastrointestinal upset, diarrhoea or other complications. One major drawback, however, is that obtaining the asymptomatic patient's informed consent for PSA screening might produce a 'chilling' effect[15,16] on the patient's willingness to submit to the screening test.

Conclusions

Antiscreening advocates might argue that a duty to *refrain* from PSA screening exists where the patient is likely to suffer net harm from screening by way of needless tests and treatments that produce harmful side effects. However, the great majority of cancers detected through PSA testing do have features, such as Gleason score and tumour volume, that suggests the likelihood of progression during the patient's lifetime.[4]

Professional accountability to the patient and to the public at large are yet to be defined; there are no clear-cut standards reflecting a duty to screen or to refrain from PSA screening. As either decision could have a substantial effect on an asymptomatic patient's health and ultimate well-being, the implications ought to be seriously considered. Whereas there may not be a duty to screen, there also may not be a duty to refrain. Let us hope that the choice will be ours.

References

1. Collins M M, Barry M J. Controversies in prostate cancer screening. Analogies to the early lung cancer screening debate. JAMA 1996; 276(24): 1976–1979
2. Hicks R J, Hamm R M, Bemben D A. Prostate cancer screening. What family physicians believe is best. Arch Fam Med 1995; 4(4): 317–322
3. McKnight J T, Tietze P H, Adcock B B et al. Screening for prostate cancer: a comparison of urologists and primary care physicians. South Med J 1996; 89(9): 885–888

4. Catalona W J, Smith D S, Ratliff T L, Basler J W. Detection of organ-confined prostate cancer is increased through prostate-specific antigen-based screening. JAMA 1993; 270(8): 948–954

5. Catalona W J, Richie J P, Ahmann F R *et al*. Comparison of digital rectal examination and serum prostate specific antigen in the early detection of prostate cancer: results of a multicenter clinical trial of 6,630 men. J Urol 1994; 151: 1283–1290

6. Brawer M K. PSA: the most useful of all tumor markers. Presented at the 2nd International Forum on Prostate Cancer, London, UK, 9–12, December 1996

7. Krahn M D, Mahoney J E, Eckman M H *et al*. Screening for prostate cancer. A decision analytic view. JAMA 1994; 272(10): 773–780

8. Woolf S H. Public health perspective: the health policy implications of screening for prostate cancer. J Urol 1994; 152: 1685–1688

9. Chodak G W. Questioning the value of screening for prostate cancer in asymptomatic men. Urology 1993; 42(2): 116–118

10. American Cancer Society. Guidelines for the cancer-related checkup: an update. Atlanta: American Cancer Society, 1993 (reported in ref. 14)

11. Mettlin C, Jones G, Averett H *et al*. Defining and updating the American Cancer Society guidelines for the cancer-related checkup: prostate and endometrial cancers. CA 1993; 43: 42–47

12. American Urological Association Executive Committee Report. Baltimore: American Urological Association, January 1992 (reported in ref. 14)

13. American College of Physicians. Clinical guideline part III: screening for prostate cancer. Ann Intern Med 1997; 126: 480–484

14. US Preventive Services Task Force: Guide to clinical preventive services: report of the US preventive services task force, 2nd edn. Baltimore: Williams and Wilkins, 1996

15. Handley M R, Stuart M E. The use of prostate specific antigen for prostate cancer screening: managed care perspective. J Urol 1994; 152: 1689–1692

16. Wolf A M, Nasser J F, Schorling J B. The impact of informed consent on patient interest in prostate-specific antigen screen. Arch Intern Med 1996; 156: 1333–1336

Chapter 17

Imaging for prostate cancer
T. J. Christmas

Introduction

The role of imaging in prostate cancer can be divided broadly into diagnosis, staging of the disease and detection of disease recurrence after definitive therapy. Imaging modalities can be used to identify tumours within the prostate to enable guidance of biopsies, to assess the local stage of the tumour and to detect metastatic disease, found most commonly within pelvic lymph nodes and bone. The exclusion of extracapsular extension (ECE) of the primary tumour and metastatic disease is particularly important prior to performing radical prostatectomy, and this can be achieved by assimilating results of imaging in combination with other data such as the serum prostate-specific antigen (PSA) and tumour differentiation within biopsies. Following radical prostatectomy, the PSA may rise in the presence of tumour recurrence. Imaging techniques can identify the site of such recurrences and hence allow a decision to be made on the use of further treatments, such as local radiotherapy or hormonal manipulation.

Enormous technical improvements have been made in all imaging modalities, which have increased the detection of prostate cancer both within and outside the prostate.

Diagnosis of prostate cancer

There is increasing evidence that early detection of prostate cancer can lead to an improved prognosis. Digital rectal examination (DRE) alone is less than 50% accurate in detecting prostate cancer.[1] False positive findings of induration or nodules may result from benign prostatic hyperplasia (BPH), prostatitis or prostatic calcification. Small prostate cancers are often impalpable. However, a combination of abnormal DRE and PSA elevation may increase the diagnostic yield. Transrectal ultrasonography (TRUS) provides an image of the internal architecture of the prostate that can aid the diagnosis of prostate cancer. The normal prostate is symmetrical and has a well-defined capsule. More than two-thirds of prostate cancers are hypoechoic on TRUS (Figure 17.1), about 30% are isoechoic and 1% are hyperechoic. It is, however, important to appreciate that only 20–25% of hypoechoic areas are malignant.[2] Other causes of hypoechoic areas within the prostate include BPH nodules, infarcts, cysts and areas of prostatitis. The most important role for TRUS is the guidance of prostate biopsies, which can be achieved using specialized equipment attached to the TRUS probe. Hypoechoic areas can be biopsied under TRUS control (Figure 17.2) and the probe can also be used to identify and biopsy suspicious areas adjacent to or outside the prostatic capsule. Abnormalities within the seminal vesicles, such as asymmetry or thickening, can be identified and biopsied under TRUS guidance.

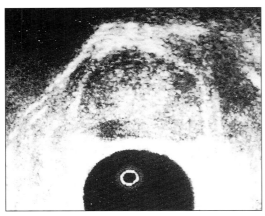

Figure 17.1. Transrectal ultrasound (TRUS) scan showing a hypoechoic area in the peripheral zone of the prostate, confirmed as adenocarcinoma on biopsy.

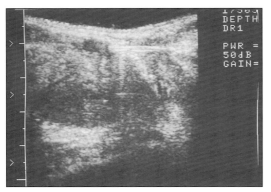

Figure 17.2. Biopsy of a peripheral zone hypoechoic area under guidance using TRUS.

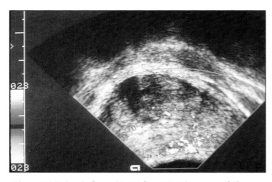

Figure 17.3. Colour Doppler TRUS scan of the prostate, showing increased vascularity of a peripheral zone area shown on biopsy to be adenocarcinoma.

Colour Doppler has been incorporated into TRUS apparatus and there is now evidence that this may increase the diagnosis of prostate cancer. Just under one-half of prostate cancers have colour Doppler flow abnormalities (Figure 17.3) and, of these, 77% have been shown to be moderately or poorly differentiated.[3] It appears that less clinically significant well-differentiated foci are less likely to have an increase in blood flow as apparent on colour Doppler. Power Doppler is able to detect smaller increases in blood flow (Figure 17.4) and is currently under evaluation to determine whether this increased sensitivity enables a greater diagnostic yield for prostate cancer. Research is currently under way to assess the additional diagnostic benefit of intravenous administration of micro-bubbles (Senovist) immediately prior to TRUS. It is possible that this might increase the acuity with TRUS by enabling clearer identification of blood vessels within the prostate.

Narrow-bore transurethral ultrasound probes have been developed for scanning the prostate from inside the prostatic urethra. The architecture and volume of the prostate can be measured with such probes.[4] However, general anaesthesia is usually required to insert the probe and its presence within the prostatic urethra can distort the image. Transurethral ultrasound appears to have no advantages over TRUS in the diagnosis of prostate cancer.

Computerized tomography (CT) scanning was the first technique to produce cross-sectional images. However, it has little or no application in the diagnosis of prostate cancer but may be of help in some men to stage the disease. The same applies to magnetic resonance imaging (MRI), which produces images of startling clarity in transverse (Figure 17.5), sagittal and oblique planes. On T2-weighted images the peripheral zone of the prostate returns high-intensity signals while prostate cancer produces lower-intensity signals. However, most other abnormalities within the prostate, such as 'adenomas', corpora amylacea and prostatitis, also return low-intensity signals; MRI should

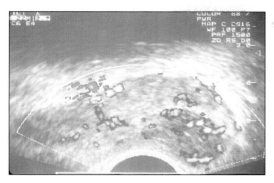

Figure 17.4. Power Doppler TRUS scan showing increased blood supply to a peripheral zone lesion later shown on biopsy to be adenocarcinoma.

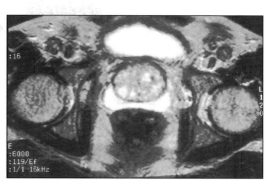

Figure 17.5. MRI scan in transverse section of a normal prostate.

not, therefore, be used routinely for the diagnosis of prostate cancer. Endoluminal MRI using a magnetic coil within the rectum can produce excellent images of the prostate but offers little over TRUS in the diagnosis of prostate cancer and is currently not able to assist with biopsy guidance.

Local staging of prostate cancer

One of the most important roles of imaging modalities is in the local staging of prostate cancer, particularly in those patients considered to be suitable candidates for radical prostatectomy. In almost all circumstances the presence of ECE is a contraindication for radical prostatectomy and hence the detection of ECE is of the utmost importance in planing treatment for men with prostate cancer. DRE is unreliable in the detection of ECE. However, TRUS may reveal extension of hypoechoic peripheral zone tumours causing bulging of the outline of the prostate, which is highly suggestive of ECE.[5] TRUS may similarly be able to demonstrate invasion of the seminal vesicles.

Although CT scanning has been shown to be of great value in staging some malignant tumours, its efficacy in the local staging of prostate cancer has been disappointingly poor. The sensitivity of CT scanning in detecting ECE with or without seminal vesicle invasion has been shown to be 18–59%;[6] hence, CT scanning is at present less accurate than TRUS in the local staging of prostate cancer. However, with technical improvements the resolution in the imaging of prostate cancer with CT scanning will improve, but it may never produce greater acuity than TRUS.

MRI scanning, although expensive, has an advantage over CT since it does not utilize ionizing irradiation. T2-weighted MRI images are able to show the internal architecture of the prostate, and usually the peripheral zone returns high-intensity signals while prostate cancer produces low-intensity signals that can be shown to extend outside the capsule in men with ECE (Figure 17.6). MRI can image the prostate in transverse axial, coronal and sagittal planes, which can enhance its ability to detect ECE from 61 to 83%. ECE is likely if there is asymmetry, irregularity of the border of the prostate, or breaching of the periprostatic fat. Seminal vesicle invasion is likely if areas of low intensity are apparent within the normally high-intensity vesicles.[7] Technological advances in both intracavity (Figure 17.7) and surface coils may well lead to increased sensitivity for the detection of ECE by MRI.[8]

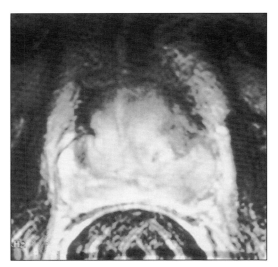

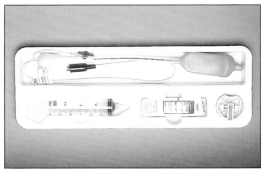

Figure 17.7. Endorectal MRI probe: the apparatus covered with a balloon is inserted into the rectum.

Figure 17.6. Endorectal MRI scan of a stage T3 prostate cancer, demonstrating invasion of the tumour through the prostate capsule.

Detection of lymph node metastases

The commonest site for lymphatic metastases from prostate cancer are the chains of lymph nodes adjacent to the obturator nerve and vessels and the external iliac vessels. The most accurate determinants for the presence of lymphatic metastases are the serum PSA and the Gleason grade of the biopsy. The incidence of lymphatic metastases in men with clinically localized prostate cancer has been reported as 5.7% (13 of 229)[9] and 2% (2 of 100) in a personal series (unpublished data). The detection of lymphatic metastases from prostate cancer is important in planning therapy since aggressive local treatments, such as radical prostatectomy, radical external beam radiotherapy and interstitial cryotherapy, are unlikely to be effective in the long term in the presence of distant lymphatic spread. Lymphangiography has been used in an attempt to detect lymphatic metastatic disease and can, in theory, detect metastases within pelvic lymph nodes that are not greatly enlarged,[10] but has been shown to identify lymphatic metastases in only 50–60% of cases. Lymphangiography has now been superseded by CT and MRI scanning. The visualization of large-volume lymph node metastases is possible with both CT and MRI, and both modalities can be utilized to guide biopsies to confirm the presence of metastatic disease. However, small-volume nodal metastases of less than 5 mm diameter are usually undetectable on both CT and MRI scanning.

Radioimmunoscintigraphy (RIS) techniques using radiolabelled monoclonal antibodies to CYT 351 have been shown to be useful in detecting lymphatic metastases from prostate cancer primary tumours.[11] Other monoclonal antibodies that are able to bind specifically to prostatic tissues are being developed and this technique may turn out to be more specific than other technologies in the detection of early metastases from prostate cancer.

The increase in metabolic activity within prostate cancer metastases permits the use of positron emission tomography (PET) scanning of men with prostate cancer. An intravenous injection of 2-deoxy-2-[fluorine-18] fluoro-D-glucose (FDG) is administered prior to performing the scan. Tissues containing metastatic prostate cancer take up the FDG 2.1–5.7 times as much as other tissues. Unfortunately, the sensitivity of PET scanning in the identification of osseous metastases is only 65% and it is therefore less accurate than conventional isotope bone scans in detecting bone metastases. However, it is more sensitive at identifying soft tissue metastases, although pelvic lymph nodes are more difficult to image owing to the activity of tracer contained within the bladder.[12]

Detection of bone metastases

When prostate cancer metastasizes to bone it may cause local pain. Plain roentgenography can be used to identify osseous metastases, which are osteosclerotic in 98% of cases (Figure 17.8); the remaining 2% being osteolytic.

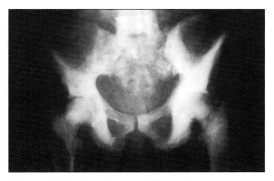

Figure 17.8. Plain X-ray of the pelvis, showing osteosclerotic prostate cancer metastases.

The commonest sites of bone metastases are the bones of the pelvis and the lumbar spine. However, osseous metastases are often very widespread and can involve any bone in the skeleton. Plain roentgenography can also demonstrate pathological fractures, which are most commonly found at the hip joint and are more likely to occur with osteolytic metastases. Bone metastases need to be at least 1.5 cm in diameter and to have replaced 50–70% of the bone to be detected on plain X-ray films.

Isotope bone scans using radiolabelled technetium can identify characteristic 'hot spots' in the skeleton in metastatic prostate cancer. However, false-positive scans may occur in the presence of recent trauma, orthopaedic surgery, osteomyelitis, Paget's disease or primary bone tumours. Isotope bone scans are more sensitive than plain roentgenography and will detect metastases of about 5 mm diameter. Hence, isotope bone scans are the investigation of choice for the detection of bone metastases, although plain roentgenography may be indicated in cases with equivocal findings. If clinical doubt about a bone lesion exists, then bone biopsy can be performed under X-ray guidance. When the serum PSA is below 20 ng/ml there is only a 0.3% chance that metastases will be detected on an isotope bone scan.[13] For this reason, some urologists no longer search for bone metastases in men with a serum PSA level of 10 ng/ml or less. An unusual but dramatic finding in men with multiple diffuse bone metastases from prostate cancer is the 'superscan', in which the entire skeleton appears to take up the isotope at high density. Other forms of RIS, using radiolabelled monoclonal antibodies to CYT-351 and CYT-356, can be used to detect bone metastases from prostate cancer.[11]

Detection of recurrence following radical prostatectomy

A rise in the serum PSA following radical prostatectomy is highly suggestive of recurrent prostate cancer. Such recurrences are detected earlier when supersensitive PSA assays accurate to 0.01 ng/ml are used. Before planning treatment for post-radical prostatectomy cancer recurrence, it is important to determine the location. In patients with a positive surgical margin the recurrence is most likely to be in the prostate bed or at the anastomosis. In men with lymphatic metastases detected at radical prostatectomy, further recurrence is most likely to be within more distant lymph nodes. Seminal vesicle invasion in the radical prostatectomy specimen increases the likelihood of disseminated disease

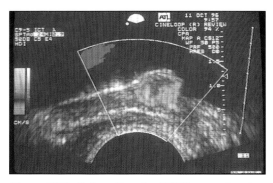

Figure 17.9. Colour Doppler TRUS scan, showing a highly vascular local recurrence after radical prostatectomy.

within the lymphatics or bone. In the face of a rising PSA, further investigation is warranted. TRUS can be used to detect recurrences within the prostate bed or at the anastomosis, which can be confirmed by biopsy. Such recurrences usually show increased blood flow on colour Doppler (Figure 17.9). Local recurrences can be successfully treated with external beam radiotherapy. Lymphatic metastases can be detected by CT, MRI or RIS. Bone metastases are unlikely to be detectable until the PSA rises to at least 20 ng/ml. Distant metastases are best treated with hormonal manipulation, although external beam radiotherapy may be appropriate for men with isolated bone metastases.

Future developments

There have been great technical improvements in the quality of images produced by TRUS, CT and MRI over the last decade; it is more than likely that further advances will be made in the future. It is hoped that such progress will not only enable more accurate local staging, particularly identification of extracapsular extension, but also detect metastases within the lymphatics at an earlier stage. If the accuracy in detecting extraprostatic disease improves, this in turn will allow more precision in selecting patients for radical local therapy and hence improve the long-term results of radical prostatectomy, external beam radiotherapy and other local treatments. The development of monoclonal antibodies specific to prostate cancer cells will allow RIS to detect even the most tiny of metastatic deposits, and it is likely that such technology will permit greater accuracy than any other imaging modality. In the future, such monoclonal antibodies might prove to be of use for both staging and therapy.

References

1. Jewett H J. Significance of the palpable prostatic nodule. JAMA 1956; 160: 838–841
2. Rifkin M D. Prostate cancer sonographic characteristics. In: Ultrasound of the prostate. New York: Raven Press, 1988: 101
3. Cheng S S, Rifkin M D, Bajas M A *et al.* Color Doppler imaging: an important adjunct to endorectal ultrasound in the diagnosis of prostate cancer. Radiology 1996; 201: 338
4. Gammelgaard J, Holm H H. Trans-urethral and trans-rectal ultrasound scanning in urology. J Urol 1980; 124: 863–868
5. Ohori M, Egawa S, Shinohara K *et al.* Detection of microscopic extracapsular extension prior to radical prostatectomy for clinically localized prostate cancer. Br J Urol 1994; 74: 72–79
6. Platt J F, Bree R L, Sdhwab R E. The accuracy of CT in the staging of carcinoma of the prostate. AJR 1987; 149: 315–318
7. Hricak H, Dooms G C, Jeffrey R B *et al.* Prostatic carcinoma: staging by clinical assessment, CT and MRI imaging. Radiology 1987; 162: 331–336
8. Schnall M D, Imai Y, Tomaszewski J *et al.* Prostate cancer: local staging with endorectal surface coil MR imaging. Radiology 1991; 178: 797–802
9. Danella J F, de Kernion J B, Smith R B, Steckel J. The contemporary incidence of lymph node metastases in prostate cancer: implications for laparoscopic lymph node dissection. J Urol 1993; 149: 1488–1491

10. Lantz E J, Hattery R R. Diagnostic imaging of urothelial cancer. Urol Clin North Am 1984; 11: 576–582
11. Feneley M R, Chengazi V U, Kirby R S *et al*. Prostatic radioimmunoscintigraphy preliminary results using technetium labelled monoclonal antibodies — CYT351. Br J Urol 1996; 77: 373–381
12. Shreeve P D, Grossman H B, Gross M D, Wahl R L. Metastatic prostate cancer: initial findings of PET with 2-deoxy-2-[F-18]fluoro-D-glucose. Radiology 1996; 199: 751–756
13. Chybowski F M, Larson Keller J J, Bergstrahl E J *et al*. Predicting radionucleotide bone scan findings in patients with newly diagnosed untreated prostate cancer: prostate specific antigen is superior to all other parameters. J Urol 1991; 145: 313–318

Chapter 18
RT–PCR molecular staging and human prostate cancer management

M. H. Sokoloff and A. S. Belldegrun

Introduction

During 1997 in the USA, a total of 334,500 new cases of prostate cancer will be diagnosed and 41,800 men will succumb to endstage disease.[1] Although advances in the diagnosis and treatment of localized disease have become well established, the optimal approach to the diagnosis and management of these lesions remains controversial, owing to the variable biological course of prostatic malignancy, imperfect staging modalities, and difficulty in predicting the biological outcome of both organ-confined and locally invasive disease.[2,3] Radical prostatectomy can cure patients with localized prostate cancer and its use in treating such tumours in younger and healthy men is generally undisputed.[4,5] Nonetheless, almost 30% of patients with pathologically organ-confined cancer will experience an early relapse with recurrent disease despite successful treatment of the primary lesion.[6,7] Additionally, current screening modalities fail to identify a significant subset of patients with locally invasive disease, and recent studies report that up to 40% of patients who were thought to have organ-confined lesions were found to be understaged subsequent to surgery.[8,9] To complicate matters further, several centres have demonstrated that the operative management of locally invasive lesions can offer a durable response in select patients.[10,11] Clearly, improved diagnostic and staging techniques are needed to identify those men with the best prognosis for surgical cure, so that all patients can be stratified to the most effective therapeutic regimens for their particular situation.

Since 1986, prostate-specific antigen (PSA) has been utilized for the clinical diagnosis of prostate cancer.[12] Although serum PSA assays have been invaluable in improving the early detection of men with curable lesions, both the specificity and sensitivity of these assays are only average and there has been much enthusiasm for the development of better tests.[12,13] Furthermore, because PSA values vary widely within a given tumour stage and overlap between different stages, the predictive value of PSA in determining pathological stage is weak.[14,15] Even with the combined use of digital rectal examination, serum PSA and transrectal ultrasound, it is not feasible to estimate reliably the stage of an individual tumour prior to surgery.[16] Another prostate-tissue-specific biomarker, prostate-specific membrane antigen (PSM), has been characterized and its future role in the diagnosis and management of prostate cancer appears promising.[17] It is ironic that, despite the comparative wealth of prostate-tissue-specific biomarkers, their application to cancer staging is relatively poor.

The haematogenous spread of prostate cancer is well established and the natural history of prostate cancer is such that, once it has metastasized from the prostatic fossa, it is considered to be incurable.[18] It has been hypothesized that those men who experience an early relapse following curative radical prostatectomy may have had disseminated disease undetected at the time of surgery. Signs and symptoms of metastatic disease occur late in the progression of prostate cancer and the presence of early metastatic spread can be missed in a patient presenting with clinically localized disease.

Several institutions, including the authors' own, have investigated the utility of using reverse transcriptase–polymerase chain reaction (RT–PCR)-based assays to detect such occult circulating prostate-tissue-derived cells, not currently identifiable by conventional imaging and screening modalities. These enquiries were founded on earlier reports in which circulating 'micrometastatic' cells were detected in patients with breast, haematological and colon cancers.[19-21] The goal is to equate the presence of these prostate-tissue-derived signals in the peripheral circulation with 'micrometastatic' disease, thereby identifying those men with clinically localized yet potentially unresectable disease (pathological stages T3, T4, N+ and M+).

RT–PCR methodology

The polymerase chain reaction (PCR) is a laboratory technique that simulates normal gene replication and synthesis.[22] *In vitro* enzymatic synthesis is used to amplify specific DNA sequences exponentially. The widespread dissemination and automation of PCR technology over the past decade has revolutionized biological and medical research. Through this technique, diminutive quantities of a gene can be reliably and rapidly detected as the desired DNA sequence is repetitively amplified. Approximately one billion copies of a single DNA molecule can be produced in a matter of hours. RT–PCR uses mRNA (instead of DNA) as the original genomic template. With RT–PCR, detection is focused on only those cells that are actively synthesizing a desired gene product, such as the PSA protein. Not only are actively synthesizing cells isolated, but the likelihood of contamination is decreased.

Figure 18.1 illustrates the methodology used to detect PSA-producing cells in the peripheral circulation by RT–PCR.[23] In this example, whole blood is processed

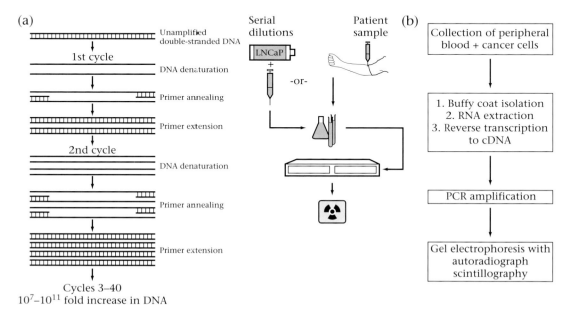

Figure 18.1. Diagram of RT–PCR technique. (a) Exponential amplification of double-stranded DNA by RT–PCR. (b) Blood is collected and then processed by centrifugation to isolate the buffy coat; mRNA is extracted and purified prior to reverse transcription to cDNA, which is subsequently amplified, separated by gel electrophoresis and quantified by scintillography (see ref. 23).

to isolate the 'buffy coat' mononuclear layer, where PSA-expressing cells reside, when present. The mRNA from *all* the cells comprising the buffy coat is collected and purified. PSA mRNA will be present only if cells actively producing PSA are present. Through the method of reverse transcription, the mRNA is converted to double-stranded complementary DNA (cDNA), which is then amplified through a series of cyclical heating and cooling phases in a programmable automated PCR-thermocycler. During the amplification process, a specific *primer* is added that will attach to and mark the gene of interest (in this case PSA), if present. The products of the RT–PCR amplification are then separated from one another on a gel, which is subsequently examined for the presence of the desired gene. Thus, a PSA signal will be present on the *gel* only if a sufficient number of cells actively synthesizing PSA are in the peripheral circulation and can be isolated in the buffy coat, and if PSA mRNA can then be isolated, purified, and made into cDNA, which will accordingly be amplified in the thermocycler and isolated on the gel. Using this technique, a single PSA-producing cell can be reliably detected in a sample of 10^7–10^8 mononuclear cells.[23]

RT–PCR and prostate cancer staging: the UCLA experience

In 1994 a phase I study was initiated at the authors' institution to investigate whether a PCR-based assay could detect occult prostate-tissue-derived cells in the peripheral circulation and thereby preoperatively differentiate men with localized prostate cancer (pT1/pT2) from those with invasive (pT3/pT4) or advanced (N+/M+) disease.[23] A total of 121 patient buffy coat specimens (including 88 with pathologically staged prostatic lesions and 33 with known hormone-refractory metastatic disease) were prospectively analysed for both PSA and PSM signals, using a reproducible, highly sensitive and specific, radioisotope primer incorporation quantitative RT–PCR-amplification technique. The sensitivity of the assay enabled the detection of the mRNA signal from a single neoplastic cell premixed in 10 ml normal whole blood, as demonstrated by the autoradiograph in Figure 18.2. This is equivalent to one tumour cell in 1×10^7 to 2×10^7 peripheral blood lymphocytes.

Of the 33 patients with advanced hormone-refractory disease, circulating PSA mRNA signals were detected in 29, establishing an 88% sensitivity for the authors' assay. Conversely, no circulating PSA mRNA signals were detected in nine cystoprostatectomy patients who had no evidence of prostate disease. Two of 10 patients with BPH had circulating PSA mRNA signals; however, one had an occult neoplasm and eventually re-presented with localized disease. With a positive circulating PSA mRNA signal being detected in only one of 19 patients with benign prostatic pathology, therefore, a specificity of 94% was achieved. In patients who underwent radical prostatectomy for clinically localized disease, positive PSA–PCR signals were detected in 59% (30/51) of patients with pT1 and pT2 lesions and in 72% (13/18) of those with pT3 disease. Positive PSA–PCR signals were also detected in 42% (5/12) of specimens with tumour at the inked apical margin, 76% (13/17) of specimens with positive surgical margins (other than apex), 66% (27/41) of specimens with capsular penetration, and 92% (12/13) of specimens with capsular perforation.

Multiple linear regression statistical analysis and analysis of variance computations were performed on the results from the 121 patient specimens. This demonstrated that neither the presence of positive PSA mRNA signals nor the quantity of these signals could reliably predict pathological stage. Analysis of independent variables was also performed in patients with pathologically staged

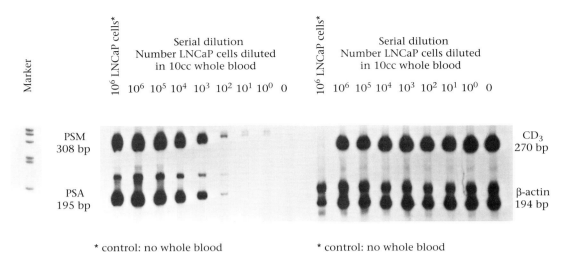

Figure 18.2. Photograph of the autoradiograph of sensitivity determination assay. CD3 expression
was used as an internal control to document the presence and absence of peripheral blood
lymphocytes in the dilutional specimens, and β-actin was used as an internal control for
quantification. PSA and PSM expression is documented on the left side of the film. With decreasing
LNCaP concentration, expression of both signals decreases, yet at a concentration of 1 LNCaP cell in
10 ml whole blood, both signals are present.

prostate cancer. This demonstrated that there was no statistically significant
relationship between PSA–PCR results and preoperative serum PSA values (Pearson
χ^2, $p = 0.560$), Gleason grade ($p = 0.357$), apical involvement ($p = 0.754$) or
capsular penetration ($p = 0.463$). There was a statistically significant relationship
between PSA–PCR and capsular perforation ($p = 0.013$) and the relationship
of PSA–PCR to positive surgical margins (other than apex) approached significance
($p = 0.115$).

PSM mRNA signals were detected in 13 of the 33 patients with metastatic
prostate cancer, none of the nine cystoprostatectomy patients, and two of the BPH
patients (the same two that had positive PSA–PCR signals, one of which had an
occult neoplastic lesion). This yields a sensitivity of 39% with a specificity of 94%.
Positive PSM–PCR signals were also detected in eight of 51 patients (16%) with
pT1 and pT2 disease and in four of the 18 patients (22%) with pT3 disease.
Neither the presence of positive PSM mRNA signals nor the quantity of these
signals could reliably predict pathological stage.

Follow-up prognostic data to evaluate for evidence of recurrent cancer has been
collected on 45 of the 69 patients who underwent radical prostatectomy. Of these
45 patients, 20 were RT–PCR–PSA negative preoperatively; 15 of these had pT2
disease (one of whom had a PSA failure at 16 months), and five had pT3 disease
(two of whom had a PSA failure at 15 month average follow-up). Of the 25
patients who were RT–PCR–PSA positive preoperatively, 19 had pT2 disease and six
had pT3 disease. Of these RT–PCR–PSA-positive patients, none of the pT2 (0/19)
and two of the pT3 (2/6) patients have had a serological or clinical failure at 14
months average follow-up. There were no significant differences in failure rates
between the PCR-positive and PCR-negative groups, indicating that the presence
of positive RT–PCR–PSA signals in the peripheral circulation of men with
pathologically confined prostate cancer did not predict PSA failure (at an average
follow-up of 14 months) using the authors' technique.

RT–PCR and prostate cancer staging: other institutional reports

Only information published in peer-reviewed journals is reviewed (Table 18.1). This in no way is meant to negate the large numbers of studies presented over the past few years at the national meetings of the AUA, AACR or ASCO.

Peripheral blood

Moreno *et al.* were the first to apply PCR technology to the identification of circulating prostate-specific signals in patients with metastatic prostate cancer, demonstrating a sensitivity of 33%.[24] This study, although significant in its pioneering nature, did not apply the technique to preoperative prostate cancer staging. Such an application was proposed by Katz and associates who detected circulating signals in 78% of patients with advanced metastatic prostate cancer and in 25 of 65 patients (38.5%) with clinically localized disease.[25] Of these 25 patients, 68% had capsular penetration and 87% had positive margins. In an ensuing analysis of 94 men undergoing radical prostatectomy, circulating PSA–PCR signals could be identified in 72% of patients with extraprostatic disease but in only 12% of those with localized disease.[26] In 1996, the same group reported that their enhanced RT–PCR assay for PSA was a better predictor of potential failure after radical prostatectomy than preoperative serum PSA or Gleason grade.[27] Jaakkola *et al.* used a similar RT–PCR technique with PSA primers in 25 men with prostate cancer.[28] Positive signals were detected in 50% of men with untreated metastatic disease. No signals were identified in any of the men with clinically localized lesions or in those patients on hormonal therapy for advanced disease. Likewise, none of the control group (including patients with BPH and renal cell carcinoma) had evidence of signals in the peripheral circulation.

Subsequent reports have not been as decisive. Seiden *et al.* evaluated the peripheral blood of 135 men with prostate cancer, using an RT–PCR–PSA assay.[29] Signals were detected in five of 65 (8%) patients with clinically localized disease,

Table 18.1. Published studies investigating detection of circulating prostate-derived signals in the peripheral circulation

Primers	Study	Control	T₁/T₂	T₃/T₄	M+	
PSA	Moreno *et al.*[24]	0	–	–	33	
	Olsson *et al.*[26]	0	12	72	88	
	Jaakkola *et al.*[28]	0	–	–	50	(untreated)
					0	(treated)
	Seiden *et al.*[29†]	0	8	–	13	(treated)
					50	(hormone refractory)
	Ghossein *et al.*[30]	0	16	33	35	
	Sokoloff *et al.*[23]	0	59	72	88	
PSM	Israeli *et al.*[33]	0	68‡	–	67	
	Loric *et al.*[34]	0	35	60	85	

*All values are percentages and all staging is pathological, unless indicated.
†Clinical stage.
‡Post-radical prostatectomy with undetectable serum PSA.

in one of 12 (8%) with increasing PSA despite definitive treatment for localized cancer, none of seven with untreated M+ lesions, one of eight (13%) with treated M+ disease, and 10 of 20 (50%) with hormone-refractory prostate cancer. Ghossein *et al.* reported on peripheral blood specimens in 107 men with prostate cancer.[30] Positive PSA signals were detected by RT–PCR in four of 25 (16%) with localized disease, two of six (33%) with clinically invasive disease, one of four (25%) with N+ and 25 of 72 (35%) with M+ disease. In neither study were circulating signals detected in the control groups.

Many of the disparities between those studies supporting and those refuting the use of RT–PCR assays to improve preoperative prostate cancer staging can be attributed to variations in technique between the different institutions. No standardization of the RT–PCR process has been established. Deviation in any phase of sample collection and fractionation, storage, reverse transcription, amplification, and product separation can have momentous effects on the ultimate result. Each centre has employed a unique selection of primers, dissimilar constituents of the PCR milieu, and varying numbers of amplification cycles. Techniques to strengthen the amplification process have included applying an assortment of radioisotope, nested, and digoxigenin-enhanced primers. Furthermore, mRNA is a very labile substrate, requiring delicate and experienced handling. Until a standardized RT–PCR technique for prostate cancer staging has been established, differences in results must be interpreted with discretion.[31]

Considerable debate has developed over the choice of PSA or PSM as the best biomarker for PCR-based prostate cancer detection assays. Both the authors' data and the Columbia University[32] experience suggest that PSM is less sensitive and less effective than PSA. Israeli and associates, however, have demonstrated better results with PSM than with PSA.[33] PSM-positive signals were detected in 48 (62%) of 77 men with prostate cancer, whereas PSA signals were detected in only seven (9%). Although circulating prostate-derived signals were detected in 72.2% of patients with pT2 disease, there was no correlation between detection of PSM signals and pathological stage. Loric *et al.* also used nested RT–PCR for PSM in 60 patients with biopsy-proven prostate cancer, and showed a greater sensitivity of PSM over PSA.[34] PSM-positive signals were detected in 85% (compared with 51% for PSA) of men with M+ disease, in 60% with pT3 lesions (compared with 20% for PSA), and in 35% with pT2 disease (compared with 5% for PSA).

Differences in PSM–PCR assay sensitivity may be explained by evaluating whether the PSM isomer utilized by each group's assay is a membrane-bound or cytosolic isomer of PSM. The authors' assay employs a membrane-bound isomer; membrane-bound proteins are more static and less likely to be replicated at an increased rate, even in the face of malignancy. Conversely, cytosolic proteins turn over at a much higher frequency and their mRNA is transcribed at a more intensified rate, especially in tumour cells. The assays utilized by Israeli and Loric detect cytosol-based PSM mRNA; their assay, therefore, has the propensity towards identifying a more vigorously replicating signal, which may account for the increase in levels.

Bone marrow

In 1994, Bretton *et al.* examined the bone marrow aspirates from 20 patients with various stages of prostate cancer.[35] Using a panel of three different immunohistochemical antibody stains, prostatic tissue-derived epithelial cells were detected in the bone marrow aspirates of none of five patients with stage T_2 in two of four patients with stage T_3, none of seven patients with stage T_4 and four of four patients with stage M+ prostate cancer. Using immunocytochemical techniques, Oberneder *et al.* isolated PSA-producing cells in 33% of patients with clinically localized prostate cancer and correlated the presence of these signals to established risk factors, including local tumour extent and tumour differentiation.[36] These reports have been corroborated by subsequent studies in which RT–PCR has demonstrated the presence of PSA-producing cells in bone marrow aspirates;[37,38] these studies included a large number of men with pathologically staged organ-confined lesions.[37] Although the presence of these signals may simply represent rudimentary functions of filtering and clearing circulating cells, the appearance of PSA-producing cells in the bone marrow strongly correlates with pathological stage. Four of 20 (20%) men with pT_2 disease had positive marrow specimens, compared with over 65% in men with extraprostatic extension (15/23). Furthermore, follow-up studies demonstrate that men undergoing radical prostatectomy with detectable marrow PSA signals have a significantly worse prognosis than their RT–PCR-negative counterparts; 5% (2/41) of the RT–PCR negative group had disease recurrence, versus 21% (8/38) of the RT–PCR-positive cohort at 19-month median follow-up.[39]

Although the RT–PCR–PSA cells were never characterized as actual metastases, these studies suggest that a subset of men with clinically localized disease probably manifest malignant cells in their bone marrow. These observations also suggest that prostate cancer has the biological potential to metastasize early, before the primary lesion exceeds the anatomical confines of the prostate.

Pelvic lymph nodes

Infiltration of neoplastic prostate cells into lymphatic channels increases the likelihood of developing distant metastatic disease.[40] Not surprisingly, men with lymph node metastases, even if microscopic, have an increased failure rate after radical prostatectomy.[41] Fortunately, with routine contemporary screening modalities, the incidence of occult lymph node spread is becoming increasingly rare and, in a large percentage of patients, the need for staging lymphadenectomy is controversial.[42] Nonetheless, several studies have investigated the use of RT–PCR to detect occult nodal metastasis in men undergoing prostatectomy.

RT–PCR can detect PSA signals in pelvic lymph nodes of men undergoing radical prostatectomy, with a greater sensitivity than traditional histological techniques.[43,44] Although no follow-up data were provided on the patients in these studies, the detection of PSA-producing cells by RT–PCR in histologically negative lymph nodes may account for early relapse and progression in post-prostatectomy patients with pathologically contained lesions. It is unclear, however, whether these prostate-derived signals represent clinically important metastatic spread or, rather, if they signify evidence of a properly functioning immune system filtering circulating prostate-derived tissue.

More provocative, however, were the results of a retrospective study of archival lymph node tissue in 36 men with pathologically localized prostate cancer and negative lymph node extension, by traditional histological and immuno-histochemical staining.[44] 16 of these men were found to have RT–PCR–PSA-positive signals; furthermore, 14 of the 16 patients with positive RT–PCR results had evidence of recurrent disease within 5 years, compared with only six of the 20 who were RT–PCR negative. This suggests that RT–PCR analysis of nodal tissue may have significant prognostic value in men considering radical prostatectomy. It has subsequently been reported that sufficient nodal tissue sampling for RT–PCR can be obtained by CT-guided fine-needle aspirate.[45] The clinical usefulness of these findings, however, remains unclear. Given the poor sensitivity of CT radiography to identify pelvic nodes accurately, either an open or a laparoscopic lymphadenectomy would be required to obtain tissue.[46] Additionally, as current RT–PCR assays are both time and labour intensive, a 'molecular staging lymphadenectomy' would have to be performed separately from the radical prostatectomy. Thus, although RT–PCR analysis of pelvic lymph node tissue may offer improved prognostic information for the patient, it currently would have questionable utility in pre-prostatectomy staging.

RT–PCR and prostate cancer staging: the controversies

Several controversial issues remain unresolved. The first involves the significance of positive circulating RT–PCR signals and whether they represent malignant spread. Tumour biology predicts that most carcinomas shed millions of cells into the circulation before the primary tumour is clinically detectable. Furthermore, the biological significance of circulating tumour cells is unclear. Intravasation of tumour cells into the circulation is just one stage of a multistep process that ultimately results in symptomatic metastatic disease. Such cells not only must enter the circulation but also must survive long enough in the bloodstream to establish a metastatic colony and to then proliferate and flourish at that site. Many studies have confirmed that even small tumours shed millions of neoplastic cells into the systemic circulation, with only a diminutive proportion developing into clinically detectable metastatic lesions.[47]

With the advent of RT–PCR, the detection of circulating prostate-derived cells has new possibilities. However, whether such signals represent hitherto undetected circulating benign cells or actively metastasizing neoplastic elements remains to be elucidated. These cells could represent early metastasis and improve the early detection of advanced disease. In the authors' study, positive PSA signals were detected in two patients with BPH, one of whom subsequently had a positive biopsy for prostate cancer. Similarly, initial reports by Israeli et al. demonstrated the presence of PSA–PCR signals in two patients with BPH;[33] both were later determined to have previously undetected prostate malignancies. Additional data from the Columbia group suggest that the presence of prostate-tissue-derived signals portends treatment failure.[48]

Further support for the argument that the presence of prostate-tissue-derived cells is indicative of metastatic disease is supplied by the majority of RT–PCR clinical studies, which report a lack of detectable circulating signals in control groups and an abundance of positive signals in patients with known advanced disease. The earlier-mentioned reports by Wood et al. of positive lymph node signals not only stress the extreme sensitivity of RT–PCR technology but have correlated RT–PCR–PSA-positive signals in lymph nodes with early relapse after radical prostatectomy.[44] Flow cytometry data suggest that RT–PCR–PSA-positive circulating cells are, in fact, neoplastic.[49] Finally, a recent report in JAMA chronicles the clinical course of an orthotopic heart transplant recipient who developed metastatic prostate cancer that is believed to have originated from nested cells in the donor bloodstream, pericardium, or myocardium.[50]

However, the presence of circulating neoplastic cells does not necessarily equate with either clinically significant metastatic disease or a poor prognosis. Several studies document that many patients with detectable circulating neoplastic cells have no clinical evidence of metastatic disease after several years of follow-up.[47,51] Furthermore, patients undergoing prostate needle biopsy, radical prostatectomy and cystoscopy often have evidence of transient circulating signals that eventually clear from the circulation.[52–54] These data suggest that non-malignant prostate-derived cells are shed into the peripheral circulation and can survive for more than a month.[55] This corroborates other studies, including the authors' own, that indicate that many RT–PCR assays have a high false-positive rate.[23] Finally, the tissue specificity of PSA has recently come under scrutiny. Several studies have documented the presence of circulating PSA signals in women and young men without prostate disease.[56] Furthermore, PSA mRNA has been detected in a variety of non-prostatic tumours, including breast, lung, ovarian, salivary gland and urethral cancers.[57-61]

The significance of capsular penetration and perforation in prostate cancer is also being questioned. In an unpublished review of over 600 consecutive radical prostatectomies at the authors' institution, patients with extracapsular penetration, yet negative surgical margins and seminal vesicle involvement, had a 10-year disease-specific survival rate greater than 70%, similar to that of those men without capsular involvement. Furthermore, data from Johns Hopkins University have documented a 70% 5-year disease non-progression rate in patients with focally positive margins after prostatectomy.[62] Therefore, instead of using PCR-based detection methods to predict capsular involvement, perhaps the focus should be on associating the presence of circulating prostate-tissue-derived signals with disease-specific survival, PSA-specific survival, or overall patient survival — studies that are currently under way at the authors' institution.

Conclusions

At present, no definitive conclusions on the utility of RT–PCR molecular staging for prostate cancer can be reached. It is a powerful scientific technique that will, no doubt, help to resolve many currently unknown aspects of prostate cancer growth and development. Because positive RT–PCR results do often correlate with known metastatic disease, and since positive results are rare in patients without prostate cancer, positive signals in a patient with pathologically localized prostate cancer could potentially indicate evidence of early metastatic disease or portend early treatment failure. However, only with prolonged follow-up and larger study populations will the true significance of circulating prostate-tissue-derived cells be determined. Until that time, in the authors' opinion, RT–PCR molecular staging assays should remain an investigational tool only and have no current role in decision-making in the clinical management of men with prostate disease.

References

1. Parker S L Tong T, Bolden S, Wingo P A. Cancer statistics, 1997. CA 1997; 40(1): 5–27
2. Lu-Yao G L, Greenberg E R. Changes in prostate cancer incidence and treatment in the USA. Lancet 1994; 343: 251–254
3. Catalona W J. Management of carcinoma of the prostate. N Engl J Med 1994; 331(15): 996–1004
4. Paulson D F, Moul J W, Walther P J. Radical prostatectomy for clinical T1–2N0M0 prostate adenocarcinoma: long term results. J Urol 1990; 144(4): 1180–1184
5. Trapasso J G, deKernion J B, Smith R B et al. Incidence and significance of detectable levels of serum prostate specific antigen after radical prostatectomy. J Urol 1994; 152(5): 1821–1825
6. Schellhammer P F. Radical prostatectomy: patterns of local failure and survival. Urology 1988; 31: 191–197
7. Lerner S P, Seale-Hawkins C, Carlton C E Jr et al. The risk of dying of prostate cancer in patients with clinically localized disease. J Urol 1991; 146: 1040–1045
8. Catalona W J, Dresner S M. Nerve-sparing radical prostatectomy: extraprostatic tumor extension and preservation of erectile function. J Urol 1985; 134: 1149–1155
9. Lu-Yao G, McLarran D, Wasson J et al. An assessment of radical prostatectomy. JAMA 1993; 269: 2633–2636

10. van den Ouden D, Davidson P J T, Hop W *et al*. Radical prostatectomy as a monotherapy for locally advanced (stage T3) prostate cancer. J Urol 1994; 151(3): 646–651
11. Ekman P. Dilemma of microscopic lymph node metastases in human prostate cancer. Eur Urol 1993; 24(S-2): 57–60
12. Crawford E D, DeAntoni E P. PSA as a screening test for prostate cancer. Urol Clin North Am 1993; 20(4): 637–646
13. Monda J M, Barry M J, Oesterling J E. PSA cannot distinguish stage T1a (A1) prostate cancer from BPH. J Urol 1994; 151(5): 1291–1295
14. Ploch N R, Brawer M K. How to use PSA. Urology (Suppl) 1994; 43(2): 27–35
15. Wirth M. Value of PSA as a tumor marker. Eur Urol 1993; 24(S-2): 6–12
16. Catalona W L. Comparison of digital rectal examination and serum prostate specific antigen in the early detection of prostate cancer. J Urol 1994; 151(5): 1283–1290
17. Israeli R S, Powell C T, Corr J G *et al*. Expression of the prostate-specific membrane antigen. Cancer Res 1994; 54: 1807–1811
18. Garnick M B. Prostate cancer: screening, diagnosis, and management. Ann Intern Med 1993; 118(4): 804–818
19. Lindemann F, Schlimok G, Dirschedl P *et al*. Prognostic significance of micrometastatic tumour cells in bone marrow of colorectal cancer patients. Lancet 1992; 340: 685–689
20. Wu A, Ben-Eyra J, Columbero A. Detection of micrometastases in breast cancer by PCR. Lab Invest 1990; 62: 109A
21. Miyomura N, Tanimoto Y, Morishima K *et al*. Detection of Philadelphia chromosome positive ALL by PCR: possible eradication of residual disease by bone marrow transplantation. Blood 1992; 52: 6110–6112
22. Templeton N S. The polymerase chain reaction: history, methods, and applications. Diagn Mol Pathol 1992; 1(1): 58–72
23. Sokoloff M H, Tso C L, Kaboo R *et al*. Quantitative polymerase chain reaction does not improve prostate cancer staging: a clinical–pathologic–molecular analysis of 121 patients. J Urol 1996; 156(5): 1560–1566
24. Moreno J G, Croce C M, Fischer R *et al*. Detection of hematogenous micrometastasis in patients with prostate cancer. Cancer Res 1992; 52: 6110–6112
25. Katz A E, Olsson C A, Raffo A J *et al*. Molecular staging of prostate cancer with the use of an enhanced reverse transcriptase–PCR assay. Urology 1994; 43(6): 765–775
26. Katz A E, de Vries G M, Begg M D *et al*. Enhanced reverse transcriptase–polymerase chain reaction for prostate specific antigen as an indicator of true pathologic stage in patients with prostate cancer. Cancer 1995; 75: 1642–1648
27. Olsson C A, de Vries G M, Raffo A J *et al*. Preoperative reverse transcriptase polymerase chain reaction for prostate specific antigen predicts treatment failure following radical prostatectomy. J Urol 1996; 155: 1557–1562
28. Jaakkola S, Vornanen T, Leinonen J *et al*. Detection of prostatic cells in peripheral blood: correlation with serum concentrations of prostate-specific antigen. Clin Chem 1995; 41: 182–186
29. Seiden M V, Kantoff P W, Krithivas K *et al*. Detection of circulating tumor cells in men with localized prostate cancer. J Clin Oncol 1994; 12(12): 2534–2639
30. Ghossein R A, Scher H I, Gerald W L *et al*. Detection of circulating tumor cells in patients with localized and metastatic prostatic carcinoma. J Clin Oncol 1995; 13(5): 1195–1200
31. Slawin K, O'Hara M, Song W *et al*. Comparison of results obtained using different RT–PCR–PSA assay method on a single set of clinical specimens. J Urol 1994; 155(5): 417A (abstr)
32. Camma C, Olsson C A, Raffo A J *et al*. Molecular staging of prostate cancer: a comparison of the application of an enhanced reverse transcriptase polymerase chain reaction assay for prostate specific antigen versus prostate specific membrane antigen. J Urol 1995; 153: 1373–1378
33. Israeli R S, Miller W H Su S L *et al*. Sensitive nested reverse transcription polymerase chain reaction detection of circulating prostatic tumor cells: comparison of prostate-specific membrane antigen and prostate-specific antigen-based assays. Cancer Res 1994; 54: 6306–6310
34. Loric S, Dumas F, Eschwege P *et al*. Enhanced detection of hematogenous prostatic cells in patients with prostate adenocarcinoma by using nested reverse transcriptase polymerase chain reaction assay based on prostate-specific membrane antigen. Clin Chem 1995; 41(12): 1693–1704
35. Bretton P R, Mulamed M R, Fair W R *et al*. Detection of occult micrometastases in the bone marrow of patients with prostate cancer. Prostate 1994; 25: 108–114

36. Oberneder R, Riesenberg R, Kriegman M *et al*. Immunocytochemical detection and phenotype characterization of micrometastatic tumor cells in bone marrow of patients with prostate cancer. Urol Res 1994; 22(1): 3–8
37. Wood D P, Banks E R, Humphreys S *et al*. Identification of bone marrow micrometastases in patients with prostate cancer. Cancer 1994; 74(9): 2533–2540
38. Melchior S, Corey E, Ross A *et al*. Highly sensitized reverse transcriptase polymerase chain reaction assay for PSA mRNA detects early tumour spread in patients with clinically localized cancer of the prostate. Proc A A C R 1996; 37: 87 (abstr)
39. Wood D P, Weinstein M, Humphries S *et al*. Prognostic significance of circulating prostate cells. J Urol 1996; 155(5): 418A (abstr)
40. Danella J F, deKernion J B, Smith R B *et al*. The contemporary incidence of lymph node metastases in prostate cancer: implications for laparoscopic lymph node dissection. J Urol 1993; 149(6): 1488–1491
41. Brawn P, Kuhl D, Johnson C *et al*. Stage D1 prostate cancer: the histologic appearance of nodal metastases and its relationship to survival. Cancer 1990; 65: 538–543
42. Petros J A, Catalona W J. Lower incidence of unsuspected lymph node metastases in 521 consecutive patients with clinically localized prostate cancer. J Urol 1992; 147(6): 1574–1575
43. Duguchi T, Doi T, Hideo E *et al*. Detection of micrometastatic prostate cancer cells in lymph nodes by reverse transcriptase-polymerase chain reaction. Cancer Res 1993; 53: 5350–5354
44. Edelstein R A, Zietman A L, de las Morenas A *et al*. Implications of prostate micrometastases in pelvic lymph nodes: an archival study. Urology 1996; 47(3): 370–375
45. Takahashi T, Hoshi S, Orikasa S *et al*. Genetic diagnosis of pelvic lymph node metastases in prostate cancer. J Urol 1996; 155(5): 378A (abstr)
46. Benson K H, Watson R A, Springer D B *et al*. The value of computerized tomography in evaluation of pelvic lymph nodes. J Urol 1992; 126(1): 63–64
47. Liotta L A, Kleinerman J, Saidel G M. Quantitative relationships of intravascular tumor cells, tumor vessels, and pulmonary metastases following tumor implantation. Cancer Res 1974; 34: 997–1004
48. Katz A E, deVries G M, Benson M C *et al*. The role of reverse transcriptase polymerase chain reaction assay for prostate-specific antigen in the selection of patients for radical prostatectomy. Urol Clin North Am 1996; 23(4): 541–550
49. Hamdy F C. Circulating PSA-positive cells correlate with metastatic prostate cancer. Br J Urol 1992; 69: 392–396
50. Loh E, Couch F J, Hendriksen L *et al*. Development of donor-derived prostate cancer in a recipient following orthotopic heart transplantation. JAMA 1997; 277(2): 133–137
51. Mansi J L, Easton D, Berger J *et al*. Bone marrow micrometastases in primary breast cancer: prognostic significance after six years follow-up. Eur J Cancer 1991; 27: 1552-1555
52. Goldman H, Weld K, Hollabaugh R *et al*. Can PSA RT–PCR be used as a prospective test to detect prostate cancer and what is the effect of prostate needle biopsy on the results of this assay? Proc AACR 1996; 37: 47 (abstr)
53. Oefelein M G, Herz B, Ignatoff J M *et al*. Longitudinal assessment by PSA–RT–PCR of circulating prostate epithelial cells following radical retropubic prostatectomy. J Urol 1996; 155(5): 552A (abstr)
54. Camma C, Olsson C A, Buttyan R *et al*. Molecular staging of prostate cancer III: effects of digital rectal exam, cystoscopy, and needle biopsy on the enhanced reverse transcriptase polymerase chain reaction. J Urol 1996; 155(5): 553A (abstr)
55. Brandt B, Junker R, Growatz C *et al*. Isolation of prostate-derived single cells and cell clusters from human peripheral blood. Cancer Res 1996; 56: 4556–4561
56. O'Hara S M, Veltri R W, Skirpstunas P *et al*. Basal mRNA levels detected by quantitative reverse transcriptase polymerase chain reaction in blood from patients without prostate cancer. Urol 1996; 155(5): 418A (abstr)
57. Diamandis E P, Yu H. New biological functions of prostate-specific antigen. J Clin Endocrinol Metab 1995; 80: 1515–1517
58. Smith M R, Biggar S, Maha H. Prostate-specific antigen mRNA is expressed in non-prostate cells: implications for detection of micrometastases. Cancer Res 1995; 55: 2640–2644
59. van Kreiken J H J M. Prostate marker immunoreactivity in salivary neoplasms. Am J Surg Pathol 1993; 17: 410–414
60. Clements A, Mukhtar A. Glandular kallikreins and prostate-specific antigen expressed in human endometrium. J Clin Endocrinol Metab 1995; 78: 1536–1540

61. Monne M, Croce C, Yu H *et al.* Molecular character of prostate-specific antigen mRNA expressed in breast tumors. Cancer 1994; 54: 6344–6347
62. Epstein J I, Carmichael M, Pizov G, Walsh P C. Influence of capsular penetration on progression following radical prostatectomy: a study of 196 cases with long-term follow-up. J Urol 1993; 150(1): 135–141

Chapter 19
Surgical treatment of localized prostate cancer: indications, technique and results

J. deKernion, A. Belldegrun and J. Naitoh

Introduction

Prostate cancer is the leading cause of cancer death in American men. In 1996, over 317,000 new cases of prostate cancer were diagnosed, and over 45,000 men died from this disease.[1] Currently, there is no chemotherapy or immunotherapy that can cure patients with prostate cancer once it has spread outside the gland. Until effective systemic treatments can be developed, the best hope of decreasing the mortality rate from prostate cancer lies in providing curative treatment while the tumour is still organ confined. The treatment choices for localized prostate cancer are limited, and include either radiotherapy or radical prostatectomy. Problematically, none of these treatment choices has demonstrated clear superiority in terms of long-term cure on disease-free survival. Each option has distinct advantages and disadvantages, and the final treatment decision is largely based on the preferences of the individual patient.

In the United States, for men who are under the age of 70, who have no significant medical co-morbidity, and who have a clinically localized prostate cancer, radical prostatectomy represents the primary form of treatment. Owing to (1) the ageing of the population, (2) the advent of prostate-specific antigen (PSA)-based prostate cancer screening, (3) the development of transrectal ultrasound, which made prostate biopsies easier to perform, and (4) the major improvements in surgical technique, the rate of radical prostatectomy has increase sixfold between 1984 and 1990.[2] However, despite the improvements in the ability to detect cancer at earlier stages, and increases in the rates of radical prostatectomy, death rates due to prostate cancer have not changed appreciably. Furthermore, biochemical (PSA-based) recurrence rates following surgery have been reported to be 20–30%, with the side effects of therapy (impotence, incontinence) potentially being worse than the symptoms caused by the cancer itself.[3–5] Although it is clear that many patients will benefit from radical prostatectomy, it is also clear that radical prostatectomy alone will not be curative in all cases and that new treatment strategies for advanced prostate cancer are needed. Additionally, since there is no biomarker that can reliably separate those patients who have indolent cancers from those patients who have biologically aggressive lesions, all patients who have prostate cancer and who have a reasonably long life expectancy should consider undergoing treatment instead of watchful waiting.

Furthermore, the choice of treatment for the patient who has a clinically localized prostate cancer has to be individualized to the characteristics of the patient, and to the grade and stage of the tumour. Currently, there is no prospective, randomized trial that has shown a definitive survival benefit for either radical prostatectomy or radiation therapy. Interpretation of these treatment results is further complicated by the knowledge that many patients will survive for an equally long period without therapeutic intervention other than endocrine therapy and symptomatic treatment of metastases. The variable biological behaviour of prostate cancer and the presence of confounding co-morbidities make objective interpretation of the available data impossible. At this time, the physician has to provide the best advice to patients, based on limited information. Until a predictive test can be established that accurately defines the aggressiveness of a specific tumour, and can determine the impact that this tumour will have on a specific patient who has specific co-morbidities, other criteria must be relied upon.

This chapter assesses the surgical treatment of prostate cancer, and also describes the indications, techniques and outcomes of radical prostatectomy. Comparisons of radical prostatectomy with watchful waiting and radiotherapy are also discussed.

Radical prostatectomy versus watchful waiting

Owing to the unpredictable behaviour of prostate cancer, and owing to the impact that patient co-morbidity and family history has on longevity, the age after which a person is not a candidate for definitive therapy (either radiotherapy or surgery) varies according to the individual patient. Besides age, tumour stage and tumour grade are other important factors that have to be entered into the decision-making algorithm. Older patients who have low-grade, low-stage tumours are ideal candidates for programmes of watchful waiting, where curative treatments are withheld under the assumption that palliative treatments (such as androgen-deprivation therapy) can control the cancer until the patient succumbs to other medical illness. Under programmes of watchful waiting, it is clear that many patients can outlive their cancers. Warner and Whitmore observed 75 patients for up to 15 years with no therapy: approximately 75% of their patients developed distant metastases during the 15 years of observation, while over 80% had local progression as well;[6] however, disease-specific survival at 15 years was 96% for B1 disease and 72% for B2 disease. Although these numbers seem quite high, it was uncertain how many of these men would have had a longer life and a better quality of life had they undergone radical prostatectomy or some other form of definitive treatment.

The Swedish literature has similarly shown high survival rates under a watchful waiting approach, especially when it was applied to elderly patients with low-grade tumours.[7,8] Adolfsson reported 10-year disease-specific survival rates of 80% for patients who were entered into a surveillance protocol, with the competing mortality rates higher than the mortality rate that occurred due to prostate cancer.[8] It has also been observed in the United States that untreated patients with low-grade tumours can have life expectancies that are similar to those of the general population.[9] However, it must be emphasized that the patients who did well in programmes of watchful waiting were highly selected, and tended to have indolent-behaving, well-differentiated tumours (Gleason sum score 2, 3 and 4 tumours). In contrast, patients who have higher-grade tumours, or patients who are younger, can show up to an 8-year loss of life expectancy under a watchful waiting programme. It is this decreased survival rate against which the outcomes of different treatment approaches must be measured. Thus, the authors and others believe that the patient who has a greater than 10-year life expectancy or who has a high-grade tumour needs treatment, whereas the patient who has a shorter life expectancy is probably better served by less aggressive approaches.[10]

Other than age, patient co-morbidity and tumour grade, the side effects of therapy must also be considered in the decision-making algorithm. Radical prostatectomy can result in wound infection, haemorrhage and deep vein thrombosis, and has a perioperative mortality rate of up to 1%.[2] In the long term, erectile dysfunction, incontinence and urethral stricture can also compromise the patient's quality of life after radical prostatectomy. For the patient for whom sexual potency is important, or where the risk of complications is great, non-surgical therapies or watchful waiting programmes may be preferred. Although newer surgical techniques that minimize periurethral dissection, and nerve-sparing procedures, can minimize the side effects of surgical treatment, the impact of radical prostatectomy on sexual function and bladder function can be significant. In contrast, watchful waiting has no immediate effects on sexual function or continence, since no treatment is initiated. However, watchful waiting programmes resulted in a trade-off, where current side effects of therapy are exchanged for future symptoms due to the potential progression of the cancer.

A review of the current literature is unlikely to answer completely each of these controversies or unambiguously to clarify the selection criteria for radical prostatectomy. It is hoped that the Prostate Intervention Versus Observation Trial (PIVOT), which will prospectively compare, over the next 15 years, a cohort of men who underwent radical prostatectomy with a matched cohort of men who are under a watchful waiting programme, will provide some useful data. However, in the interim, the physician will have to advise the patient regarding therapeutic options using the most current information available.

Radical prostatectomy versus radiotherapy

Even more controversial than the choice between treatment and watchful waiting, is the choice between surgical treatment and radiotherapy. Unfortunately, there is no conclusive evidence to show that one modality offers a long-term, significant survival advantage over the other. Radiotherapy does have certain advantages when compared with radical prostatectomy: there is no need for hospitalization, and the risks of a surgical procedure and the discomfort of an incision are avoided. The incontinence risk is lower than with surgery, although impotence can still be a problem over time. However, the side effects of treatment, the protracted time course of radiotherapy (daily treatments over several weeks), and questions about its efficacy relative to surgical treatment are factors that make radiotherapy a far from ideal treatment option for all patients.

The complications of radiotherapy have been well defined, although variations in the dosage of radiation given and the fractionation of the treatment dosage will also affect the complications rates (Table 19.1). Proctitis has occurred in up to 30% of patients while they are undergoing treatment, with 1–2% having long-term rectal problems including stenosis or chronic proctitis. Cystitis and gross haematuria are additional side effects that can occur during radiotherapy to the pelvis. Fortunately, most of these irritative symptoms will resolve after treatment, with only 2% of men having severe, long-term problems following external beam radiotherapy.[11] Erectile dysfunction can also be associated with radiotherapy, with approximately 50–66% of potent men becoming impotent after treatment.[11] Unlike erectile dysfunction associated with surgery, impotence following radiotherapy trends to be progressive after treatment, and can occur months to years after the therapy.

Although the side effects and long-term complications of radiotherapy and radical prostatectomy have been well characterized, it is impossible to compare the efficacy of these different treatments directly, as the patient populations who

Table 19.1. Complications of external beam radiotherapy

Complications	Short-term incidence rate of complication (%)	Percentage of patients with long-term symptoms
Rectal bleeding	3.8 – 14.9	0 – 2.7
Diarrhoea	10 – 12	0.4 – 2
Incontinence	0 – 1.4	0 – 1.5
Haematuria	5.8 – 10.8	1 – 2.7
Erectile dysfunction*	–	55 – 66
Urethral stricture/bladder neck contracture	1.5 – 8.3	0 – 8.0

*For patients who were evaluated ≥ 5 years after treatment.
(From ref. 11 with permission.)

undergo radiotherapy versus surgery are not equivalent. Historically, patients who underwent radiotherapy tended to be older and had more locally advanced tumours. Comparison between surgery and radiotherapy series is also difficult, as radiotherapy studies have always been based on clinical stage whereas surgical series have been based on pathological stage. However, the tendency of the surgeon to underestimate the clinical disease stage has been somewhat counterbalanced by a similar tendency for the radiotherapist to overestimate the clinical extent of the tumour.

Clinical trials have been performed in order to compare the efficacy of radiotherapy versus surgery, but the results have not provided definitive answers to this controversy. Kupelian recently reported the 5-year follow-up rates of two comparable groups of men who underwent either radical prostatectomy or radiotherapy.[12] At the 5-year point, biochemical recurrence rates (as defined by a detectable PSA in the radical prostatectomy group, or a rising PSA following radiotherapy) were similar in both groups. Although this evidence suggests that the short-term results of radiotherapy and surgery are equivalent, the longer-term results are not yet available.

However, there is preliminary evidence to suggest that cancer control rates may not be as good with radiotherapy as with surgery. A comparison of progression rates of patients who underwent radical prostatectomy with a similar group of men who underwent radiotherapy showed that 22% of the patients who underwent surgery had PSA progression at 5 years, whereas 39% of the radiotherapy patients had PSA progression. Furthermore, PSA-based failure rates of radiotherapy have been reported to be as high as 50% at 5 years, with 20–50% of men still having histological evidence of prostate cancer, based on prostate biopsies performed 2 years after radiotherapy.[13] A structured literature review by Goluboff and Benson also suggested that long-term PSA recurrence rates are higher in patients treated with radiotherapy than in patients treated with radical prostatectomy. For studies that had patients with 15 years of follow-up, the biochemical (PSA-based) relapse-free rates ranged between 19 and 46% in the radiotherapy patients, whereas they were between 40 and 75% in the patients who underwent radical prostatectomy.[14] Thus, it is currently not known whether radiotherapy can control prostate cancer as effectively as radical prostatectomy, although the long-term data seem to favour surgical outcomes. It is hoped that the results of further studies by the Prostate Outcome Research Team (PORT) may help to clarify this controversy, as they compare the different treatment approaches while trying to control for tumour stage and grade, and for patient age and co-morbidity.

In summary, the majority of patients will probably have their disease controlled with radiotherapy, although the long-term (greater than 10-year) disease-free rates may be better with surgery. There are no perioperative or anaesthetic risks associated with radiotherapy; recuperation time back to normal activity is quicker with radiotherapy, and the risk of incontinence is lower. In the authors' opinion, radiotherapy is an effective treatment option for any patient who has prostate cancer, although they tend to recommend radical prostatectomy for the younger patient with prostate cancer, or for the patient who has a high-grade tumour. Additionally, since nerve-sparing surgery provides a better chance of preserving erectile function than radiotherapy, the patient who wants to preserve his potency will probably be better served with surgery if bilateral nerve sparing is feasible. In either case, patients who have low-grade tumours and low PSA levels (which probably reflect small tumour volumes) will do well with either treatment approach.

Management of clinical stage T1a and T1c prostate cancer

Stage T1a prostate cancer is very uncommon, especially if strict criteria are used to define it. The authors define clinical stage T1a prostate cancer as a tumour that is unsuspected and detected after a transurethral resection of the prostate (TURP), where less than 5% of the TURP specimen contains only well-differentiated tumour, and where subsequent prostate biopsies fail to show any residual tumour after TURP. It is assumed in the stage T1a patients that the TUR alone was curative, on the basis of the belief that there is no residual cancer located elsewhere in the gland.

Clearly, many patients with clinical stage T1a disease are cured after TURP alone. Walsh and colleagues showed that only 24% of patients with stage T1a tumour had substantial tumour found at the time of radical prostatectomy, although over 90% of the specimens did contain residual foci of prostate cancer.[15] Although the clinical significance of those foci were unclear, it has also been shown that progression of disease in patients with T1a tumour is uncommon, and occurred in only 16% of the patients reviewed by Epstein et al.[16]

However, it is also now recognized that many patients with tumours in the transition zone of the prostate can have additional, and possibly more aggressive, prostate cancers in the peripheral zone that are undetectable by TURP. It is hoped that the use of serial PSA determinations, transrectal ultrasound (TRUS) evaluations, and multiple needle biopsies will be able to identify those patients who have clinical stage T1a tumours that need treatment, versus those patients who have been 'cured' by the TURP alone.

Terris et al. detected residual cancer in almost 50% of the patients with clinical T1a disease when extensive TRUS-guided biopsies of the prostate were performed.[17] Those authors further determined that a PSA greater than 2.5 ng/ml indicated the presence of residual cancer following TURP, while Carter et al. determined that patients who had a post-TURP PSA of less than 1 ng/ml had a decreased risk of progression.[18] The use of serial PSA measurements (PSA velocity) may also be of benefit in the management of patients with stage A disease.

The authors' current approach to evaluate the patient with stage T1a disease is to perform TRUS-guided prostate biopsies of the prostate following TURP to look for significant amounts of residual cancer. However, if the patient has a considerable volume of residual tissue following TURP, then a more thorough

TURP would be considered, in addition to the ultrasound-guided needle biopsies of the prostate. If the re-sampling is negative, patients are followed carefully with serial digital rectal examination (DRE) and monitoring of PSA levels at 6-month intervals. Any significant change in the PSA or the DRE indicates the need for further biopsies to rule out the presence of a more significant tumour that needs treatment.

The decision for treatment, and the type of treatment, are then determined on the basis of the patient's age, tumour grade, PSA level, and presence or absence of medical co-morbidity. The older patient with stage T1a tumour, even through the prostate may harbour other microfoci of tumour, is not likely to die of prostate cancer and therefore should not undergo aggressive diagnostic evaluation and treatment. In contrast, the young, healthy patient will be considered for more aggressive evaluation and therapy, given the likelihood that progression of disease may occur if given enough time.

The increased use of PSA for early detection of prostate cancer has resulted in the detection of a large number of tumours that are non-palpable and were diagnosed only on the basis of the elevated PSA (stage T1c). The primary justification of PSA-based screening programmes is based on the ability of the test to detect cancer before any palpable change has occurred in the prostate. It is hoped that the tumours that are detected through PSA-based screening programmes will be clinically significant, but, simultaneously it is also hoped that these cancers have a greater probability of being organ confined and will therefore be more curable by surgical removal.

Although PSA screening will allow for the earlier detection of prostate cancer before the cancer becomes palpable, the major concern raised with PSA-based screening was the possibility that many indolent cancers would also be detected. Potentially, PSA-based screening could result in the overtreatment of patients who had lesions that would never have caused harm or decreased life expectancy. On the basis of studies of prostates that were removed incidentally during radical cystectomy, Stamey defined a prostate tumour as clinically insignificant if it occupied less than 0.3 cm of a core biopsy, if it was confined to one biopsy core, and if it was of low Gleason grade.[19] Although such criteria are helpful to determine the necessity of treatment in the case of an individual tumour, some patients with a 'clinically insignificant' tumour on biopsy will be found to have more tumour than expected at the time of radical prostatectomy. Although it is hoped that such patients will be detected with serial PSA determinations, the validity of this supposition is unknown at this time.

However, it is apparent that the majority of cancers found from PSA-based screening programmes do not fit the definition of clinically insignificant, as defined by Stamey. The importance of PSA-detected tumours was clearly shown in the screening studies of Catalona et al.: increased PSA was the only indication of tumour in 44% of the total number of tumours detected in this series.[20] Furthermore, although the majority of the PSA-detected tumours were pathologically organ confined, most of them were also of significant volume. Elgamal et al. also showed that stage T1c tumours are of a clinically significant size, with the prostate tumours having a median volume of 1.6 cm^3.[21]

Additionally, it has been shown that stage T1c tumours are often pathologically more advanced than might be suspected on the basis of clinical staging. Douglas et al. detected pathological involvement of the periprostatic fat in 44% of clinical stage T1c cases, seminal vesicle extension in 8% and insignificant tumour in only 5%.[22] At the present authors' institution, 72 patients with stage T1c tumour were studied: the mean Gleason score was 5.6, and 25% had a Gleason score equal to or greater than 7. Thus, it appears to be the case that most PSA-detected tumours are clinically significant, are amenable to surgical treatment, and have a significant risk for tumour progression under programmes of watchful waiting. However, it is also important to remember that between 10 and 16% of patients with stage T1c disease had clinically insignificant cancers found at the time of radical prostatectomy, as judged by the finding of small-volume tumours of low Gleason grade in the pathological specimen.[23,24] Thus, in the future, the inclusion and exclusion criteria for treatment of patients with clinical stage T1c prostate cancer will have to become better defined, and will have to be more thoroughly tested.

The management of T1c tumours, like that of all other prostate cancers, is influenced by patient age, patient co-morbidity, PSA level and tumour grade. The authors generally recommend definitive treatment for young patients, even for those patients who have small foci of well-differentiated tumour. For patients in their 60's and 70's who have low-grade tumours, or for those patients who have significant medical co-morbidity, the authors tend to adopt a less aggressive approach, provided that a second set of prostate biopsies, including transition zone biopsies, shows no significant tumour volume and no tumour with a component of Gleason score 4 or 5.

Management of stage T1b and T2 prostate cancer

Although there is debate as to whether patients with non-palpable tumour should be treated at all, few disagree that young patients with clinical stage T1b and T2 cancer should be offered some form of definitive treatment. Historically, the problem with DRE-based screening programmes was the inability to detect prostate cancer while it was still small, non-palpable and therefore organ confined. Furthermore, significant understaging of clinically palpable lesions can occur, because such tumours invariably have a large volume and also because of the insensitivity of the DRE. It has been shown that up to 66% of patients who underwent radical prostatectomy for presumed stage B disease had penetration into the capsule, invasion through the capsule, or involvement of the seminal vesicles.[25] These results are similar to those previously reported in other series.

The authors recently analysed the outcomes of the last 367 patients who underwent radical prostatectomy at their institution, representing those patients who were diagnosed and treated in the era of mass PSA screening. Patients who had neo-adjuvant hormone treatment were excluded from this analysis. The mean follow-up of the entire group is 13 months. A summary of the data is given in Table 41.2. The incidence of positive nodes in recent years was 3%, which reflects an improved understanding of prostate cancer behaviour and better patient selection for radical prostatectomy, and is also due to the large number of lower-volume PSA-detected tumours that have been treated in this recent series. Only 10% of the patients have had a clinical recurrence (as defined by a positive DRE, a positive biopsy of the vesico-urethral anastomosis, or a positive bone scan) of their prostate cancer at 5 years. However, when the definition of cancer recurrence after radical prostatectomy is defined as a PSA of more than 0.4 ng/ml, biochemical recurrence rates have been much higher than the clinical recurrence rates reported before (Table 19.2). Other recently published radical prostatectomy series[3,4,26–28] have reported similar recurrence rates (Table 19.3).

Although the overall 5-year biochemical (PSA) relapse rates in all of these series seem high, the authors have also noted that the average PSA levels of patients undergoing radical prostatectomy have been declining steadily over the last 7 years. Accompanying this decline is a concomitant increase in the percentage of

Table 19.2. Probability of remaining free of PSA recurrence after radical retropubic prostatectomy diagnosed in the era of PSA screening according to pathological stage (367 patients)

	Pathological stage			
	T2	T3A/B	T3C	Overall
Percentage of patients free of biochemical recurrence	82	63	25	72

Table 19.3. Probability of remaining free of biochemical recurrence following radical prostatectomy

Series	Pathological stage of tumour	Percentage of patients free of biochemical recurrence at 5 years
Cleveland Clinic[4]	Overall series	61
	Specimen-confined disease	80
	Pathological stage 3 disease	37
Mayo Clinic[26]	Overall series	70
Washington University[27]	Organ-confined disease	90
	Pathological stage T3A/T3B	75
	Pathological stage T3C	33
Duke University[3,28]	Organ-confined disease	85

patients in the authors' series who underwent radical prostatectomy and had pathologically organ-confined disease (Figures 19.1 and 19.2). With the increasing application of PSA screening in the population, and an increased understanding of the clinical usefulness of PSA as a marker for the diagnosis and staging of prostate cancer, patient selection for radical prostatectomy has steadily improved. The authors expect that the improved selection of patients who undergo radical prostatectomy, in combination with the improved cancer detection that is provided by PSA screening, will eventually translate into improvements in PSA-based recurrence rates following surgical therapy.

However, it also must be remembered that the clinical significance of many of these PSA recurrences is unclear. Whereas approximately 33% of all of the authors' patients have had a relapse, as judged by a detectable PSA of more than 0.4 ng/ml only 10% of the patients have developed clinically detectable relapses to date. It may be the case that the majority of these patients will not need any further treatment, and that they will outlive their cancers despite the biochemical relapse. The rate of PSA rise after surgery, independent of any other factor, seems to predict best which patients will develop clinical recurrence once the PSA became detectable following surgery.[29] Patients who had PSA doubling times of less than 6 months had a clinical recurrence rate of 20–35%, whereas patients who had a doubling time of over 18 months had only a 15% clinical recurrence rate. Thus, patients who had a slow doubling time had a low risk of developing clinical recurrence despite the presence of a rising post-prostatectomy PSA. In contrast, patients whose PSA is rising rapidly may benefit from early, adjuvant treatment. This experience parallels the experience that has been reported by others.[30]

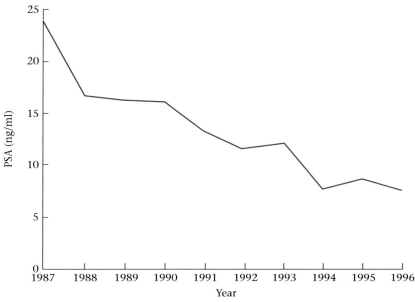

Figure 19.1. Average preoperative PSA in the authors' series of patients: trend from 1987 to 1996.

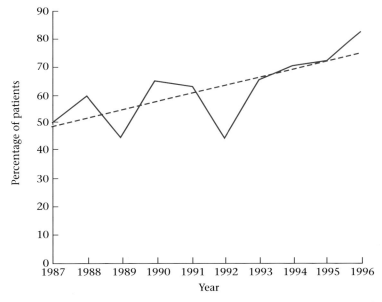

Figure 19.2. Percentages of patients in the authors' series (1987–1996) with tumours that were pathologically organ confined: —— percentage of patients; ----- linear trend.

In summary, the ability of prostatectomy to control disease must be balanced against the impact that the therapy has on the patient's *quality* of life, not to mention the fact that there is still no study that definitively shows that radical prostatectomy can even increase the *quantity* of life. At this time, radical prostatectomy appears to be the most effective method for eradicating localized prostatic cancer. Local recurrence rates have been shown to be very low after surgical treatment.[5] However, long-term questions regarding quality-of-life issues and overall longevity remain unanswered.

Surgical management of patients with locally advanced disease

Patients with clinical stage T3 (stage C) prostate cancer are not considered to be ideal candidates for radical prostatectomy, since the probability that surgery alone can cure these patients is low. Van den Ouden reported results in 100 patients who underwent radical prostatectomy alone for clinical stage T3 prostate cancer.[31] Of these patients, 48% had positive nodes and 2% had T4 tumours. Only one-third of these patients were clinically free of tumour within 4 years, with local recurrence occurring in approximately 30% of patients. Biochemically defined (i.e. PSA based) recurrence rates probably would have been even higher.

Unfortunately, radiotherapy had also had only limited efficacy in treating patients with locally advanced prostate cancer. For these reasons, neo-adjuvant hormone-deprivation therapy has been tried in an attempt to decrease the size of the tumour prior to both surgery and radiotherapy, with the idea that decreasing the size of the tumour will make it more amenable to treatment. Unfortunately, neo-adjuvant hormone therapy has not been effective in 'downstaging' tumours, with the rate of PSA recurrence following radical prostatectomy unchanged when the results were compared with those of a group of patients who did not receive neo-adjuvant therapy.[32]

However, reduction of tumour volume with neo-adjuvant therapy prior to radiation therapy may improve local control and disease-free survival, since the volume of tumour is decreased, which then increases the relative dosage of radiation that can be given to the tissue. Pipepich *et al.* found that local control, disease-free survival, and PSA-disease-free survival were 71, 43 and 26% for radiotherapy alone versus 84, 61 and 46% in the group receiving neo-adjuvant hormones.[33] Whether this beneficial response will translate into longer overall survival is unknown.

Multiple studies have been performed involving patients with locally advanced prostate cancer, in an attempt to determine whether either radiotherapy or surgery offers a better chance of long-term disease-free survival. Unfortunately, despite these efforts, concrete conclusions about the efficacy of each treatment approach still cannot be drawn. There is only one preoperative randomized study to date that has directly compared surgery versus radiotherapy in patients with clinical stage T3 tumours. The National Prostate Cancer Project (NPCP) protocol (Gibbons R. P. G, personal communication, June 1996) has now accrued long-term follow-up, with no difference found in either overall survival or progression-free survival between the two groups. In contrast, a recent series from the Mayo Clinic did show a higher than usual rate of progression-free survival after prostatectomy for T3 tumours, but selection bias in this non-randomized protocol could have accounted for the differences that were noted.[34]

At this time, decisions regarding management of the patient with T3 prostate cancer must be based on the known prognostic factors that influence overall survival and tumour progression. For the most part, radical prostatectomy will not help these patients, since up to 50% of patients with a clinical T3 lesion will have lymphatic metastasis at the time of surgery, and since surgery overall has not been proved to be superior to radiotherapy in the management of these tumours. However, owing to the more indolent behaviour of low-grade lesions, young, symptomatic patients who have locally advanced tumours (especially those patients who have low-grade tumours) can, in the authors' opinion, obtain a survival benefit from surgical therapy. A review of the authors' results has shown that over 80% of patients who have low-grade (Gleason grade less than 7) T3C tumours remained free of PSA relapse after 5 years of follow-up.

The management of patients who are discovered to have pelvic lymph node metastases is also controversial. Interpretation of the data is confounded by the administration of immediate endocrine therapy in many patients, as well as by the wide variety of endocrine treatments that have been used in these patients. The authors' institution recently reviewed a series of consecutive patients who underwent radical prostatectomy, despite the presence of microscopic lymph node metastases: the 10-year cause-specific survival in these patients was 80% if they received immediate endocrine therapy.[35] The Mayo Clinic reported similar findings, with their data demonstrating that patients who had diploid tumours had the greatest benefit: only a few of these patients had tumour recurrence.[36] These studies have been cited as support for radical surgery in patients with node-positive disease, especially in younger patients where treatment options are limited for providing long-term control of the disease.

The overall prognosis for this group of patients depends upon the volume of the tumour (including the volume of nodal metastases), tumour grade, PSA level, ploidy, and the presence of significant medical co-morbidities in the patient. It is generally believed that aggressive regional or local management of patients with grossly enlarged lymph nodes is unwarranted. However, some patients with microscopic positive nodes, especially in cases where the tumour is low grade, will remain clinically free of disease following aggressive surgical therapy. Thus, the authors do not routinely perform frozen sections of the pelvic lymph nodes during radical prostatectomy to check for occult metastatic disease if the nodal packet is grossly normal, and will proceed with radical prostatectomy unless there is gross adenopathy secondary to the presence of metastatic cancer.

In summary, the incidence of lymph node metastases has markedly decreased in recent years, owing to better patient selection. Patients with PSA over 25 ng/ml and/or any Gleason grade 4 or 5 tumour should have a lymph node dissection. Otherwise, pelvic lymph node dissection is unnecessary, even in patients who are undergoing radical retropubic prostatectomy. The authors follow those general guidelines, and perform frozen sections of the pelvic lymph nodes only in patients who have a high probability of metastases, or in patients with palpable nodes. If gross adenopathy is present, the authors generally do not proceed with prostatectomy, but do proceed with endocrine therapy.

Technique of radical prostatectomy

The resurgence of radical prostatectomy for localized prostatic cancer is due to the known risk of local recurrence following radiotherapy, as well as to improvements in the technique of radical prostatectomy. These improvements have decreased the morbidity of therapy and have made the surgical treatment of prostate cancer more acceptable to the patient.

The surgeon can approach the prostate through either a perineal or a retropubic approach. The traditional radical perineal prostatectomy is a less arduous operation, and is associated with less blood loss and a generally shorter hospitalization.[37,38] In the published series, the risk of impotence and rectal perforation may be greater with perineal prostatectomy than with radical retropubic prostatectomy, although no randomized comparative studies have been performed.[39,40] Potency sparing may not be as feasible in perineal surgery as in retropubic surgery, although modifications in the technique have attempted to improve the ability to save the nerves.[41]

Another disadvantage of perineal prostatectomy is the inability to evaluate the pelvic lymph nodes at the time of surgery. In general, the pelvic lymphadenectomy must be performed as a separate procedure in patients when there is a high-stage or a high-grade tumour. Fortunately, node dissection of any type is seldom essential for the majority of patients who undergo surgical therapy, owing to the low risk of nodal metastasis that is seen in current series, and owing to the improved ability to stage patients accurately prior to surgery.

The choice of surgical technique between the perineal and retropubic approach is more often based on the training and experience of the surgeon than on the specific advantages or disadvantages of each approach. However, it is safe to conclude that perineal prostatectomy can be feasibly performed in patients with smaller prostate glands (< 40 g) and where there is a wide separation between the ischial tuberosities, whereas patients who need lymph node dissections, who have larger prostate glands, or who have a strong desire to preserve their neruovascular bundles, are better served by retropubic prostatectomy.

Technique of radical perineal prostatectomy

Radical perineal prostatectomy is performed through a small horseshoe incision made at the base of the scrotum. Since the dorsal venous complex is not divided during surgery, the amount of blood that can be lost from this procedure is less than that lost during radical retropubic prostatectomy. Recuperation time is also shorter, given the lack of a midline abdominal incision, with hospital stays ranging from 2 to 3 days. Although the hospital stay has traditionally been shorter for perineal prostatectomy than for retropubic prostatectomy, recent developments of clinical care pathways and the widespread use of non-narcotic pain medications postoperatively have decreased the hospital stay for retropubic prostatectomy patients to the point where it is almost identical to that for those undergoing perineal prostatectomy.

The main disadvantage of perineal prostatectomy is the inability to access the pelvic lymph nodes for accurate staging, which requires a separate procedure to sample this nodal tissue if metastatic disease is suspected. Initial enthusiasm for laparoscopic approaches for lymph node dissection[42] in combination with perineal prostatectomy has subsided, owing to the fact that current preoperative parameters such as clinical stage, PSA and tumour Gleason score can provide prognostic information about the probability of lymph node metastasis. In fact, owing to better patient selection, the rate of positive lymph nodes found during radical prostatectomy in most series has decreased to less than 5%. As such, lymph node dissections in the majority of patients who undergo prostatectomy are unnecessary.

Other limitations to perineal prostatectomy include the difficulties that can be encountered if the prostate is large or if the pelvic anatomy is not favourable. Additionally, access to the seminal vesicles can be difficult, and nerve sparing is more difficult because the neurovascular bundles are difficult to visualize through the perineal approach.

For perineal prostatectomy, the patient is placed in an exaggerated lithotomy position. The rectum is irrigated clear with antibiotic solution, and then the patient is prepped and draped in a sterile manner. An O'Connor drape with a sterile finger cot allows for intra-operative access to the rectum. Palpation of the rectum intra-operatively allows for identification of the anterior rectal wall during surgery, and it facilitates dissection. A curved Lowsley retractor is placed transurethrally into the bladder to allow for manipulation of the prostate during the dissection.

A horseshoe incision is made around the rectum, running between the ischial tuberosities and anterior to the rectum. The central tendon of the perineum is cut, and then the ischiorectal fossae are bluntly developed lateral to the prostate. The prostate is then positioned by the Lowsley retractor so that it protrudes into the incision, after which the anterior rectal wall is gently dissected away from the posterior aspect of the prostate. Care is taken to avoid rectal injury, with occasional palpation of the rectum lumen during dissection allowing for identification of the anterior rectal wall. After short division of the recto-urethral muscle, the rectum falls posteriorly, which then provides for full exposure of the posterior aspect of the prostate. Denonvilliers' fascia is then opened vertically (the 'Pearly Gates'), and the investing fascia around the prostate is pushed laterally, which should allow for preservation of the neurovascular bundles. Further dissection laterally with a right-angle clamp allows for identification and dissection of the pedicles to the prostate, which can then be ligated and divided.

The urethra and the apex of the prostate are then identified. After the posterior wall of the urethra is opened, the Lowsley retractor is removed to allow for complete transection of the urethra, with a straight Lowsley retractor placed in the prostate to allow for further manipulation of the prostate. Blunt dissection pushes the dorsal venous complex off the anterior surface of the prostate. Palpation of the Lowsley retractor blades in the bladder allows for identification of the bladder neck. An incision is made along the anterior bladder neck until the bladder is entered. Indigo carmine can then be given intravenously to allow for identification of the ureteral orifices. Under direct vision, the lateral and posterior bladder neck are divided to free the prostate from the bladder, with care taken to avoid ureteral injury. As the dissection proceeds behind the bladder, the seminal vesicles and vas deferens are identified and removed in continuity with the prostate. Anastomotic sutures are then placed in the urethral stump, and the vesico-urethral anastomosis is then completed over a 24 Fr Foley catheter.

Penrose drains are then placed around the anastomosis, after which the incision is closed. The patient postoperatively is started on clear liquids, and is ambulated on the first day after surgery. The Penrose drains, in general, can be removed just prior to the patient's discharge home on the second hospital day, with the Foley catheter remaining in place for 2 weeks.

Complications of radical perineal prostatectomy

Many of the complications that can follow perineal prostatectomy are similar to those that can follow retropubic prostatectomy. Incontinence and impotence rates are similar to those seen following retropubic prostatectomy (see below), although some authors believe that perineal approaches result in higher impotence rates due to difficulties with nerve sparing in this procedure. Blood loss is less with perineal approaches, since the dorsal vein complex is not divided, and recuperation time is probably quicker with a perineal incision versus a midline lower abdominal incision, although data to substantiate this claim do not exist, to the authors' knowledge. However, there are some complications that are unique to perineal prostatectomy: rectal injury rates appear to be higher with perineal approaches, and can be as high as 11%;[40] furthermore, the exaggerated lithotomy position has been reported to result in transient lower back pain postoperatively, as well as episodes of nerve palsy or compartment syndrome of the lower extremities due to prolonged surgical time or due to incorrect positioning of the legs.[43,44]

Technique of radical retropubic prostatectomy

Since the development of the anatomical radical prostatectomy by Walsh and Donker, the procedure has become the gold standard by which all other techniques for prostate removal must be measured.[45,46] Multiple modifications have been developed in order to improve the technique, since the outcomes of potency and continence after surgery have not been perfect. Tubularization of the bladder neck, preservation of intraprostatic urethral length, and various 'no-touch' approaches around the rhabdosphincter of the urethra are all recent developments aimed at decreasing the severity of incontinence that is seen following surgery.[47,48]

In recent years, the standard Walsh procedure has also been modified in several ways in order to improve ultimate urinary continence as well as to decrease the time to return of urinary continence postoperatively. Additionally, by creating a postoperative clinical care pathway that emphasizes early ambulation, early oral intake and minimal use of narcotic pain medications, the average hospital stay in the authors' institution following radical prostatectomy has been decreased to 2.4 days.

The authors have devised multiple modifications to the standard Walsh procedure in order to improve postoperative continence: these have involved (1) preserving all the layers of the urethra, including the outer spongy and muscular layer, (2) preserving maximum urethral length and (3) preserving retropubic urethral support. In this technique, dissection around the urethra is minimized. The puboprostatic ligaments are left intact, and a large absorbable suture ligature is placed around the dorsal venous complex just above the prostatic apex to control back-bleeding and to allow for better definition of the apex.

After creation of a midline, lower abdominal incision, bilateral pelvic lymph node dissection is performed. If there is no obvious spread of cancer to the lymph nodes, then prostatectomy is performed. The surface of the prostate is exposed, and the dorsal vein complex overlying the prostate is bunched together with a Babcock clamp. A large chromic suture ligature is then placed around the dorsal vein just above the prostatic apex to control back-bleeding and to allow for definition of the apex. A stitch is also placed distally in the dorsal vein to assist in control of bleeding while the vein is divided. The dorsal vein tissue is divided carefully, staying close to the anterior surface of the prostate. The dissection is continued posteriorly until the urethra is identified.

A right-angle clamp is then placed under the superficial pelvic fascia on each side of the prostate, and the fascia is divided. The neurovascular bundles are then identified and mobilized posteriorly from the level of the apex to the bladder neck. This facilitates safe division of the urethra and recto-urethral muscle. This apex of the prostate is then identified and mobilized away from the pelvic floor musculature, and the urethra is divided. After division of the urethra, the posterior wall of the urethra and the recto-urethral muscle are identified and incised close to the prostate apex. The lateral pedicles of the prostate are then ligated and divided, after which dissection is carried behind the bladder neck. Opening of Denonvilliers' fascia behind the bladder allows for exposure of the seminal vesicles and the vas deferens, which are then mobilized. The bladder neck is then opened, and the prostate is separated from the bladder neck and removed with the seminal vesicles.

Anastomotic sutures are then placed in the urethral stump, and the vesico-urethral anastomosis is then completed over a 16 Fr Foley catheter. Closed suction drains are then placed around the anastomosis, after which the incision is closed.

The patient postoperatively is started on clear liquids on postoperative day 1, and is ambulated on the first day after surgery. Ketorolac is used for pain control in order to minimize the ileus that can occur if narcotic pain medications are used. The drains are removed just prior to the patient's discharge home on the second hospital day, with the Foley catheter remaining in place for 2 weeks.

Complications of radical prostatectomy

The major complications of radical prostatectomy include stricture, rectal perforation, impotence and urinary incontinence. Previous studies have reported varying incidences of these complications, but the more contemporary series clearly show a paucity of significant complications. Lange and Reddy reported their complication rate in a series of 150 patients who underwent radical retropubic prostatectomy:[49] an anastomotic stricture occurred in 1%, rectal perforation in 1% and only 1% had total or severe urinary stress incontinence. Four patients developed deep vein thrombosis and there was one death. Andriole et al. also recently summarized the early complication rates following radical prostatectomy from a series derived from Washington University (Table 19.4).[50]

Preservation of potency during nerve-sparing radical prostatectomy, as initially described by Walsh and Donker,[45] has further extended the use of this procedure in patients with localized prostate cancer. Preservation of potency has been shown to depend primarily upon the age of the patient and the size of the tumour: Walsh reported 84% potency rates in patients aged 50–60 years and 60% in patients aged 60–70 years;[46] in contrast, men over the age of 70 were rarely potent.

Tumour stage, and ability to preserve the nerve bundles, were other important factors that predicted postoperative preservation. Patients who had small stage B lesions had a 71% incidence of potency, compared with a rate of 56% postoperative potency in patients who had stage B2 lesions. Removal of one of the bundles decreased the overall postoperative potency rate to 69%. Catalona and Basler confirmed these findings, reporting potency rates of 63% in all aged men after bilateral nerve-sparing, and 41% in patients who underwent unilateral nerve-sparing procedures.[51] Complete continence was noted in 94% of the patients in this series. It is clear that patient selection, as well as the attention paid by the surgeon to nerve sparing, both affect the results of nerve-sparing prostatectomy.

In the authors' series, potency results were related to the age of the patient and to the ability to save both nerve bundles. In patients who had normal erectile function preoperatively, 80% of men under the age of 50 were able to have erections

Table 19.4. Early complications following radical prostatectomy

Complication	No.*
Deep vein thrombosis/embolism	34 (2.5)
Myocardial infarction/arrhythmia	19 (1.4)
Wound infection/haematoma	17 (1.3)
Lymph leak/prolonged drainage	8 (0.6)
Foley catheter malfunction	5 (0.4)
Rectal injury	3 (0.3)
Death within 30 days of surgery	3 (0.2)

*n = 1342; percentages in parentheses.
(From ref. 50 with permission.)

satisfactory for sexual intercourse if bilateral nerve sparing was done. For men aged 50–60 years, 55% retained normal postoperative sexual function (Table 19.5).

A concern that has been raised about nerve-sparing procedures is that they increase the risk of cancer recurrence by decreasing the margin of normal tissue that is removed around the prostate during surgery. It is the authors' opinion that this risk is minimized by the application of nerve sparing to only those patients who have small tumours, and by judicious selection of patients for unilateral or bilateral nerve-sparing procedures. In view of the low potency rates in men aged 70 or over, the utility of nerve sparing should be questioned in that patient population as well.

With the modified apical dissection as described above, the time needed to regain bladder control has significantly decreased. As shown by survey data, 55% of the authors' patients were either totally continent or used a single, small pad daily from the time of catheter removal. By 3 months, 72% of the patients were completely continent, with only 6% of the incontinent patients using more than one pad per day. Overall, for patients with a minimum of 3 months of follow-up, 75% were completely continent, 20% used one pad per day, 4% had moderate incontinence, and only 0.6% had total urinary incontinence after surgery.

The cost and the morbidity of radical prostatectomy have also been reduced significantly, mainly owing to the initiation of a clinical pathway that standardizes intra-operative and postoperative care of the patients who undergo radical prostatectomy. Through use of this pathway, refinements in surgical technique, early ambulation, replacement of narcotic analgesics with ketorolac, and the elimination of epidural anaesthesia and narcotic postoperative analgesics, the length of the hospital stay has been decreased by 28%, and hospital costs were reduced by 25%.[52] Currently, the average hospital stay following radical prostatectomy is 2.4 days. Other centres have noted similar savings with the implementation of similar clinical care pathways.[53] For radical prostatectomy to remain a viable option for treating prostate cancer in this era of cost containment, measures to improve the efficiency of treatment and to decrease the morbidity of treatment must be pursued.

Patient satisfaction is also a major issue, even in this era of cost containment. The quality-of-care group at the authors' institution sent questionnaires to 100 patients who were on this clinical care pathway, inquiring specifically about level of pain control and level of satisfaction. Virtually all patients had excellent pain control and little discomfort postoperatively. Furthermore, 95% felt that their length of stay in hospital was adequate and they would not have requested any longer hospitalization. Only one patient felt he definitely should have had another day in hospital. Furthermore, no patients were readmitted for

*Table 19.5. Postoperative potency rates by age**

Age (years)	Percentage of patients potent postoperatively	
	Bilateral nerve sparing	Unilateral nerve sparing
40–49	80 (20)	–
50–59	55 (33)	33 (33)
60–69	26 (34)	0 (100)

*Including only patients who had normal potency preoperatively, and who had at least 1 year of follow-up.
†Percentages of patients partially potent, in parentheses.

complications, and the rate of other complications was minimal and not greater than that observed in the past.

Conclusions

Radical prostatectomy provides the most effective local control of prostate cancer. However, radical prostatectomy and aggressive prostate cancer screening have yet to result in a decrease in the mortality rate from this disease. The burden of proof is on the urologic community to show that the surgical treatment of prostate cancer can decrease the morbidity and mortality from this disease, while doing so with few side effects to the patient. Survival after surgery depends upon many factors, but death from prostate cancer in patients undergoing surgery for organ-confined tumours is rare. Severe complications, including significant urinary incontinence, are also rare following anatomical radical prostatectomy. Potency-sparing procedures are appropriate and effective in many patients, but should be restricted to younger, sexually active patients who have low-stage disease. Unfortunately, radical prostatectomy alone is not curative for many patients with prostate cancer, and may represent the overtreatment of some men who had otherwise biologically indolent lesions. These deficiencies in the ability to manage the patient with prostate cancer point to the urgent need to develop more effective treatment strategies for the patient with disseminated disease, and to develop better biomarkers that can distinguish the patient who has an indolent cancer from the patient who has a potentially lethal lesion.

References

1. Scardino P T, Hanks G E. Does screening for prostate cancer make sense? Sci Am 1996; 275: 114–115
2. Lu-Yao G L, McLerran D, Wasson J, Wennberg J E. An assessment of radical prostatectomy. Time trends, geographic variation, and outcomes. The Prostate Patient Outcomes Research Team. JAMA 1993; 269: 2633–2636
3. Paulson D F, Moul J W, Walther P J. Radical prostatectomy for clinical Stage T1-2N0M0 prostatic adenocarcinoma: long-term results. J Urol 1990; 144: 1180–1184
4. Kupelian P, Katcher J, Levin H et al. Correlation of clinical and pathologic factors with rising prostate-specific antigen profiles after radical prostatectomy alone for clinically localized prostate cancer. Urology 1996; 48: 249
5. Trapasso J G, deKernion J B, Smith R B, Dorey F. The incidence and significance of detectable levels of serum prostatic specific antigen after radical prostatectomy. J Urol 1994; 152: 1821
6. Warner J, Whitmore W F Jr. Expectant management of clinically localized prostatic cancer. J Urol 1994; 152: 1761
7. Johansson J E, Adami H O, Andersson S O et al. High 10-year survival rate in patients with early, untreated prostatic cancer. JAMA 1992; 267: 2191
8. Adolfsson J, Ronstrom L, Lowgahen T et al. Deferred treatment of clinically localized low grade prostate cancer: the experience from a prospective series at the Karolinska Hospital. J Urol 1994; 152(5 pt 2): 1757
9. Albertsen P C, Fryback D G, Sturer B E et al. Long-term survival among men with conservatively treated localized prostate cancer. JAMA 1995; 274: 626
10. Catalona W J. Editorial: Expectant management and the natural history of localized prostate cancer. J Urol 1994; 152(5, pt 2): 1751
11. Shipley W U, Zietman A L, Hanks G E et al. Treatment related sequelae following external beam radiation for prostate cancer: review with update in patients with stages T1 and T2 tumour. J Urol 1994; 152(2 pt 2): 1799
12. Kupelian P. Beam or scalpel for prostate cancer? Urol Times 1997; 25(1): 28
13. Scardino P T, deKernion J B, Carroll P R et al. The management of clinically localized prostate cancer. AUA News 1996; 1(4): 22

14. Goluboff E T, Benson M C. External beam radiation therapy does not offer long-term control of prostate cancer. Urol Clin North Am 1996; 23(4): 617

15. Epstein J I, Oesterling J E, Walsh P C. The volume and anatomical location of residual tumor in radical prostatectomy specimens removed for Stage A1 prostate cancer. J Urol 1988; 139: 975

16. Epstein J, Paull G, Eggleston J, Walsh P. Prognosis of untreated stage A1 prostate carcinoma: a study of 94 cases with extended follow-up. J Urol 1986; 136: 837

17. Terris M K, McNeal J E, Stamey T A. Transrectal ultrasound imaging and ultrasound guided prostate biopsies in the detection of residual carcinoma in clinical Stage A carcinoma of the prostate. J Urol 1992; 147: 864

18. Carter H, Partin A, Epstein J et al. The relationship of prostate specific antigen levels and residual tumor volume in stage A prostate cancer. J Urol 1990; 144: 1167

19. Dietrick D D, McNeal J E, Stamey T A. Core length in ultrasound-guided systematic sextant biopsies: a pre-opertive evaluation of prostate cancer volume. Urology 1995; 45(6): 987

20. Catalona W J, Richie J P, Ahmann F R et al. Comparison of digital rectal examination and serum prostate specific antigen (PSA) in the early detection of prostate cancer: results of a multicenter clinical trial of 6630 men. J Urol 1994; 151: 1283

21. Elgamal A A, Van Poppel H P, Voorder W M V et al. Impalpable invisible stage T1c prostate cancer: characteristics and clinical relevance in 100 radical prostatectomy specimens — a different view. J Urol 1997; 157(1): 244

22. Douglas T, Sesterhenn I, Moul J, McLeod S. The significance of PSA-detected non-palpable adenocarcinoma of the prostate. J Urol 1995; 153(4): abstr 92

23. Oesterling J E, Suman V J, Zincke H, Bostwick D G. PSA detected (clinical stage T1c or B0) prostate cancer. Pathologically significant tumors. Urol Clin North Am 1993; 20: 687

24. Epstein J I, Walsh P C, Carmichael M, Brendler C B. Pathologic and clinical findings to predict tumor extent of nonpalpable (stage T1c) prostate cancer. JAMA 1993; 271: 687

25. Mukamel E, Hanna J, deKernion J. Pitfalls in pre-operative staging in prostate cancer. Urology 1987; 30: 318

26. Zincke H, Oesterling J E, Blute M L et al. Long-term results after radical prostatectomy for clinically localized (Stage T2C or lower) prostate cancer. J Urol 1994; 152: 1850

27. Catalona W J, Smith D S. 5-year recurrence rates after anatomic radical retropubic prostatectomy for prostate cancer. J Urol 1994; 152: 1837

28. Paulson D F. Impact of radical prostatectomy in the management of clinically localized disease. J Urol 1994; 152: 1826

29. Dorey F, Franklin J, deKernion J B, Smith R B. Use of multiple PSA values for predicting clinical disease recurrence after radical retropubic prostatectomy. J Urol 1996; 155(suppl): 487A

30. Frazier H A, Robertson J E, Humphrey P A, Paulson D F. Is prostate specific antigen of clinical importance in evaluating outcome after radical prostatectomy? J Urol 1993; 149: 516

31. Van den Ouden D, Davidson P J T, Hop W, Schroder F H. Radical prostatectomy as a monotherapy for locally advanced (stage T3) prostate cancer. J Urol 1994; 151: 646

32. Soloway M S, Sharifi R, Wajsman Z et al. Randomized prospective study — radical prostatectomy alone vs radical prostatectomy preceded by androgen blockade in cT2b prostate cancer. J Urol 1996; 155: 976A

33. Pilepich M V, Krall M, Al Sarral M et al. RTOG #8610. ASCO Proceedings, 1993;

34. Blute M, Lerner S, Bergstralh E J, Eickholt J T. Extended experience with radical prostatectomy (RP) for clinical stage T3 prostate cancer (PC): outcome and contemporary morbidity. J Urol 1995; 153(4): abstr 338

35. deKernion J, Neuwirth H, Stein A et al. Prognosis of patients with stage D1 prostate carcinoma following radical prostatectomy with and without early endocrine therapy. J Urol 1990; 144: 700

36. Myers R P, Larson-Keller J J, Bergstralh J J et al. Hormonal treatment at time of radical retropubic prostatectomy for stage D1 prostate cancer: results of long-term follow-up. J Urol 1992; 147: 910

37. Levy D A, Resnick M I. Laparoscopic pelvic lymphadenectomy and radical perineal prostatectomy: a viable alternative to radical retropubic prostatectomy. J Urol 1994; 151: 905

38. Frazier H A, Robertson J E, Paulson D F. Radical prostatectomy: the pros and cons of the perineal versus retropubic approach. J Urol 1992; 147: 888

39. Takla N, Graham S, Witt M. The incidence of erectile dysfunction following radical perineal nerve sparing prostatectomy: a retrospective review of 76 cases. J Urol 1994; 151(suppl): 355A

40. Lassen P M, Kearse W S. Rectal injuries during radical perineal prostatectomy. Urology 1995; 45(2): 266

41. Weiss J P, Schlecker B A, Wein A J, Hanno P M. Preservation of periprostatic autonomic nerves during total perineal prostatectomy by intrafascial dissection. Urology 1985; 26(2): 160

42. Lerner S E, Chamberlin J W, Fleischman J et al. Combined laparoscopic pelvic lymph node dissection and modified Belt radical perineal prostatectomy for localized prostatic adenocarcinoma. Urology 1994; 43(4): 493

43. Bruce R G, Kim F H, McRoberts W. Rhabdomyolysis and acute renal failure following radical perineal prostatectomy. Urology 1996; 47(3): 427

44. Katirji M B, Lanska D J. Femoral mononeuropathy after radical prostatectomy. Urology 1990; 36(6): 539

45. Walsh P C, Donker P J. Impotence following radical prostatectomy: insight into etiology and prevention. J Urol 1982; 128: 492

46. Walsh P. Radical prostatectomy, preservation of sexual function, cancer control. Urol Clin North Am 1987; 14: 663

47. Gaker D L, Gaker L B, Stewart J F, Gillenwater J Y. Radical prostatectomy with preservation of urinary continence. J Urol 1996; 156: 445

48. Steiner M S, Burnett A L, Brooks J D et al. Tubularized neourethra following radical retropubic prostatectomy. J Urol 1993; 150: 407

49. Lange P, Reddy P. Technial nuances and surgical results of radical retropubic prostatectomy in 150 patients. J Urol 1987; 138: 348

50. Andriole G L, Smith D S, Rao G et al. Early complications of contemporary radical retropubic prostatectomy. J Urol 1994; 152 (5 pt 2): 1858

51. Catalona W J, Basler J W. Return of erections and urinary continence following nerve sparing radical retropubic prostatectomy. J Urol 1993; 150: 905

52. Litwin M S, Smith R B, Thind A et al. Cost-efficient radical prostatectomy with a clinical care path. J Urol 1996; 155: 989

53. Koch M O, Smith J R. Clinical outcomes associated with the implementation of a cost-efficient programme for radical retropubic prostatectomy. Br J Urol 1995; 76: 28

Chapter 20
Controversies in the management of clinically localized prostate cancer

M. S. Soloway

Introduction

There is no shortage of controversy with regard to the management of men who present with apparent localized prostate cancer. Although there has been a tremendous increase in interest in this subject, with an accompanying explosion of data, there are few prospective randomized trials that help to direct the clinician and patient to reach a decision on appropriate management. Once the diagnosis has been established, the clinician usually has the following information: the prostate-specific antigen (PSA) level; the degree of differentiation of the tumour and the Gleason grade and sum; the number and approximate location of biopsies; the amount of tumour in each of the biopsy cores; the findings of the digital rectal examination (DRE), and, when appropriate, radiographic studies to help determine whether the tumour has metastasized. The clinician and the patient then have a lengthy discussion regarding the various treatment alternatives. Depending on the patient's age and comorbidity, his expected survival will be approximated. This will be important in suggesting treatment: if the Gleason score is 6 or less and the PSA is less than 10 ng/ml the 10-year disease-specific survival rate approaches 90%, whereas if the Gleason score is 7 or more and the PSA is more than 10, the survival will be lower.

Much has been made of the relatively long natural history of prostate cancer and the high incidence of cancer in prostates obtained at autopsy or cystoprostatectomy performed for bladder cancer. The contrast between incidental and clinical cancers has led to the approach of 'watchful waiting'. The advantages to be expected from 'watchful waiting' include delaying or omitting the quality-of-life impact that may accompany therapy, and the excellent palliation achieved with androgen deprivation at the time of progression. The competing causes of death, particularly for men who are more than 70 years old, and the lack of proof that early treatment decreases prostate cancer mortality, provide support for this approach. On the other hand, the disadvantages for watchful waiting in an otherwise healthy man are as follows: (1) most prostate cancers progress, given sufficient time; (2) androgen deprivation therapy significantly alters quality of life, and (3) disease progression causes morbidity. In addition, the 'window of curability' is not an indefinite period and one cannot be assured that initiation of therapy upon progression will provide an opportunity for cure.

Some suggest that, by using prognostic criteria (e.g. the PSA, PSA density, biopsy information, the Gleason score), patients with minimal prostate cancer can be identified and therapy omitted. Although in general this may be true, the lack of correlation is sufficiently high to make it difficult to counsel the individual patient regarding the benefits of a conservative (non-intervention) approach. To highlight the lack of reliability of the DRE, the author analysed a group of consecutive patients who had a DRE that was felt to be abnormal. Of the 78 men,

74 had a unilateral firm area thought to be consistent with prostate cancer. Following a radical prostatectomy and 2–3 mm sectioning of the prostate, adenocarcinoma was found from both the right and left sides of the prostate in two-thirds of the patients; often, the palpable tumour crossed the midline. Analysing the location of biopsies and using this information in an attempt to identify the location of tumour is not much more helpful. This was reviewed in 133 patients: 83 (62%) had a positive biopsy on one side only, whereas 50 (38%) had biopsies positive for tumour from both the right and left sides of the prostate. In patients who had only unilateral positive biopsies, 69% had tumour in both the right and left sides of the prostate when the prostatectomy specimen was examined. In only 48% of the patients with bilateral tumour was the tumour predominantly on the side with the positive biopsy. Thus, the information derived from the biopsies and the DRE is far from precise, making clinical staging inaccurate.

Perceptions of urologists in the United States

On numerous occasions the author has asked large groups of US urologists what would be their advice to a 60-year-old healthy man with a PSA of 8 ng/ml, a normal DRE and a biopsy that demonstrated Gleason score 6 adenocarcinoma: the overwhelming majority recommend radical prostatectomy. When the same urologists are questioned about their perceptions of the cure rate for radiation therapy in such a patient, 60% feel that there is only a 20% chance that the patients will have a PSA less than 1.5 ng/ml at 10 years; 20% suggest that there is a 50% chance of being free of disease. If these urologists are then asked to assess the likelihood that the same patients will have an undetectable PSA 10 years after radical prostatectomy, 50% believe there is a 70% chance that the patient will be 'cured' and 30% believe there is a 50–50 chance.

Thus, there is a perception among US urologists that total prostatectomy is superior to radiation therapy. The answer to this question, in the author's view, does not differ greatly when it is posed to urologists in Canada, South America or much of Western Europe. The greater than 50% increase in the number of radical prostatectomies performed in the United States over the last 5 years attests to this perception.

The Cleveland Clinic recently evaluated their experience of radical prostatectomy and radiation therapy and found that, if they used the pretreatment PSA to stratify patients, the likelihood of being free of disease did not differ significantly between these two treatments.[1] Randomized prospective trials are the only way to provide a meaningful answer for urologists and for their patients; they must examine not only cause-specific survival but quality of life and cost issues. Unfortunately, these two treatment methods have never been compared in a properly randomized setting.

Since clinicians lack sufficient data to decide optimal therapy it is important that they openly discuss management decisions with their colleagues and, of course, their patients. This provides a forum for each clinician to hear alternative viewpoints and make his or her decision based on available evidence. The author has had the opportunity to chair many conferences, during which, members of the audience have been asked for their opinions (the audiences have consisted mainly of urologists). An interactive keypad response system has been used to quantify the responses to specific questions, thus giving an idea of the practice patterns and opinions of many urologists on specific issues with regard to the work-up and management of prostate cancer. Much of this information has not been documented elsewhere.

Protocol

After the diagnosis of prostate cancer, the clinician must decide whether to perform a bone scan. Several studies indicate that the likelihood of a true positive bone scan for a patient with a PSA of less than 10 ng/ml approaches zero.[2] It is not until the PSA level is above 20 ng/ml that the chance of a positive bone scan increases substantially. Nonetheless, a majority of urologists in the United States obtain a bone scan in all newly diagnosed patients. It is the author's view that a bone scan is not necessary if an asymptomatic patient has an apparent clinically organ-confined prostate cancer and the PSA is less than 10 ng/ml.

An MRI or CT scan rarely adds important information for the patient whose PSA is less than 10–15 ng/ml. These studies are not accurate in determining the local stage (T). A positive node in a patient with a PSA of less than 10 ng/ml is rare. In addition, there are false negatives and false positives, and the likelihood that these radiographic studies will benefit the patient and change management is low.

Some suggest that it is not cost effective to ask the patient to donate blood prior to total prostatectomy; however, most US urologists ask the patient to donate one or two units of blood to minimize the chance of homologous blood during total prostatectomy. Pre-surgery autologous donation has blossomed in the United States because of the patient's concern about acquiring hepatitis or HIV infection.

General anaesthesia is most commonly used; however, approximately 20% of urologists use an epidural, either alone or in addition to a general anaesthetic. There are several advantages to avoiding a general anaesthetic: these include less postoperative pain, a possible reduction in intraoperative blood loss, and avoidance of the pulmonary side effects of general anaesthetic agents. Increasingly, many clinicians prescribe a non-narcotic for postoperative analgesia.

Radical retropubic prostatectomy is the procedure of choice for most urologists. Only 5% of prostatectomies are performed by the perineal approach.

If a total prostatectomy is performed, the surgeon must decide whether to perform a pelvic lymph node dissection. Rarely is this a complete pelvic lymph node dissection: most urologists prefer a modified dissection in which lymph nodes adjacent to and underneath the external iliac vein and surrounding the obturator nerve are removed. The node dissection extends to the bifurcation of the external and internal iliac artery and vein. A pelvic lymph node dissection is for staging; few would argue that the procedure is therapeutic. The primary reason not to perform a pelvic lymph node dissection is that it prolongs the surgery. The morbidity associated with a modified pelvic lymph node dissection is minimal. Approximately 70% of urologists routinely perform a pelvic lymph node dissection and the majority send the lymph nodes for frozen section. Most will abandon the procedure if the lymph nodes contain tumour. In the author's experience the likelihood of positive lymph nodes for the patient with a PSA less than 15 ng/ml and a clinical T1–T2 prostate cancer is less than 1% and, thus, although I usually perform a modified bilateral pelvic lymph dissection I rarely request frozen sections.

Surgical technique

The technique of radical prostatectomy is being refined and modified. There are some differences in technique that engender discussion. The surgeon must decide whether to preserve the neurovascular bundles, with the hope of retaining potency. Critical to this issue is obtaining an adequate history from the patient, and possibly from his sexual partner to determine the adequacy of erections prior to surgery. Information from the biopsy and DRE is also necessary. If it is likely that the tumour extends beyond the capsule, the neurovascular bundle should not be separated from the lateral aspect of the prostate on the tumour-bearing side, since this will increase the chance of tumour at the surgical margin. The likelihood that a patient will achieve normal erections following prostatectomy varies, depending upon his age, the adequacy of preoperative erections, and at least in part on the preservation of the neurovascular bundle(s). Success ranges from 20 to 80% if at least one bundle is preserved. Most urologists feel that there may be some risk of not excising all the tumour if a nerve-sparing procedure is performed. None the less, most would be willing to take this risk if the patient is less than 65 years old, has a T1c or T2a tumour, has a PSA of less than 10 ng/ml, indicates that he has normal erectile function, and is anxious to preserve potency.

The most important technical factor in preserving continence is the careful dissection of the urethra, distal to the apex of the prostate.[3] Once the distal urethra has been transected, the prostate is mobilized. The inferior vascular pedicles are divided, the ampullae of vas are transected and the seminal vesicles freed of vascular attachments. The prostate is further mobilized by dividing the lateral pedicles. The bladder neck must be transected. The two common techniques are either wide excision of the bladder neck, with subsequent reconstruction, or preservation of the bladder neck and the proximal urethra as it enters the prostate. Those favouring wide excision indicate their desire to ensure removal of all the malignancy. Careful technique, with eversion of the mucosa and narrowing the neck of the bladder to 20–22 Fr, provides good results. Those advocating bladder neck preservation indicate the lack of evidence that this adversely affects prognosis. There is a very low chance that the bladder neck is the only site of a positive margin. In the author's opinion, bladder neck preservation reduces the chance of an anastomotic stricture and improves the early return of continence. Urologists are equally divided on the approach to the bladder neck.

The emphasis on reducing the cost of medical care has greatly influenced the management of the patient who is to have a radical prostatectomy. In the United States, patients are admitted on the day of surgery. Non-narcotic analgesics are often used perioperatively to reduce the duration of postoperative ileus. Ambulation and a liquid diet are initiated the morning following surgery. Patients are discharged on the second or third postoperative day, thus occupying a hospital bed for only two or three nights. Patient education and home health care are critical to the success of this approach.

The morbidity associated with total prostatectomy has been dramatically reduced over the last few years. Careful attention to the dissection of the urethra distal to the apex of the prostate and accurate anastomosis of the bladder neck/urethra to the distal urethra have resulted in a marked decrease in the likelihood of significant urinary incontinence. Some degree of stress urinary incontinence occurs in approximately 15% of patients; total incontinence should be less than 1%. The primary morbidity associated with total prostatectomy is erectile dysfunction. The most frequent morbidities associated with external beam radiation therapy are diarrhoea and proctitis. Erectile dysfunction and irritative bladder symptoms occur but are not immediate: their onset may be months or years following radiation therapy.

Androgen deprivation prior to radical prostatectomy or radiation therapy

The prognostic factors associated with the success of total prostatectomy or radiation therapy have been largely determined. Good prognostic factors are a PSA of less than 10 ng/ml, a Gleason score of 6 or less, absence of Gleason grade 4–5, and clinical stage T1c or T2a. Patients with clinical stage T2b, T2c or T3, a PSA greater than 10 ng/ml and Gleason grade 4–5 cancer have a high likelihood of failure with monotherapy, be it radiation or total prostatectomy. In an effort to address the higher chance of failure in these subgroups, combination therapy has been tried. The approaches that have been investigated include androgen deprivation, prior to total prostatectomy or radiation therapy, and adjuvant therapy. The adjuvant therapy may consist of radiation therapy following total prostatectomy or androgen deprivation following either prostatectomy or radiation therapy.

There have been several prospective, randomized trials that have used 3–4 months of androgen deprivation prior to radical prostatectomy:[4,5] all of them indicate that tumour at the inked surgical margin is lower with preoperative androgen deprivation; in most studies the difference has been statistically significant. On the basis of these initial results, approximately 50% of urologists in the United States use androgen deprivation prior to radical prostatectomy, primarily in patients with clinical stage T2b or if the PSA is above 10–15 ng/ml and the decision is made to proceed with total prostatectomy. It is hoped that, with the use of androgen deprivation prior to radical prostatectomy, there will be a decrease not only in positive margins but also in the use of adjuvant radiation; a decrease in the local recurrence is also hoped for. Obviously, the goal is to improve overall and disease-specific survival. The results of these studies have not, to date, demonstrated an improvement in progression-free survival: the US and Canadian multi-institutional trials have not shown an advantage in the time to relapse, using PSA as a surrogate for recurrence;[4,5] these studies are not mature, however, the mean follow-up being only 2 years.

Some have advocated longer periods of androgen deprivation, in the belief that this approach is reasonable and that cells sensitive to androgen can be eradicated with a longer duration of androgen deprivation. Prospective randomized trials comparing 3 vs 8 or 9 months of androgen deprivation are in progress.

The use of androgen deprivation, for 2–3 months prior to and 2 months during, external beam radiation therapy has been analysed by the United States Radiation Therapy Oncology Group (RTOG).[6] Their initial report included over 400 patients with clinical T3–T4 prostate cancer and indicated a statistically significant benefit in terms of local failure and disease-free survival for those patients who received androgen deprivation before and during radiation therapy. The decreased size of the prostate may allow improved blood flow and less tumour cell hypoxia and, thus, improved radiosensitivity. Many radiation oncologists and urologists now feel that this should be routine. Current RTOG protocols have instituted preoperative androgen deprivation as standard therapy for patients with clinical T3 and T4 prostate cancer. There is now a randomized trial for T1–T2 prostate cancer to determine whether the benefit achieved in T3–T4 prostate cancer will also be found in those with less extensive apparently localized prostate cancer.

References

1. Kupelian P, Katcher J, Levin H *et al*. Correlation of clinical and pathologic factors with rising prostate specific antigen profiles after radical prostatectomy alone for clinically localized prostate cancer. Urology 1996; 48: 249–260

2. Oesterling J. Prostate specific antigen: a critical assessment of the most useful tumor marker for adenocarcinoma of the prostate. J Urol 1991; 145: 907–923

3. Stamey T, Villers A, McNeal J *et al*. Positive surgical margins at radical prostatectomy: importance of the apical dissection. J Urol 1990; 143: 166–173

4. Goldenberg S L, Klotz L H, Srigley J *et al*. Randomized, prospective, controlled study comparing radical prostatectomy alone and neoadjuvant androgen withdrawal in the treatment of localized prostate cancer. Canadian Urologic Oncology Group. J Urol 1996; 156: 873–877

5. Soloway M S, Sharifi R, Wajsman Z *et al*. Randomized prospective study comparing radical prostatectomy alone versus radical prostatectomy preceded by androgen blockade in clinical stage B2 (T2bNxM0) prostate cancer: the Lupron Depot Neo-Adjuvant Prostate Cancer Study Group. J Urol 1995; 154: 424–428

6. Pileptich M V, Krall J M, Al-Sarraf M *et al*. Androgen deprivation with radiation therapy compared with radiation therapy alone for locally advanced prostate cancer. A randomized comparative trial of the Radiation Therapy Oncology Group. Urology 1995; 45: 616–623

Chapter 21
A radical prostatectomy: the patient's perspective

A. D. C. Turner

Just 12 months ago today, at the age of 63, I became a patient being made ready for a radical prostatectomy, and it would be no idle phrase to say that, from that moment on, it changed my life.

Thinking back, I suppose after the natural disquiet about surviving the operation itself, as I went down to theatre my thoughts were an intermingling of the way my wife looked as I left her, how much pain I would have to take, how I would cope with incontinence if it were to become a long-term problem, and just how bad the sexual dysfunction was likely to be. I would suggest that would be about the average mix of emotions for the average radical prostatectomy patient.

Today, I feel good. The prostate-specific antigen (PSA) reading last week was 0.01 ng/ml. I have no incontinence, and never did have from the moment the catheter came out, and sexual function of a kind has returned. So, yes, I'm lucky. And I hope it stays that way. But I dare say, in common with so many people who have gone through a life-threatening experience, my attitude to life and living has altered, and my perspective about what is important has unquestionably been reconstructed. Radical surgery tends to focus the mind.

However, I was lucky from the start. I had very good advice from a urologist who was treating me for kidney stones and in the course of his investigations rather chanced upon my prostatic cancer. A PSA of 8.8 ng/ml, and rising, was the only symptom before the biopsy showed some tumours. Yes, a quite typical presentation. I subsequently saw one of the finest consultants in the country — I had one of the best anaesthetists in London. I went to one of the country's top private hospitals — the London Clinic. I had adequate insurance cover. I had an employer who was totally sympathetic and wanted me back. And, crucially, in my case, I was married to an extremely experienced nursing sister, originally trained at Guys, with clinical teaching experience and a mass of practical bedside nursing 'savvy' and competence. How many of your patients have been that fortunate?

Additionally, I chose thoroughly to research the condition. I read articles. I took pages from the Internet. I asked lots of questions. I thought about it all, and weighed up the pros and cons. I made my decision based on as much state-of-the-art knowledge and information as I could get. And I decided that thinking positively would be all to the good.

I joined the committee of the Prostate Research Campaign UK, and have been helped thereby, and have tried to offer what help I can in return.

However, the experience that has affected me most of all has not been the operation itself, which went smoothly and well, but a decision by Roger Kirby to refer many of his patients to me so that, prior to their decision, they could talk with me and ask endless questions — many of which were extremely and necessarily intimate and potentially embarrassing, but enabling them to get a better feel for what this operation would mean at the time — and thereafter.

Surgeons do not have the time, nor, I suspect, the inclination, to talk a patient through the 'nitty gritty' of things which for you and the nurses are routine matters — certainly of importance, but not all that relevant to the success of the actual operation.

You may have done dozens, scores, hundreds, of radical prostatectomies, or have overseen a great deal of radiation treatment, but how many of you have gone through the operation or undergone the treatment for yourselves? How can you really know, or how can you be expected to know, how deeply nearly all men feel about 'things down below', when those things go wrong, despite the fact that you deal with the 'down below' probably every working day of your professional lives?

There are those 15 minutes in the surgery or the consulting room when the news about prostatic cancer, and what can and needs to be done, is imparted to an otherwise healthy man, exactly as it was for me one particular Thursday when Roger Kirby first met me. And then it's on to the next patient.

You are trained to be careful. You are trained to read the body language. You are trained to talk with sensitivity. You are trained to assess your patients and treat them as individuals. You are trained to conduct fine surgery and you are urged to keep abreast of the research in your sphere. But what's missing in the mix is proper and necessary alleviation of the fear, the ignorance, the confusion, the sheer terror, the sinking of hope, the psychological effect of the news, the blow to natural macho instincts, the worry about whether the man's job will be affected... the list is long. And just how important and genuinely helpful is that element in the mix, is what I believe Roger Kirby and I have found out about this year.

He gives his men my home telephone number and tells them I may be able to help them because I have gone through what it is he has in mind for them. They call me. Some have been the great and the good. We talk sometimes for an hour. Sometimes the call is late, when the spouse has gone to bed. I tell them everything. I tell them about Roger Kirby. I tell them about Peter Amoroso, the anaesthetist with whom he will probably work. I tell them about the 24-hour intensive care period. I talk to them about the food in the hospital, and why it helps to have the lighter diet. I talk about wind and the importance the nurses attach to that. I talk about bowel movements and holding on to your tummy. I discuss the catheter and its inconvenience and management. I tell them about pain control. I tell them what visitors ask. I talk about how important it is to keep drinking. Of course these are all fundamental things for you. But people forget more than half you tell them. And sometimes they put up a psychological barrier to taking it in anyway.

I explain how little time Mr Kirby will be able to spend with them once the operation is over. I advise them to write down the questions they want to ask him, and to make him stay and answer them!

I tell them about wearing loose clothing when they get home. I talk about suitable exercise. I tell them not to worry too much about what will almost certainly be temporary incontinence, if, indeed, they experience any.

I reassure them that when they wake up and see what their scrotum looks like, it really will deflate and all that bruising will disappear before long. We talk about the operation and drain scars. We discuss what it's like to have the stitch and the catheter out. They just don't know about these aspects.

We talk about sexual dysfunction and the ways to overcome an aspect, which without a single exception, worries all of them. We talk about what's available to help in that respect. We talk about relationships after the operation. You might be surprised how openly some of those men will talk. Some of them have been gay or bisexual, and even Roger may not know that. I explain that it will be a year before the healing inside is complete. I urge them to take 2 months off work if they are still employed. I do all I can to persuade them to listen to their bodies.

I could go on and on. There is no limit to the time we talk, and the time they want. I write to them on the day they go into hospital. I keep in touch with some of them when they are there and when they come out. I leave it with them to maintain any regular contact, although I do telephone occasionally to see how they are getting on. Some of them remain frightened.

'Have you some mission?' one man asked me. The answer is that I have no mission other than to recognize that we are all in this together.

What I want to leave you surgeons and doctors with is the thought that simple, and reasonably sensitive, but nevertheless straight-talking, counselling has an exceptionally positive effect on these men. They make better patients. They get better quickly, and their mind-sets are more positive. And they and I both learn from each other, which helps the next caller.

You need to find lots of folk like me who see it in this light. Build a team of counsellors for your patients; you owe it to them, believe me!

Chapter 22
Three-dimensional conformal radiation therapy in the management of localized prostate cancer

M. J. Zelefsky

Introduction

With the advent of sophisticated new computer-based technologies, the ability to deliver high-precision radiotherapy has now become a reality in the form of three-dimensional conformal radiotherapy (3D-CRT). Over the last 5 years there has been an ever-increasing volume of information related to emerging developments in 3D technology, treatment planning and its early results in the treatment of prostate cancer. The purpose of this chapter is to review the role of 3D-CRT in the treatment of clinically localized prostate cancer as well as the technological and treatment planning considerations that are critical for its implementation.

Rationale for conformal radiotherapy

The 3D approach to the treatment of prostate cancer is designed to overcome some of the reasons for the failure to eradicate prostatic tumours locally with conventional radiotherapeutic techniques. In many cases the traditional approaches to tumour localization and treatment planning appear now not to have encompassed precisely the entire prostatic target within the volume receiving the high doses of irradiation.[1,2] This may have been a function of suboptimal imaging techniques for defining the target volume, insufficient accuracy of the methods available for dose calculation, or both. Furthermore, several retrospective studies have indicated a direct relationship between local tumour control and treatment dose for carcinoma of the prostate.[3,4] Hanks *et al.*[3] reviewed the local outcome of 624 patients with stage C prostate cancer from the Patterns of Care study outcome survey. The actuarial 7-year local recurrence rate was 36% for patients receiving 60–64.9 Gy, 32% for 65–69.9 Gy, and 24% for those who received 70 Gy or higher. However, although higher doses appear to be necessary for improved local tumour control, the proximity of the prostate to critical normal structures (the bladder and the rectum) has limited the ability to deliver effective dose levels (in excess of 70 Gy) when conventional radiotherapeutic techniques have been used.[3-8]

3D-CRT applies sophisticated computer-aided techniques to plan and deliver the prescribed radiation dose to a given tumour volume, conforming its pattern of distribution to the entire 3D configuration of the targeted tumour. The new techniques of 3D imaging and 3D treatment planning provide complete anatomical and dose information for the entire tumour volume and its surrounding normal tissues.[9,10] Since 3D dose computations are highly labour-intensive and require large numbers of dose computation points, the implementation of this technique depends on the availability of efficient computer algorithms and fast computer hardware. Furthermore, rapid computer-aided calculations and displays of dose distributions are critical for interactive modes of 3D treatment planning and plan evaluation. The application of 3D-CRT was, therefore, not possible until several years ago, because the highly complex software required for 3D treatment planning and for computer-controlled radiation delivery systems was not available. The recent introduction of high-performance workstations, and the new computer-aided treatment delivery machines with multileaf collimators and on-line real-time imaging systems, have made the planning and implementation of 3D-CRT feasible for prostatic cancer and several other types of malignancies. In addition to the decreased risk of missing or underdosing the tumour target, reduction of normal tissue complications is also achievable, potentially permitting a significant escalation of the tumour dose, regarded as the most effective approach to overcome the relative resistance of prostatic tumour clones to the lethal effects of radiation.

3D treatment planning and treatment delivery techniques

Although 3D treatment-planning systems vary in their details, they are based on similar principles. In this chapter, the Memorial Sloan-Kettering Cancer Center (MSKCC) system.[9-11] is used as a model. Most current 3D prostate treatment plans are coplanar, using multiple lateral and oblique fields. At MSKCC, patients are treated in the prone position. To ensure that the patient can be positioned for planning and treatment in a reproducible fashion, individualized thermoplastic casts are produced for each patient. Conventional simulators are used to determine the positioning of the patient, to define a provisional isocentre, and to produce reference localization skin marks. The patient is scanned in the planned treatment position within the immobilization device. To produce high-resolution 3D reconstructions, consecutive CT images with a 0.5 cm slice thickness are obtained from approximately 3.0 cm above the superior aspect of the seminal vesicles to 3.0 cm below the prostate. Additional CT images with a slice thickness of 1.0 cm are obtained above and below these levels, from the lower abdomen to the upper thighs.

Prostate and seminal vesicle positional variability is minimized by instructing the patient to empty his bladder before the simulation CT scan and to repeat this routine at the same time interval before each treatment session. If the planning CT scan shows that the bladder or the rectum are full, the treatment-planning procedure is repeated after the contents of these organs are emptied. It is likely that careful attention to these details will reduce tumour underdosage due to daily variations in prostate location and geometry.

The planning target volume is defined on each relevant CT slice by drawing a 1.0 cm margin around the CT-identifiable prostate tissue, extending from 1.0 cm cephalad to the superior aspect of the seminal vesicles to 1.0 cm caudal to the apex of the prostate, except posteriorly at the interface with the rectum where only a 0.6 cm margin is used. The normal organs, including the bladder wall, rectal wall, small bowel, osseous structures, and the outer surface of the skin, are identified by drawing contours around these structures on every CT slice where they appear. The target volume and normal organ images are reconstructed in 3D and displayed with the beam's eye view (BEV) technique,[12] using wire-frame graphics to delineate surfaces and colour to differentiate between structures (Figure 22.1).

Dose distributions are calculated using a pencil beam convolution algorithm with pixel-by-pixel inhomogeneity corrections, as previously described.[13-15] The

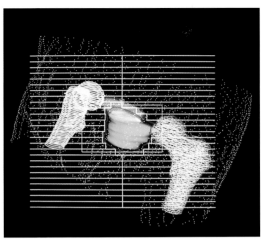

Figure 22.1. Beam's eye-view (BEV) display of a six-field coplanar prostate plan beam arrangement.

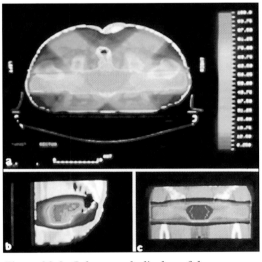

Figure 22.2. Colour-wash display of dose distributions for the transverse, sagittal and coronal planes of a six-field coplanar three-dimensional plan for a patient who received a cumulative dose of 75.6 Gy prescribed to the planning target volume.

target dose is prescribed to the maximum isodose surface distribution that completely encompasses the target volume. The dose inhomogeneity within the target volume with the author's 3D treatment technique varies from 4 to 7%. The adequacy of target coverage and the doses to the surrounding normal tissues are evaluated by examining isodose distributions on midplane axial, sagittal and coronal CT images (Figure 22.2) and by dose–volume histograms (DVHs).[16] DVH displays condense the dose-distribution data and present the volume (or the percentage of the total organ volume) receiving at least the dose D (or the percentage of the total dose). One DVH is generated for the tumour and one for each organ involved in the treatment plan, and the compilation of the curves is used for evaluating or comparing treatment plans. Rectal wall, bladder wall, and small bowel DVHs are used to determine the indication for neo-adjuvant hormonal therapy to reduce the size of the prostate. When the volume of any of these structures receiving the prescription dose exceeds limits that place the patient at a presumed increased risk of treatment-related toxicity (> 30% for rectal wall, ≥ 50% for bladder wall, and ≥ 65% for adjacent small bowel), a 3-month course of androgen-deprivation therapy is given before proceeding with radiation therapy. Significant reductions in the respective volumes irradiated have been observed in nearly 90% of patients treated with this approach.[17]

To date, the author has observed one instance of grade 3 genitourinary toxicity (0.5%) among over 200 patients who received neo-adjuvant hormonal therapy prior to radiotherapy; apart from this, no moderate or severe late rectal, bladder or bowel complications have been observed in this group.

3D treatment techniques generally require large numbers of beams daily to improve the ratio of tumour dose to normal tissue dose. Therefore, the practical application of 3D-CRT is facilitated by the use of newly designed treatment machines that are capable of rapidly delivering large numbers of arbitrarily shaped fields under automated computer control. In addition, automated beam-shaping using multileaf collimation (MLC) is also an important component of 3D treatment delivery systems.[18,19] Currently available multileaf collimators are already capable of automatically shaping the apertures of each treatment field in rapid succession under computer control. Thus, multiple radiation fields can be delivered within times that are comparable to those for traditional techniques, despite the increased number of fields and complex treatment manoeuvres.

A recent major development in the delivery of conformal radiotherapy that has further improved the associated precision of this form of therapy is the availability of intensity-modulated radiotherapy (IMRT). The technology of intensity modulation allows for the use of customized intensity patterns of the irradiation beam from each field of therapy. The intensity of the beam profile is designed by the treatment planner or the optimization program to minimize further the dose to the normal tissues while further enhancing conformality of the prescribed radiation dose to the target. Several approaches have been used to implement intensity-modulated-based therapy. At the MSKCC dynamic multileaf collimation (DMLC) has been used. With the ability to vary the aperture of the machine head at any point in time during the delivery of therapy from one field, dose distributions can be created that vary in intensity over the width of the field. This unique system enables convex or concave isodose distributions to be created, as well as low-dose areas in close proximity to high-dose regions. The latter may be exploited in particular in the prostate–rectal interface region where, ideally, the maximum dose should be delivered to the target without exceeding the tolerance of the rectum. The author's preliminary experience with IMRT has also revealed improved homogeneity of the dose distribution compared with non-IMRT based plans (Figure 22.3).[20]

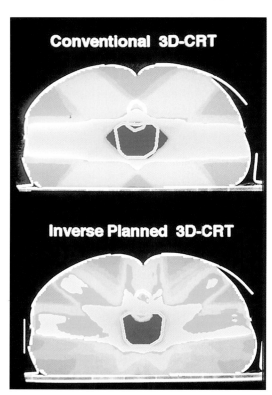

Figure 22.3. Comparison of a 'standard' conformal isodose distribution planned for a cumulative dose to 81 Gy and an intensity-modulated conformal plan for the same dose. Note the enhanced conformality with the latter approach.

Tolerance of CRT

As indicated earlier, the implementation of the 3D-CRT approach permits an increase in tumour dose to overcome the relative radiation resistance of prostatic tumour clones, without increasing the risk of normal organ complications. The long-term tolerance profiles in patients with localized prostate cancer treated with 3D-CRT at MSKCC have been highly encouraging.[21] In this experience, the treatment volume included the entire prostate and seminal vesicles, but did not encompass the regional pelvic lymph nodes. Pelvic lymph node irradiation has been omitted because of the absence of proof of benefit from this type of treatment.[22]

Initially, the 3D-CRT doses were 64.8–70.2 Gy, given in daily increments of 1.8 Gy, as classically used with conventional 2D techniques. After baselines for acute tolerance and 2-year late complications for the 3D approach at these dose levels had been established, a phase 1 prospective dose-escalation study was begun in patients with stage T2c–T3 tumours. When 40 patients were treated with 75.6 Gy and no late toxicity was observed after a minimum follow-up time of 1 year, this dose became available to patients with lower-stage disease, whereas the dose for T2c–T3 patients was further escalated to 81.0 Gy. A restriction imposed in designing the treatment plan for 81.0 Gy limited the rectal dose to no more than 75.6 Gy. To meet this requirement, the last 9.0 Gy (five daily treatment fractions) were delivered using a separate six- to eight-field coplanar beam arrangement with the rectum completely blocked in each field (Figure 22.4). The seminal vesicles were also excluded if there was no clinical evidence for involvement by tumour.

Acute toxicity and late treatment-related complications were graded according to the RTOG morbidity scoring scale.[5] Conformal therapy at these dose levels has been well tolerated. An earlier analysis in 432 patients showed that 85% of patients had either no or mild (grade 1) acute rectal (GI) toxicity and 61% of patients had either no or mild (grade 1) acute urinary (GU) toxicity. Grade 2 acute GI and GU toxicity requiring short-term medication to alleviate symptoms was observed in 15% and 39%, respectively. Only one patient (0.2%) had higher grade (grade 3) acute morbidity. These incidences of grade 2 or higher acute toxicity are about one-half of that expected with conventional approaches.[23]

Late GI and GU complications of treatment by the radiation dose have been previously reported and are summarized in Tables 22.1 and 22.2. Late toxicity has been absent or minimal (grade 0 or 1) in nearly 95% of patients. The 3-year actuarial grade 2 late GI and GU complication rates were 4% and 6%, respectively. No intermediate or severe toxicities (grade 3 or higher) have been encountered in

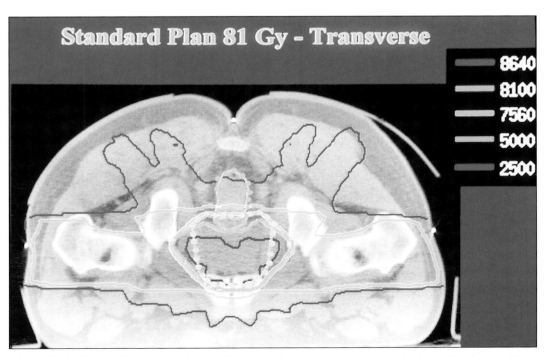

Figure 22.4. Cumulative isodose distribution for coplanar beam arrangement planned to deliver 81 Gy to the planning target volume (PTV). In order to maintain the dose constraint to the anterior rectal wall, a limited volume of the PTV at the prostate–rectal interface receives a gradient of dose from 75.6 to 81 Gy.

Table 22.1. Late GI toxicity according to prescribed dose of radiation

Prescribed dose (Gy)	Number of patients*				
	Grade 0	Grade 1	Grade 2	Grade 3	Grade 4
All	364 (84)	50 (13)	17 (5)	0	1 (0.4)
64.8–70.2	244 (85)	37 (13)	6 (2)	0	1 (0.6)
75.6–81.0	120 (83)	13 (12)	11 (11)	0	0
75.6 only	79 (81)	11 (14)	8 (12)	0	0
81.0 only	41 (89)	2 (5)	3 (7)	0	0

*Values in percentages are percentage actuarial toxicity at 2 years from completion of therapy.

Table 22.2. Late GU toxicity according to prescribed dose of radiation

Prescribed dose (Gy)	Number of patients*				
	Grade 0	Grade 1	Grade 2	Grade 3	Grade 4
All	375 (87)	44 (12)	11 (2)	2 (0.3)	0
64.8–70.2	254 (88)	29 (12)	4 (1)	1 (1)	0
75.6–81.0	121 (84.0)	15 (12)	7 (5)	1 (1)	0
75.6 only	82 (84)	9 (10)	7 (7)	0	0
81.0 only	39 (85)	6 (14)	0	1 (4)	0

*Values in parentheses are percentage actuarial toxicity at 2 years from completion of therapy.

the 98 patients receiving 75.6 Gy within a median follow-up of 22 months. In that report, the median follow-up among the 46 patients given 81.0 Gy was 19 months. The 3-year actuarial likelihood of grade 2 late GI toxicity for patients who received 64.8–70.2 Gy was 3.5%, compared with 10% for those treated with 70.2–81 Gy ($p = 0.004$). Similarly, the 3-year actuarial likelihood of grade 2 late GU toxicity for patients who received 64.8–70.2 Gy was 4%, compared with 12% for those treated with doses of 70.2–81 Gy ($p = 0.02$). Two patients developed a grade 3 urethral stricture at doses of 70.2 and 81 Gy, and one patient (0.4%) developed a grade 4 late rectal complication. The latter patient, who received only 64.8 Gy, had a history of ulcerative colitis, which is considered to be a predisposing risk factor for rectum-related toxicity. The median times for development of grade 2–4 GI and GU complications were 15 and 13 months, respectively.[21]

Other centres in the United States have reported the tolerance of high-dose CRT.[24–27] Sandler *et al.*[24] reported the rectal toxicity profile of 721 patients with localized prostate cancer treated with CRT at the University of Michigan Medical Center. Radiotherapy doses ranged from 59.4 to 80.4 Gy; the median follow-up was 20 months. As these doses were routinely prescribed to the isocentre, the doses delivered were, in general, lower than those used at MSKCC, in which the irradiation is prescribed to the 100% isodose line, which completely encompasses the planning target volume (PTV). In that study, 12 patients (2%) were reported to have developed grade III proctitis and two developed grade IV toxicity. The latter two patients were treated with doses of 69 and 76 Gy. Multivariate analysis revealed the dose to be the most important predictor of grade 3–4 rectal toxicity. The actuarial incidence of grade 3–4 rectal toxicity among patients who received doses of more than 68 Gy was 9% at 3 years compared with 2% among patients who received lesser doses.

Schultheiss *et al.*[25] analysed factors contributing to late toxicity among 616 patients who were treated with conformal and conventional radiation techniques. In that study patients who developed rectal bleeding and required less than three cautery procedures were characterized as having grade 2 toxicity; 13 patients developed GI toxicity of grade 3 or above with an actuarial incidence at 5 years of 2.7%; six patients developed GU late toxicity of more than grade 3, with a 3.4% actuarial incidence at 5 years. Late toxicity strongly correlated with the central axis dose. In a recent analysis by Lee *et al.*[26] the 18-month actuarial incidences of grade 2–3 late rectal toxicity were 7, 16 and 23% for central axis doses of less than 74, 74–76 and more than 76 Gy, respectively ($p = 0.05$). These investigators also noted the importance of lateral rectal wall shielding in reducing the toxicity after high-dose CRT. Among patients who received doses of 76 Gy or higher, the addition of rectal shielding for the last 10 Gy reduced the incidence of grade 2–3 toxicity from 22 to 7% ($p = 0.003$).

The low incidence of late toxicity in the MSKCC experience is probably related to several factors. In these patients, dose–volume histograms are routinely analysed prior to therapy to ensure that doses to normal tissues do not exceed imposed constraints within the conformal treatment plan. Among patients where more than 30% of the rectal wall, 50% of the bladder wall or 65% of the adjacent small bowel received the prescription dose, a 3-month course of neo-adjuvant androgen-ablative therapy is used for volume reduction before radiotherapy, with the intention of minimizing potential toxicity of therapy. Among 213 patients treated with neo-adjuvant androgen-ablative therapy at the author's institution, no grade 3–4 toxicity has been observed after high-dose radiotherapy (median dose 75 Gy), despite the fact that these patients had bulky tumours prior to therapy.[28] Others have also demonstrated the efficacy of pretreatment volume reduction with neo-adjuvant hormonal therapy (NHT) for locally advanced prostatic tumours prior to high-dose CRT.[29,30]

Treatment in the prone position may also contribute to a lower incidence of chronic rectum-related toxicity. In a prospective comparison of patients planned in both the prone and supine treatment position, less rectal volume was observed in the prone than in the supine position.[31] These differences were most pronounced in the region of the seminal vesicles. This latter phenomenon is probably related to the changes of configuration of the PTV and, in particular, the changes noted within the geometry of the seminal vesicles, where these structures fall backwards in the supine postion, wrapping themselves in some cases around portions of the rectal wall. In that study, treatment position also had a significant effect on the volume of bowel in the high-dose region. Treatment position had no effect, however, on the volume of bladder in close proximity to the high-dose region.[31]

Other technical considerations that contribute to the excellent tolerance profile in this study are the meticulous attention to tighter margins used at the prostate–rectal interface, and the author's general approach of not using pelvic fields. Careful attention to the rectal wall dose is critical for the safe application of high-dose CRT. This was also realized by the investigators at the Fox Chase Cancer Center, and led them to add rectal shielding when delivering high-dose CRT.[26] In a report of 257 patients who received isocentre doses in the range of 75 Gy, 88 patients had rectal shielding blocks added to the lateral fields for the last 10 fractions of a four-field plan. The investigators estimated that the dose reduction to the anterior rectal wall was approximately 4–5 Gy. Using this approach, the observed incidence of grade 2–3 rectal toxicity was reduced from 22 to 7%. Among patients who received isocentre doses of 74–76 Gy, the 18 month actuarial rate of grade 2–3 GI late toxicity was 19% for those who were not treated with a lateral rectal shielding approach, compared with 10% for those treated with this approach ($p < 0.001$).[26]

Outcome with conformal therapy for localized prostate cancer

In a multivariate analysis of 432 patients treated at the MSKCC with 3D-CRT, variables were identified that affected prostate-specific antigen (PSA) relapse-free survival.[21] In that report, PSA relapse was defined as two consecutive PSA-rising values from a post-treatment nadir of 1.0 ng/ml or less. The pretreatment PSA (≤ 20 ng/ml vs > 20 ng/ml), stage ($\leq$ T2c vs $\geq$ T3), and Gleason score (≤ 6 vs ≥ 7) were each found to be significant, independent variables that affected to a similar degree the risk of subsequent chemical relapse. These factors were combined to categorize patients further into risk groups. Three prognostic groups were identified: these were a favourable group with PSA of 20 ng/ml, or less and Gleason score of 6 or less; an intermediate group characterized by a PSA of 20 ng/ml, or less, and Gleason score of 7 or more, or PSA above 20 ng/ml and Gleason score of 6 or less; and an unfavourable group with PSA of more than 20 ng/ml and Gleason score of 7 or more. Figure 22.5 shows the combined predictive value of pretreatment PSA and Gleason score on the biochemical outcome of patients with stage T1c–T3 disease.[21]

The rate of PSA normalization to levels of 1.0 ng/ml or less, from abnormal pretreatment levels, was used as an early surrogate endpoint to evaluate the initial response to treatment. Figure 22.6 represents an analysis of patients, with pretreatment PSA levels of 20 ng/ml or less, who did not receive NHT prior to radiotherapy. Patients who received 70.2 Gy and higher had a significantly higher rate of PSA normalization than did patients treated with lower doses. In a more recent analysis, the time to PSA normalization to levels of 1.0 ng/ml or less was more rapid and more frequently achieved among patients who received higher

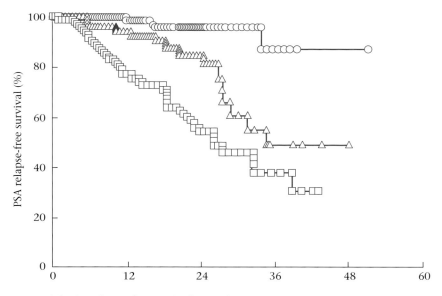

Figure 22.5. Actuarial PSA relapse-free survival according to prognostic risk groups: ○, *favourable (n = 155);* △, *intermediate* (n = 155); □, *unfavourable* (n = 122). *Differences between groups: favourable vs intermediate,* p = 0.0003; *intermediate vs unfavourable,* p = 0.0001.

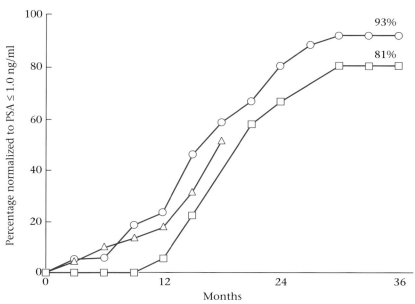

Figure 22.6. Actuarial likelihood of PSA normalization to levels of 1.0 ng/ml or less, according to the radiation prescription dose. Significant difference between high-dose versus low-dose radiotherapy was observed, p < 0.01. Patients had stage T1–T3 prostate cancer, Gleason score ≤ 6 and initial PSA ≤ 20 ng/ml; no NHT before radiotherapy. □, *64.8–66.6 Gy (52);* ○, *70.2 Gy (99);* △, *≥ 75.6 Gy (38).*

radiotherapy doses. This analysis included 740 patients with clinically localized prostate cancer. Of these patients, 214 (29%) were treated with neo-adjuvant androgen ablation prior to therapy and were excluded from this analysis. Among the 526 evaluable patients, the clinical stages were as follows: T1C = 128 (24%); T2A = 76 (15%); T2B = 116 (22%); T2C = 99 (19%) and T3 = 107 (20%). The prescription dose to the PTV was 64.8–68.4 Gy in 87 patients (17%); 70.2 Gy in 191 (36%); 75.6 Gy in 209 (40%) and 81 Gy in 39 (7%). The median pretreatment PSA value was 11.2 ng/ml (range 0.3–114). The median follow-up was 20 months (range 6–76 months). A total of 154 (29%) patients continued to show declining PSA levels within the first 2 years after therapy, and 130 patients (25%) failed to normalize to PSA levels of 1.0 ng/ml or below. Among patients who received doses of 75.6 Gy or more, the likelihood of achieving a PSA nadir of 1.0 ng/ml or less at 24 and 36 months was 86 and 93%, respectively, compared with 74 and 80%, respectively, among those who received lower doses ($p < 0.001$). A dose of 75.6 Gy or more was the strongest independent predictor for a PSA nadir level of 1.0 ng/ml or less ($p < 0.001$) followed by pretreatment PSA levels of 10 ng/ml or less ($p < 0.001$) and stage ($p = 0.01$), whereas the Gleason score had no significant impact.

Higher radiation doses delivered with CRT have also translated into improved PSA-relapse-free survival rates. Hanks *et al.*[32] reported the biochemical freedom from disease in 375 patients treated with a CRT technique to doses ranging from 66–79 Gy. PSA relapse was defined as a PSA of 1.5 ng/ml or more, and rising; the median follow-up was 21 months. Patients who received more than 71 Gy had a significantly higher PSA-relapse-free survival than did patients who received lower doses. In that report, the 2-year PSA control rates were 85% for patients who received more than 71 Gy, compared with 72% for those who received lower doses ($p = 0.007$). These differences were noted for patients with pretreatment PSA levels above 10 ng/ml. Among patients with pretreatment PSA levels of 10 ng/ml or less, there was no apparent benefit from higher radiotherapy doses.[21]

Future directions in 3D-CRT

Experience from several centres has demonstrated a promising potential for 3D-CRT in the management of localized carcinoma of the prostate. A reduction in both acute and late radiation morbidity and the feasibility of safely escalating the radiation dose to unprecedented levels have already been demonstrated. Subsequent studies must be designed to test whether high-dose CRT will improve local tumour control and the long-term disease-specific outcome in patients with prostatic carcinoma. On the basis of the relationship between the pretreatment PSA, Gleason score and subsequent biochemical (PSA) outcome, treatment strategies must be individualized according to their prognostic risk factors. Patients who have favourable prognostic characteristics have a strong likelihood of having organ-confined disease, and excellent results can be achieved with local therapy, such as surgery or radiotherapy, alone. Patients with intermediate risk features have a higher risk of extracapsular disease. This subgroup may be the most suitable cohort for staging lymphadenectomy to determine their eligibility for high-dose 3D-CRT.

Patients with locally advanced disease, with high-risk features suggestive of the presence of micrometastases, represent a cohort of patients least likely to benefit from local therapy alone. These patients may benefit from combined-modality treatment programmes such as neo-adjuvant or adjuvant hormonal therapy in combination with radiotherapy. Recently, the results of two large randomized trials have been reported, which examined the issue of integrating NHT in an adjuvant setting for patients' locally advanced prostatic disease.[33–34] The Radiation Therapy Oncology Group (RTOG) conducted a phase III randomized trial comparing conventional radiotherapy alone (with doses of 70 Gy) with radiotherapy followed by adjuvant hormonal therapy for at least 2 years.[33] The 5-year results demonstrated improved local control (based on digital rectal examination), distant-metastasis-free survival and PSA relapse-free survival in the arm that received adjuvant hormonal therapy, although no survival benefit was found. Bolla et al.[34] reported the preliminary results of a similar study conducted by the European Organization for Research and Treatment of Cancer: in this study a survival advantage was also noted at 5 years. These encouraging data will, nevertheless, require further follow-up to substantiate that these improvements observed with the integration of hormonal therapy will be maintained in the long term. In these high-risk patients, longer courses of androgen-ablative therapy (in the neo-adjuvant and/or adjuvant setting) or effective systemic therapies may be needed to improve survival. Because of the relatively poor results for patients with pretreatment PSA levels of more than 20 ng/ml, even in combination with androgen-ablative therapy, the author and colleagues are currently treating patients in a phase I study in their institution with estramustine and vinblastine in combination with 3D-CRT, in an effort to address the strong likelihood of micrometastases in this cohort of patients with a poor prognosis.

References

1. Ten Haken R K, Perez-Tamayo C, Tesser R J et al. Boost treatment of the prostate using shaped fixed fields. Int J Radiat Oncol Biol Phys 1989; 16: 193–200
2. Sandler H M, McShan D L, Lichter A S. Potential improvement in the results of irradiation for prostate carcinoma using improved dose distribution. Int J Radiat Oncol Biol Phys 1991; 22: 361–367
3. Hanks G E, Martz K L, Diamond J J. The effect of dose on local control of prostate cancer. Int J Radiat Oncol Biol Phys 1988; 15: 1299–1305

4. Perez C A, Pilepich M V, Zivnuska F. Tumor control in definitive irradiation of localized carcinoma of the prostate. Int J Radiat Oncol Biol Phys 1986; 12: 523–531
5. Lawton C A, Won M, Pilepich M V et al. Long-term treatment sequelae following external beam irradiation for adenocarcinoma of the prostate: analysis of RTOG studies 7506 and 7706. Int J Radiat Oncol Biol Phys 1991; 21: 935–939
6. Smit W G J M, Helle P A, Van Putte W L J et al. Late radiation damage in prostate cancer patients treated by high dose external radiotherapy in relation to rectal dose. Int J Radiat Oncol Biol Phys 1990; 18: 23–29
7. Greskovich F J, Zagars G K, Sherman N E, Johnson D E. Complications following external beam radiation therapy for prostate cancer: an analysis of patients treated with and without staging lymphadenectomy. J. Urol 1991; 146: 798–802
8. Zagars G K, von Eschenbach A C, Johnson D E, Oswald M J. Stage C adenocarcinoma of the prostate: an analysis of 551 patients treated with external beam radiation. Cancer 1987; 60: 1489–1499
9. Fuks Z, Leibel S A, Kutcher G E et al. Three dimensional conformal treatment: a new frontier in radiation therapy. In: DeVita V T Jr, Hellman S, Rosenberg S A (eds) Important advances in oncology. Philadelphia: JB Lippincott, 1991: 151–172
10. Fuks Z, Hellman S. Three-dimensional conformal radiotherapy. In: DeVita V T Jr, Hellman S, Rosenberg S A (eds) Cancer principles and practice of oncology, 4th edn. Philadelphia: J.B. Lippincott, 1992: 2614–2624
11. Leibel S A, Zelefsky M J, Kutcher G J et al. Three-dimensional conformal radiation therapy in localized carcinoma of the prostate: interim report of a phase 1 dose escalation study. J Urol 1994; 152: 1792–1798
12. Goitein M, Abrams M, Rowell D et al. Multi-dimensional treatment planning: II. Beam's eye-view, back projection, and projection through CT sections. Int J Radiat Oncol Biol Phys 1983; 9: 789–797
13. Mohan R. Three-dimensional radiation therapy treatment planning. Australas Phys Eng Sci Med 1989; 12: 73–91
14. Mohan R, Chui C S. Use of Fourier transforms in calculating dose distributions for irregularly shaped fields for three dimensional treatment planning. Med Phys 1987; 14: 70–77
15. Chui C S, Mohan R. Extraction of pencil beam kernels by the deconvolution method. Med Phys 1988; 15: 138–144
16. Drzymala R E, Mohan R, Brewster L et al. Dose–volume histograms. Int J Radiat Oncol Biol Phys 1991; 21: 71–78
17. Zelefsky M J, Leibel S A, Burman C A et al. Neoadjuvant hormonal therapy improves the therapeutic ratio in patients with bulky prostatic cancer treated with three-dimensional conformal radiation therapy. Int J Oncol Biol Phys 1994; 29: 755–761
18. LoSasso T J, Chui C S, Kutcher G J et al. The use of multi-leaf collimator for conformal radiotherapy in carcinomas of the prostate and nasopharynx. Int J Radiat Oncol Biol Phys 1993; 25: 161–170
19. Mageras G S, Podmaniczky K C, Mohan R. A model for computer-controlled delivery of 3D conformal treatments. Med Phys 1992; 19: 945–953
20. Ling C C, Burman C, Chui C S et al. Conformal radiation treatment of prostate cancer using inversely planned intensity-modulated photon beams produced with dynamic multileaf collimation. Int J Radiat Oncol Biol Phys 1996; 35: 721–730
21. Zelefsky M J, Leibel S A, Kutcher G J et al. The feasibility of dose escalation with three-dimensional conformal radiotherapy in patients with prostatic carcinoma. Cancer J Sci Am 1995; 1: 142–150
22. Leibel S A, Fuks Z, Zelefsky M J, Whitmore W F Jr. The effects of local and regional treatments on the metastatic outcome in prostatic carcinoma with pelvic lymph node involvement. Int J Radiat Oncol Biol Phys 1994; 28: 7
23. Marks L B, Anscher M S. Radiotherapy for prostate cancer: should the seminal vesicles be considered target? Int J Radiat Oncol Biol Phys 1992; 24: 435–440
24. Sandler H M, McLaughlin P W, Ten Haken R K et al. Three dimensional conformal radiotherapy for the treatment of prostate cancer: low risk of chronic rectal morbidity observed in a large series of patients. Int J Radiat Oncol Biol Phys 1995; 33: 797–801
25. Schultheiss T E, Hanks G E, Hunt M A, Lee W R. Incidence of and factors related to late complications in conformal and conventional radiation treatment of cancer of the prostate. Int J Radiat Oncol Biol Phys 1995; 32: 643–649

26. Lee W R, Hanks G E, Hanlon A *et al*. Lateral rectal shielding reduces late rectal morbidity following high dose three-dimensional conformal radiation therapy for clinically localized prostate cancer: further evidence for a significant dose effect. Int J Radiat Oncol Biol Phys 1996; 35: 251–257

27. Hartford A C, Niemierko A, Adams J A *et al*. Conformal irradiation of the prostate: estimating long-term rectal bleeding risk using dose–volume histograms. Int J Radiat Oncol Biol Phys 1996; 36: 721–730

28. Zelefsky M J, Harrison B S. Neoadjuvant androgen ablation prior to radiotherapy for prostate cancer: reducing the potential morbidity of therapy. Urology 1997; 49: 38–45

29. Forman J D, Kumar R, Haas G *et al*. Neoadjuvant hormonal downsizing of localized carcinoma of the prostate: effects on the volume of normal tissue irradiation. Cancer Invest 1995; 13: 8–15

30. Yang F E, Chen G T, Ray P *et al*. The potential for normal tissue dose reduction with neoadjuvant hormonal therapy in conformal treatment planning for stage C prostate cancer. Int J Radiat Oncol Biol Phys 1995; 33: 1009–1017

31. Zelefsky M J, Happersett L, Leibel S A *et al*. The effect of treatment positioning on normal tissue dose in patients with prostate cancer treated with 3-dimensional conformal radiotherapy. Int J Radiat Oncol Biol Phys 1997; 37: 13–19

32. Hanks G E, Lee W R, Hanlon A L *et al*. Conformal technique dose escalation in prostate cancer: improved cancer control with higher doses in patients with pretreatment PSA > 10 ng/ml. Int J Radiat Oncol Biol Phys 1996; 35: 861–868

33. Pilepich M V, Sause W T, Shipley W U *et al*. Androgen deprivation with radiation therapy compared with radiation therapy alone for locally advanced prostatic carcinoma: a randomized comparative trial of the Radiation Therapy Oncology Group. Urology 1995; 45: 616–623

34. Bolla M, Gonzalez D, Warde P *et al*. Controlled clinical trial in high metastatic risk carcinoma of the prostate comparing pelvic radiotherapy alone to pelvic radiotherapy plus LHRH analogue. Int J Radiat Oncol Biol Phys 1996; 36: 227

Chapter 23
The way ahead for radiotherapy in prostate cancer

D. Dearnaley

Introduction

Prostate cancer detection has increased by an estimated 30–50 thousand cases per year in the USA as a result of biochemical testing using prostate-specific antigen (PSA),[1] so that prostate cancer (CAP) is now the most commonly diagnosed male malignancy in North America. In Europe and the UK the uptake of PSA testing has been slower, Schröder suggesting that 20% of European men undergo regular PSA testing compared with 70% in the USA.[2] The figure in the UK is probably much lower and is reflected in the ratio of prostate cancer incidence to mortality in the UK (12,496 cases diagnosed in 1988; 9629 deaths in 1992) compared with the USA (projected incidence in 1994, 200,000 cases; deaths in 1990, 35,000).[3,4] The considerable majority of the 'newly' diagnosed cancers are of early stage and potentially curable. In the UK, a rapidly increasing rate of CAP diagnosis over the next 5–10 years and a corresponding demand for potentially curative treatment options should be anticipated. In both the UK and North America, radical radiotherapy has been the most commonly used curative modality,[5] although the proportion of men in the USA (particularly those aged 70 years or less) undergoing radical prostatectomy has risen rapidly.[6] The increase in diagnosis in CAP has substantial implications for the provision of services to deliver radiotherapy or perform prostatectomy: for example, the demand for radiation treatment has increased three- to fourfold in some centres[7,8] and there is, therefore, an increasing urgency to determine the optimal selection of patients for radical local treatment and to decide on the most effective and appropriate radiation therapy techniques.

The seminal paper by Chodak and colleagues[9] on 'watch and wait' management of T1/2 CAP has shown that tumour grade is of overriding importance in determining outcome. Although cause-specific mortality was only 13% at 10 years for Grade 1 or 2 tumours compared with 66% in men with grade 3 cancers, metastases occurred in 19, 42 and 74%, respectively, of patients with grade 1/3 cancers, 10 years after diagnosis, clearly demonstrating the progressive nature of disease in men with a reasonable life expectancy. A retrospective analysis by Schröder and Chodak (data presented at British Prostate Group Symposium 1996), studied 2558 men treated with total prostatecomy compared with 815 managed with a 'watch and wait' policy. For those patients with high-grade localized tumours, surgical treatment gave a 78% 10-year survival compared with 34% for men treated by a watch and wait policy ($p = 0.004$). On multivariate analysis, expectant management predicted poor survival. Such data need confirmation from prospective randomized studies. Patient recruitment continues in Sweden and North America, although, unfortunately, in the UK the Medical Research Council study comparing radiotherapy with prostatectomy or expectant management has failed because of poor recruitment.

Results of external beam radiotherapy treatment for localized prostate cancer

The long-term results of external beam radiotherapy for CAP derived from reports from the Patterns of Care Surveys, Radiation Therapy Oncology Group (RTOG) studies and large single-institute series[5,10–14] are shown in Table 23.1. Results from the Royal Marsden NHS Trust in 388 clinically staged patients treated between 1970 and 1989 showed broadly similar results, with 5/10-year actuarial local control rates of 88/77% for T1, 80/65% for T2 and 74/68% for T3 cancers. It should be noted that these series do not contain patients who have had pathological lymph node staging and, as might be expected, the 10-year cause-specific mortality in 104 patients with T1B–T2 N0 surgically staged disease treated in RTOG trial 7706 was 90%, and 87% of patients were clinically free of local recurrence.[15] The survival in this group of patients exceeded that of an age-matched control population and, in general, for patients with T1 and T2A disease, overall results are generally similar to those reported after radical prostatectomy.[16]

It is clear from these studies that results for more advanced T2C, T3–4 tumours have been less favourable. Survival of these patients is affected by the presence of undiagnosed metastatic disease, and understaging of pelvic lymph nodes at the time of initial treatment. Additionally, however, a general finding is that large tumours have poorer local control, failure rates rising from 25% for tumours palpably less than 25 cm^2 to more than 50% for tumours with a product of their diameters greater than 25 cm^2.[17] Most local recurrences are detected by digital rectal examination (DRE) and the true rate determined by post-radiation biopsy is probably higher. There is general agreement that a positive biopsy 24 months after radiotherapy indicates persisting disease.[18] The reported rates of positive biopsy specimens vary considerably and the true incidence of positive biopsy results in patients with normal DRE is uncertain.[19] Reported incidences of positive biopsy vary from 18%–45% post-treatment and increases with disease bulk from 15% for men with B1 disease (<1.5 cm nodule) to 68–79% for men with bulky stage B or C cancer.[20,21]

Table 23.1. External beam radiotherapy for CAP: long-term results from Patterns of Care Surveys, RTOG studies and large single-institute series

| | | Percentage survival | | | | | | | | |
| | | Local recurrence | | | No evidence of disease | | | Overall | | |
Stage	No. of patients	5 year	10 year	15 year	5 year	10 year	15 year	5 year	10 year	15 year
T_1N_x	583	3–6	4–8	17	84–85	52–68	39	83–95	52–76	41–46
T_2N_x	1117	12–14	17–29	32–35	66–90	27–85	15–42	74–78	43–70	22–36
T_3N_x	2292	12–26	19–31	25–56	32–60	14–46	17–40	56–72	32–42	23–27

Data from refs 5, 10–14.

Prostate-specific antigen (PSA) and external beam radiotherapy

It is becoming clear that PSA estimation, both before and after irradiation, can give useful information to guide prognosis and selection of patients for treatment, as well as being a very sensitive indicator of disease recurrence. Hancock and colleagues[22] studied 110 patients with T1–T3 CAP with a mean follow-up of 12.6

years and found long-term biochemical control of 72% for T1 cancers, 54% for T2A cancers, falling to 22% and 28% for bulkier T2 and T3 cancers, respectively. A favourable outcome was also seen in patients with cancers that had a low Gleason score, who had a 75% rate of biochemical control compared with only 18% for Gleason sum 7 and 0% for Gleason sum 8 or 9. It has also been shown that pretreatment PSA levels are of critical importance.[23-25] For example, Hanks and colleagues[25] found that, of 120 patients with PSA more than 20 ng/ml at presentation, only 28% remained biochemically free of progressive disease at 4 years, although 81% still had no evidence of distant metastases. The nadir level of PSA following radiotherapy also appears to be a powerful predictor of outcome, although it remains uncertain whether 1.0 ng/ml or 0.5 ng/ml gives optimal discrimination.[26,27] Groups from Harvard and DeKalb have suggested that it is important to achieve nadir values of 0.5 ng/ml. Zietman and colleagues[23] showed that 63% of 314 men with T1/2 NxM0 carcinomas were free of biochemical progression after radical radiotherapy at 5 years. If the PSA nadir was 0.5 ng/ml or less, then biochemical recurrence-free rate was 90% compared with 46% if the PSA nadir was higher. The likelihood of reaching a PSA nadir was clearly related to initial PSA but not to Gleason score. Critz and colleagues,[28] using a combination of external beam radiotherapy and interstitial treatment, described a group of 536 patients with T1, T2 N0 cancers: 80% achieved a nadir of 0.5 ng/ml or less and 5- and 10-year biochemical disease-free survival rates were 95 and 84%, respectively, compared with 29% at 5 years for those with a higher nadir level; all patients with a nadir of more than 1.0 ng/ml ultimately failed. In the future, presenting levels of PSA may be useful in determining which patients are most suitable for treatment using dose-escalation techniques. For example, Hanks and colleagues[25] analysed 375 consecutive patients treated with conformal radiotherapy techniques. Dividing patients into those who received above or below 71 Gy showed an advantage in biochemical disease-free recurrence for those patients presenting with PSA levels more than 10 and 20 ng/ml, but not for those with PSA levels below 10 ng/ml at the time of presentation. In the future, PSA levels in combination with clinical staging and Gleason score will be used to stratify patients for appropriate treatment and PSA will be valuable as a proxy endpoint in studies looking at different treatment combinations and radiotherapy techniques.

The importance of local tumour control

Long-term clinically judged local tumour control is good for patients with stage T1 cancers (83% at 15 years) but becomes increasingly less secure with increasing T stage, falling to 65–68% for T2 and 44–75% for T3 cancers (Table 23.1). As above, prostate biopsy may show higher rates of recurrence than can be detected clinically and biochemical (PSA) failure rates are certainly significantly higher.[24] Review of Royal Marsden Hospital patients showed 57% metastasis-free survival at 5 years in patients with clinically local controlled disease compared with 26% of patients with local recurrence ($p < 0.01$), and local control remained highly significant ($p < 0.001$) when included as a time-dependent variable in a multivariate analysis of outcome (survival and development of metastases). These findings are in accordance with other series that have documented distant metastases developing in 19–41% of patients with stages A–C disease and local control of disease compared with 57–83% for patients who have developed local failure.[16] Local failure has been reported to be the most important determinant on multivariate analysis in predicting the development of metastatic disease for all stages of disease;[29] additionally, this study demonstrated that distant metastases developed on average later in patients with local failure than in those patients who had local control of disease, strongly suggesting that local failure itself was an important determinant of outcome. Yorke and collegues[30] estimated, using Monte Carlo simulation techniques, that 50% of the metastases in patients with local recurrence were due to local treatment failure.

Complications after radiotherapy

Radiation-induced complications are dose limiting, and current 'standard' radiotherapy doses and fractionation schedules have been derived from years of clinical experience to give acceptable morbidity. Acute side effects from radiotherapy to the pelvis include proctitis causing rectal discomfort and diarrhoea, cystitis producing dysuria and frequency of micturition, and occasional skin reactions. Reported incidence ranges from 70 to 90% for mild, from 20 to 45% for moderate and from 1 to 4% for severe or prolonged reactions.[31–33] Such side effects depend upon the volume of tissue treated (pelvis or prostate only)[34] and also relate to treatment technique. Acute side effects are expected to settle within 4–6 weeks of completing radiotherapy treatment.

Late complications may develop months or years after treatment and are potentially of more concern. Late gastrointestinal side effects include persistent rectal discharge, tenesmus, rectal bleeding and rectal stricture. Major late genitourinary complications include chronic cystitis, bladder ulcers, urinary incontinence and urethral stricture and impotence.

Results from over 1000 patients treated in recent single-institute series suggest an overall moderate complication rate of 16–19%, with severe complications requiring surgical correction in 1–3% of patients.[12,35,36] The Patterns of Care study group has defined major complications as those requiring hospital admission for investigation or management. Of 619 patients treated, 4.5% had such complications (gastrointestinal 2.6%, urological 1.8%) and complications were related to treatment technique, being higher in patients treated with only anterior/posterior radiation fields or in whom only one radiation field was treated each day. Doses above 70 Gy were also associated with increased complications.[37] This series was updated with a 10-year follow-up;[38] at that time, 2% of patients had needed surgical correction of complications, a further 2% had developed a major complication not requiring surgery and two patients had died from treatment related side effects. The actuarial 5- and 10-year complication-free rates were 93 and 86%, respectively. A further series of 313 patients with stage T1 tumours had a similar complication rate, with less than 2% requiring surgical correction. An increase in the overall complication rate from 6 to 11% was noted for patients treated with doses below and above 65 Gy, respectively.[39] The remaining complication is impotence, which has been estimated to occur in between 30 and 40% of treated patients, usually developing during the 6 months after treatment.[40] In a recent randomized study by the RTOG,[41] 76% of men who were sexually potent before treatment reported return of sexual function. In a report of conformal radiotherapy,[42] 62% of men reported return of sexual function. 'Quality-of-life' questionnaires may lead to a higher estimate of sexual dysfunction,[43] although this may be little different from an age-matched control population.[44]

Methods to improve the results of radiotherapy

As described above, the local control of CAP becomes increasingly uncertain with increasing tumour stage and tumour bulk. Potential methods to improve results are shown in Table 23.2. Retrospective studies have shown a dose–response

Table 23.2. Methods to improve local control with radiotherapy in CAP

Increased radiation dose	Conformal radiotherapy
	Interstitial irradiation
Particle beam radiotherapy	Protons
	Neutrons
Combined-modality treatment with androgen deprivation	Neoadjuvant
	Adjuvant
Combined-modality treatment with total prostatectomy	

relationship for CAP. For stage C disease, Perez *et al.*[45] reported figures of 38% local recurrence for doses of less than 60 Gy compared with 20% for 60–70 Gy and 12% for more than 70 Gy. Similar figures have been reported from the Patterns of Care Studies Group[46] for 1348 stage B and C patients. The actuarial 5-year local recurrence rate for stage C patients was 37% for doses of less than 60 Gy, 36% for 66–64 Gy, 28% for 65–69 Gy and 19% for doses of more than 70 Gy. Dose escalation, therefore, seems justified. However, as discussed above, radiotherapy-induced side effects restrict attempts to increase the delivered radiation dose above 70 Gy using conventional photon irradiation, with rectal bleeding increasing from 12 to 20%.[47] There are few clinical data concerning volume–complication relationships for either rectum or bladder, but there is an expectation of decreased side effects using either conformal radiotherapy or interstitial treatment approaches. The calculation of dose/volume histogram (DVH) and normal tissue complication probability (NTCP)[48,49] will eventually permit refinement of mathematical models of radiation toxicity and it is essential that clinical and medical physics data are collected prospectively. One such study,[50] including 41 patients, has suggested that there is a dose–volume relationship for rectal bleeding. A high probability of complications ranged between 60 CGE (Cobalt Grey Equivalent) delivered to 70% of the anterior rectal wall and 75 CGE to 30%. A further complicating factor is that inherent radiosensitivity may vary between patients,[51–53] and tests to detect sensitive patient populations would be most helpful in deselecting patients from radical radiotherapy treatments, particularly those using dose-escalation techniques.

Conformal radiotherapy

Prostate cancer has become the focus of attention for conformal radiotherapy, particularly in the USA. Accurate patient positioning, computed tomography (CT) planning with three-dimensional reconstruction of volumes of interest, clear definition of treatment margins, and meticulous verification procedures of the shaped fields produced by customized shaped blocks or multileaf collimation (MLC), are necessary components of this approach.[5,54] Multiple planar and complex non-coplanar beam orientations have been designed,[55,56] although clear advantages over more simple arrangements, particularly with more moderate degrees of dose escalation, are not overwhelming.[57–60] The amount of normal tissue treated to the 90% isodose may be reduced by 42%, with 46 and 41% reductions in the volumes of bowel and bladder, respectively.[61] Dose-escalation studies have been reported by three North American groups.[56,62,63] Using

meticulous planning and immobilization techniques, doses of 75 Gy have been
well tolerated (albeit with a relatively short follow-up) and, currently, doses in
excess of 80 Gy are being delivered. Further National Cancer Institute-sponsored
dose-escalation trials are under way, comparing doses of 68.4, 73.8 and 79.8 Gy, in
a multicentre phase II study.

In the UK, the Institute of Cancer Research and the Royal Marsden NHS Trust
have commenced a randomized study comparing 74 Gy with 64 Gy in
conjunction with the use of neoadjuvant androgen deprivation,[8] and it is planned
for the Medical Research Council Radiotherapy Working Party to adopt this study
formally in the near future. These exciting advances in external beam
radiotherapy are considered in fuller detail in Chapter 22.

Interstitial radiotherapy

Interstitial radiotherapy has been used for treatment of CAP since the beginning
of the twentieth century. Isotopes used are shown in Table 23.3. Theoretically, this
approach is attractive, as the radiation dose may be limited to conform to the
prostate. However, older retropubic techniques of insertion frequently gave
suboptimal dose distributions. The transperineal approach using transrectal
ultrasound (TRUS)-guided seed placement is required.[64] Isotopes currently used
include iodine-125, palladium-103 and Iridium-192. Iridium-192 gives radiation at
a high dose rate and a temporary implant is inserted using a perineal template.
Considerable skill with this approach is required and damage to the anterior rectal
wall is not uncommon. Iodine-125 and palladium-103 have very low photon
energies (Table 23.3). This has the advantage that the range of treatment is
limited, reducing the dose to rectum and bladder. These isotopes are used to give a
permanent implant so that treatment can be undertaken quickly and potentially
on an outpatient basis. The associated risk using lower-energy photons is that seed
placement has to be accurate to avoid areas of potential underdosage.[65,66] Iodine-
125 treats at a low dose rate and the more recently available palladium-103 may
be more effective against rapidly proliferating high-grade tumours.

Results of contemporary studies have been summarized,[64] showing local
control rates of 83–100%, positive post-treatment biopsies in 3–48% of cases and
PSA control in 85–94% of patients, with relatively short follow-up ranging from
12 to 15 months. The largest series of patients (318) have been treated in Seattle,[67]
and recent analysis of complications showed that 13% of patients required
medical or surgical intervention. Permanent sequelae were seen in 8%, the
majority affecting the urinary tract (7%), and 5% of patients had stress
incontinence, which was common (17%) if transurethral resection of the prostate
(TURP) had been performed, but was not seen in the 130 men without a history of
TURP. Recently, Wallner and colleagues[66] reported on 92 patients with clinical
stage T1/T2 disease treated with iodine-125 prostate implants to a minimum

Table 23.3. Isotopes for interstitial treatment of CAP

Isotope	Half-life (days)	Energy (MeV)
Iodine-125	60	0.027–0.032
Palladium-103	17	0.02
Gold-98	2.7	0.41
Iridium-192	74	0.38

radiation dose of 140–160 Gy. Freedom from biochemical failure at 4 years was 63% and, on multivariate analysis, the strongest predictor of failure was pretreatment PSA level (less than or greater than 10 ng/ml) followed by Gleason score and stage. In this series, of 56 patients who were sexually active before implantation, 85% retained potency at 3 years and interstitial radiation may well be the optimal treatment method for maintenance of potency.

Interstitial treatment may also be combined with external beam radiotherapy. Dattoli and colleagues[68] treated 73 'high-risk' patients with stage T2A–T3 disease. High risk was defined on the basis of T2B or greater disease, a Gleason score of 7 or more or PSA of more than 15 ng/ml. Limited-field pelvic irradiation (41 Gy) was followed by a boost using palladium-103 to a dose of 80 Gy. At 3 years, biochemical control was maintained in 79% of patients. The strongest predictors of failure were acid phosphatase, PSA and Gleason score. Treatment-related morbidity was reported to be mild and the actuarial potency rate at 3 years was 77%.

Interstitial treatment has not been formally compared with either conventional or conformal radiotherapy or total prostatectomy. Its use is limited to a few centres that have gained the necessary technical expertise. Implant treatment alone should be limited to patients with T1/T2 disease with Gleason scores of 7 or less who have not undergone prior TURP. Prostate volume much above 45–50 cm^3 technically makes implantation more difficult and dose distribution poorer. For this group of patients, additional neoadjuvant androgen deprivation can be considered to reduce prostate volume prior to implantation.

Particle beam radiotherapy

The ultimate method of improving radiation dose distributions using external beam treatment is to use particle therapy with, for example, protons or pions (negative pimesons). This type of irradiation has a highly advantageous dose distribution, as energy is deposited in a 'Bragg peak' over a small area. This physical property allows a high dose to be given to the target area, with a sharp fall-off in dose to the surrounding tissues. Energies in the region of 250 MeV are required to treat deep-seated lesions and so far these have been available in only a few centres.[69] However, a randomized trial has already been undertaken in Massachusetts.[70] Results have shown a small improvement in the rate of local control (77% versus 60% at 8 years; $p = 0.089$), particularly for poorly differentiated tumours, but this has not been translated into certain benefit for metastasis-free or overall survival. However, the study has produced very important information on dose–volume relationships for complications. The incidence of rectal bleeding increased from 16 to 34% as the dose increased from 67.2 Gy to 75.6 CGE and, at the higher dose level, 20% of men had this complication if less than 40% of the anterior rectal wall was treated, compared with 72% when more than 40% was irradiated. Theoretical studies have looked at the potential advantage of proton beam therapy over modern conformal photon beam irradiation.[71] A small advantage only was seen for proton beam therapy within two opposing fields, compared with three- or six-field photon beam irradiation (Figure 23.1). Approximately one-third of cases had benefit from a proton beam plan; any advantage in the remaining patients was limited because of the need to include the anterior rectal wall in the target volume. In practice, therefore, real advantages for proton beam therapy may be limited for CAP treatment.

Neutron beams have no inherent advantages for dose distribution compared with photons, but they do have a higher linear energy transfer (LET), which may lead to increased efficacy against hypoxic radioresistant tumours. Preliminary

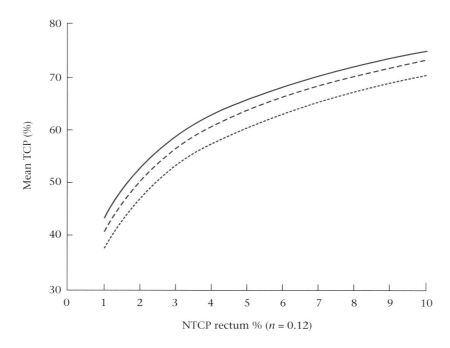

Figure 23.1. Comparison of proton and photon beam conformal radiotherapy in 20 patients using mathematical modelling techniques (from refs 104–106). Tumour control probability (TCP) is on average slightly improved for a given rectal normal tissue complication probability (NTCP) using high-energy protons compared with conformal photon beam techniques (reproduced from ref. 71 with permission.) Proton beam therapy (——); 3-field photon beam therapy (----); 6-field photon beam therapy (.........).

studies in stage C and D1 CAP have been performed using mixed neutron–photon irradiation.[72] Subsequently, a randomized study has been reported to show that neutron therapy improves local control and PSA normalization rates in comparison with photon beam therapy.[73] Clinical or biochemical failure occurred in 32 and 45% of patients on the photon arm, compared with 11 and 17% in the neutron group — but at the expense of significantly increased (11% vs 3%) grade 3 complications that were technique dependent. There was a strong indication that the use of beam shaping using MLC (in a similar manner to conformal radiotherapy using photons) reduces late radiation toxicity. In the subgroup of patients treated at the University of Washington using an MLC, no excess side effects were seen, although improvements in local control were maintained.[74]

The technology to produce particle beam therapy is very expensive and it is unlikely that these techniques will gain wide acceptance, unless prospective randomized studies show unequivocal and clear advantages.

Combined-modality treatment using androgen deprivation and radiotherapy

Neoadjuvant androgen deprivation offers potential advantages in two ways (Figure 23.2). First, combined-modality treatment may lead to increased tumour cell kill (androgen deprivation probably causes apoptosis whereas radiotherapy induces mitotic cell death) and hence improvements in local control. Secondly, initial shrinkage of the prostate and prostate cancer can lead to a beneficial modification of radiation treatment volume. Reducing the radiation target volume may favourably affect the therapeutic ratio, either by reducing radiation sequelae

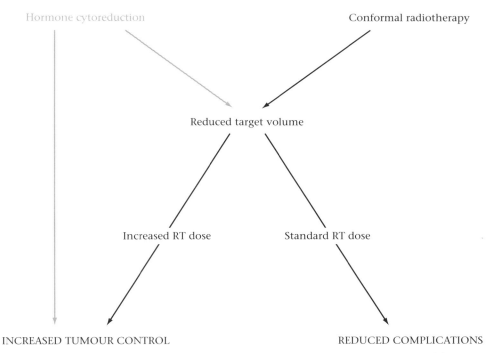

Figure 23.2. Theoretical advantages of neoadjuvant androgen deprivation in combination with radiotherapy.

for a standard radiation dose or by permitting dose escalation, which should increase tumour control probability while maintaining acceptable levels of radiation complications. In addition to these potential benefits from additive local effects, adjuvant hormonal therapy may have advantages in 'spatial cooperation' — an improvement in the therapeutic results that is achieved by one modality treating disease spatially missed by the other.[75] Such benefit has clearly been demonstrated for the use of adjuvant hormone therapy in breast cancer,[76,77] but has not been adequately addressed in prostate cancer. The addition of neoadjuvant systemic treatments in, for example, breast,[78] lung[79] and head and neck cancer,[80] has been shown to improve the local and overall treatment results at these sites. Cytotoxic chemotherapy has been the appropriate systemic modality for these tumour types but frequently interacts with irradiation to enhance toxicities; androgen deprivation is the appropriate systemic treatment for prostate cancer and no enhanced toxicities have been observed in the studies outlined below.

Studies at the Royal Marsden Hospital,[61,81,82] using 3–6 months of initial luteinizing hormone-releasing hormone (LHRH) analogue treatment, have demonstrated a 50% reduction in prostate volume, with an associated 40% potential reduction in radiotherapy treatment volume. Preliminary results show that 70% of patients with initially bulky T2–T4 cancers (pretreatment median PSA 30 ng/ml) remain in biochemical remission 18 months after completion of therapy.[83] A prospective randomized study has been undertaken by the RTOG in North America.[41] In protocol 8610, 457 men with bulky stage B2/C CAP were randomized to receive goserelin and flutamide for 2 months before and during radiotherapy, or to receive radiotherapy alone. With a median potential follow-up of 4.5 years, the cumulative incidence of local progression at 5 years was 46% for combined-modality treatment compared with 71% for radiotherapy alone ($p < 0.001$). The 5-year incidence rates of distant metastases were 34 and 41%, respectively ($p = 0.09$). Biochemical progression-free survival rates showed an advantage with the combined-modality group, with 36% progression free at 5 years compared with 15% in patients treated with irradiation alone.

Radiotherapy and adjuvant androgen deprivation

It is well accepted that adjuvant hormone therapy has a significant effect on both recurrence and survival in breast cancer. There is now increasing evidence that a similar benefit may be seen in CAP, and relevant studies are summarized in Table 23.4. The RTOG has studied adjuvant LHRH analogues commenced at the time of radiotherapy. In protocol 85–31,[84] 977 men with clinical or pathological stage T3 or T4 disease or with evidence of lymph node involvement were randomized between prostate and pelvic irradiation with either adjuvant LHRH analogues or LHRH analogues to be started on relapse. There was a significant reduction in clinical local failure of disease, from 32% on radiotherapy alone to 17% with LHRH analogue treatment ($p < 0.001$), a reduction of distant metastases from 29 to 19% ($p < 0.001$), improvement of biochemical control of disease from 17 to 49% ($p < 0.001$) and a 5% improvement in survival (but this did not reach statistical significance). A similar trial perfomed by the European Organization for Research and Treatment of Cancer (EORTC) group recruited 415 patients with poorly differentiated T1/T2 disease or T3/T4 tumours. Patients were randomized to receive radiotherapy alone to the prostate and pelvis or additional LHRH analogue therapy for 3 years. After a median follow-up of 33 months, 5-year estimates of local control were improved from 75 to 95% with combined-modality treatment, and metastasis-free survival from 56 to 89% ($p < 0.001$), with an overall improvement in survival of 56–78% ($p = 0.001$).[85] In addition, the Medical Research

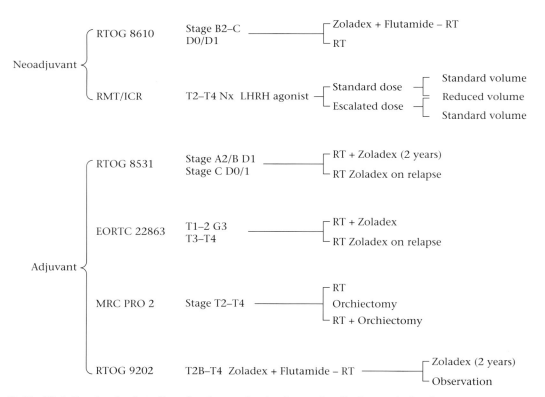

Table 23.4. Randomized studies of androgen deprivation and radiotherapy in local prostate cancer.

Council has recently reported results of a relatively small three-arm study comparing radiotherapy, orchiectomy and combined-modality treatment using radiotherapy combined with orchiectomy. A total of 277 patients were randomized and results show a significant lengthening of time for the development of metastases in the orchiectomy group.[86,87] Furthermore, there was a gain in local control and survival, with approximately 10% improvement in overall survival in the orchiectomy and radiotherapy group compared with the group treated with radiotherapy alone, but this difference failed to reach statistical significance. The current RTOG study protocol 92-02 of patients with T2B–T4 cancers evaluates treatment with initial neoadjuvant LHRH agonist and radical radiotherapy with a subsequent randomization to continue LHRH therapy for 2 years or to discontinue androgen deprivation. The results of this comprehensive set of clinical studies should give guidance as to the value of both adjuvant and neoadjuvant approaches to combined-modality therapy. However, for patients with advanced localized disease or high-grade tumours, there remains doubt concerning the contribution of radiotherapy and whether these patients might be managed effectively with hormonal treatment alone. This question is being addressed in a study (NCIC CTG PR3) coordinated by the National Cancer Institute in Canada, which randomizes patients with T3 and T4 N0 CAP to either maximum androgen blockade alone or maximum androgen blockade in combination with full radical radiotherapy. It is appropriate that this set of studies should include quality-of-life measures as well as disease-related endpoints, as each modality of treatment can bring its own particular set of toxicities.

The role of radiotherapy in pathological T3 disease

Pathological analysis of total prostatectomy specimens in stage T2 cancer shows pT3 disease in 30–50% of cases.[88–90] Retrospective review of the literature has suggested that local recurrence occurred in 23% of patients treated without postoperative radiotherapy compared with 3% of patients with irradiation.[91] Subsequent reports have supported the idea that immediate adjuvant radiotherapy reduces the incidence of local recurrence[92–94] and, following postoperative radiotherapy, recurrence rates have been shown to be 5% or less.[93,95–97] If radiotherapy is delayed until after evidence of local recurrence, higher radiation doses are required and treatment morbidity may be greater for less certain local control (70%).[97] A recent report on 46 patients with PSA relapse alone showed biochemical disease control (PSA ≤ 0.3 ng/ml) in 59% of patients, with actuarial freedom from recurrence of 50% at 5 years.[98] It has been suggested that radiation therapy improves long-term outcome by controlling local regional disease.[94,99–101] A recent report[102,103] of 288 patients managed at the Mayo Clinic showed a significant improvement in biochemical disease control (PSA ≤ 0.3 ng/ml) in those patients given postoperative radiotherapy, but (as yet) no difference in the distant failure rate at 5 years, of 8% versus 10% ($p = 0.09$). It cannot, therefore, be assumed that improved local disease control will necessarily translate into therapeutic gain, and postoperative radiotherapy treatment runs the risk of producing an increase in side effects from the combined-modality approach. It is, therefore, appropriate that randomized studies are undertaken to define clearly the role of postoperative radiotherapy in pT3 disease. Recently, there have been two such studies. In RTOG Protocol 91-19, patients with pT3 disease (capsular invasion, positive margins, positive seminal vesicles) were randomized to immediate radiotherapy (60–64 Gy) or observation. The EORTC Protocol No. 22911, which is still in progress, randomizes similar patients between radiotherapy (60 Gy) or observation and aims to recruit a total of 700 patients. Results from these comprehensive studies should guide the selection of patients for such treatment.

Conclusions

As for cancer arising at other sites, radiotherapy alone is capable of sterilizing the primary tumour and can improve loco-regional control in conjunction with radical surgery. However, assessment of the real value of radical treatment to the patient is made difficult because of both the long natural history of disease in many patients and the competing causes of death. The rapid increase in diagnosis of localized carcinoma of the prostate, due to increased public awareness and PSA testing, highlights the requirement for improving patient selection and minimizing treatment-related side effects.

Local control may be improved by increasing tumour dose by a variety of methods including 'conformal' radiotherapy, particle beam therapy or interstitial treatment. Late damage to rectum and bladder/urethra limits dose escalation, and high degrees of technical skill are required if these approaches are to be implemented safely.

Neoadjuvant androgen deprivation has been shown to be complementary to radiotherapy and to improve local control without significant excess (and probably with reduced) toxicity. As in breast cancer, adjuvant treatment may improve recurrence-free and overall survival at the cost of long-term hormone side effects. Alternative hormonal strategies to LHRH and maximal androgen blockade would be of interest. Ongoing clinical studies will address some of these issues, but enthusiasm for 'high tech' therapies should not obscure the overall aims of treatment, which can be assessed accurately only in prospective randomized studies, with endpoints including overall survival and quality-of-life assessments, as well as biochemical data on disease control.

For the future, improved understanding of the biology of prostate cancer may lead to optimal patient selection for treatment. Optimization of dose and radiotherapy techniques using DVH and TCP/NTCP considerations should improve uncomplicated tumour control probabilities. The role of normal tissue sensitivity testing deserves further study, and the indications for and duration of neoadjuvant and adjuvant hormone therapy must be clarified. Finally, new modalities should be tested and integrated as they become available.

References

1.   Mettlin C. The status of prostate cancer early detection. Cancer 1993; 72(suppl 3): 1050–1055
2.   Schröder F H. Screening for prostate cancer (letter). Lancet 1994; 343(8910): 1438–1439
3.   Cancer Research Campaign. Cancer of the prostate. Factsheet 20(1), 1994
4.   Boring C C, Squires T S, Tong T. Cancer statistics, 1993. CA 1993; 43(1): 7–26
5.   Hanks G E. Treatment of early stage prostate cancer: radiotherapy. In: DeVita V T, Hellman S, Rosenberg S A (eds) Important advances in oncology. Philadelphia: J B Lippincott, 1994: 225–239
6.   Lu-Yao G L, McLerran D, Wasson J, Wennber J E. An assessment of radical prostatectomy. Time trends, geographic variation, and outcomes. The Prostate Patient Outcomes Research Team. JAMA 1993; 269: 2633–2636
7.   de Jong B, Crommelin M, van der Heijden L H, Coebergh J W W. Patterns of radiotherapy for cancer patients in south-eastern Netherlands, 1975–1989. Radiother Oncol 1994; 31: 213–221
8.   Dearnaley D P. Radiotherapy for prostate cancer: the changing scene. Clin Oncol 1995; 7(2): 147–150

9. Chodak G W, Thisted R A, Gerber G S *et al*. Results of conservative management of clinically localized prostate cancer. N Engl J Med 1994; 330(4): 242–248

10. Hanks G E, Hanlon A, Owen J B, Schultheiss T E. Patterns of radiation treatment of elderly patients with prostate cancer. Cancer 1994; 74(suppl 7): 2174–2177

11. Goffinet D R, Baghaw M A. Radiation therapy of prostate carcinoma: thirty-year experience at Stanford University. In: Schröder F H, ed. *EORTC Genitourinary Group Monograph 8. Treatment of Prostatic Cancer — Facts and Controversies*. New York, Chichester, Brisbane, Toronto, Singapore: Wiley-Liss Inc, 1990: 209–222

12. Zagars G K, von Eschenback A C, Johnson D E, Oswald M J. Stage C adenocarcinoma of the prostate: an analysis of 551 patients treated with external beam radiation. Cancer 1987; 60(7): 1489–1499

13. Zagars G K, von Eschenbach A C, Johnson D E, Oswald J M. The role of radiation therapy in stages A2 and B adenocarcinoma of the prostate. Int J Radiat Oncol Biol Phys 1988; 14: 701–709

14. Perez C A, Pilepich M V, Garcia D *et al*. Definitive radiation therapy in carcinoma of the prostate localized to the pelvis: experience at the Mallinckrodt Institute of Radiology. NCI Monogr 1988; 7: 85–94

15. Hanks G E, Asbell S, Krall J M *et al*. Outcome for lymph node dissection negative T-1b, T-2 (A-2, B) prostate cancer treated with external beam radiation therapy in RTOG 77-06. Int J Radiat Oncol Biol Phys 1991; 21(4): 1099–1103

16. Leibel S A, Zelefsky M J, Kutcher G J *et al*. The biological basis and clinical application of three-dimensional conformal external beam radiation therapy in carcinoma of the prostate. Semin Oncol 1994; 21(5): 580–597

17. Pilepich M V, Krall J M, Sause W T *et al*. Prognostic factors in carcinoma of the prostate—analysis of RTOG study 7506. Int J Radiat Oncol Biol Phys 1987; 13(3): 339–349

18. Crook J, Robertson S, Collin G *et al*. Clinical relevance of trans–rectal ultrasound, biopsy and serum prostate-specific antigen following external beam radiotherapy for carcinoma of the prostate. Int J Radiat Oncol Biol Phys 1993; 27(1): 31–37

19. Zietman A L, Shipley W U, Willett G C. Residual disease after radical surgery or radiation therapy for prostate cancer. Clinical significance and therapeutic implications. Cancer 1993; 71: 859–869

20. Scardino P T, Bretas F. Interstitial radiotherapy. In: Bruce AW, Trachtenberg J (eds) Adenocarcinoma of the prostate. London: Springer-Verlag, 1987: 145–158

21. Freiha F S, Bagshaw M A. Carcinoma of the prostate: results of post-irradiation biopsy. Prostate 1984; 5(1): 19–25

22. Hanks G E, Hanlon A L, Hudes G *et al*. Patterns-of-failure analysis of patients with high pretreatment prostate-specific antigen levels treated by radiation therapy: the need for improved systemic and locoregional treatment. J Clin Oncol 1996; 14(4): 1093–1097

23. Zietman A L, Tibbs M K, Dallow K C *et al*. Use of PSA nadir to predict subsequent biochemical outcome following external beam radiation therapy for T1–2 adenocarcinoma of the prostate. Radiother Oncol 1996; 40(2): 159–162

24. Horwitz E M, Vicini F A, Ziaja E L *et al*. Assessing the variability of outcome for patients treated with localised prostate irradiation using different definitions of biochemical control. Int J Radiat Oncol Biol Phys 1996; 36(3): 565–571

25. Hanks G E, Lee W R, Hanlon A L *et al*. Conformal technique dose escalation for prostate cancer: biochemical evidence of improved cancer control with higher doses in patients with pretreatment prostate-specific antigen ≥10 ng/ml. Int J Radiat Oncol Biol Phys 1996; 35(5): 861–868

26. McLaughlin P W, Sandler H M, Jiroutek M R. Prostate-specific antigen following prostate radiotherapy: how low can you go? (Editorial). J Clin Oncol 1996; 14(11): 2889–2892

27. McNeil C. PSA levels after radiotherapy: how low must they go? J Natl Cancer Inst 1996; 88(12): 791–792

28. Critz F A, Levinson A K, Williams W H, Holladay D A. Prostate-specific antigen nadir: the optimum level after irradiation for prostate cancer. J Clin Oncol 1996; 14(11): 2893–2900

29. Fuks Z, Leibel S A, Wallner K E *et al*. The effect of local control on metastatic dissemination in carcinoma of the prostate: long term results in patients treated with I^{125} implantation. Int J Radiat Oncol Biol Phys 1991; 21(3): 537–547

30. Yorke E D, Fuks Z, Norton L *et al*. Modeling the development of metastases from primary and locally recurrent tumors: comparison with a clinical data base for prostatic cancer. Cancer Res 1993; 53: 2987–2993

31. Duncan W, Warde P, Catton C N *et al.* Carcinoma of the prostate: results of radical radiotherapy (1970–1985). Int J Radiat Oncol Biol Phys 1993; 26(2): 203–210
32. Amdur R J, Parsons J T, Fitzgerald L T, Million R R. Adenocarcinoma of the prostate treated with external-beam radiation therapy: 5-year minimum follow-up. Radiother Oncol 1990; 18(3): 235–246
33. Mithal N P, Hoskin P J. External beam radiotherapy for carcinoma of the prostate: a retrospective study. Clin Oncol 1993; 5(5): 297–301
34. Sagerman R H, Chun H C, King G A *et al.* External beam radiotherapy for carcinoma of the prostate. Cancer 1989; 63(12): 2468–2474
35. Aristizabal S A, Steinbronn D, Heusinkveld R S. External beam radiotherapy in cancer of the prostate. Radiother Oncol 1984; 1: 309–315
36. Forman J D, Zinreich E, Ding-Jen L *et al.* Improving the therapeutic ratio of external beam irradiation for carcinoma of the prostate. Int J Radiat Oncol Biol Phys 1985; 11: 2073–2080
37. Leibel S A, Hanks G E, Kramer S. Patterns of care outcome studies: results of the national practice in adenocarcinoma of the prostate. Int J Radiat Oncol Biol Phys 1984; 10(3): 401–409
38. Hanks G E, Diamond J J, Krall J M *et al.* A ten year follow-up of 682 patients treated for prostate cancer with radiation therapy in the United States. Int J Radiat Oncol Biol Phys 1987; 13(4): 499–505
39. Hanks G E, Krail J M, Martz K L *et al.* The outcome of treatment of 313 patients with T-1 (UICC) prostate cancer treated with external beam irradiation. Int J Radiat Oncol Biol Phys 1988; 14(2): 243–248
40. DeWit L, Ang K K, van der Schueren E. Acute side effects and late complications after radiotherapy of localised carcinoma of the prostate. Cancer Treat Rev 1983; 10: 79–89
41. Pilepich M V, Krall J M, al-Sarraf M *et al.* Androgen deprivation with radiation therapy compared with radiation therapy alone for locally advanced prostatic carcinoma: a randomised comparative trial of RTOG. Urology 1995; 45: 616–623
42. Roach M I, Chinn D M, Holland J, Clarke M. A pilot survey of sexual function and quality of life following 3D conformal radiotherapy for clinically localized prostate cancer. Int J Radiat Oncol Biol Phys 1996; 35(5): 869–874
43. Helgason A R, Fredrikson M, Adolfsson J, Steineck G. Decreased sexual capacity after external radiation therapy for prostate cancer impairs quality of life. Int J Radiat Oncol Biol Phys 1995; 32(1): 33–39
44. Fransson P, Widmark A. Self-assessed sexual function after pelvic irradiation for prostate carcinoma. Comparison with an age-matched control group. Cancer 1996; 78(5): 1066–1078
45. Perez C A, Walz B J, Zivnuska F R. Irradiation of carcinoma of the prostate localized to the pelvis: analysis of tumor response and prognosis. Int J Radiat Oncol Biol Phys 1980; 6(5): 555–563
46. Hanks G E, Martz K L, Diamond J J. The effect of dose on local control of prostate cancer. Int J Radiat Oncol Biol Phys 1988; 15(6): 1299–1305
47. Pilepich M V, Asbell S O, Krall J M *et al.* Correlation of radiotherapeutic parameters and treatment related morbidity — analysis of RTOG study 77–06. Int J Radiat Oncol Biol Phys 1987; 13(7): 1007–1012
48. Emami B, Lyman J, Brown A *et al.* Tolerance of normal tissue to therapeutic radiation. Int J Radiat Oncol Biol Phys 1991; 21: 109–122
49. Kutcher G J, Burman C, Brewster L *et al.* Histogram reduction method for calculating complication probabilities for three-dimensional treatment planning evaluations. Int J Radiat Oncol Biol Phys 1991; 21: 137–146
50. Hartford A C, Niemierko A, Adams J A *et al.* Conformal irradiation of the prostate: estimating long-term rectal bleeding risk using dose–volume histograms. Int J Radiat Oncol Biol Phys 1996; 36(3): 721–730
51. Johansen J, Bentzen S M, Overgaard J, Overgaard M. Relationship between the in vitro radiosensitivity of skin fibroblasts and the expression of subcutaneous fibrosis, telangiectasia, and skin erythema after radiotherapy. Radiother Oncol 1996; 40(2): 101–109
52. Burnet N G, Nyman J, Turesson I *et al.* The relationship between cellular radiation sensitivity and tissue response may provide the basis for individualising radiotherapy schedules. Radiother Oncol 1994; 33: 228–238
53. Brock W A, Tucker S L, Geara F B *et al.* Fibroblast radiosensitivity versus acute and late normal skin responses in patients treated for breast cancer. Int J Radiat Oncol Biol Phys 1995; 32: 1371–1379

54. Rosenthal S A, Roach III M, Goldsmith B J *et al*. Immobilization improved the reproducibility of patient positioning during six-field conformal radiation therapy for prostate carcinoma. Int J Radiat Oncol Biol Phys 1993; 27(4): 921–926
55. Ten Haken R K, Perez-Tamayo C, Tesser R J *et al*. Boost treatment of the prostate using shaped, fixed fields. Int J Radiat Oncol Biol Phys 1989; 16(1): 193–200
56. Leibel S A, Heimann R, Kutcher G J *et al*. Three-dimensional conformal radiation therapy in locally advanced carcinoma of the prostate: preliminary results of a phase I dose-escalation study. Int J Radiat Oncol Biol Phys 1994; 28(1): 55–65
57. Mesina C F, Sharman R, Rissman L S *et al*. Comparison of a standard four-field boost technique with a customized non-axial external beam technique for the treatment of adenocarcinoma of the prostate. Int J Radiat Oncol Biol Phys 1993; 27(suppl 1): 193
58. Sailer S L, Rosenman J G, Symon J R *et al*. The tetrad and hexad: maximum beam separation as a starting point for noncoplanar 3-D treatment planning: prostate cancer as a test case. Int J Radiat Oncol Biol Phys 1994; 30(2): 439–446
59. Sandler H, McLaughlin P W, Ten Haken R *et al*. 3D conformal radiotherapy for the treatment of prostate cancer: low risk of chronic rectal morbidity observed in a large series of patients. Int J Radiat Oncol Biol Phys 1993; 27(suppl 1): 135
60. Neal A J, Oldham M, Dearnaley D P. Comparison of treatment techniques for conformal radiotherapy of the prostate using dose–volume histograms and normal tissue complication probabilities. Radiother Oncol 1995; 37(1): 29–34
61. Dearnaley D P, Nahum A, Lee M *et al*. Radiotherapy of prostate cancer. Reducing the treated volume. Conformal therapy, hormone cytoreduction and protons. Br J Cancer 1994; 70(suppl 22): 16
62. Sandler H M, Perez-Tomayo C, Ten Haken R K, Lichter A S. Dose escalation for stage C (T3) prostate cancer: minimal rectal toxicity observed using conformal therapy. Radiother Oncol 1992; 23(1): 53–54
63. Epstein B E, Hanks G E. Radiation therapy techniques and dose selection in the treatment of prostate cancer. Semin Radiat Oncol 1993; 3(3): 179–186
64. Russell K J. Current research directions in the radiation therapy of localised prostate cancer. In: Dawson N A, Vogelzang N J (eds) Prostate cancer. New York: Wiley, 1994: 133–149
65. Wallner K E. Iodine[125] brachytherapy for early stage prostate cancer. New techniques may achieve better results. Oncology 1991; 5: 115–122
66. Wallner K E, Roy J, Harrison L. Tumour control and morbidity following transperineal Iodine[125] implantation for stage T1/T2 prostatic carcinoma. Int J Radiat Oncol Biol Phys 1996; 14(2): 449–453
67. Russell K J, Blasko J C. Recent advances in interstitial brachytherapy for localised prostate cancer. In: Lange P H, Paulson D F (eds) Problems in urology: therapeutic strategies in prostate cancer. Hagerstown, MD: Lippincott, 1993; 7: 260–279
68. Dattoli M, Wallner K, Sorace R *et al*. 103Pd brachytherapy and external beam irradiation for clinically localized, high-risk prostatic carcinoma. Int J Radiat Oncol Biol Phys 1996; 35(5): 875–879
69. Nahum A E, Dearnaley D P, Steel G G. Prospects for proton-beam radiotherapy. Eur J Cancer 1994; 30A(10): 1577–1583
70. Shipley W U, Verhey L J, Munzenrider J E *et al*. Advanced prostate cancer: the results of a randomized comparative trial of high dose irradiation boosting with conformal protons compared with conventional dose irradiation using photons alone. Int J Radiat Oncol Biol Phys 1995; 32(1): 3–12
71. Lee M, Wynne C, Webb S *et al*. A comparison of proton and megavoltage x-ray treatment planning for prostate cancer. Radiother Oncol 1994; 33(3): 239–253
72. Griffin D T W. Fast neutron irradiation of locally advanced prostate cancer. Semin Oncol 1988; 15(4): 359
73. Russell K J, Caplan R J, Laramore G E *et al*. Photon versus fast neutron external beam radiotherapy in the treatment of locally advanced prostate cancer: results of a randomized prospective trial. Int J Radiat Oncol Biol Phys 1994; 28(1): 47–54
74. Austin-Seymour M, Caplan R, Russell K *et al*. Impact of a multileaf collimator on treatment morbidity in localised carcinoma of the prostate. Int J Radiat Oncol Biol Phys 1994; 30(5): 1065–1071
75. Steel G G. Combined radiotherapy–chemotherapy: principles. In: Steel G G, Adams G E, Horwich A (eds) The biological basis of radiotherapy, 2nd edn. Oxford: Elsevier Science, 1989: 267–289

76. Early Breast Cancer Trialists' Collaborative Group. Systemic treatment of early breast cancer by hormonal, cytotoxic, or immune therapy (Part I). Lancet 1992; 339(8784): 1–15

77. Early Breast Cancer Trialists' Collaborative Group. Systemic treatment of early breast cancer by hormonal, cytotoxic, or immune therapy (Part II). Lancet 1992; 339(8785): 71–85

78. Powles T J, Hickish T F, Makris A et al. Randomized trial of chemoendocrine therapy started before or after surgery for treatment of primary breast cancer. J Clin Oncol 1995; 13(3): 547–552

79. Sause W T, Scott C, Taylor S et al. Radiation Therapy Oncology Group (RTOG) 88–08 and Eastern Cooperative Oncology Group (ECOG) 4588: preliminary results of a phase III trial in regionally advanced, unresectable non-small-cell lung cancer. J Natl Cancer Inst 1995; 87(3): 198–205

80. Munro A J. An overview of randomised controlled trial of adjuvant chemotherapy in head and neck cancer. Br J Cancer 1995; 71(1): 83–91

81. Shearer R J, Davies J H, Gelister J S K, Dearnaley D P. Hormonal cytoreduction and radiotherapy for carcinoma of the prostate. Br J Urol 1992; 69(5): 521–524

82. Dearnaley D P, Shearer R J, Ellingham L et al. Rationale and initial results of adjuvant hormone therapy and irradiation for localised prostate cancer. In: Motta M, Serio M (eds) Sex hormone and antihormones in endocrine dependent pathology: basic and clinical aspects. Amsterdam: Elsevier Science, 1994: 197–208

83. Dearnaley D P. Radiotherapy of prostate cancer: established results and new developments. Semin Surg Oncol 1995; 11(1): 50–59

84. Pilepich M V, Caplan R, Byhardt R W et al. Phase III of androgen suppression using goserelin in unfavourable prognosis carcinoma of the prostate treated with definitive radiotherapy (Report of RTOG Protocol 85–31). Proc Am Soc Clin Oncol 1995; 14: 239

85. Bolla M, Gonzalez D, Warde P et al. Immediate hormonal therapy improves locoregional control and survival in patients with locally advanced prostate cancer. Results of a randomised phase III clinical trial of the EORTC Radiotherapy and Genito-Urinary Tract Cancer Cooperative Groups. Proc Am Soc Clin Oncol 1996; 15: 238

86. Fellows G J, Clark P B, Beynon L L et al. Treatment of advanced localised prostatic cancer by orchiectomy, radiotherapy, or combined treatment. A Medical Research Council Study. Br J Urol 1992; 70(3): 304–309

87. Dearnaley D P, Horwich A, Shearer R J. Treatment of advanced localised prostatic cancer by orchidectomy, radiotherapy or combined treatment. A Medical Research Council Study. Br J Urol 1992; 72(5(I)): 673–674

88. Lange P H, Narayan P. Understaging and undergrading of prostate cancer. Argument for postoperative radiation as adjuvant therapy. Urology 1983; 21(2): 113–118

89. Eggleston J C, Walsh P C. Radical prostatectomy with preservation of sexual function: pathological findings in the first 100 cases. J Urol 1985; 134(6): 1146–1148

90. Feneley M R, Gillatt D A, Hehir M, Kirby R S. A review of radical prostatectomy from three centres in the UK: clinical presentation and outcome. Br J Urol 1996; 78(6): 911–920

91. Hanks G E, Dawson A K. The role of external beam radiation therapy after prostatectomy for prostate cancer. Cancer 1986; 58: 2406–2410

92. Ray G R, Bagshaw M A, Freiha F. External beam radiation salvage for residual or recurrent local tumor following radical prostatectomy. J Urol 1984; 132(5): 926–930

93. Bahnson R R, Garnett J E, Grayhack J T. Adjuvant radiation therapy in stage C and D, prostatic adenocarcinoma: preliminary results. Urology 1986; 27(5): 403–406

94. Eisbruch A, Perez C A, Roessler E H, Lockett M A. Adjuvant irradiation after prostatectomy for carcinoma of the prostate with positive surgical margins. Cancer 1994; 73(2): 384–387

95. Lange P H, Lightner D J, Medini E et al. The effect of radiation therapy after radical prostatectomy in patients with elevated prostate specific antigen levels. J Urol 1990; 144(4): 927–933

96. Lange P H, Moon T D, Narayan P, Medini E. Radiation therapy as adjuvant treatment after radical prostatectomy: patient tolerance and preliminary results. J Urol 1986; 136: 45–49

97. Anscher M S, Prosnitz L R. Radiotherapy vs. hormonal therapy for the management of locally recurrent prostate cancer following radical prostatectomy. Int J Radiat Oncol Biol Phys 1989; 5(17): 953–958

98. Schild S E, Buskirk S J, Wong W W *et al.* The use of radiotherapy for patients with isolated elevation of serum prostate specific antigen following radical prostatectomy. J Urol 1996; 156(5): 1725–1729

99. Carter G E, Lieskovsky G, Skinner D G, Petrovich Z. Results of local and/or systemic adjuvant therapy in the management of pathological stage C or D1 prostate cancer following radical prostatectomy. J Urol 1989; 142: 1266–1271

100. Cheng W S, Frydenberg M, Bergstralh E J *et al.* Radical prostatectomy for pathologic stage C prostate cancer: influence of pathologic variables and adjuvant treatment on disease outcome. Urology 1993; 42(3): 283–291

101. Freeman J A, Lieskovsky G, Cook D W *et al.* Radical retropubic prostatectomy and post-operative adjuvant radiation for pathological stage C (PcN$_0$) prostate cancer from 1976 to 1989: intermediate findings. J Urol 1993; 149(5): 1029–1034

102. Schild S E, Wong W W, Grado G L *et al.* The results of radical retropubic prostatectomy and adjuvant therapy for pathological stage C prostate cancer. Int J Radiat Oncol Biol Phys 1996; 34(3): 535–541

103. Schild S E. Regarding postoperative radiotherapy for pathologic stage C prostate cancer: In response to Dr Lawrence and Mr Collins. Int J Radiat Oncol Biol Phys 1996; 36(3): 757–759

104. Kutcher G J, Burman C. Calculation of complication probability factors for non-uniform normal tissue irradiation: the effective volume method. Int J Radiat Oncol Biol Phys 1989; 16(6): 1623–1630

105. Lyman J T. Complication probability as assessed from dose–volume histograms. Radiat Res 1985; 22: 355–359

106. Webb S, Nahum A E. A model for calculating tumour control probability in radiotherapy including the effects of inhomogeneous distributions of dose and clonogenic cell density. Phys Med Biol 1993; 38: 653–666

Chapter 24

Monotherapy with anti-androgens

G. R. P. Blackledge

Introduction

Endocrine therapy remains the fundamental systemic treatment for prostate cancer with the principle of androgen deprivation having been established half a century ago.[1] Androgen deprivation can take many forms, from surgical castration to combined therapy with a luteinizing hormone releasing hormone (LHRH) agonist and an anti-androgen. All give approximately similar results in terms of outcome, including response rate, palliation and survival.[2] Advantages for combined therapy have been claimed, but these are likely to be small and have been demonstrated only in some of the randomized trials evaluating this approach.[3] The major differences between different forms of therapy are in their tolerance, convenience, psychological acceptability, reversibility and compliance. On the basis of these issues, monotherapy with anti-androgens may offer an alternative to established androgen deprivation therapies, although like all treatments there will be disadvantages as well as potential advantages. The potential advantages of anti-androgen monotherapy include convenience, psychological acceptability, tolerability advantages and reversibility. Potential disadvantages include the chance that it may not be as effective as other therapies because of the risk of non-compliance, and elevation of testosterone because of hypothalamic pituitary testicular feedback. Other disadvantages include side effects not seen with other therapies and the psychological effect of the need to take daily oral treatment. The relative advantages and disadvantages of anti-androgen monotherapy and its potential roles are discussed in this chapter.

How do anti-androgens work?

The non-steroidal anti-androgens have been shown to block the binding of androgens to the androgen receptor at the prostate cancer cell level.[4–6] Both testosterone and dihydrotestosterone, which is metabolized at a cellular level from both testosterone and other androgens, are blocked by the non-steroidal anti-androgens. This has the effect of down-regulating cell growth and replication, and may lead to apoptosis. Of the four commercially available anti-androgens, one — cyproterone acetate — is a steroidal anti-androgen; the other three — flutamide, bicalutamide and nilutamide — are non-steroidal anti-androgens with a similar core structure.[7] All anti-androgens are orally bioavailable and require chronic administration for optimal effects.

Potential roles for anti-androgen monotherapy

The classic role for hormonal therapy of any kind is in the treatment of advanced disease, where the disease has either extended outside the prostate gland and is locally advanced, or where there is evidence of metastases. The palliative benefits of hormone therapy have been long established and, although there are no definitive trials comparing hormonal therapy with supportive care only, it is highly likely that hormonal therapy contributes a small survival advantage in this setting.

Increasingly, fewer patients with prostate cancer are presenting with metastatic disease, because of earlier diagnosis; therefore, hormonal therapy is now being evaluated and used earlier in the management of disease. In particular, hormonal therapy has been used to cytoreduce locally advanced disease prior to radical local treatment,[8] and data are also emerging to indicate that androgen deprivation can contribute to improved survival when given as an adjuvant following radical local treatment.[9]

In patients who progress following diagnosis at an earlier stage, hormonal therapy can again be employed and there is increasing evidence that different forms of androgen deprivation can be sequenced to give an optimal palliative benefit.[10]

Most of the published studies of anti-androgen monotherapy have been in patients with established advanced disease. The results of such studies are reviewed below.

Anti-androgen monotherapy in advanced disease

Trials with flutamide

Flutamide was first evaluated in Phase II studies in patients with advanced prostatic cancer without previous endocrine therapy.[11] Favourable response rates were seen in a majority of patients and some responses were reported of being of a significant duration. Around one-third to one-half of patients experienced mild gynaecomastia and some patients suffered from diarrhoea that, in a number of patients, required discontinuation of drug treatment.[12] In one study by Delaere and Van Thillo,[13] sexual potency was evaluated in 15 patients, 10 of whom remained sexually active during treatment. The conclusion of these studies[11–13] is that flutamide monotherapy was perceived to be relatively safe and effective in patients with advanced prostatic cancer.

A number of randomized studies have also been carried out with flutamide against a variety of comparators. A study reported by Neri and Kassem[14] compared two doses of flutamide (250 mg tid, $n = 39$; 500 mg tid, $n = 42$) and diethylstilboestrol (DES, stilboestrol; 1 mg daily, $n = 44$).

About one-half of the patients in each of the arms experienced a partial remission, with a further one-quarter of the patients having clinical improvement that did not achieve the criteria for partial remission. The time to response (around 10 weeks) was similar in all three arms and the duration of response of around 6–9 months was also similar in both arms, with no statistical differences existing between the three groups.

A survival analysis of this small randomized trial did not detect a difference between the three arms of the trial.

The drugs were relatively well tolerated, with the most common side effect being gynaecomastia and breast tenderness; this occurred in 35% of patients who were treated with flutamide and 43% of those treated with DES. Cardiovascular problems were more frequent with treatment with DES. Other side effects were infrequent.

A Japanese trial compared flutamide monotherapy at a dose of 125 mg tid with chlormadinone acetate, a progestogenic anti-androgen available only in Japan.[15] The results of this study, which recruited 87 patients, suggested that rates of response [prostate-specific antigen (PSA) decrease] were equivalent between the two arms of the trial. The serum testosterone level decreased in the chlormadinone acetate group and remained within normal limits in the flutamide group. Eight of the 47 patients receiving flutamide reported gynaecomastia, and diarrhoea and hepatic toxicity were observed in both groups, but only rarely. The conclusions of this study were that flutamide was as effective as chlormadinone acetate in its activity against advanced prostate cancer, but without decreasing testosterone levels.

A further study reported by Boccon-Gibod et al. from France compared flutamide 250 mg tid with bilateral orchiectomy.[16] 54 patients were randomized to flutamide and 50 patients to orchiectomy. There was no difference in terms of progression-free survival or survival with a minimum follow-up of 24 months, with patients whose PSA was less than 120 ng/ml at entry faring best. Gynaecomastia was the most common side effect in patients receiving flutamide, compared with hot flushes for patients who had undergone orchiectomy. Gastro-intestinal (GI) disorders (nine patients) and hepatitis (one patient) were seen in the flutamide arm, and flutamide was stopped because of side effects in three patients. The conclusion from this study is that flutamide is a reasonable option for patients with D2 prostate cancer, provided that PSA at entry is below 129 ng/ml and the patient has agreed to be submitted to a close monitoring of PSA, testosterone and liver enzymes.

The final randomized trial was recently reported by Chang et al.[17] where 48 patients were randomized to receive DES and 44 patients received flutamide. Patient characteristics were evenly distributed between the two treatments. The overall response rate was similar (DES 62%, flutamide 50%) and grade III or worse cardiovascular or thromboembolic toxicity developed in 33% of patients on DES and in 17.6% of patients on flutamide ($p = 0.051$). Other toxicities were similar between the two treatment arms. However, DES produced a significantly longer time to treatment failure (26.4 vs 9.7 months; $p = 0.016$) and longer survival than flutamide (43.2 vs 28.5 months; $p = 0.040$).

The conclusion from this study was that, as primary hormonal therapy of stage D2 prostate cancer, DES caused more serious cardiovascular and thromboembolic complications than flutamide. Despite this, flutamide was not as active an initial agent as DES.

Bicalutamide

Bicalutamide was initially studied in Phase I and Phase II studies. Dose ranging in these studies from doses of 10–50 mg suggested that 50 mg gave a better response in terms of objective response and PSA fall.[18] This dose was therefore evaluated further in three randomized trials. In the first of these trials, conducted in Scandinavia, patients were randomized between bicalutamide and bilateral orchiectomy.[19] With a median follow-up of 31 months there was a significant difference in terms of progression-free survival and overall survival in favour of castration. Hot flushes were more common in the castration arm, whereas gynaecomastia was the most common side effect seen in patients receiving bicalutamide. Quality-of-life assessment in this trial showed significant differences between the groups in favour of orchiectomy for pain, bed disability, social functioning and emotional well-being. The differences favoured bicalutamide in terms of sexual interest and sexual functioning.

A second trial comparing bicalutamide (50 mg once daily) with castration was carried out in the UK, Austria and the Netherlands.[20] In this trial, which recruited 119 patients to bicalutamide and 126 patients to medical or surgical castration, no significant differences were seen in terms of progression-free survival and survival between the two arms. When quality of life was assessed there was a significant difference in favour of castration in overall health at month 6, whereas there was benefit for bicalutamide in terms of sexual interest and sexual function. The side effect profile was similar to that seen in the Scandinavian trial. The authors of this study concluded that it had demonstrated equivalence between the two arms and confirmed the excellent tolerability profile of bicalutamide, particularly with respect to the low incidence of GI side effects and the retention of sexual interest and function.

A third trial, comparing bicalutamide (50 mg once daily) with castration, was carried out in North America;[21] 243 patients were randomized to bicalutamide and 243 patients to medical or surgical castration. Treatment failure and time to progression occurred more frequently in the patients receiving bicalutamide but, with a medium survival follow-up of 86 weeks, there was no difference in survival. Changes in quality-of-life variables, including emotional wellbeing, overall health and social functioning, sexual functioning and sexual interest, were all significantly improved in favour of bicalutamide. The tolerability profiles of both arms were similar to those reported in the other trials and the authors concluded that, although a dosage of 50 mg bicalutamide once daily was not as effective as castration, the favourable quality-of-life outcomes and the low incidence of non-hormonal adverse events provide reasons to evaluate bicalutamide as a single therapeutic agent at higher doses.

A number of studies have evaluated bicalutamide at higher doses with a variety of comparators. The first of these randomized over 1200 patients either to bicalutamide 150 mg daily or castration (medical or surgical) in a 2:1 randomization.[22] Patients could enter this study if they had either evidence of metastatic disease or locally advanced disease with a PSA elevated to more than five times the upper limit of normal. At an interim analysis there was evidence that, although symptom control and quality of life measures were superior in patients receiving bicalutamide with evidence of metastatic disease, time to progression and survival were shorter than with patients who had undergone castration.[23] In patients without evidence of metastatic disease, relatively few events had occurred but there were fewer deaths in patients who had received bicalutamide than in those patients who had been castrated. The tolerability profile of bicalutamide at a dose three times higher than had previously been evaluated was identical to those reported in previous studies, with gynaecomastia being the most common side effect and other side effects being seen uncommonly, and rarely requiring withdrawal from therapy.

Two other studies have recently been reported in which bicalutamide 150 mg daily has been compared with two forms of combined therapy. In the first study, reported by Delli Ponti et al.,[24] bicalutamide was compared with flutamide plus goserelin in patients with locally advanced or metastatic prostate cancer; 108 patients received bicalutamide and 112 patients received the combination therapy. With a median follow-up time of 20 months, there is no difference in terms of time to progression or survival between the two arms of the trial. Diarrhoea and hot flushes were more common in the patients receiving combination therapy, whereas gynaecomastia was more common in the bicalutamide patients. Treatment was discontinued owing to side effects in 2% of patients receiving bicalutamide and in 16.5% of patients receiving combination therapy. Of 52 patients, 20 maintained normal erections in the bicalutamide group compared with five of 60 in the combination group ($p < 0.001$). The authors conclude that bicalutamide monotherapy was well tolerated and as effective as total androgen deprivation independently of disease stage, and also that bicalutamide was better tolerated than flutamide and, when used as monotherapy, allowed a better quality of life.

In a further study, which compared bicalutamide 150 mg with nilutamide plus surgical or medical castration, there was no difference in terms of time to progression, subjective response and quality of life, apart from an increased sexual interest in bicalutamide patients at 12 months.[25] At a median follow-up time of 2.7 years, 37% of patients receiving bicalutamide and 39% of patients receiving combination therapy had died. Patients receiving bicalutamide were more likely to experience gynaecomastia and breast pain, whereas hot flushes, visual disorders and alcohol intolerance were more common in patients receiving combination treatment. The authors conclude from this trial that bicalutamide was superior to combination treatment regarding time to treatment failure; this superiority was due to a better safety profile, with no difference in terms of time to progression and no survival differences being detected, with just over one-third of the patients having died.

Ongoing trials of anti-androgen monotherapy

It can be seen from the description of the trials above that, whereas some of the trials have not detected a difference between the gold standard therapy of castration and anti-androgen monotherapy, some trials suggest that there is a shortfall in terms of survival. In every trial in which it has been assessed, there are clear potential benefits in terms of retention of sexual interest and function for the anti-androgen arm. Nonetheless, even in a palliative situation, a potential shortfall in survival, no matter how small, would need to be considered quite carefully by an individual clinician and patient before they agreed to anti-androgen monotherapy. For these reasons, higher doses of anti-androgens have been evaluated. In particular, there is an ongoing trial evaluating higher doses of bicalutamide. The trial design is shown in Figure 24.1 which is essentially a

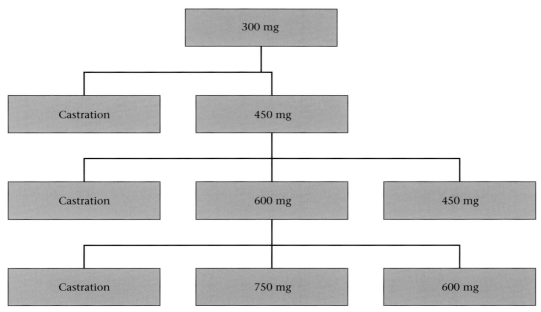

Figure 24.1. Design of a randomized ascending-dose study of bicalutamide. All patients have cancer of the prostate and raised prostate-specific antigen. Each dose above 450 mg is randomized against castration and against previous dose.

randomized ascending-dose study focusing primarily on tolerability, pharmacokinetics and PSA fall as a surrogate of activity. The number of patients entered into this trial is shown in Table 24.1.

At the current time, the reductions in PSA for doses of 450 mg and 600 mg are at least as great as those seen with castration, and the tolerability profiles of these higher doses appear to be similar to those seen at doses of 50 and 150 mg. This study will continue to provide data relating to clinical endpoints and also to quality-of-life information. This study suggests, however, that if dose escalation can be achieved with an anti-androgen, then effects equivalent or superior to standard therapy may be possible.

Anti-androgens have also been investigated as second-line therapy. Fossa et al.[26] evaluated flutamide (250 mg tid) in patients in whom previous hormonal therapy had failed. Subjective responses were seen in five of 25 fully evaluable patients and the 40% or greater decrease in pretreatment PSA levels was observed in seven of 24 patients. This finding correlated with improved survival. Toxicity was mainly GI and resulted in discontinuation of flutamide in five patients.

In an ongoing study evaluating bicalutamide 200 mg in patients in whom previous therapy had failed, Scher and Kolvenbag[27] observed that further PSA, and symptomatic, responses can be observed even when combination therapy has failed, and a flutamide withdrawal response has also shown evidence of progression. These data would strongly suggest that sequential therapy in patients at progression could contribute to improved palliation and possibly an extension of the patient's life.

Finally, there is increasing evidence that androgen deprivation following radical local treatment may improve survival. Bolla et al.[9] have evaluated the role of an LHRH agonist following radiotherapy and have shown a statistically significant improvement in terms of local recurrence, time to progression and survival.

Castration, by whatever means, may be an unacceptable therapy in patients who might have been cured by primary local treatment; there is, therefore, real potential for a monotherapy anti-androgen treatment that would have the same clinical effects but would also retain quality of life. With this in mind, three studies are currently ongoing that will recruit a total of 7500 patients, evaluating the role of bicalutamide as an adjuvant therapy following primary local treatment. These trials began recruiting in September 1995 and recruited more than 3000 patients within the first 12 months. It is anticipated that the first data from these trials will be available in 1999.

Table 24.1. Number of patients entered at each dose level to the ascending-dose bicalutamide trial

Phase	300 mg	450 mg	600 mg	Castration
300 mg	21	–	–	–
450 mg	–	48	–	54
600 mg	–	45	40	35
Totals	21	93	40	89

Discussion

All trials that have evaluated anti-androgen monotherapy have shown clear evidence of activity and, in general, the non-steroidal anti-androgens are well tolerated. The real issue around anti-androgen monotherapy is whether a sufficient dose response can be achieved and also whether comparative efficacy can be proved unequivocally to be comparable with standard therapy in the form of castration. At present, although there are some trials that do not show a difference, there are other trials that have shown a deficit for anti-androgen monotherapy. It is, therefore, clear at the present time that any decision to treat a patient with anti-androgen monotherapy must be taken with the fully informed consent of the patient. It is possible that, with careful PSA monitoring, an early change to conventional therapy could be considered if, for example, the PSA had not fallen by at least 90% or into the normal range after 12 weeks of treatment.[28] This could then allow the patient the potential of retention of sexual function and a convenient regimen with the benefits of an effective regimen.

It is worth exploring why anti-androgen monotherapy may not be as effective in terms of time to progression and survival as castration. A number of factors may influence this, the first of which relates to compliance. All anti-androgens are oral and need to be taken between one and three times a day. Numerous studies have demonstrated that there are very few patients who are completely compliant with any oral drug regimen and, therefore, the level of anti-androgen blockade may vary slightly in patients receiving oral therapy.[29]

The next possible reason for a shortfall in efficacy could be the fact that there is, for all the non-steroidal anti-androgens, hypothalamic pituitary testicular feedback that results in an elevation of testosterone of around 1.6 times the baseline level.[30] This is in contrast to patients who receive castration treatment, where testosterone falls to castrate levels. This increase in the agonist for the androgen receptor may be in part responsible for the lack of comparative efficacy that has been seen in some studies.

A final factor that may influence the efficacy of anti-androgen monotherapy is the bulk of disease. There are suggestions, from the studies evaluating bicalutamide, 150 mg, and the escalating high-dose study of bicalutamide, that patients with low-volume disease may have a better outcome (compared with castration) than in patients with metastatic disease. This, in turn, could be related to the number of androgen receptors that require blockade in a patient with bulky disease, in comparison with a patient with less bulky disease where there would be fewer androgen receptors that required blockade. This theory is currently being tested in a prospective study evaluating the binding of anti-androgen to locally confined disease against metastatic disease, using positron emission tomography.

The development of anti-androgens has offered the clinician further choice in the treatments that can be used for androgen deprivation in prostate cancer. All clinicians and their patients should be prepared to discuss the optimal management of a patient on an individual basis, allowing the patient an informed choice of appropriate therapy based on that patient's priorities. For patients in whom the convenience of an oral therapy and the wish to retain libido and sexual function are dominant issues, anti-androgen monotherapy, based on currently available evidence, already offers a real option. Higher doses of anti-androgens may provide therapeutic equivalence with standard therapies, and their tolerability profile and convenience as oral therapies may allow them to be established as the treatment of choice as adjuvant therapy in locally confined prostate cancer.

References

1. Huggins C, Hodges C V. Studies on prostatic cancer: I. The effect of castration of estrogen and of androgen injection on serum phosphatases in metastatic carcinoma of the prostate. Cancer Res 1941; 1: 293–297
2. Perez C A, Fair W R, Ihde D C. Carcinoma of the prostate. In: DeVita V T Jr, Hellman S, Rosenberg S A (eds) Cancer: principles and practice of oncology, 3rd edn. Philadelphia: Lippincott, 1989: 1049–1052
3. Prostate Cancer Trialists' Collaborative Group. Maximum androgen blockade in advanced prostate cancer: an overview of 22 randomised trials with 3283 deaths in 5710 patients. Lancet 1995; 346: 265–269
4. Neri R, Florance K, Koziol P, Van Cleave S. A biological profile of a non-steroidal anti-androgen, SCH 13521. Endocrinology 1972; 91: 427–437
5. Decensi A U, Boccardo F, Guarneri D et al. Monotherapy with nilutamide, a pure nonsteroidal antiandrogen, in untreated patients with metastatic carcinoma of the prostate. The Italian Prostatic Cancer Project. J Urol 1991; 146: 377–381
6. Kennealey G T, Furr B J. Use of the nonsteroid antiandrogen Casodex in advanced prostatic carcinoma. Urol Clin North Am 1991; 18: 99–110
7. Neri R O. Antiandrogens: preclinical and clinical studies. 4th International Prostate Cancer Update, Beaver Creek, 27–30 Jan 1994. Urology 1994; 44(6A): 53–60
8. Flamm J, Fischer M, Holtl W, Pfluger H, Tomschi W. Complete androgen deprivation prior to radical prostatectomy in patients with stage T3 cancer of the prostate. Eur Urol 1991; 19: 192–195
9. Bolla M, Gonzalez D, Warde P et al. Immediate hormonal therapy improves locoregional control and survival in patients with locally advanced prostate cancer. Results of a randomized Phase III clinical trial of the EORTC radiotherapy and genitourinary tract cancer co-operative groups. 32nd Annual Meeting of the American Society of Clinical Oncology, Philadelphia, 18–21 May 1996. Proceedings of the American Society of Clinical Oncology 1996; 15: 238 (Abstr 591)
10. Scher H I, Kelly W K. Flutamide withdrawal syndrome: its impact on clinical trials in prostate cancer. J Clin Oncol 1993; 11: 1566–1572
11. Sogani P C, Vagaiwala M R, Whitmore W F. Experience with flutamide in patients with advanced prostatic cancer without prior endocrine therapy. Cancer 1984; 54: 744–750
12. Lundgren R. Flutamide as primary treatment for metastatic prostatic cancer. Br J Urol 1987; 59: 156–158
13. Delaere K P J, Van Thillo E L. Flutamide monotherapy as primary treatment in advanced prostatic carcinoma. Semin Oncol 1991; 18(5, Suppl 6): 13–18
14. Neri R, Kassem N. Biological and clinical properties of antiandrogens. Prog in Cancer Res Ther 1984; 31: 507–518
15. Akaza H, Usami M, Kotake T et al. A randomized Phase II trial of flutamide vs chlormadinone acetate in previously untreated advanced prostatic cancer. Jpn J Clin Oncol 1993; 23: 178–185
16. Boccon-Gibod L, Fournier G, Bottet P et al. Flutamide versus orchidectomy in patients with metastatic prostate cancer. 11th Congress of the European Association of Urology 1994; Berlin, 13–16 July 1994 (abstr 25)
17. Chang B A, Yeap B, Davis T et al. Double-blind, randomized study of primary hormonal treatment of stage D2 prostate carcinoma: flutamide versus diethylstilbestrol. J Clin Oncol 1996; 14: 2250–2257
18. Soloway M S, Schellhammer P F, Smith J A et al. Bicalutamide in the treatment of advanced prostatic carcinoma. A phase II noncomparative multicenter trial evaluating safety, efficacy and long-term endocrine effects of monotherapy. J Urol 1995; 154(6): 2110–2114
19. Iversen P, Tveter K, Varenhorst E on behalf of the Scandinavian Casodex Cooperative Group. Randomised study of Casodex 50 mg monotherapy vs orchiectomy in the treatment of metastatic prostate cancer. Scand J Urol Nephrol 1996; 30(2): 93–98
20. Kaisary A V, Tyrrell C J, Beacock C et al. A randomised comparison of monotherapy with 'Casodex' 50 mg daily and castration in the treatment of metastatic prostate carcinoma. Eur Urol 1995; 28: 215–222
21. Chodak G, Sharifi R, Kasimis B et al. Single-agent therapy with bicalutamide: a comparison with medical or surgical castration in the treatment of advanced prostate carcinoma. Urology 1995; 46(6): 849–855

22. Kaisary A V. Current clinical studies with a new nonsteroidal antiandrogen, Casodex. Prostate 1994; Suppl 5: 27–33.
23. Tyrrell C, Kaisary A V, Iversen P *et al*. A randomised comparison of 'Casodex' 150 mg versus castration in the treatment of advanced prostate cancer. 32nd Annual Meeting of the American Society of Clinical Oncology, Philadelphia, 18–21 May 1996. Proceedings of the American Society of Clinical Oncology 1996; 15: 192 (abstr 411)
24. Boccardo F, Rubagotti A, Miglietta L *et al*. Bicalutamide (B) monotherapy versus flutamide (F) plus goserelin (G) in prostate cancer (CA) patients (pts). Preliminary results of an Italian Prostate Cancer Group (PONCAP) study. 33rd Annual Meeting of the American Society of Clinical Oncology (ASCO), Denver, 17–20 May, 1997. Proceedings of the American Society of Clinical Oncology 1997; 16: 317a (Abstr 1128)
25. Chatelain C, Fourcade R O, Delchambre J. Bicalutamide (Casodex) versus combined androgen blockade: Open French multicentre study in patients with metastatic prostate cancer. (In Press)
26. Fossa S D, Hosbach G, Paus E. Flutamide in hormone-resistant prostatic cancer. J Urol 1990; 144: 1411–1414
27. Scher H I, Kolvenbag G J C M. The antiandrogen withdrawal syndrome in relapsed prostate cancer. New avenues and perspectives in the management of advanced prostate cancer, Paris, 1 September 1996. Eur Urol 1997; 31(Suppl 2): 3–7
28. Furr B J A, Blackledge G P. Is there a place for antiandrogen monotherapy? In: Motta M, Serio M (eds) Sex hormones and antihormones in endocrine dependent pathology: basic & clinical aspects, Proceedings of an International Symposium, Milan, 10–14 Apr 1994. Excerpta Medica International Congress Series 1064. Amsterdam: Elsevier, 1994: 157–175
29. Kaisary A V. Compliance with hormonal treatment for prostate cancer. Br J Hosp Med 1996; 55: 259–366
30. Mahler C, Van Cangh P, Bouffioux C *et al*. Endocrine effects of 'Casodex', a new non-steroidal antiandrogen. In: Murphy G, Khoury S, Chatelain S, Denis L (eds) Recent advances in urological cancers diagnosis and treatment. 2nd International Symposium on Recent Advances in Urologic Cancer, Paris, 27–29 Jun, 1990: 42–45

Chapter 25

Combined androgen blockade: clinical basis

D. Crawford

Introduction

Combined or maximum androgen blockade (MAB), which involves the addition of a pure anti-androgen to surgical or medical castration, is fast becoming the preferred treatment for advanced prostate cancer. However, this area of therapy is one surrounded by controversy and its superiority over castration alone is questioned in some quarters. This is in spite of the favourable findings of a handful of prospective, large-scale, double-blinded and controlled studies assessing the efficacy of flutamide and nilutamide plus castration against that of castration alone. A recent meta-analysis conducted by the Prostate Cancer Trialists' Collaborative Group[1] has served to fuel such controversy still further and a further meta-analysis is planned by the same group for 1997. This chapter considers the clinical and statistical findings of landmark studies addressing the efficacy of MAB, as well as looking at the rationale underlying MAB. Maximum androgen blockade is a term used to describe the ablation of all sources of androgen; that is, the addition of anti-androgen to castration reduces androgen availability by competitively inhibiting testosterone- and dihydrotestosterone (DHT)-binding at the androgen receptor level. In the case of alternative measures of achieving androgen blockade, finasteride — a 5α-reductase type 2 inhibitor — reduces conversion of less active androgen precursors of adrenal origin at the stage of testosterone, so preventing formation of the more potent androgen DHT, of which testosterone is the direct precursor. The action of this inhibitor is at the level of the prostate where the enzymatic machinery for the synthesis of 40% of total androgen production is in place. With the recent elucidation of the genes corresponding to enzymes regulating androgen formation in the prostate, the probability of genetic approaches to inhibition of DHT synthesis at this level in the future are likely to become a reality. Monotherapy with castration or luteinizing hormone-releasing hormone (LHRH) agonists, or surgical castration, addresses only the issue of testicular androgens, so leaving the prostate open to stimulation by intraprostatic androgens that promote growth of androgen-hypersensitive cells. Such therapy, involving castration and blockade at the prostate level, is variously termed combined androgen blockade (CAB) or total androgen blockade as well as MAB. The preferred term in this chapter is CAB.

Regulation of prostate growth

Both normal and cancerous prostatic cell growth is stimulated by the active androgen DHT the origin of which was once thought to be solely from the testis in the form of its precursor — testosterone. Although the testis and ovaries are the exclusive source of androgens and oestrogens in lower mammals, it is now well appreciated that this is not the case in higher primates. In man, androgen formation also takes place in the peripheral tissues, including the prostate, and it is now appreciated that the prostate contributes significantly to DHT formation. The greatest source of androgens in the intact male is the testis, the testosterone from which is converted in peripheral tissues, including the prostate, to the active metabolite DHT. In 1941, Huggins and Hodges[2] established the sensitivity of prostate cancer to androgens, but surgical castration or administration of high-dose oestrogen therapy[3,4] became the cornerstone of treatment for advanced prostate cancer, before the advent of CAB about 11 years ago. Despite the use of orchiectomy as standard first-line treatment for metastatic prostate cancer, its use has not been shown to substantially increase patient survival and relapse is inevitable.[5]

With the recognition that the adrenals secrete significant quantities of inactive DHT precursors [dehydroepiandrosterone (DHEA), its sulfate DHEA-S and androstenedione (Δ^4-dione)] which are converted into DHT in the prostate (Figure 25.1.) the term intracrinology, which refers to the synthesis of *active* steroids locally within peripheral tissues, evolved. The adrenal steroid precursors described must be locally transformed within the prostatic cells to stimulate prostatic growth. Within the prostate, transformation of adrenal precursors, as well as testosterone from the testis, into the active androgen DHT takes place and DHT in turn interacts with androgen receptors, so initiating cell growth (Figure 25.1). The

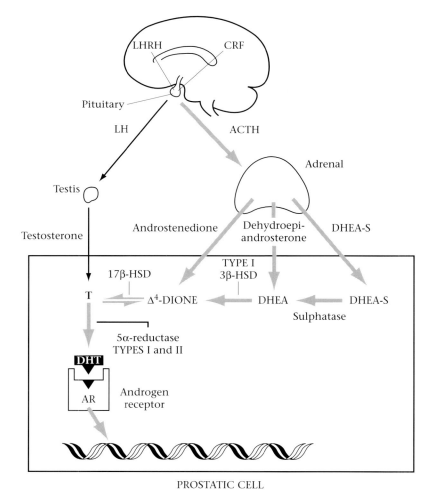

Figure 25.1. Intracrine activity of the human prostate; CRF, corticotrophin-releasing factor. (From ref. 6 with permission.)

greater part of androgen-mediated activity is the result of the potent action of DHT at the receptor level; however, testosterone can also bind to the androgen receptor, but has a far lower affinity for the receptor and a less potent action than DHT.

Castration by surgical means or with LHRH superagonists results in a 95% reduction in serum testosterone concentration; at first sight this erroneously suggests that 95% of androgen production is from the testis. Measurement of circulating serum testosterone is an insufficient means of assessing the level of active androgen available to the prostate, in the light of the fact that steroid precursors to the active androgen DHT are secreted by the adrenals; intraprostatic concentration of DHT, which is around 40% of that in intact men,[6] is the only useful indicator of androgenic activity in prostatic tissue.

In addition to the awareness that the prostate synthesizes its own androgens by transformation of the inactive adrenal precursors alluded to above, the structure of the three enzyme families (3β-hydroxysteroid dehydrogenase/Δ^5–Δ^4 isomerase, 17β-hydroxysteroid dehydrogenase and 5α-reductase) required for the biosynthesis of androgens within the prostate have been elucidated and their corresponding genes have been found to be expressed in prostatic tissue. For each case two types of isoenzyme and gene have been identified, denoted type 1 and type II. These are distributed differently and, for example, type II 5α-reductase is the main form found in the prostate.

Rationale for combined androgen blockade

The rationale for CAB is based on the hypothesis of Labrie et al.[7] regarding mixed populations of cells with a wide range of phenotypes in advanced tumours. According to this theory the androgen-dependent cells contained within the tumour have differing androgen requirements for the maintenance of cell growth and cell function. In conventional treatment, monotherapy with orchiectomy or an LHRH agonist achieves ablation of testicular androgens only. An initial response may occur, owing to the suppression or destruction of prostatic cancer cells with high or moderate androgen dependence. However, as discussed above, androgen precursors of adrenal origin are converted into (albeit lower) levels of androgen in the prostate, but these are present in sufficient quantity to stimulate tumour cells that have a lower androgen requirement. As a result, these selective clones continue growing and ultimately mutate into androgen-independent cells.

Combination therapy aims to block androgens of both testicular and adrenal origin simultaneously and, in so doing, to suppress or destroy both androgen-hypersensitive cells as well as cells with moderate to high androgen dependence. As illustrated in Figure 25.1, androgens exert their effect within the target cell by binding to a specific nuclear receptor protein. Blocking the androgen receptor prevents the interaction of DHT and testosterone with the receptor. Orchiectomy or medical castration with a variety of LHRH agonists completely blocks testicular testosterone secretion (which accounts for about 60% of DHT within the prostate). The rationale for CAB is to block the action of any remaining androgens within the prostate; these are of adrenal origin and account for 40% of DHT within the prostate. To achieve adrenal-androgen blockade successfully, an anti-androgen is used in combination with orchiectomy or an LHRH agonist. The ideal anti-androgen should have a high specificity and affinity for the androgen receptor and, in blocking the receptor, should prevent access of DHT to the receptor. By this means the androgens influence genetic expression, and prostate cancer cell growth should be greatly reduced (Figure 25.2).

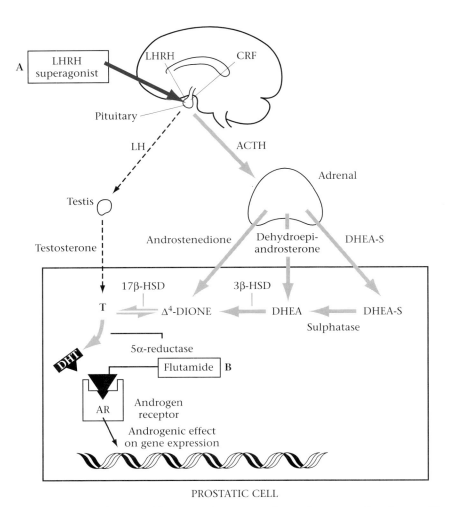

Figure 25.2. Combination therapy with an LHRH superagonist and a pure anti-androgen. (From ref. 6 with permission.)

To achieve maximal blockade of androgens within the prostate, the anti-androgen, as well as having high specificity and affinity for the receptor, should also lack any androgenic, glucocorticoid, progestational, oestrogenic, or other antihormonal or hormonal activity. Few of the compounds so far developed meet these criteria; of the anti-androgens available, the pure or non-steroidal anti-androgens are of most use, but they are by no means perfect in terms of affinity for the androgen receptor. It is on this basis, as discussed later (see 5α-reductase type 2 inhibitors, page 260), that extra efforts are being made to reduce intraprostatic levels of DHT, which has the higher affinity for the androgen receptor and thus out-competes the currently available anti-androgens. Cyproterone acetate (CPA), which was the first available anti-androgen, is a steroidal derivative (progestin derivative) with intrinsic androgenic as well as anti-androgenic activity; its overall anti-androgenic activity is lower than that of pure (non-steroidal) anti-androgens, such as flutamide and nilutamide. The first non-steroidal anti-androgen to be discovered was flutamide,[8] after which two of its analogues, nilutamide[9] and bicalutamide,[10] were developed. To date, only non-steroidal compounds have been demonstrated to have only anti-androgenic activity. However, as discussed later, there is evidence that CPA may be of use in combination with LHRH to avoid the flare phenomenon associated with LHRH agonists during the first few days of use.

LHRH agonists

For many patients, orchiectomy is an unacceptable treatment option and alternative means of hormonal manipulation involving low-dose oestrogens are associated with marked toxicity.[11] LHRH agonists are now used as an alternative to orchiectomy and a variety of analogues are available.

Testosterone is a product of the Leydig cells of the testis. The secretion of testosterone is stimulated by the direct action of luteinizing hormone (LH) on high-affinity LH receptors located on the Leydig cells. LH secretion from the pituitary is in turn stimulated by LHRH which is produced in the hypothalamus and delivered to the pituitary via the pituitary portal blood vessels. As a result, LHRH indirectly regulates the secretion of testosterone from the testis. LHRH agonists virtually abolish testosterone secretion, owing to their continuous presence at the level of the pituitary, leading to a loss in responsiveness to their action. That is to say, the pituitary's LHRH receptors become downregulated or desensitized as a result of continuous exposure to LHRH or its agonists. This downregulating effect is not immediate but follows an initial stimulation of LH secretion, which in turn leads to a transient increase in testosterone secretion lasting between 5 and 12 days. For this reason LHRH agonists should not be administered on their own in patients with bone pain or urinary obstructive symptoms, because of the risk of tumour growth being exacerbated during this initial period of increased testosterone secretion. Biochemical manifestations of tumour activity in the form of raised levels of serum alkaline phosphatase and prostate-specific antigen (PSA) have been noted during this period of raised androgen levels[12,13] and are thought to be due to this transient increase in testosterone levels.[14] The flare phenomenon, as it has become known, can be seriously life-threatening in symptomatic patients with a high tumour burden.[12,14] According to Mahler,[14] the initial and temporary damaging effect that is occasionally observed when using LHRH agonists as monotherapy can be prevented by simultaneously administering oestrogens, steroidal anti-androgens (CPA), ketoconazole, or pure anti-androgens (flutamide, nilutamide or bicalutamide). As discussed below, the flare phenomenon may be circumvented completely, according to early reports of studies utilizing novel LHRH *ant*agonist agents.

The use of LHRH agonists as monotherapy cannot be expected to improve the prognosis of cancer to any greater extent than does orchiectomy, because their effects are limited to testicular androgen blockade and no more.

Other combinations

LHRH antagonists

As mentioned previously, the use of LHRH agonists results in a transient release of LH, with the subsequent LH-dependent production of testosterone from the testis; this transient course of events occurs before downregulation of the pituitary LHRH receptors is achieved and results in the risk of tumour flare-up.

LHRH *ant*agonists block LHRH receptors, so avoiding the transient stimulation that occurs with LHRH agonists in monotherapy. As a result, androgen ablation is achieved immediately. The usefulness of such antagonists in the treatment of advanced prostate cancer is already being reported;[15] they appear to be useful as primary single therapy for the treatment of metastatic prostate cancer. Controlled clinical trials assessing the efficacy of such antagonists in combination with anti-androgens is warranted.

5α-reductase type II inhibitors

One of the problems with the anti-androgens currently available is that their affinity for the androgen receptor is relatively low, so significant levels of DHT are able to engage with the androgen receptor. By decreasing the levels of DHT available at the androgen receptor the efficacy of pure anti-androgens could (theoretically) be enhanced. In the light of the fact that testosterone has a far lower affinity for the androgen receptor than DHT, and is far less potent, a logical point of blockade would be at the stage of conversion of testosterone to DHT. The enzyme catalysing this stage is 5α-reductase type II; 5α-reductase type II inhibitors are being assessed for their effectiveness in facilitating the better action of pure anti-androgens. However, this remains controversial.

Bologna et al.[16] have demonstrated that one such 5α-reductase type II inhibitor (finasteride) has a direct inhibitory effect on prostate cancer cell lines. Additionally, Fleshner and Trachtenberg[17] have shown that a combination of flutamide and finasteride decreases the size of the rat ventral prostate. However, using finasteride as monotherapy, Presti et al.[18] have not found clinical response to be dramatic. Although finasteride blocks the conversion of testosterone to DHT within the prostate, it does not decrease serum concentrations of testosterone; owing to the low affinity of the androgen receptor for testosterone, an escape is seen and growth of the tumour continues to be stimulated. In theory, the combination of finasteride and flutamide could effectively control tumour growth while at the same time maintaining serum concentrations of testosterone and decreasing the side effects associated with hormonal manipulation. In a small non-randomized study, Fleshner and Trachtenberg[19] found that administration of a combination of finasteride and flutamide to sexually active patients with stage C and D1 cancer led to a durable response, lasting up to 24 months, the chemical response, measured by serum PSA levels, was evident in 22 of the 23 patients treated. Sexual function was maintained in 86% of the participants. This form of combination therapy appears to control tumours (stage D1) well and has the added advantage of preserving sexual function.

Effectiveness of CAB in the treatment of prostate cancer

In order to test the theory that CAB is superior to conventional treatment of prostate cancer, using orchiectomy alone, a large number of controlled trials have been conducted, many of which are still in progress; for others the results are still awaited. These randomized trials involve a CAB arm generally utilizing one of four anti-androgens — flutamide, nilutamide, bicalutamide or CPA — the latter is steroidal and generally considered less effective than the other three, which are pure, non-steroidal anti-androgens, as discussed earlier. For both the CAB and castration-only arms a variety of LHRH antagonists have been utilized or, alternatively, bilateral orchiectomy has been performed. Many trials of this sort have been unable to demonstrate any advantage of CAB therapy over monotherapy, but such studies have often been of insufficient statistical power, or have reported results prior to sufficient follow-up. The importance of allowing sufficient follow-up in order to reach significance is reflected in the first published results of the EORTC 30853 study, which, at the time, showed no difference in survival rates between 320 patients randomized to bilateral orchiectomy or CAB with the LHRH agonist goserelin plus flutamide;[20] however, as reiterated later in this chapter, the analysis and publication of more mature data revealed an improvement in survival of 7 months ($p = 0.02$). Three well-known studies, of which EORTC 30853 is one, in which the design of the trials is considered to be good, have provided optimistic results regarding the efficacy of combination therapy in the treatment of prostate cancer in cases of minimal disease. These are considered further in due course.

For advanced disease, orchiectomy alone has been the standard therapy against which all combination therapies involving anti-androgens, oestrogens, or 5α-reductase inhibitors are compared. A variety of the combinations used in CAB studies are considered below and the results, where available, summarized with emphasis on response rate, time to progression, symptomatic benefit and survival.

Surgical castration and anti-androgens

Orchiectomy and flutamide

Results from the SWOG-INT 0105 trial, in which orchiectomy and flutamide CAB has been compared with orchiectomy alone, indicate that there is no statistically significant advantage of combination therapy over orchiectomy alone in terms of time to progression or survival.[21] In this large study involving 1387 patients, chemical response rates, measured by PSA, were 81 and 61% for CAB and for orchiectomy only, respectively. For patients treated with combination therapy, time to progression was 21 months; however, on analysis of a subset of patients with minimal metastatic skeletal deposits, time to progression was found to be 49 months. For the same subset of good-risk patients, survival for patients in the CAB arm was 52 months as opposed to 31 months when considering bad-risk patients in the analysis. The negative findings of this study to date are disappointing, and bolster further the arguments of the Prostate Cancer Trialists' Collaborative Group[1] regarding their meta-analysis of 25 CAB studies. This meta-analysis is considered further in due course.

Orchiectomy and nilutamide

In this multinational trial involving 457 men with stage D2 cancer, orchiectomy plus nilutamide was compared with orchiectomy alone. Regression and stabilization was 78% for combination therapy vs 63% with orchiectomy.[22] Median interval to objective progression was 20.8 and 14.9 months for CAB and orchiectomy, respectively. Differences in response and progression rates between combination therapy and orchiectomy alone were statistically significant. For combination therapy and placebo, median survival time was 27.3 and 24.2 months, respectively. Cancer-specific survival time (death due to cancer) was 30 and 37 months for orchiectomy alone and combination therapy respectively (NS). Combination therapy was associated with statistically significant pain relief compared with castration alone, and PSA levels were also reduced.

Orchiectomy and CPA

Results of trials comparing this combination with orchiectomy alone have not yet been published. However, the initial results and a further survival analysis[23,24] from the largest clinical trial using this combination — EORTC protocol 30805 — have shown that, in the combination arm, progression and survival rates did not differ from those in the monotherapy arm. These reports[23,24] did not address data relating to response rate, median interval to progression or duration of survival, quality of life or symptom improvement.

Medical castration (using an LHRH agonist) plus anti-androgen

Leuprolide and flutamide vs leuprolide alone (SWOG-INT 0036)

Following encouraging results from an early CAB study conducted by Labrie *et al.*,[25] a larger trial (SWOG-INT 0036),[26] addressing the shortfalls of Labrie's trial (the trial was non-randomized and involved only a small number of patients) was initiated. A total of 643 patients were involved in this randomized, double-blind, placebo-controlled multicentre trial designed to compare the tolerability and efficacy of CAB, using the anti-androgen flutamide and the LHRH agonist leuprolide, against the use of leuprolide alone. The median age of patients was 67 years (range 42–98 years). The patients involved in the trial, who all had histologically confirmed metastatic prostate cancer that had been previously untreated, were stratified for extent of disease and performance status and then randomized in a 1:1 ratio between the CAB and LHRH-only treatment arms, after which they were followed-up until there was evidence of progression.

As indicated in Figure 25.3, those patients randomized to CAB had a median length of survival of 35.6 months compared with those in the leuprolide and placebo group who had a median length of survival of 28.3 months ($p = 0.03$); this represents a 26% extension of overall survival in the CAB group of patients. Progression-free survival time increased from 14 to 17 months ($p = 0.039$) in the patients randomized to CAB (Figure 25.4).

When considering a subset of 82 patients (14%) with only minimal disease (defined here as the presence of metastases in the axial skeleton and/or the retroperitoneal lymph nodes, good performance status and relatively low PSA levels) the benefit of CAB appeared to be even greater. In these patients median survival was 61 and 42 months for the CAB and placebo arm, respectively, as shown in Figure 25.5; time to progression was increased from 19 to 48 months in the CAB arm, as shown in Figure 25.6.

No benefit was seen from CAB in relation to those patients with severe disease ($n = 38$) and poor performance status (ECOG PS > 3). However, survival advantages ranging from 6 months to 2 years were achieved in patients with a good performance status.

Further analysis of results relating to survival benefits to those patients in the placebo arm of the trial who were treated with flutamide after progression

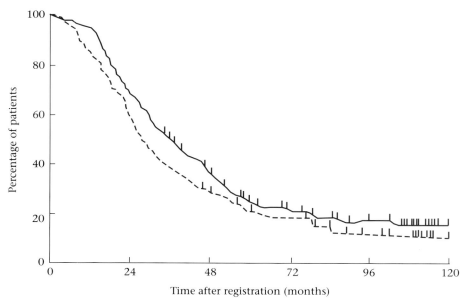

Figure 25.3. Overall survival: National Cancer Institute Intergroup Study 0036; leuprolide with flutamide (——— ; at risk, 303; deaths, 259; median 35 months) or placebo (- - - - ; at risk, 300; deaths, 267, median 29 months); p = 0.03.

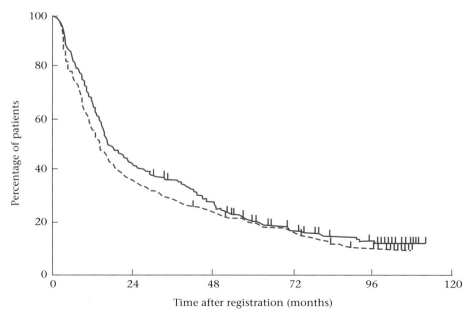

Figure 25.4. Progression-free survival: National Cancer Institute Intergroup Study 0036; leuprolide with flutamide (——; at risk, 303, events, 266; median 17 months) or placebo (- - - -; at risk, 300; events, 274; median 14 months); p = 0.04.

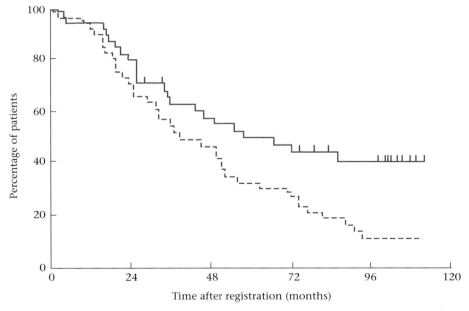

Figure 25.5. Overall survival in good prognosis: National Cancer Insitute Intergroup Study 0036; leuprolide with flutamide (——; at risk, 41; deaths, 23; median 61 months) or placebo (- - - -; at risk, 41; deaths, 37; median 42 months); p = 0.04.

revealed no survival benefit; this finding reflects the poor prognosis following progression.

Goserelin plus flutamide vs bilateral orchiectomy (EORTC 30853)

In reporting Phase III results of the EORTC trial 30853, Denis *et al.*[27] demonstrated a 7-month improvement in survival for patients treated with the LHRH agonist goserelin plus the anti-androgen flutamide compared with patients treated with

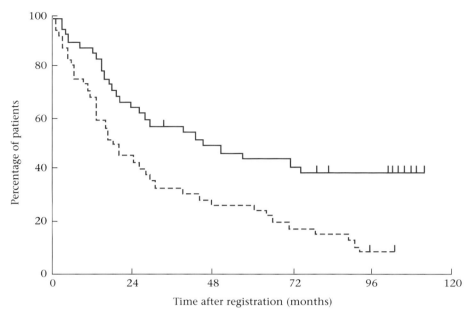

Figure 25.6. Progression-free survival in good prognosis: National Cancer Institute Intergroup Study 0036; leuprolide with flutamide (———; at risk, 41; events, 25; median 48 months) or placebo (- - - -; at risk, 41; events, 39; median 19 months); p = 0.03.

bilateral orchiectomy (median duration of survival was 34.4 months on CAB and 27.1 months with orchiectomy). Median time to subjective progression was 21.75 months for CAB and 13 months for orchiectomy alone. Average time to objective progression for patients treated with CAB and orchiectomy alone was 33.25 and 21.25 months, respectively. The time to first objective or subjective progression was 11.5 months for orchiectomy and 17.75 months for CAB. For orchiectomy and CAB, disease-specific survival was 28.8 and 43.9 months, respectively (p = 0.007). Compared with the total treatment group, those patients having a good or intermediate prognosis had improved overall survival. A similar trend was observed in the SWOG-INT 0036 trial, discussed below, in which patients with minimal disease had a clear survival advantage over those with advanced disease.

Busereline acetate plus CPA vs orchiectomy alone

Klijn *et al.*[28] were unable to show any advantage of the above combination over orchiectomy alone or any benefit in outcome when using CPA for only 2 weeks (in combination with long-term busereline) to counteract the flare phenomenon. No differences over monotherapy (busereline alone or orchiectomy) were detected with respect to time to progression or duration of survival, response rate or degree of pain relief.

Of the studies described above, three in particular appear to confirm the benefits of CAB in advanced disease, these being the SWOG INT 0036[26] study involving flutamide and leuprolide, the EORTC 30853 trial of Denis *et al.*,[27] involving goserelin acetate and flutamide vs bilateral orchiectomy, and the trial of Janknegt *et al.*[22] involving orchiectomy and nilutamide. However, there are many more trials in which the findings have been apparently less encouraging.

CAB therapy: a controversial treatment option

In spite of the three favourable CAB studies described above (SWOG INT 003626, EORTC 3085327, Janknegt *et al.*[22]), there continues to be a good deal of controversy surrounding the issue of CAB therapy. Most recently a meta-analysis of 25 CAB trials published in the *Lancet* has fuelled the debate concerning the efficacy of CAB further, and in some quarters there is particular concern regarding the way in which this analysis, which concluded unfavourably regarding CAB, was conducted.[29] Such critics maintain that the SWOG-INT 0036 and EORTC 30853 studies of CAB 'demonstrate statistically that the use of an anti-androgen with castration is the treatment of choice to prolong life in advanced cancer'[29] and that the data from these trials were diluted in the meta-analysis (by the introduction of heterogeneity due to the inclusion in the analysis of patients with non-metastatic disease and pooling of data from studies with different classes of anti-androgen) to such an extent that the clearly demonstrated benefits of CAB in the treatment of advanced prostate cancer were masked. Furthermore, critics comment that the statistical power of the analysis was insufficient, owing to the inclusion of immature studies, some of which were not even designed to measure survival.

Owing to the fact that many of the studies relating to CAB have been unable to provide 'convincing and consistent evidence of improved survival', the Prostate Cancer Trialists' Collaborative Group[1] undertook its meta-analysis of randomized trials to test pharmacological or surgical castration against CAB. Statistically, the analysis was unable to demonstrate that, in terms of survival, CAB therapy is superior to castration alone and, from the trialists' findings, it might be concluded that, if any difference does exist, it is likely to be small. However, one of the many criticisms of this analysis is that criteria other than survival, such as symptom relief and length of symptom-free survival, which are potential benefits, were not assessed. Only overall survival was considered in this analysis, which involved 25 trials initiated prior to December 1989. Data on individual patients were available from 22 of the 25 trials, which included 5710 patients with advanced prostate cancer (87% M1). Of these, 3283 (57%) patients had died. Although median follow-up was at 40 months, the trials included in the meta-analysis had been initiated between 1981 and 1989; hence, there was a significant variation in trial maturity and the percentage of deaths ranged from 18.4 to 79.3%.

In the studies included in the analysis three different anti-androgens were used in the CAB arm, two of which were non-steroidal (nilutamide and flutamide) and one of which was a steroid (CPA). Bilateral orchiectomy or one of three different LHRH agonists (administered as a nasal spray, a daily subcutaneous injection or as a monthly depot) were used in the control arm or as part of the CAB arm in each of the trials included in the analysis.

Overall mortality was 56.3 and 58.4% for patients in the CAB or castration group, respectively. Five-year survival estimates for the CAB and castration group were 26.2 and 22.8%, respectively. These results, although corresponding to a 6.4% reduction in the annual odds of death, were not significantly different statistically, even though they appear to favour CAB. Only in those studies using non-steroidal anti-androgens in the CAB arm were the differences in favour of CAB; however, even excluding the studies involving the steroidal anti-androgen, CPA from the analysis did not enable statistical significance, in terms of gain in survival, to be achieved.

Apart from the lack of consideration in this analysis for the potential benefits of treatment on length of symptom-free survival and ability to relieve symptoms, other criticisms have been made regarding its validity. Blumenstein[30] questions how trial maturity heterogeneity associated with this analysis influences the statistical power of the meta-analysis. Denis[31] points out that comparison between treatments, as well as analysis of subgroups, is made impossible owing to a lack of knowledge regarding prognostic factors.

The meta-analysis just described lends support, to some extent, to the hypothesis that, in patients with minimal disease (i.e. metastatic patients with a low tumour burden), CAB is of particular benefit. The meta-analysis revealed no difference in mortality during the first 2 years, but after this time a difference in mortality in favour of CAB appeared. This observation favours the hypothesis posited above in the light of the fact that, typically, patients suffering from minimal disease do not contribute to mortality before 2 years. In the light of this observation and from the findings of subgroup analyses in the EORTC 30853[27] and SWOG-INT 0036[26] studies, in which benefits of CAB appear to be associated with minimal disease, the instigation of new studies designed to address this issue specifically is in order, as is the extension of the follow-up period in existing studies to assess the possibility of favourable outcomes associated with CAB, as opposed to castration alone, particularly in patients with minimal disease.

In the EORTC 30853[27] and SWOG-INT 0036[26] studies, described above, the benefits of CAB were particularly evident among those patients with minimal disease and good performance status. However, differences have not been validated statistically. This poses the question of whether the benefits of CAB are confined to such subgroups of patients and as to whether the above two studies incorporated a greater percentage of patients with minimal disease. Hazard ratios for different prognostic groups, published in the EORTC 30853 study, strongly suggest that in patients with severe disease and poor performance, gain in survival disappears. Survival curves from the SWOG-INT 0036 study suggest the same, although there does appear to be some difference in favour of CAB.

If, as some of the evidence suggests, patients with minimal disease respond well to CAB in terms of gains in survival it might be reasonable to suppose that there should be a similarly favourable response to CAB in those patients with only locally advanced prostate cancer. However, in a study conducted by Tyrrell et al.,[32] in which 246 of the total recruits had locally advanced disease only, differences in objective response and overall survival between the two treatment arms (CAB vs goserelin acetate alone) could not be detected. However, at the time of this interim analysis median survival had not yet been reached. The potential for CAB in the treatment of localized prostate cancer is considered further at a later point in this chapter.

Timing of treatment

The timing of androgen ablation remains a controversial issue and, although patients who are symptomatic should be treated immediately, there is disagreement regarding treatment of those patients with advanced disease who remain asymptomatic. One of the main stumbling-blocks in the case of minimal disease is that, although survival may be improved with CAB, it is associated with significant impairment of quality of life and considerable economic cost.[33] According to Labrie et al.,[34] the diagnosis of prostate cancer at a clinically localized stage has been made possible in almost all patients following recent advances in the rational use of serum PSA levels and transrectal ultrasonography. This should, theoretically, allow screening programmes to detect and so to treat the disease at an earlier stage. Ideally, this would be the case, because in the region of 50% of patients present with disease at a stage too far advanced for curative therapy; these patients have a poor prognosis, with a life expectancy in the region of 2 years.

The efficacy of CAB in checking the growth of cancerous cells is greatest at the level of the prostate. In patients with stage D2 cancer undergoing CAB as initial treatment, the disease is well and quickly controlled at this level. After the initial response to CAB, progression is most evident in the bones (approximately 98% of cases), as compared with a very rare rate of progression at the level of the prostate (2% of cases) (see Labrie *et al.*[35]). The only opportunity for curing prostate cancer presents itself at an early stage, at which disease is localized and confined to the prostate. Following radical prostatectomy, patients with disease confined to the prostate, as determined at final histopathological staging following surgery, should have a life expectancy equivalent to that of similarly aged men without prostate cancer.[36] Although it is well recognized that early, pre-emptive treatment is essential if progression to metastases is to be avoided, there has been a delay in the wide acceptance of radical prostatectomy owing to the fact that, in the past, inadequate diagnostic techniques have frequently resulted in the diagnosis of localized, organ-confined disease when, in fact, it was at a more advanced stage. This latter fact becomes evident when the specimen is analysed following surgery.

A variety of studies have suggested that the incidence of cancer-positive surgical margins can be reduced by utilizing neo-adjuvant combination therapy for some months before radical prostatectomy[37–44] or radiotherapy.[45] In the light of this, it should be pointed out that although CAB is fast becoming the standard treatment for *advanced* disease, its use as part of any therapeutic strategy aimed at early, organ-confined, stages of the disease should be evaluated in clinical trials.

Labrie *et al.* [see Labrie *et al.*,[35] reporting on a prospective randomized study designed to determine potential advantages of neo-adjuvant therapy using flutamide and Lupron (an LHRH superagonist)] concluded that neo-adjuvant combination therapy leads to both downsizing and downstaging of prostate cancer. In patients randomized to receive flutamide and Lupron for 3 months prior to radical prostatectomy, the incidence of cancer-positive surgical margins was 13.0% (10 of 77) compared with 38.5% (25 of 65) ($p = 0.006$) in the control group. In the treatment group, 42.9% (33 of 77) of patients had an improved histopathological stage compared with only 7.7% (5 of 65) in the control arm. Worsening of the stage (upstaging) was detected in 40 of 65 patients (61.5%) in the control group whereas upstaging was dramatically decreased in the treatment group in whom upstaging was only detected in 15 of 77 patients (19.5%).

As already discussed above the response to CAB in the SWOG-0036[26] study was most favourable in that subgroup of patients with minimal disease. In that subset there was a 19.5- month advantage in the CAB group (median survival was 61 and 42 months for the CAB and placebo arm, respectively); however, when considering the treatment group as a whole the median overall survival advantage was only 7.3 months. Similar findings in patients with good performance status were made in the EORTC 3085327 study, which utilized goserelin and flutamide in the CAB arm, as discussed earlier. These findings support the view that CAB therapy should not be delayed and that treatment should be initiated as soon as metastasis has been diagnosed. In a re-evaluation of the survival data from the VACURG study,[46] it was concluded that a survival benefit was derived from the initiation of hormonal therapy at the time of diagnosis; the patients in this study had high-grade tumours (Gleason score 7–10) and stage D disease. Additionally, retrospective analyses have demonstrated prolonged progression-free intervals and a trend for longer survival in patients having surgically proven stage D1 disease.[47,48] However, there is as yet no definitive evidence that all patients have prolonged survival with early hormonal therapy. Theoretical risks associated with early CAB therapy include the possibility that androgen-independent clones could be selected for, so leading the disease into a phase for which there is no efficient alternative therapy. Addressing the issue of early vs late treatment of metastatic prostate cancer, Labrie *et al.*[35] stratified a cohort of prostate cancer patients (stage

D2; soft tissue or bony metastasis), receiving flutamide and the LHRH agonist gonadotrophin-releasing hormone (GnRH) ethylamide, according to bone lesion incidence; they concluded that a relatively small increase in bone lesion numbers has 'a major negative impact on survival'. In patients with one to five bone metastases, median survival had not been reached by 8 years, whereas, in patients stratified to the group with six to ten bone lesions, survival was reduced dramatically to 3.56 years. Median survival was 2.36 years for those patients with 11–40 bone lesions and where disseminated disease was evident survival was reduced to 1.76 years.

As alluded to earlier, androgen hypersensitive tumours with resistance to antihormonal therapy develop where low androgen levels, comparable to those evident in men who have undergone orchiectomy, exist.[49] On the basis of this knowledge, and in the light of the findings of SWOG-INT 0036,[26] combination therapy should be considered as first-line treatment rather than second-line treatment following failure of standard therapy. In SWOG-INT 0036, patients in the control arm were treated with flutamide after they started to progress, but no survival benefit was evident and this reflects the invariably poor prognosis in advanced stages of the disease. That is to say, the efficacy of CAB is much reduced (if not, indeed, lost) when used as second-line treatment at the time of relapse following first-line treatment with monotherapy.

Anti-androgen withdrawal syndrome

Kelly and Scher[50] were the first to note that when anti-androgen — in this case, flutamide — is withdrawn from patients receiving CAB therapy, after signs of disease progression become evident, there is a marked improvement in chemical and biological response. Since this observation, what has become known as the 'anti-androgen withdrawal syndrome' has also been noted with other pure anti-androgens as well as steroidal anti-androgens, and with oestrogens.[51] The syndrome is associated with prolonged treatment with any form of anti-androgen in combination with orchiectomy or medical castration. The quality of the response seems to be associated with the duration of anti-androgen treatment, but the response is not apparent when anti-androgens are used as monotherapy. After evidence of disease progression, and subsequent withdrawal of anti-androgen, between 25 and 56% of patients undergo a symptomatic improvement, and more than a 50% reduction in PSA from baseline is seen in 28–80% of patients. The patients most likely to respond in this way are those with the highest PSA values and those who have undergone lengthy treatment with CAB.[51,52] Looking at the apparently stimulatory effect of flutamide on LNCaP prostate cancer cell lines, Moul et al.[52] demonstrated the existence of a mutated androgen receptor that responded to anti-androgen as if it were an agonist rather than an antagonist; that is to say, these receptors are stimulated by anti-androgen in a dose-related manner. This mutation has been reported in hormonally independent and metastatic prostate cancer tissue. Synthesis of androgen receptors is induced by castration,[53] and amplification of receptors has been reported in 30% of prostate cancer specimens;[54] such amplification in association with mutation may explain the positive response observed when withdrawing anti-androgens at the time of disease progression. Whether this phenomenon is a set-back to CAB therapy or is a therapeutically advantageous aspect if exploited correctly is yet to be understood, but it would seem that it provides another means of improving survival. The possibility that such a response to withdrawal has played a part in CAB studies in which a survival benefit has been demonstrated cannot be excluded and in future

CAB trials this phenomenon will have to be accounted for. There are authors who suggest that the differences in survival noted in the combination arm of some CAB trials may be explained by the anti-androgen withdrawal syndrome. When looking at retrospective studies of CAB therapy, such as the meta-analysis involving 25 CAB trials conducted by the Prostate Cancer Trialists' Group, various questions come to mind. In trials for which a survival benefit for CAB was demonstrated, was anti-androgen treatment withdrawn when disease progression was detected? Was withdrawal of anti-androgen at progression less usually practised in those CAB trials that were negative? When looking at other interim endpoints used in CAB trials, such as time to progression, the argument for the role of anti-androgen withdrawal response in any positive outcome in favour of CAB appears to be negated. Interim results showing improvement of time to progression, for example, have also improved in positive CAB studies; such measurements are usually made before any manoeuvre to withdraw anti-androgen is made — as one would expect, since the onset of progression, at which time withdrawal would be considered, is the endpoint of the time to progression measurement.

Conclusions

Although the controversy associated with CAB continues, and the Prostate Cancer Trialists' meta-analysis as it stands points toward limited survival benefits for patients with advanced disease, the two studies discussed in this chapter with subsets of patients having minimal disease must be viewed as encouraging. Should larger studies with this category of patient be undertaken to achieve sufficient statistical power to provide the all-important significant response? Preliminary results of the SWOG-INT105 study, which stratified patients according to extent of disease and performance status, were disappointing and unhelpful to the cause of the CAB enthusiast.

However, for the future it would seem that, as a result of the techniques now available for earlier diagnosis of prostate cancer, more patients will present with a lower tumour burden. Much of the ground covered in this chapter suggests that this is the population most likely to benefit from CAB treatment, and we might look forward to a significantly reduced mortality rate from advanced disease, for which the prognosis is currently so bad.

References

1. Prostate Cancer Trialists' Collaborative Group. Maximum androgen blockade in advanced prostate cancer: an overview of 22 randomized trials with 3283 deaths in 5710 patients. Lancet 1995; 346: 265–269
2. Huggins C, Hodges C V. Studies on prostatic cancer. The effect of castration, of estrogen and of androgen injection on serum phosphatases in metastatic carcinoma of the prostate. Cancer Res 1941; 1: 293–297
3. Veterans Administration Cooperative Urological Research Group (VACURG). Treatment and survival of patients with cancer of the prostate. Surg Gynecol Obstet 1967; 124: 1011–1017
4. Mettlin C, Natarajan N, Murphy G P. Recent patterns of care of prostatic cancer patients in the United States: results from the surveys of the American College of Surgeons Commission on Cancer. Int Adv Surg Oncol 1982; 5: 277–321
5. Paulson D, Howe G B Jr, Hinshaw W et al. Radiation therapy versus delayed androgen deprivation for stage C carcinoma of the prostate. J Urol 1984; 131: 901–902
6. Labrie P, Belanger A, Dupont A et al. Science behind total androgen blockade: from gene to combination therapy. Clin Invest Med 1993; 16: 475
7. Labrie F, Dupont A, Belanger A et al. New approach in the treatment of prostate cancer: complete instead of partial withdrawal of androgens. Prostate 1983; 4: 579

8. Hamada N, Neumann F, Junkman K. Intrauterine antimaskuline beinflussing von rattenfetendurch ein stark gestagen wirksames steroid. Steroid Acta Endocrinol 1995; 44: 330–388

9. Labrie F, Dupont A, Belanger A *et al*. New hormonal therapy in prostatic carcinoma; combined treatment with an LHRH agonist and an antiandrogen. Clin Invest Med 1982; 5: 267–275

10. Fur B J A, Valcaccia B, Curry B *et al*. ICI 176 334. A novel nonsteroidal peripherally selective antiandrogen. J Endocrinol 1987; 113: R7–9

11. Cox L E, Crawford E D. Estrogens in the treatment of prostate cancer. J Urol 1995; 154: 1991–1998

12. Schroeder F H, Lock T M T W, Chadha D R *et al*. Metastatic cancer of the prostate managed with buserelin versus busereline plus cyproterone acetate. J Urol 1987; 137: 912–918

13. Kuhn J M, Billebaud T, Navratil H *et al*. Prevention of the transient adverse effects of gonadotropin-releasing hormone analogue (buserelin) in metastatic prostatic carcinoma by administration of an antiandrogen (nilutamide). N Engl J Med 1989; 321: 413–418

14. Mahler C. Is disease flare a problem? Cancer 1993; 72(suppl 12): 3799–3802

15. Gonzalez-Barcena D, Vadillo-Buenfil M, Cortez-Morales A *et al*. Luteinizing hormone-releasing Hormone antagonist Cetrorelix as primary single therapy in patients with advanced prostatic cancer and paraplegia due to metastatic invasion of spinal cord. Urology 1995; 45: 275–281

16. Bologna M, Muzi P, Biordi L *et al*. Pinasteride dose-dependently reduces the proliferation rate of the LnCap human prostatic cancer cell line in vitro. Urology 1995; 45: 282–290

17. Fleshner N E, Trachtenberg J. Sequential androgen blockade: a biological study in the inhibition of prostatic growth. J Urol 1992; 148: 1928–1929

18. Presti J C Jr, Fair W R, Andriole G *et al*. Multicenter, randomized, double-blind, placebo controlled study to investigate the effect of finasteride (MK-906) on stage D prostate cancer. J Urol 1992; 148: 1201–1212

19. Fleshner N E, Trachtenberg J. Combination finasteride and flutamide in advanced carcinoma of the prostate: effective therapy with minimal side effects. J Urol 1995; 154: 1642–1646

20. Labrie F. Endocrine therapy of prostate cancer. Endocrinol Metab Clin North Am 1991; 20: 845–872

21. Crawford E D, Eisenberg M A, McLeod D G *et al*. Comparison of bilateral orchiectomy with or without Flutamide for the treatment of patients with stage D2 adenocarcinoma of the prostate: Results of NCI intergroup study 0105 (SWOG and ECOG). J Urol 1997; 157: 336. (abstr 1311)

22. Janknegt R A, Abbou C C, Bartoletti R *et al*. Orchiectomy and Anandron (nilutamide) or placebo as treatment of metastatic prostatic cancer in a multinational double-blind randomized trial. J Urol 1993; 149: 77–83

23. Robinson M R G, Hetherington J. The EORTC studies: is there an optimal endocrine management for M1 prostatic cancer?. World J Urol 1986; 4: 171–175

24. Robinson M R G. A further analysis of European Organization for Research and Treatment of Cancer Protocol 30805. Orchidectomy versus orchidectomy plus cyproterone acetate versus low-dose diethylstilbestrol. Cancer 1993; 72 (suppl 12): 3855–3857

25. Labrie C, Belanger A, Labrie F. Androgenic activity of dehydroepiandrosterone and androstenedione in the rat ventral prostate. Endocrinology 1988; 123: 1412–1417

26. Crawford E D, Eisenberg M A, McLeod D G *et al*. A controlled trial of leuprolide with and without Flutamide in prostatic carcinoma. N Engl J Med 1989; 321: 418–424

27. Denis J, Carneiro de Moura J L, Bono A *et al*. Goserelin acetate and flutamide versus bilateral orchiectomy: a phase III EORTC Trial (30853). Urology 1993; 42: 119–129

28. Klijn J G M, de Voogt E D, Studer U E *et al*. for the European Organization for Research and Treatment of Cancer — Genitourinary Group. Short-term versus long-term addition of cyproterone acetate to buserelin therapy in comparison with orchidectomy in the treatment of metastatic prostate cancer. Cancer 1993; 72(suppl 12): 3858–3862

29. Waxman J, Pandha H, Labrie F *et al*. Anti-androgens in treatment of prostate cancer. Lancet 1995; 1030–1031

30. Blumenstein B A. Overview analysis issues using combined androgen deprivation overview analysis as an example. Urol Oncol 1995; 1: 95

31. Denis, L. Endocrine treatment — should it be total (maximal) blockade? In: Peeling W B (ed) Questions and uncertainties about prostate cancer. Oxford: Blackwell Science, 1996: 246

32. Tyrrell C J, Altwein J E, Klippel F *et al.* A multicentre randomized trial comparing the luteinizing hormone-releasing hormone analogue goserelin acetate alone and with flutamide in the treatment of advanced prostate cancer. J Urol 1991; 146: 1321

33. Robson M, Dawson N. How is androgen-dependent metastatic prostate cancer best treated? Hematol Oncol Clin North Am 1996; 10(3): 727–747

34. Labrie F, Candas B, Cusan L *et al.* Diagnosis of advanced or noncurable prostate cancer can be practically eliminated by prostate-specific antigen. Urology; 1996: 212–217

35. Labrie F, Belanger A, Dupont A *et al.* Science behind total androgen blockade: from gene to combination therapy. Clin Invest Med 1993; 16: 475–492

36. Rheaume E, Lachance Y, Zhao H F *et al.* Structure and expression of a new cDNA encoding the almost exclusive 3β-hydroxysteroid dehydrogenase/Δ^5-Δ^4 isomerase gene and its expression in mammalian cells. J Biol Chem 1990; 265: 20469–20475

37. Labrie F, Belanger A, Simard J *et al.* Combination therapy for prostate cancer. Cancer 1993; 71: 1059–1067

38. Monfette G, Dupont A, Labrie F. Temporary combination therapy with flutamide and tryptex as adjuvant to radical prostatectomy for the treatment of early stage prostate cancer. In: Labrie F, Lee F, Dupont A (eds) Early stage prostate cancer: diagnosis and choice of therapy. New York: Excerpta Medica, 1989: 41–51

39. McHugh T A. The influence of transrectal ultrasound of the prostate on a private urology practice. In: Labrie F, Lee F, Dupont A (eds) Early stage prostate cancer: diagnosis and choice of therapy. New York: Excerpta Medica, 1989: 37–40

40. Labrie F, Dupont A, Cusan L *et al.* Downstaging of localized prostate cancer by neoadjuvant therapy with flutamide and Lupron. Clin Invest Med 1993; 16: 499–509

41. Lee F, Littrup P J, Torp-Pedersen S T *et al.* Prostate cancer. comparison of transrectal US and digital rectal examination for screening. Radiology 1988; 168: 389–394

42. Pinault S, Tetu B, Gagnon J *et al.* Transrectal ultrasound evaluation of local prostate cancer inpatients treated with LHRH agonist and in combination with flutamide. Urology 1992; 39: 254–261

43. Tetu B, Srigley J R, Boivin J C *et al.* Effect of combination endocrine therapy (LHRH agonist and flutamide) on normal prostate and prostatic adenocarcinoma. Am J Surg Pathol 1991; 15: 111–120

44. Schulman C C, Sassine A M. Neoadjuvant hormonal deprivation before radical prostatectomy. Clin Invest Med 1993; 16: 523–531

45. Pilepich M V, Krall J, Al-Sarraf M *et al.* A phase III trial of androgen suppression before and during radiation therapy (RT) for locally advanced prostatic carcinoma: preliminary report of RTOG protocol 8610. Proc Am Soc Clin Oncol 1993; 12: 229 (abstr 703)

46. Byar D P, Corle D. Hormone therapy for prostate cancer: Results of the Veterans Administration Cooperative Urological Research Group's studies of cancer of the prostate. NCI monograph 1988; 7: 165–170

47. Zincke H, Bergstralh E J, Larson-Keller J J *et al.* Stage D1 prostate cancer treated by radical prostatectomy and adjuvant hormonal treatment. Evidence for favorable survival in patients with DNA diploid tumors. Cancer 1992; 70(suppl): 311–323

48. Kramolowski E V. The value of testosterone deprivation in stage D 1 carcinoma of the prostate. J Urol 1988; 139: 1242–1244

49. Wu L, Einstien M, Geissler W M *et al.* Expression cloning and characterization of human 17b-hydroxysteroid dehydrogenase type II, a microsomal enzyme possessing 20a hydroxysteroid dehydrogenase activity. J Biol Chem 1993; 268: 12964–12969

50. Kelly W K, Scher H L. Prostate specific antigen decline after antiandrogen withdrawal. J Urol 1993; 149: 607–609

51. Scher H I, Zhang Z F, Nanus D, Kelly W K. Hormone and antihormone withdrawal: implications for the management of androgen-independent prostate cancer. Urology 1996; 47(suppl lA): 61–69

52. Moul J W, Srivastava S, McLeod D G. Molecular implications of the antiandrogen withdrawal syndrome. Semin Urol 1995; 13: 157–163

53. Hiipakka R A, Liao S. Androgen physiology. In: DeGroot L J (ed) Endocrinology, 3rd edn. Philadelphia: Saunders, 1995: 2336–2347

54. Visakorpi T, Hytinen E, Koiviston P *et al.* Amplification of androgen receptor gene associated with tumor recurrence in prostate cancer patients receiving androgen withdrawal therapy. In: Basic and clinical aspects of prostate cancer. Philadelphia: American Association for Cancer Research, 1994: A41 (abstr)

Chapter 26

Intermittent androgen suppression for the treatment of prostate cancer

N. Bruchovsky, L. Goldenberg and M. Gleave

Introduction

The therapeutic use of castration began in the 1890s, more than 40 years before testosterone was identified as the chemical factor elaborated by the testis. Men suffering from senile enlargement of the prostate responded well to therapy, with rapid glandular atrophy reported in 87% of cases.[1] However, the procedure was associated not only with a troubling high mortality rate of 18% but also with psychic disturbances and shock out of proportion to the extent of mutilation.[2] The therapeutic use of castration gained momentum in the 1940s, when it was applied with remarkable success to the treatment of metastatic prostate cancer.[3] Owing to the high response rate and frequency of profound remissions, there was little incentive to examine the less obvious physiological changes that accompanied androgen ablation and affected the sense of well-being. In addition to loss of libido and potency, the adverse effects on bone (osteoporosis), muscle (atrophy), breast (gynaecomastia), blood (anaemia), lipids (low high-density lipoproteins), and mood (depression) remain a source of distressing clinical symptoms.

Although no other treatment exists that equals or surpasses castration in checking the growth of prostate cancer, for reasons that remain unknown the cell death process induced by androgen ablation fails to eliminate the entire malignant-cell population.[4] Another limitation of conventional androgen ablation is that it increases the rate of progression of prostate cancer to an androgen-independent state and, after a variable period of time averaging 24 months, the tumour inevitably recurs with increasing serum prostate-specific antigen (PSA) levels and is characterized by androgen-independent growth. Intermittent androgen suppression, a form of ablative therapy delivered in pulses, offers periodic relief from the adverse physiological effects of castration and may temporarily retard the progression of a tumour to androgen independence.

Clinical development of intermittent regimens of androgen suppression

The intermittent regulation of serum testosterone levels for therapeutic purposes was first attempted with cyclic administration of oestrogenic hormone by Klotz.[5] Several practical advantages of the intermittent regimen were foreseen, including interval restoration of plasma testosterone with resumption of sexual activity, a decreased risk of cardiovascular complications, and, in accordance with Noble's findings,[6] a possible salutory inhibition of tumour growth at testosterone levels above those achieved by castration. In the pilot study undertaken, 19 patients with advanced prostate cancer received diethylstilbestrol (DES) (stilboestrol) until a clinical response was clearly demonstrated and then it was withheld until symptoms recurred. One additional patient was treated with flutamide using a similar schedule. The mean duration of the initial therapy was 30 months (range 2–70 months). Subjective improvement was noted in all patients during the first 3 months of treatment. When the treatment was stopped, 12 of 20 patients relapsed after a mean interval of 8 months (range 1–24 months) and all subsequently responded to re-administration of drug. Therapy-induced impotency was reversed in nine of 10 men within 3 months of the break in treatment. An improved quality of life was achieved owing to reduced intake of DES, and no adverse effects on survival were apparent.

Akakura[7] examined the strategy of restoring apoptotic potential with multiple rounds of androgen withdrawal and replacement. Advantage was taken of the reversible feature of combination therapy employing luteinizing hormone-releasing hormone (LHRH) agonists and antiandrogens to alternate patients between periods on and off treatment. In four of stage C and three of stage D patients with prostate cancer, androgen withdrawal was initiated with cyproterone acetate (100 mg/day) and DES (0.1 mg/day) and then maintained with cyproterone acetate in combination with the LHRH agonist, goserelin acetate (3.6 mg/month). After 6 or more months of suppression of serum PSA into the normal range, treatment was interrupted for 2–11 months. After recovery of testicular function, androgen-withdrawal therapy was resumed when serum PSA increased to a level of about 20 µg/litre. This cycle was repeated sequentially to a total of two to four times over treatment periods of 21–47 months with no loss of androgen dependence.

In extending the preliminary experience with this approach, Goldenberg[8] investigated the effects of cyclic androgen withdrawal and replacement therapy in a group of 47 patients with prostate cancer [clinical stages: D2 (14), D1 (10), C (19), B2 (2) and A2 (2)], with a mean follow-up time of 125 weeks. Treatment was initiated with combined androgen blockade and continued for at least 6 months until a serum PSA nadir was observed. Medication was then withheld until the serum PSA increased to a mean value between 10 and 20 µg/litre. This cycle of treatment and no treatment was repeated until the regulation of serum PSA became androgen independent. The consistent pattern of PSA response and recovery achieved with this approach is illustrated in Figure 26.1 for the first two cycles. An updated analysis of the results on 51 patients is given in Table 26.1.

The length of four consecutive treatment cycles was 21, 19, 18 and 13 months and the overall mean percentage time off therapy was 45, 46, 48 and 40 months, respectively. The mean PSA at the start of each cycle of treatment was 150, 14, 12 and 28 µg/litre. The mean time to achieve a PSA nadir was 5, 4, 5 and 5 months and this was less than or equal to 2.0 µg/litre in 88% or more of the patients.

Serum testosterone returned to the normal range within 8 weeks (range: 1–26 weeks) of stopping treatment. The off-treatment period in all cycles was associated with an improvement in sense of well-being, and the recovery of libido and potency in the men who reported normal or near-normal sexual function before the start of therapy. In seven patients with stage D2 disease, the cancer progressed to an androgen-independent state. The mean and median times to progression were 128 weeks and 108 weeks. Seven patients have died, one from a non-cancer-related illness, with mean and median overall survival times of 210 weeks and 166 weeks. These studies demonstrated that the androgen-dependent state of prostate cancer can be maintained by intermittent androgen suppression, affording the possibility of multiple apoptotic regressions under well-regulated conditions.

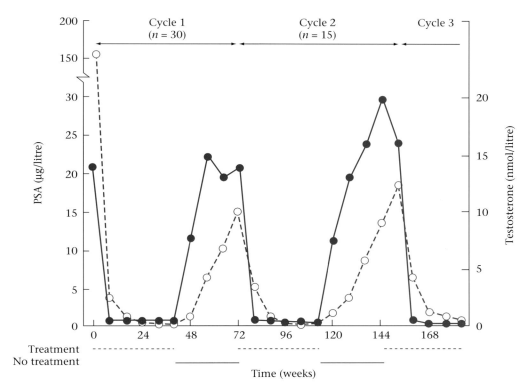

Figure 26.1. Intermittent androgen suppression. Composite results on 47 patients with prostate cancer, 30 of whom have completed one cycle of treatment, 15, two cycles and two who are still on the first cycle. A cycle consists of a period of treatment followed by a period of no treatment (modified from ref. 8 with permission.)

Table 26.1. Intermittent androgen suppression: analysis by cycle

	Complete cycle			
	1	2	3	4
Number of patients	51	19	8	2
Mean PSA at start (µg/litre)	150	14	12	28
Mean time to PSA nadir (months)	5	4	5	5
PSA nadir 2.0 µg/litre (% of patients)	95	89	88	100
Mean length of cycle (months)(range)	21 (9–54)	19 (10–39)	18 (10–26)	13 (11–16)
Mean time off therapy (months)	10	9	8	5
Mean time off therapy (%)	45	46	48	40

When should therapy be interrupted?

In theory, androgen withdrawal should be continued as long as necessary to maximize the apoptotic regression of tumour, but stopped before there is any development of the androgen-independent phenotype. After institution of androgen-withdrawal therapy, serum PSA levels initially may decrease rapidly, owing to the cessation of androgen-regulated PSA gene expression, and then more slowly as a result of the apoptotic elimination of PSA-producing cells.

A favourable response to treatment is indicated by an initial decrease in serum PSA, often into the normal range, within the first 10 weeks followed by a slower decline to lower levels over the succeeding 30–40 weeks. At least 32 weeks of treatment are necessary in order to bring the serum PSA into the normal range in the majority of patients with stage D2 prostate cancer.[9]

A decrease of serum PSA to a stable or decreasing nadir in a normal range is an important aspect of response to therapy. If the serum PSA remains above 4 µg/litre between 24 and 32 weeks of treatment, the median survival time is only 18 months.[9] On the other hand, if the serum PSA is below 4 µg/litre between 24 and 32 weeks of therapy, the median survival time is much greater, at 40 months. Only those patients whose serum PSA has reached a stable or decreasing value in the normal range at 24 and 32 weeks should be considered eligible for intermittent androgen suppression. The procedure that is followed for deciding whether patients with stage D2 prostate cancer are eligible for interruption of therapy is summarized in Figure 26.2.

The therapeutic induction period should be the same length with disease in earlier stages. Gleave[10] found that the time required for serum PSA to reach a nadir in a group of 50 men with clinically confined prostate cancer after institution of neoadjuvant androgen-withdrawal therapy was often longer than 6 months. Using a lower limit of sensitivity of 0.2 µg/litre, the serum PSA reached a nadir in only 34% of the patients after 3 months, 60% after 5 months, 70% after 6 months, and 84% at 8 months. In 16% the serum PSA was still decreasing at 8 months. The percentage of patients with a nadir serum PSA level of equal to or less than 0.2 µg/litre increased from 14% at 2 months, to 34% at 3 months, 56% at 5 months and 66% at 8 months. No evidence of outgrowth of androgen-independent clones was found in the radical prostatectomy specimens. These

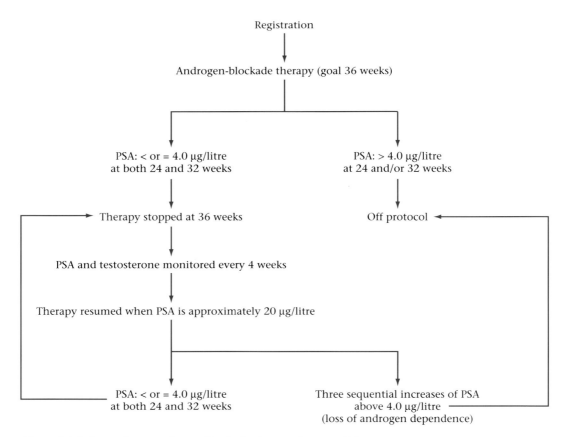

Figure 26.2. Intermittent androgen-blockade therapy for stage D2 prostate cancer.

observations support the idea that the androgen-withdrawal phase of the treatment cycle can be extended to 9 months to obtain a maximum response without altering the androgen-dependent state of the tumour.

When should therapy be resumed?

The optimal time to reinstitute androgen-ablation therapy remains undefined and empirical. In patients with advanced prostate cancer, the serum PSA at the time of diagnosis may range in values from the upper limit of the normal range to a level of several thousand µg/litre. In those patients with a pretreatment serum PSA of less than 20 µg/litre, it would be reasonable to start the second cycle of treatment when the serum PSA increases to the pretreatment level again. If the serum PSA at presentation is greater than 20 µg/litre, the authors' practice is to start the second cycle when the serum PSA increases to approximately 20 µg/litre as indicated in Figure 26.2. In an ideal response to intermittent androgen suppression, the patient is on therapy for an overall period of 8–9 months. The serum PSA is observed to decrease to the lower limit of detection, 0.1 µg/litre, after 24 weeks of therapy; the same value is measured after 32 weeks of therapy, thus indicating that the serum PSA has reached a stable nadir in the normal range. Therapy is then interrupted after 36 weeks, marking the start of the off-treatment period; the serum testosterone recovers to normal within 8–14 weeks. However, in contrast to the rate of recovery of serum testosterone, the increase in serum PSA in the majority of cases will be slower, affording a no-treatment period of 8–9 months.

PSA guidelines

In theory, intermittent androgen suppression should be suitable for the long-term management of inoperable, incompletely excised or locally recurrent prostate cancer, especially after failure of external beam radiation. The standard regimen developed for stage D2 prostate cancer (Figure 26.2) has been adapted for use in the treatment of patients with initially localized prostate cancer who have failed either radical prostatectomy, or irradiation, or radical prostatectomy and irradiation, as demonstrated by a rising serum PSA.

Although intermittent androgen suppression was originally envisaged for the treatment of advanced prostate carcinoma with minimal tumour burden, the application of this approach has broadened to include other potential indications,

Table 26.2. Serum PSA guidelines in intermittent androgen suppression

Stage	Condition	Serum PSA (µg/litre)				
		At start of cycle 1	24 weeks	32 weeks	To initiate cycle 2	Refractory disease 3 increases above
A2, B or C	Untreated	~6	0.2 or <0.2	0.2 or <0.2*	~1	0.2
D1 or D2	Untreated	>20	4 or <4	4 or <4*	~20	4
B2 or C	Failed irradiation	>6	4 or <4	4 or <4*	~10	4
A2, B or C	Failed prostatectomy	0.8 to 1	0.2 or <0.2	0.2 or <0.2*	~1	0.2
A2, B or C	Failed prostatectomy, failed irradiation	>1	1 or <1	1 or <1*	~1	1

*Stable or decreasing value relative to result at 24 weeks.

as suggested in Table 26.2. Since no single set of PSA trigger points could be uniformly applied to all such conditions of prostatic malignancy, how best to stratify patients and assess response to treatment on the basis of serum PSA determinations is an open question. Furthermore, PSA is monitored on the assumption that measured values are related to volume of tumour.[11-13] However, this may not be true in every case, since the level of PSA in the serum is the end result of one or more cellular reactions. The following possibilities should be kept in mind: first, the synthesis of PSA may be inhibited by androgen withdrawal without any associated apoptotic cell death; second, the synthesis of PSA may continue unabated in the absence of androgen, but if the malignant cell population is greatly reduced through apoptosis, the overall production of PSA would decline; third, the reduction of PSA may reflect a combination of arrested synthesis and accelerated cell death. Although current evidence is compatible with the latter interpretation, more information is needed from clinical trials of intermittent androgen suppression before the full meaning of any therapy-related PSA response (decrease or increase) can be judged with accuracy.

Quality-of-life and survival

There is little doubt that quality of life can be improved by cyclic androgen suppression. Recovery of sexual function is possible and a greater sense of well-being is experienced during the off-treatment periods. Other advantages include the preservation of the androgen-dependent state of the tumour, reduced expense of treatment, less cumulative drug toxicity and the potential for augmenting intermittent androgen suppression with other treatment modalities such as 5α-reductase inhibitors, differentiation agents, cytotoxic chemicals and possibly gene therapy. However, whether intermittent androgen suppression alters survival in a beneficial or adverse way is unknown and will have to be determined in future randomized clinical trials. In 14 men treated for stage D2 prostate cancer by Goldenberg,[8] the median time to progression and survival were in keeping with results expected with continuous androgen blockade.

Although the ultimate safety and the value of intermittent androgen suppression in extending survival are unproven, multiple cycles of therapy have now been achieved in a small number of men with advanced disease, as illustrated in Figure 26.3. Panel A depicts four complete cycles of treatment over 250 weeks in a 57-year-old patient with local progression of previously irradiated stage C disease and a solitary metastasis in the lumbar spine. Panel B depicts three cycles of therapy over 310 weeks in a 69-year-old man with stage C disease associated with a high initial serum PSA; this patient had no previous treatment. Panel C depicts four cycles of treatment over a period of 340 weeks in a 56-year-old man with early stage D2 disease and no previous treatment. Panel D depicts four cycles of therapy over a period of 180 weeks in a 51-year-old man with previously untreated stage D1 disease.

At the present time it is not known whether there are any patient characteristics, pathological features or PSA-related response criteria that can be used to predict the length or number of cycles possible. As more patients are entered into trials of intermittent androgen suppression, this information should become available.

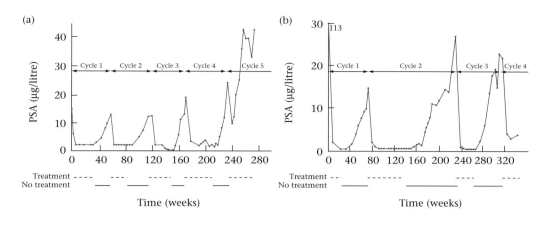

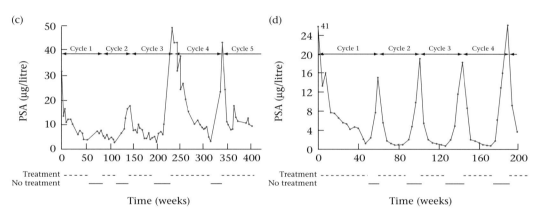

Figure 26.3. Multiple cycles of intermittent androgen suppression: (A) patient with local progression of previously irradiated stage C adenocarcinoma and a metastasis in the lumbar spine (refractory disease in fifth cycle); (B) patient with stage C adenocarcinoma and no previous treatment (now in fourth cycle); (C) patient with stage D2 adenocarcinoma having metastases in the thoracic spine and pelvis and no previous treatment (now in fifth cycle); (D) patient with stage D1 adenocarcinoma and no previous treatment (now in fifth cycle). ©N. Bruchovsky

Dilemmas

There are situations that may arise during the course of therapy, compelling a change in the method of treatment. Circumstances of this nature are listed in Table 26.3 with suggestions for remedial action.

Table 26.3. Dilemmas in intermittent androgen suppression

Problem	Clinical response
Failure of serum PSA to nadir within specified range	Increase dose of anti-androgen or switch to another anti-androgenic agent
Rapid increase in serum PSA following interruption of therapy	Use finasteride during the off-treatment period of the next cycle
Very slow increase in serum PSA following interruption of therapy	Continue to observe but check for other signs of tumour progression
Increase in serum PSA while testosterone is suppressed	Avoid secondary flare reaction, escalate dose of anti-androgen, substitute another anti-androgen, start chemotherapy
PSA trigger points for different indications	See Table 26.2

Other applications

Relapse after neoadjuvant therapy

A better understanding of the biology of prostate cancer and the results of reverse transcription–polymerase chain reaction (RT–PCR) testing for PSA mRNA in blood have highlighted the fact that the risk of systemic spread is already appreciable at the time of initial diagnosis.[14–18] Under such conditions, the results of radical prostatectomy will be less than optimal, although it may still be indicated for control of local–regional disease. Preoperative treatment with a reversible androgen withdrawal agent affords the possibility of downstaging the primary tumour, reducing the incidence of positive surgical resection margins, and eradicating micrometastases. Preliminary evidence suggests that long-term treatment of 8 months is superior to a shorter regimen of 3 months.[10] The same principle has been used in the cytoreduction of prostate cancer prior to external beam irradiation, with beneficial effects.[19] Androgen withdrawal therapy is usually interrupted approximately at the time when the surgical or radiation procedure is carried out. This means that tumour cells that escape removal and remain *in situ* may well recover apoptotic potential when serum testosterone becomes normal again. Repeated use of androgen withdrawal is then possible in the event of recurrent disease.

Chemoprevention

Reference has been made recently to evidence that hormonal therapy may indirectly influence the thymus, affording an improved immune response and the possibility of tumour rejection. Oliver and Gallagher[20] have pointed out that, perhaps, this has provided a scientific rationale to justify the use of intermittent androgen suppression. In their preliminary experience with cyclic therapy, treatment was stopped in six patients with early tumours whose acid phosphatase and PSA values were normal after 3–6 months of androgen suppression. Three of these patients remained progression free at 16, 18 and 24 months. From this experience, Oliver and Gallagher inferred that the use of intermittent hormone therapy might offer a new approach to the management of patients with small tumours in whom repeated treatment for 3 months only might be justified.

In a radical departure from conventional approaches, the same investigators suggested that intermittent hormone therapy might be considered for chemoprevention of prostate cancer. Given its slow growth rate in the early stages, they believe that it would be acceptable to treat for a short interval of 3 months or less every 5–10 years. This would be attractive in instances of familial prostate cancer for an individual at risk; even if the serum PSA value is normal, the response could be measured with a hypersensitive assay for PSA and the treatment continued until the serum level falls below the lowest limit of detection.

Future directions

There is increasing acceptance of the view that surgical castration or any equivalent therapy that brings about a state of continuous androgen deprivation in a patient with prostate cancer, borders on overtreatment, at least in some men. This impression follows from increasing numbers of observed lengthy remissions following relatively short periods of androgen-withdrawal therapy. By interrupting therapy and restoring normal levels of testosterone, it is possible to reduce the undesirable long-term physiological effects of castration. These include atrophy of skeletal muscles, osteoporosis, fall in haemoglobin, sense of chronic fatigue and weakness, depression, and loss of libido and potency. Castration is also detrimental to the biological condition of prostate cancer, in that it fosters tumour progression and leads to androgen-independent growth. In contrast, intermittent androgen-withdrawal therapy, which takes advantage of the reversible features of LHRH agonists and anti-androgens, offers potential for long-term control of prostate cancer while minimizing the physiological and possibly the biological side effects associated with one-time castration. For this reason, the intermittent therapy option will be incorporated increasingly into the formulation of long-range treatment strategies. These will attempt to increase the probability of cure by introducing such measures as extended periods of neoadjuvant therapy before radical prostatectomy or irradiation. Where a potentially curative approach fails, emphasis then will be given to therapies that can maintain the disease in a chronic condition. Intermittent therapy will assume a prominent role at this juncture, especially if methods of producing extended cycles can be developed.

It is possible that the intermittent therapy option will become an alternative to radical prostatectomy or irradiation for the primary treatment of localized prostate cancer in men who are reluctant to submit to these procedures, or in older men with a life expectancy of less than 10 years.

References

1. White J W. The results of double castration in hypertrophy of the prostate. Ann Surg 1895; 22: 1–80
2. Cabot A T. The question of castration for enlarged prostate. Ann Surgery 1896; 24: 265–309
3. Huggins C, Hodges C V. Studies on prostate cancer: I. Effect of castration, estrogen, and androgen injection on serum phosphatases in metastatic carcinoma of the prostate. Cancer Res 1941; 1: 293–297
4. Bruchovsky N, Rennie P S, Coldman A J et al. Effects of androgen withdrawal on the stem cell composition of the Shionogi carcinoma. Cancer Res 1990; 50: 2275–2282
5. Klotz L H, Herr H W, Morse M J et al. Intermittent endocrine therapy for advanced prostate cancer. Cancer 1996; 58: 2546–2550
6. Nobel R L. Sex steroids as a cause of adenocarcinoma of the dorsal prostate in Nb rats, and their influence on the growth of transplants. Oncology 1977; 34: 138–141
7. Akakura K, Bruchovsky N, Goldenberg S L et al. Effects of intermittent androgen suppression on androgen-dependent tumours: apoptosis and serum prostate specific antigen. Cancer 1993; 71: 2782–2790
8. Goldenberg S L, Bruchovsky N, Gleave M E et al. Intermittent androgen suppression in the treatment of prostate cancer: a preliminary report. Urology 1995; 45: 839–845
9. Bruchovsky N, Goldenberg S L, Akakura K et al. Luteinizing hormone-releasing hormone agonists in prostate cancer: elimination of flare reaction by pretreatment with cyproterone acetate and low-dose diethylstilbestrol. Cancer 1993; 72: 1685–1691
10. Gleave M E, Goldenberg S L, Jones E C et al. Biochemical and pathological effects of 8 months of neoadjuvant androgen withdrawal therapy before radical prostatectomy in patients with clinically confined prostate cancer. J Urol 1996; 155: 213–219
11. Stamey T A, Kabalin J N, McNeal J E et al. Prostate specific antigen in the diagnosis and treatment of adenocarcinoma of the prostate. II. Radical prostatectomy treated patients. J Urol 1989; 141: 1076–1083
12. Partin A W, Carter H B, Chan D W et al. Prostate specific antigen in the staging of localized prostate cancer: influence of tumor differentiation, tumor volume and benign hyperplasia. J Urol 1990; 143: 747–752
13. Gleave M E, Hsieh J T, Wu H-C et al. Serum PSA levels in mice bearing human prostate LNCaP tumors are determined by tumor volume and endocrine and growth factors. Cancer Res 1992; 52: 1598–1605
14. Seiden M V, Kantoff P W, Krithivas K et al. Detection of circulating tumor cells in men with localized prostate cancer. J Clin Oncol 1994; 12: 2634–2639
15. Wood D P Jr, Banks E R, Humphreys S et al. Sensitivity of immunohistochemistry and polymerase chain reaction in detecting prostate cancer cells in bone marrow. J Histochem Cytochem 1994; 42: 505–511

16. Jaakkola S, Vornanen T, Leinonen J *et al.* Detection of prostatic cells in peripheral blood: correlation with serum concentrations of prostate-specific antigen. Clin Chem 1995; 41: 182–186

17. Katz A E, de Vries G M, Begg M D *et al.* Enhanced reverse transcriptase–polymerase chain reaction for prostate specific antigen as an indicator of true pathologic stage in patients with prostate cancer. Cancer 1995; 75: 1642–1648

18. Ghossein R A, Scher H I, Gerald W L *et al.* Detection of circulating tumor cells in patients with localized and metastatic prostatic carcinoma: clinical implications. J Clin Oncol 1995; 13: 1195–1200

19. Pilepich M V, Krall J M, Al-Sarraf M *et al.* Androgen deprivation with radiation therapy compared with radiation therapy alone for locally advanced prostatic carcinoma: a randomized comparative trial of the Radiation Therapy Oncology Group. Urology 1995; 45: 616–623

20. Oliver R T D, Gallagher C J G. Intermittent endocrine therapy and its potential for chemoprevention of prostate cancer. Cancer Surv 1995; 23: 191–207

Chapter 27
Immediate versus deferred treatment for advanced disease

D. Kirk

Introduction

The arguments concerning the merits of early rather than late treatment of advanced prostate cancer were discussed at a previous meeting of the Prostate Cancer Charitable Trust in 1994.[1] The philosophy behind the Medical Research Council's trial comparing immediate versus deferred treatment for advanced prostate cancer was described. Preliminary results from this study are now available and have been published.[2] These results are considered here in the context of the arguments presented in the previous publication.[1]

The Veterans Administration Cooperative Research Group (VACURG) studies,[3] which included randomized control groups treated initially with a placebo but started on active treatment on progression, led to the acceptance of the principle of deferred treatment. In men with locally advanced non-metastatic disease, deferring treatment until metastases occurred appeared not to be detrimental for survival, and this absence of survival difference between active and placebo groups in the VACURG studies provided the justification for deferring treatment in asymptomatic men. In patients who already have metastatic disease, as an extension of the same principle, treatment is deferred until they develop pain. Byar,[3] in his review in 1973, was able to state only that 'These data support the concept that treatment can be delayed'. The potential advantages of deferring treatment are that any side effects resulting from treatment will occur for a shorter period of time, and, particularly, that death from an unrelated cause might occur before the patient develops symptoms requiring treatment — indeed, the patient who dies without requiring treatment represents a successful outcome of a deferred-treatment policy. In the VACURG studies, even in those with metastatic disease, only 50% of patients dying did so from prostate cancer.[3] It seemed that unless early treatment could be shown to have advantages, deferment until an indication arises might be preferable.[4] Thus, to justify early treatment, the question to be answered is 'Does immediate treatment prolong survival?' To justify delayed treatment, the question is 'How many men will die before they need treatment if it is deferred?'

Although these are critical points, other issues are also cited in favour of early treatment,[1,4,5] including the following:

1. The evidence that deferring treatment has no effect on survival is not conclusive;
2. Local progression in the absence of treatment increases the number of patients requiring transurethral resection of the prostate (TURP) for recurrent outflow obstruction;
3. Catastrophic events, such as spinal cord compression, pathological fractures and ureteric obstruction, may occur in untreated patients;

4. Treatment should be more effective while tumour bulk is smaller;
5. Prostate cancer may become less hormone sensitive as it progresses.

Although deferred treatment avoids the side effects of hormone treatment, it has been argued that new developments such as luteinizing hormone-releasing hormone (LHRH) analogues have reduced the disadvantages of hormone therapy and there has been a swing back towards early treatment.[6] On the other hand, as these new treatments are expensive, they have added an economic component to the argument. Impotence still remains a problem for many patients, not least the younger man for whom, paradoxically, deferring treatment is probably least appropriate. Into this debate came the suggestion by Crawford and his colleagues,[7] that any benefit from maximal androgen blockade appeared most marked in those with least disease, reviving the old argument about loss of hormone sensitivity as prostate cancer progresses that was used by Nesbit and Baum[8] in 1950 at the time of the first debate on timing of treatment.

This discussion was based for many years on the results of the VACURG studies, which were rapidly becoming obsolete, which involved a rather elderly selected group of patients (mainly World War I survivors) and which were never actually designed to answer this question.[4] Retrospective reviews of anecdotal series gave conflicting results.[9,10] What was needed was hard evidence from a prospective controlled study designed specifically to answer the question 'In asymptomatic advanced prostate cancer, should hormone therapy be commenced on diagnosis or can it be deferred until clinically significant progression occurs?' Such a study has been sponsored by the British Medical Research Council.[11] Recruitment into the study ended in 1993, with 938 patients entered (Table 27.1), and the first results have been published recently.[2]

Table 27.1. MRC immediate vs deferred treatment study: patients with follow-up information available

	Treatment			
M stage	Immediate		Deferred	
M0	256	(256)*	244	(247)
Mx†	83	(83)	90	(91)
M1	130	(130)	131	(131)
Total	469	(469)	465	(469)

*Total numbers recruited, in parentheses.
†Patients who did not undergo bone scan, but with no other evidence of metastatic disease.
(From ref. 2 with permission.)

Study protocol

The study was designed to assess the impact of hormonal treatment started at the time of diagnosis on the course of the disease, compared with delaying treatment until clinical progression occurred. Participants were encouraged to manage patients according to their clinical practice. Entry and follow-up were simplified as much as possible, and only data considered relevant to the main issue were collected. Eligibility was largely governed by Peto's uncertainty principle — if the clinician had genuine uncertainty as to whether the patient would benefit from immediate hormone treatment, and no clear reason to defer treatment, and provided that this concurred with the informed view of the patient, he was eligible for entry. Similarly, indications for treatment in deferred patients were at the discretion of the participant.

After the trial had started, it was discovered that many British urologists did not have ready access to nuclear medicine facilities and that some patients entered as 'non-metastatic' had not had this confirmed by a bone scan. In classifying patients' metastatic status, these patients were categorized as 'Mx' (Table 27.1).

The absence of stringent follow-up schedules in the protocol has been criticized, but reflecting normal clinical practice in the UK at the time of the trial makes the results more applicable to everyday urology than those of a trial conducted within an artificially rigorous framework. The data have been analysed on an 'intention to treat' basis. Thus, the trial reflects the effect of a policy either of immediate or of deferred treatment applied in routine urological practice in the UK in the late 1980s.

Results

Of those patients with metastases (M1) randomized to deferred treatment, 50% had been treated 9 months after randomization compared with 27 months in those with non-metastatic disease. Approximately 10% of all the patients randomized to deferred treatment died from other causes before treatment was indicated, mostly patients over the age of 70 and mainly with non-metastatic disease at presentation (Table 27.2). On the other hand, some 5% died *from prostate cancer* without receiving treatment. Surprisingly, most of these had M0 disease, but the majority were aged over 75 at randomization.

As would be expected, progression from M0 to M1 disease was significantly more rapid in patients with deferred treatment (Figure 27.1). In addition, in those with M1 disease at randomization, bone pain occurred earlier. The philosophy of deferred treatment accepts this, progression being the indication for treatment. However, *local* progression also was more rapid, and twice the number of patients (141 vs 65; 2 $p < 0.00001$) in the deferred arm needed a TURP during follow up. This proportion was similar in M0 and M1 patients.

As indicated earlier, a major concern with deferred treatment is leaving the patient exposed to serious complications. As shown in Table 27.3, the incidence of spinal cord compression, pathological fracture, ureteric obstruction and extraskeletal

Table 27.2. MRC immediate vs deferred treatment study: death from other causes before treatment (deferred patients)

Age at randomization (years)	No. randomized	No. of deaths
< 60	10	1
60–64	41	0
65–69	80	4
70–74	116	10
75–79	136	20
80 +	82	16
M stage		
M0	247	29
Mx	91	16
M1	131	6

(From ref. 2 with permission.)

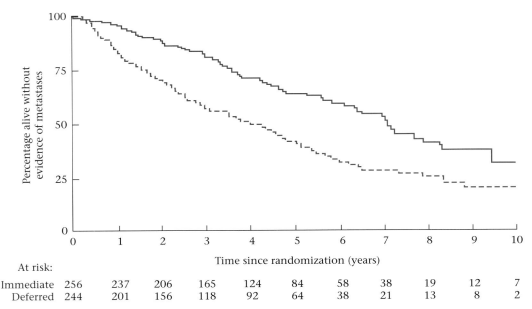

At risk:

Immediate	256	237	206	165	124	84	58	38	19	12	7
Deferred	244	201	156	118	92	64	38	21	13	8	2

Figure 27.1. MRC immediate vs deferred treatment study: progression to M1 disease. Patients entered as M0, immediate (——) vs deferred (-----) treatment (2p < 0.001). (From ref. 2 with permission.)

Table 27.3. MRC immediate vs deferred treatment study: major complications

		Treatment	
Complication	M stage	Immediate (*n* = 469)	Deferred (*n* = 465)
Pathological fracture	M0	3	6
	Mx	1	4
	M1	7	11
	Total	11	21
Cord compression	M0	3	3
	Mx	1	6
	M1*	5	14
	Total**	9	23
Ureteric obstruction[†]	M0	22	28
	Mx ***	1	12
	M1	10	15
	Total**	33	55
Extra skeletal metastases	M0	17	26
	Mx	7	9
	M1	13	20
	Total*	37	55

Asterisks indicate significant differences between treatments (*2p < 0.05; **2p < 0.025; *** 2p < 0.005), otherwise statistically non-significant.
[†]Excludes seven patients receiving local radiotherapy to the prostate.
(From ref 2. with permission.)

metastases are all more frequent in deferred patients. Although true statistical significance applies only to the overall differences, it seems clear that it is the patient who has metastatic disease at presentation who is most at risk. It should be noted that spinal cord compression often occurred *after* treatment had been started for another indication, possibly reflecting a greater disease load that might have been prevented by immediate treatment.

There is, overall, a clear difference in the numbers and rate of *prostate cancer* deaths in those randomized to deferred treatment (Figure 27.2a). Although overall survival from all causes of death is just statistically significant (Figure 27.2b), the difference is clearly much greater when only prostate cancer deaths are considered. From the statistician's viewpoint (R. Peto, personal communication) it is more correct to consider prostate cancer deaths not as part of the overall deaths, but to compare them with non-cancer deaths as independent events (Figure 27.3). Owing to the small numbers, the excess of non-cancer deaths in the immediate arm is not significant and, indeed, as data have matured, this discrepancy has become less marked.

The mortality outcome depends on metastatic status. For those with M0 disease, confirmed by a negative bone scan, both overall and prostate cancer

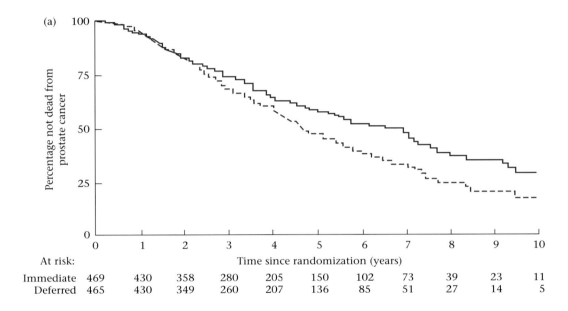

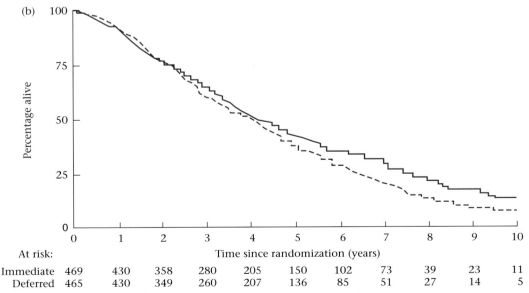

Figure 27.2. MRC immediate vs deferred treatment study: (a) survival curves for prostate cancer deaths; all patients, immediate (────) vs deferred (‗ ‗ ‗ ‗) treatment (2p = 0.001); (b) survival curves, death from all causes; all patients, immediate (────) vs deferred (‗ ‗ ‗ ‗) treatment (2p = 0.02). (From ref. 2, with permission.)

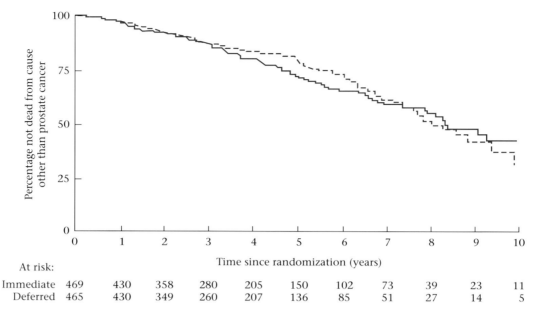

At risk:

Immediate	469	430	358	280	205	150	102	73	39	23	11
Deferred	465	430	349	260	207	136	85	51	27	14	5

Figure 27.3. MRC immediate vs deferred treatment study: survival curves, for deaths from causes other than prostate cancer; all patients, immediate (———) vs deferred (-----) treatment (2p = 0.5; NS). (From ref. 2, with permission).

survival was clearly better in the immediate treatment group (Figure 27.4), whereas in those with metastatic disease no difference in survival can be identified (Figure 27.5). Thus, as far as survival is concerned, the man with metastatic disease may not benefit from immediate treatment.

Of all patients who died during the study, 67% did so from prostate cancer, a proportion rising to 78% in those with M1 disease on entry. The relevant figures in the VACURG studies were 41 and 50% respectively.[3] Clearly, improvements in life expectation now make prostate cancer a more potent cause of death, and reduce the chance of a man avoiding the need for treatment — reflected in the fact that few men entered under the age of 70 died from other causes before treatment was started (Table 27.2).

Discussion

Although 70% of patients entered into the study have now died, in some aspects the data remain immature and others will always remain open to debate. The results will be considered in the context of the issues raised earlier in this chapter. Overall, in these patients, immediate treatment has produced an improvement in survival. This requires qualification in two respects: first, the improvement in survival is highly significant for cancer deaths, but only just reaches significance for all causes of death: second, the improved survival is only apparent in those with M0 disease confirmed on entry. The second point is discussed in detail later; the first is to be expected in a disease that affects elderly men. In effect, the improved survival resulting from delay in *cancer* death allows some of the patients to live longer, only to die from another cause. Indeed, the rate of non-cancer deaths (Figure 27.3) implies that 50% of these patients would have died within 7 years even if they had not had prostate cancer, and the impact on overall survival is as good as can be expected (R. Peto, personal communication). The advantages of deferring treatment are that, for those with M0 disease, on average, treatment will not be needed for 27 months, whereas for those with metastases mean treatment delay is 9 months. About 10% of men will escape treatment before they

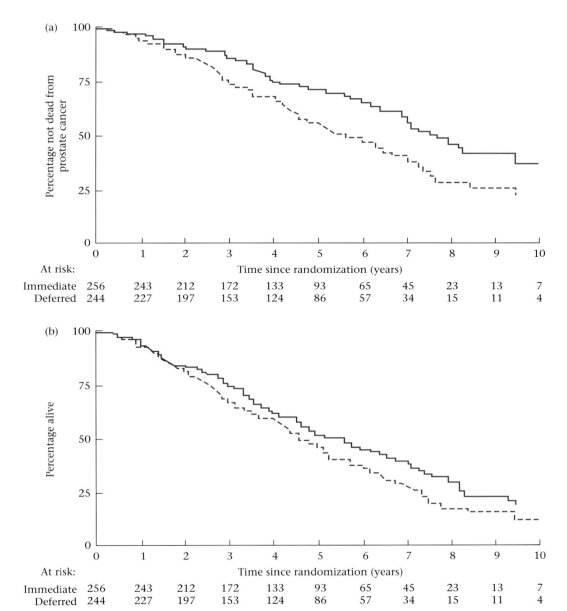

Figure 27.4. MRC immediate vs deferred treatment study: (a) survival curves for prostate cancer deaths; patients entered as M0 (2p = 0.0003, immediate (———) vs deferred (-----)); (b) survival curves, death from all causes; patients entered as M0 (2p = 0.02, immediate (———) vs deferred (-----)). (From ref. 2, with permission.)

die from other causes, although this is unlikely in men under the age of 70, or with metastatic disease. On the other hand, 5% of men will die from prostate cancer before receiving treatment — a problem found by others in the practice of deferred treatment.[10]

As far as the other issues raised earlier are concerned, it is clear that, untreated, local disease will progress and substantially increase the need for a further TURP. Local progression to ureteric obstruction, and the most serious consequences of metastatic disease — spinal cord compression and pathological fracture — are more common if treatment is deferred, especially in those with metastatic disease. There seems to be an absolute increase in the occurrence of these complications, rather than that they simply occur sooner in the deferred group. It is also apparent

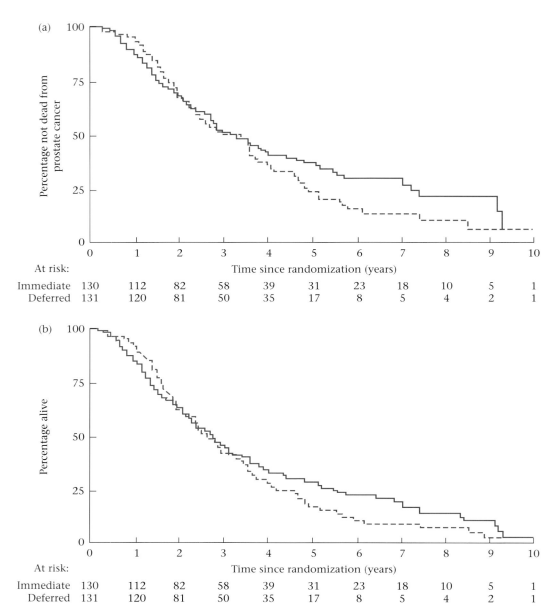

Figure 27.5. MRC immediate vs deferred treatment study: (a) survival curves for prostate cancer deaths; patients entered as M1 (2p = 0.2; NS, immediate (———) vs deferred (- - - -)); survival curves, death from all causes; patients entered as M1 (2p = 0.2; NS, immediate (———) vs deferred (- - - -)).

that many of the instances of spinal cord compression occur after treatment has been started for other reasons; perhaps the delay in treatment has, indeed, allowed tumour bulk to increase and be less readily controlled by treatment when it is started.

Why is a survival benefit from immediate treatment seen only in those with non-metastatic disease? This may in part be due to the smaller numbers of patients with metastases at entry into the study, and the shorter interval to treatment; a difference might have become apparent with larger numbers of M1 patients. Furthermore, of those dying from cancer before receiving deferred treatment, many were M0 on entry, and this may have contributed to the difference. However, assuming some of the difference is biological, this result has a bearing on the question of hormone sensitivity. A patient with M0 disease on average is not treated for over 2 years, and is treated because his disease has progressed; a loss of hormone sensitivity on progression would explain the detrimental effect on survival. The man with metastases already has advanced disease and will be treated within a few months; a change in hormone sensitivity is unlikely and hence no survival difference is apparent. These results do provide confirmation of the hypothesis of loss of hormone sensitivity suggested by circumstantial evidence from earlier studies.[7,8]

In practical terms, these results give little comfort to the supporters of deferred treatment. For those with metastatic disease, the majority are not going to escape treatment, usually within a few months, and on these grounds, it seems reasonable to recommend that deferred treatment is not considered for men under 70. Although no clear adverse effect on survival is apparent in those with M1 disease, there will be an increased chance that during this relatively short survival period a further TURP will be required, as happened to 31 of 131 (24%) deferred M1 patients, compared with 11 of 130 (8%) treated immediately. The chances of sustaining spinal cord compression or other complications seem greater. As 224 of 261 patients with metastatic disease already have died, it is likely that the overall incidence of these complications will remain higher in the deferred group.

In patients with non-metastatic disease, the advantages of deferring treatment are greater. Treatment will, on average, be delayed for over 2 years and, in those over 70, there is a reasonable chance that they might avoid treatment in their lifetime. However, these benefits are at the expense of a definite chance of dying earlier from prostate cancer than if treatment had been started immediately, and of requiring further treatment for local recurrence although, at this stage of follow-up, an increased risk of more serious complications is less apparent in M0 patients.

It is important to emphasize that this study is not without significant deficiencies. Its very simplicity does mean that data available on the patients are limited. The study started before prostate-specific antigen (PSA) measurement was widely available and it is impossible to determine whether a subgroup of patients suitable for deferred treatment could be identified by PSA level at diagnosis or by PSA velocity over the early months of follow-up.[12] Similarly, there are no quality-of-life data available to quantify the side effects of hormone treatment against the clear benefits of hormone treatment in slowing disease progression. As a result, the author feels that these data, although contributing significantly to the argument about timing of treatment, must be discussed carefully and the final outcome of the study must await full maturity when most of the patients have died.

Is deferred treatment still acceptable? Hot flushes and loss of potency may still be significant problems for some men. The author has a policy of discussing management issues with the patient and, even after introducing the results of the MRC study into such conversations, some men are still reluctant to start treatment when they have no appreciable symptoms. In such cases, the author's practice is to advise regular monitoring of PSA. If this suggests rapid tumour progression, treatment is then started. Otherwise, accepting that a stable PSA is not entirely reliable,[13] careful follow-up is mandatory. It is essential, if treatment is deferred, that the patient and his general practitioner are fully aware of the situation. However, it is the author's impression that the climate is already swinging away from deferred treatment and that the results of the MRC study will be taken as confirmation of this.

Acknowledgements

More than 60 British urologists contributed to the MRC Study, which would not have been conceived without the statistical input from Professor Richard Peto. The data collection was performed by the staff of the Clinical Trial Service Unit, Oxford, ably assisted by the author's research secretaries, Mrs Jean Breakey, Mrs Anne McGregor and Ms Louise Neeson Jurcsyk. The statistical analysis of the trial data has been capably performed by Dr Jillian Boreham. Without these and many others, the results described in this chapter would not have been obtained.

References

1. Kirk D. Immediate versus deferred treatment for advanced disease. In: Oliver R T D, Belldegrun A and Wrigley P M F (eds) Preventing prostate cancer: screening versus chemoprevention. Cancer Surveys 23. New York: Cold Spring Harbor Laboratory Press, 1995: 183–190
2. The Medical Research Council Prostate Cancer Working Party Investigators Group. Immediate versus deferred treatment for advanced prostatic cancer: initial results of the Medical Research Council Trial. Br J Urol 1997; 79: 235–246.
3. Byar D P. The Veterans Administration Cooperative Research Group's studies of cancer of the prostate. Cancer 1973; 32: 1126–1130
4. Kirk D. Trials and tribulations in prostatic cancer. Br J Urol 1987; 59: 375–379
5. Kirk D. Deferred treatment for advanced prostatic cancer. In: Waxman J, Williams G (eds) Urological oncology. Sevenoaks: Edward Arnold,1991: 117–125
6. Kozlowski J M, Ellis W J, Grayhack J T. Advanced prostatic carcinoma. Early versus late endocrine therapy. Urol Clin North Am 1991; 15: 15–24
7. Crawford E D, Eisenberger M A, McLeod D G et al. A controlled trial of leuprolide with and without flutamide in prostatic carcinoma. N Engl J Med 1989; 321: 419–424
8. Nesbit R M, Baum W C. Endocrine control of prostatic cancer. Clinical survey of 1818 cases. JAMA 1950; 143: 1317–1320
9. Parker M C, Cook A, Riddle P R et al. Is delayed treatment justified in carcinoma of the prostate? Br J Urol 1985; 57: 724–728
10. Carr T W, Handley R C, Travis D et al. Deferred treatment of prostate cancer. Br J Urol 1988; 62: 249–253
11. Kirk D. Prostatic carcinoma. Br Med J 1985; 290: 875–876
12. Armitage T G, Cooper E H, Newling D W W et al. The value of measurements of serum prostate specific antigen in patients with benign prostatic hyperplasia and untreated prostate cancer. Br J Urol 1988; 62: 584–589
13. Josefsen D, Waehre H, Paus E, Fossa S D. Increase in serum prostate specific antigen and clinical progression in pN+ M0 prostate cancer. Br J Urol 1995; 75: 502–506

Chapter 28
Optimizing combined androgen blockade in prostate cancer
F. Labrie

Introduction

Prostate cancer is the second most frequent cause of cancer death in men in the Western world, and its medicosocial impact is close to that of breast cancer in women. In fact, it was predicted that 40,400 men would die from prostate cancer in the United States in 1996.[1] As population ages, the incidence of prostate cancer is expected to increase further, with graver consequences and an increased financial burden for the health care system, thus indicating the urgent need for improvement in diagnosis and treatment of this disease. The annual health care costs, largely related to treatment of advanced and terminal disease, are estimated at US$4.5 billion in the United States.[2]

The best-known and unanimously recognized characteristic of prostate cancer is its high sensitivity to androgen deprivation. In fact, among all hormone-sensitive cancers, prostate cancer shows the best response to endocrine therapy. Accordingly, since 1941, the standard and exclusive treatment of advanced metastatic disease has been androgen deprivation.[3] The two most relevant questions concerning endocrine therapy are (1) what is the best endocrine therapy in 1997 and (2) when should treatment be started? The results of recent clinical trials indicate that there are good reasons to believe that hormone therapy, in addition to remaining the first-line treatment of advanced disease, should now be part of any treatment of early-stage disease; endocrine therapy should thus be part of therapy or the single therapy of any patient treated for prostate cancer.

What are the sources of androgens regulating prostatic growth?

Before deciding on the best endocrine therapy, it is important to review briefly the most recent information about the endocrinology of the prostate. Until recently, it was believed that 95% of androgens were of testicular origin.[4] This erroneous opinion was based on the misleading observation that plasma levels of testosterone are 95% reduced following orchiectomy[3] or treatment with a luteinizing hormone-releasing hormone (LHRH) agonist,[5] thus leading to the belief that the 95% decrease in the serum testosterone concentration seen after castration was equivalent to the elimination of 95% of all androgens. As described below, this conclusion has to be drastically changed, since castration eliminates only 50–60% and not 95% of androgens in men of prostate cancer age. As indicated in more detail later, measurement of serum testosterone alone is not a reliable parameter of the intracellular action of androgens. Moreover, although castration leads to a positive response in 60–80% of patients with advanced prostate cancer, thus improving quality of life, such treatment has never been shown to prolong life.[6]

Relative importance of testicular and adrenal androgens

Although castration (orchiectomy or treatment with an LHRH agonist) causes a 95% reduction in serum testosterone concentration, a much smaller effect is seen on the only meaningful indicator of androgenic action in the prostate, namely the concentration of dihydrotestosterone (DHT) in the prostatic tissue itself. In fact, after elimination of testicular androgens by medical or surgical castration, the intraprostatic concentration of DHT remains at about 40% of that measured in intact men (Figure 28.1a). As another measure of the importance of adrenal androgens in adult men, the serum levels of the main metabolites of androgens, namely androstane-3α, 17β-diol-glucuronide (3α-diol-G) and androsterone-glucuronide (ADT-G), are reduced by only 50–70% following castration, thus reflecting the high level of adrenal precursor steroids converted into DHT in peripheral tissues (including the prostate) in castrated men (Figure 28.1b). Contrary to the wrong belief that the testes are responsible for 95% of total androgen production in men, as suggested by simple measurement of circulating serum testosterone, it is now well established that the prostatic tissue efficiently transforms the inactive steroid precursors dehydroepiandrosterone sulphate (DHEA-S) and DHEA, into the active androgen DHT. In fact, the prostate synthesizes its own androgens from adrenal precursors in quantities comparable to those of testicular origin.

It is important to recognize that, although LHRH agonists offer a more acceptable method of castration that is free of the important side effects of high doses of oestrogens, it cannot be expected that the prognosis of prostate cancer

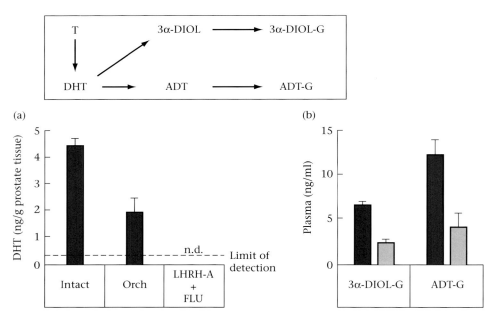

Figure 28.1. (a) Effect of orchiectomy (Orch) and combination therapy (addition of flutamide to orchiectomy or treatment with an LHRH superagonist) on the concentration of DHT in human prostatic cancer tissue. Note that orchiectomy has only a partial inhibitory effect (approximately 60% reduction), whereas the addition of flutamide to castration decreases intraprostatic DHT to undetectable levels (n.d.). The lower limit of sensitivity of DHT measurement is 0.2 ng DHT/g tissue. About 40% of DHT thus remains in the prostatic cancer after castration, thus illustrating the need to block such a high level of androgens of adrenal origin left free to stimulate growth of prostate cancer after castration. (b) Effect of castration (■, intact; ▩, castrated) on serum levels of the main metabolites of DHT, namely, androsterone-glucuronide (ADT-G) and androstane-3α,17β-diol-glucuronide (3α-diol-G).

will be improved beyond the results achieved with orchiectomy, because the effects of LHRH agonists are also limited to blockade of testicular androgens and have no influence on the secretion of DHEA-S and DHEA by the adrenals.

Enzymes responsible for androgen formation in the prostate

To stimulate prostatic growth, the adrenal steroid precursors DHEA-S and DHEA must be taken up by the prostatic tissue and be locally transformed into active androgens. As illustrated in Figure 28.2, the formation of the active androgen DHT

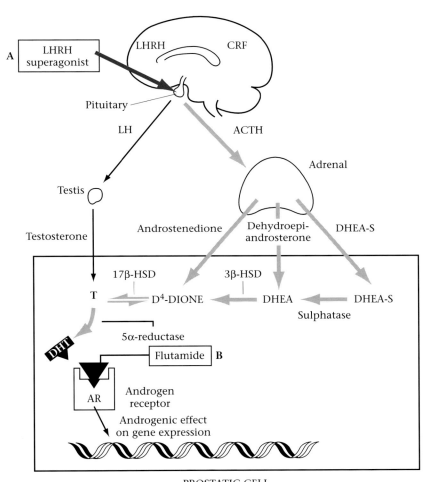

Figure 28.2. Schematic representation of the effect of combination therapy with an LHRH agonist and a pure anti-androgen (flutamide) on prostate cancer growth and of the biosynthetic steps involved in the formation of the active androgen dihydrotestosterone (DHT) from testicular testosterone as well as from the adrenal precursors dehydroepiandrosterone (DHEA), DHEA sulphate (DHEA-S), and androstenedione (Δ^4-dione) in human prostatic tissue. (17β-HSD, 17β-hydroxysteroid dehydrogenase; 3β-HSD, 3β-hydroxysteroid dehydrogenase/Δ^5-Δ^4-isomerase. The testis secretes testosterone (T), which is transformed into the more potent androgen DHT by 5α-reductase in the prostate. Instead of secreting T or DHT directly, the adrenal secretes large amounts of DHEA and DHEA-S which are transported in the blood to the prostate and other peripheral tissues. These inactive precursors are then transformed locally into the active androgens T and DHT. The genes encoding DHEA sulphatase, 3β-HSD, 17β-HSD and 5α-reductase are all expressed in the prostatic cells, thus providing 40–50% of total DHT in this tissue. The anti-androgen blocks the access of DHT to the androgen receptor, thus greatly reducing the influence of androgens on genetic expression and prostate cancer cell growth, while testicular testosterone secretion is completely blocked by the LHRH agonist or surgical castration (orchiectomy).

from DHEA involves three enzymatic activities, these are: 3β-hydroxysteroid dehydrogenase/Δ^5–Δ^4 isomerase (3β-HSD), 17β-hydroxysteroid dehydrogenase (17β-HSD), and 5α-reductase. Alternatively, DHEA can be transformed into androst-5-ene-3β,17β-diol (5-diol) by 17β-HSD, whereas 3β-HSD catalyses the conversion of the latter into testosterone.

The structure of two 3β-HSD, five 17β-HSD and two 5α-reductase human enzymes has been elucidated.[7–9] The expression of genes encoding each of these three categories of enzymatic activities has been demonstrated in the human prostate, thus providing the basis for the high level of DHT formation from DHEA in this tissue.[7] This new field of endocrinology has been called intracrinology.[10] This area offers great promise for future therapeutic developments, since it relates to the formation of active steroids in peripheral (intracrine) tissues from inactive adrenal precursors. These steroids, made locally, act directly in the cells where their synthesis takes place, without being released in the extracellular compartment, thus requiring much smaller amounts of steroids and avoiding unnecessary exposure of other tissues. These intracrine tissues, such as the human prostate, can thus control the synthesis and the inactivation of androgens according to the local needs.[10]

Combination endocrine therapy in metastatic disease

On the basis of the knowledge that the testes and the adrenals contribute about equally to androgen formation in men, combination therapy was developed to block simultaneously testicular and adrenal androgens at the start of therapy in advanced prostate cancer[11] (Figure 28.2). The benefits of combination therapy, first described in 1982, have been confirmed by all four large-scale, double-blind and placebo-controlled randomized studies[12–15] (Table 28.1). In fact, these pivotal studies have confirmed and demonstrated the important advantages of combination therapy using a pure anti-androgen and an LHRH agonist (or orchiectomy) on all the objective and subjective parameters measured. Of particular importance is the observation that the simple addition of flutamide added, on average, 7.3 (ref. 13) and 15.1 (ref. 14) months of life, whereas the use of an analogue of flutamide (Eulexin), namely, nilutamide (Anandron), added 5.4 (ref. 12) and 4.1 (ref. 15) months of life, respectively (Table 28.1). Studies that have not shown a benefit of combination therapy have had methodological problems such as too few patients, inclusion of other than stage D$_2$ patients, and no double-blind or placebo control.[16–18]

In three of the combination therapy studies,[13–15] the anti-androgen was added to the control arm at the time of progression, this addition leading to little or no significant benefit. Such results clearly demonstrate the absolute need to use combination therapy at the start of treatment instead of at the time of relapse following failure of standard therapy. The above-indicated observations argue extremely strongly against a two-step approach for the treatment of prostate cancer. It is thus clear that combination therapy should always be applied as first-line therapy because the same treatment loses much of its efficacy when used as second-line therapy at the time of relapse following monotherapy.

This approach of maximal androgen blockade at start of therapy is well supported by the well-known observation that patients relapsing after castration or treatment with oestrogens, LHRH agonists or an anti-androgen alone have a poor or nil response to adrenalectomy, hypophysectomy or flutamide.[11] Moreover, strong support for the harmful effect of exposure of prostate cancer cells to low androgen levels is provided by the observation that low serum testosterone levels

Table 28.1. Combination therapy with a pure anti-androgen and castration in stage D2 disease: double-blind, randomized, placebo-controlled and prospective studies

Study	No. of patients	Best response	No response	Pain relief	PSA or PAP normalization	Duration of response (months)	Death due to cancer (months)	Death from all causes (months)
Béland et al.[12]*	194	46% vs 20% $p < 0.01$	20% vs 38% $p < 0.01$	$p < 0.05$	$p < 0.05$	Positive trend		24.3 vs 18.9 (5.4) $p < 0.05$
National Cancer Institute[13]†	602	$p < 0.05$		$p < 0.05$	$p < 0.05$	16.9 vs 13.8 (3.1)[a] $p < 0.05$		35.6 vs 28.3 (7.3) $p < 0.05$
Janknegt et al.[15]*,‡	423	41% vs 24% $p < 0.001$	22% vs 36% $p < 0.002$	$p < 0.05$	$p < 0.05$	19.0 vs 14.9 (4.1) $p = 0.006$	37.1 vs 29.8 (7.3)	27.3 vs 24.2 (4.1)
European Organization for Research and Treatment of Cancer[14]‡	327	–	–	$p < 0.05$	$p < 0.05$	30.7 vs 19.6 (11.1) $p = 0.008$	43.9 vs 28.8 (15.1) $p = 0.007$	34.4 vs 27.1 (7.3) $p = 0.02$

*Nilutamide and orchiectomy *vs* orchiectomy as control.
†Flutamide and luteinizing hormone-releasing hormone (LHRH) agonist *vs* LHRH agonist as control.
‡Flutamide and LHRH agonist *vs* orchiectomy as control.
NS, not significant; PAP, prostatic acid phosphatase; PSA, prostate-specific antigen.
[a] = Data in parentheses = difference in months.

are associated with shorter survival following androgen deprivation.[19] In fact, low pretreatment serum testosterone levels before the start of endocrine therapy are associated with a poor prognosis, this variable being even more important than the extent of bone metastases.[19] Such clinical data are well supported by the laboratory findings that low levels of androgens comparable to those found after castration in men induce the development of androgen-hypersensitive tumours that are resistant to antihormonal therapy.[20]

Since partial blockade of androgens (orchiectomy, LHRH agonist or anti-androgen alone) leads to shorter survival,[11–15] it appears unethical to use any therapy having lower androgen-blocking capacity than the combination therapy with a pure anti-androgen in association with surgical or medical castration. The choice of a pure anti-androgen is important in order to achieve maximal androgen blockade. It should be mentioned that, using pure anti-androgens, a prolongation of life could be demonstrated in prostate cancer,[11,13–15] whereas no such benefit could be obtained in metastatic breast cancer where treatment of early disease but not of metastatic disease has shown increased survival.[21]

Redefining advanced disease

It is clear, however, that treatment of prostate cancer at the advanced metastatic stage with even the best treatment available — namely combination therapy using a pure anti-androgen — although providing major benefits in terms of disease-free survival, decreased pain, improved quality of life and even prolongation of life, cannot provide a cure. Fortunately, major progress has been achieved during recent years, by many groups, in the diagnosis and treatment of early-stage prostate cancer, and much information has been obtained on the natural history of the disease. The recent developments in the rational use of serum prostate-specific antigen (PSA) and transrectal ultrasonography (TRUS) of the prostate now permit the diagnosis of prostate cancer at a clinically localized stage in almost all patients.[22] Previously, 'watchful waiting', or deferred treatment, has been suggested as an alternative for patients diagnosed as having localized prostate cancer. However, the observation that, at all ages below 75 years, men with non-metastatic prostatic cancer who do not receive immediate curative therapy have a greater than 50% risk of dying from the disease,[23] poses very serious doubts about deferred treatment. Figure 28.3 illustrates the best estimate of local progression, distant metastases and death from prostate cancer for patients with clinically localized prostate cancer choosing deferred treatment when diagnosed at different ages.

Unfortunately, despite the use of the most efficient diagnostic procedures available, prostate cancer has already migrated outside the prostate at time of first diagnosis in approximately 50% of cases (Figure 28.4). Consequently, the most serious limitation to the curative approaches of clinically localized prostate cancer is that, in approximately 50% of cases, the cancer is found to have already migrated outside the prostate at histopathological examination of the surgical specimen, thus making the surgery performed of doubtful utility.[24–30] As an example, only 51% of 157 stage T1c (non palpable prostate cancers diagnosed by needle biopsy) were organ-confined (no capsular penetration) with 17% having positive margins.[31] Moreover, of 439 cases of stage T2 (palpable) cancer, organ-confined disease was limited to 34% and surgical margins were positive in 43%. In another study,[32] 70% of 60 stage T1c cancers were organ-confined but 23% had positive margins. Such data indicate that a large proportion of stage T1c tumours become incurable by surgery before they are diagnosed.

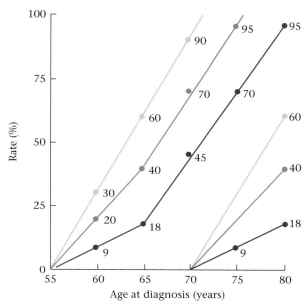

Figure 28.3. Estimate of rates of local progression (——), distant metastases (——) and death (from prostate cancer) (——) in patients diagnosed as having clinically localized prostate cancer at the ages of 55 and 70 years, and receiving deferred treatment or watchful waiting. (From ref. 76 with permission.)

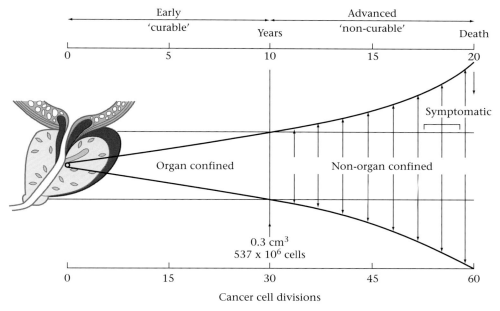

Figure 28.4. Estimated critical volume of prostate cancer. At a volume larger than 0.3 cm³, 537 × 10⁶ cells or 30 cancer cell divisions, there is high risk of extracapsular extension and micrometastases. (From ref. 76 with permission.)

Since the critical volume of prostate cancer, before cancer cells migrate outside the prostate, is estimated at 0.3 cm³ (~ 7.5 mm in diameter, if spherical, or 0.5 ng PSA/ml), early diagnosis becomes of crucial importance to avoid incurable disease. However, this critical volume of tumours is at the limit of sensitivity of the available diagnostic procedures, namely PSA assays, digital rectal examination and TRUS of the prostate, even when the procedures are combined. Consequently, it has to be concluded that screening is not sensitive enough to detect clinically insignificant cancers. In fact, even with the best screening procedures, about 50% of cancers are not confined to the prostate at time of diagnosis.[22] Our knowledge of the threshold of biological significance of prostate cancer has thus changed dramatically (Figure 28.4). With this information, we should now consider prostate cancer outside the prostate as advanced disease, thus indicating the need for an earlier diagnosis and/or an efficient treatment of micrometastases.

Combined androgen blockade in association with surgery or radiotherapy

A means of increasing the proportion of patients with organ-confined disease and cancer-negative margins was suggested by the well-known clinical observation that patients with metastatic prostate cancer treated by combination therapy, using a pure anti-androgen associated with medical or surgical castration, show a much more rapid and marked regression of their cancer in the prostatic area than at distant metastatic sites.[11,33,34] Moreover, it is well recognized that, when recurrence of the disease occurs in a patient with advanced prostate cancer treated with combination therapy, progression of the cancer at the level of the prostate is a rare event whereas, as a rule, the bones are the usual site of progression. Since prostate cancer localized in the prostatic area is so highly sensitive to androgen deprivation, it seemed logical to use combination therapy to downstage prostate cancer in men diagnosed as having localized disease before radical surgical prostatectomy, cryosurgery, radiotherapy or brachytherapy, and to use adjuvant endocrine therapy to cause further apoptosis or cell death of the micrometastases not under the control of surgery or radiotherapy or brachytherapy.[35–38]

Radical prostatectomy and androgen blockade

A few randomized trials have studied the potential benefits of combination therapy using flutamide and an LHRH agonist administered for 3 months before radical prostatectomy.[38–42] The first randomized trial analysed the rates of organ-confined and specimen-confined disease and compared the definite stage at histopathological examination of the surgical specimen with the clinical stage estimated at diagnosis.[38,39] In that study, neoadjuvant combination therapy before radical prostatectomy decreased cancer-positive surgical margins from 33.8% in the control group to only 7.8%, thus giving 92.2% of patients with negative margins at surgery (Figure 28.5b). Although, on average, the final stage determined by histopathological examination of the surgical specimen was more advanced than predicted at initial diagnosis in 33.8% of control patients, the opposite was noted in the group of men who received the 3-month neoadjuvant combination therapy; in this group, the final stage at surgery, instead of being more advanced, was less advanced than that at diagnosis in an average of 21.1% of men for a net 54% improvement of staging in favour of combination therapy. The most important endpoint, organ-confined disease, on the other hand, increased from 49.3 to 77.8% of patients after 3 months of combination therapy, for a 57.8% increase in the incidence of organ-confined disease (Figure 28.5a). No cancer was found in six (6.7%) prostatectomy specimens from the treated group.

Almost superimposable results have been obtained by Soloway et al.[40] and Fair et al.,[43] while Schulman et al.,[41] in a population of patients showing more advanced disease, have also found comparable results. In fact, Soloway et al.[40] reported that, among 303 men with clinical stage T2b prostate cancer, patients treated for 3 months with flutamide and lupron showed an increase in organ-confined disease, from 47% in those who had radical prostatectomy alone to 78%

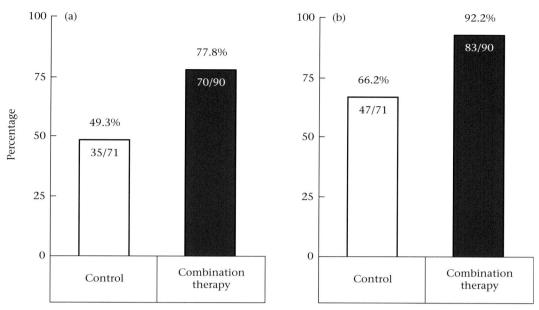

Figure 28.5. Effect of 3-month neo-adjuvant combination therapy with flutamide and an LHRH agonist on (a) organ-confined disease and (b) specimen-confined disease in localized prostate cancer (T1/T2). (From ref. 38 with permission.)

in patients who had neoadjuvant combination therapy for only 3 months. Moreover, the rate of positive margins decreased from 48 to 18% in the same groups.

Other studies also showed that combination endocrine therapy decreases the total volume of the prostate and of the cancer.[36,42,44–48] Several studies confirmed that neoadjuvant androgen deprivation markedly reduces the incidence of positive margins.[43,49–51]

Radiation therapy and androgen blockade

Particularly important data have been obtained with the association of radiation therapy and androgen blockade. Thus, in 456 evaluable patients, the cumulative incidence of local progression at 5 years was 46% in patients who received combination therapy with flutamide 2 months before and 2 months during radiotherapy (group 1), compared with 71% in the group of men who had radiotherapy alone.[35] Progression-free survival rates, including normal serum PSA at 5 years, were 36% in group 1 versus 15% in patients who received radiotherapy alone. No significant effect was observed on survival. In such a population of locally advanced disease (70% stage T3, T4 or C and 30% T2 or stage B2), the short 4-month treatment with combination therapy led to an impressive increase in local control and disease-free survival compared with pelvic irradiation alone. Recent evaluation of Radiation Therapy Oncology Group (RTOG) data has shown prolongation of life in stage T3 patients who received androgen blockade associated with radiation therapy, compared with radiation therapy alone.

For the first time, improved survival has been demonstrated recently in localized prostate cancer. In fact, treatment with an LHRH agonist, at the onset of radiation therapy for a period of 3 years, not only improved local control by 27% (compared with control) but also increased survival by 39%.[52] At median follow-up of 33 months, estimated local control was achieved in 95% of men who received endocrine therapy versus only 75% of those who had radiation therapy alone. On the other hand, the survival rate was 78% in the endocrine-treated patients compared with 56% in the patients who had radiation therapy alone.[52] The LHRH agonist was administered monthly for 3 years, beginning on the first day of radiotherapy, whereas the steroidal mixed anti-androgenic–androgenic compound cyproterone acetate was administered for 1 month only at the start of therapy. Such findings are extremely important since, hitherto, treatment of localized prostate cancer was thought by many to bring no significant advantage to prostate cancer patients,[53] thus making it possible to recommend deferred treatment with its well-recognized high level of risk of death from prostate cancer.[54]

As support for the data of Pilepich et al.,[35] Bolla et al.[52] and Laverdière et al.,[37] similar prostate tumour destruction was found with lower doses of radiation therapy in castrated rats than in intact animals receiving the same radiation therapy. Moreover, optimal results were obtained when radiation therapy was applied at the time of maximal response to androgen deprivation.[55]

Importance of combined androgen blockade

Because the aim of androgen blockade is to cause a maximal reduction in prostatic androgen levels in order to induce maximal atrophy, apoptosis, and death of prostate cancer cells, combination therapy using a pure anti-androgen[11,33,56] in association with an LHRH agonist is the most logical approach. The use of an LHRH agonist alone, an anti-androgen alone, or an inhibitor of androgen formation alone, is not recommended because partial blockade of androgens is likely to induce the development of tumours resistant to androgen blockade.[57–59] This would be of major concern to patients having incomplete removal of the cancer cells at radical prostatectomy or cryosurgery or incomplete cell kill by radiation therapy or brachytherapy, since those patients would be left with cancer cells potentially less sensitive to combined androgen deprivation administered later at the time of recurrence of the disease. It is, in fact, well known that the addition of flutamide to castrated patients in progression shows limited efficacy compared with its use as first treatment.[11,13]

An example of the importance of combined androgen blockade is provided by the observation that treatment with an LHRH agonist and flutamide decreased positive surgical margins from 39% in control patients to 24%, whereas 45% of positive surgical margins were found after treatment with cyproterone acetate alone, a therapy equivalent to castration.[49] Moreover, whereas a 47.4% decrease in prostate size was observed at 6 months of combination therapy using castration and flutamide, a decrease of only 30.9% was observed when flutamide was used alone over the same period.[60]

Effect of combined androgen blockade alone in localized disease

As mentioned above, prostate cancer is the most sensitive of all cancers to hormone deprivation. It is also clear that the responsiveness to androgen deprivation is greatest at the earliest stage of disease. It thus seems logical to concentrate our efforts on finding the optimal duration of treatment and on the optimal efficacy of combined androgen blockade applied at a clinically localized stage of prostate cancer.

In this context, it seems important to summarize data recently obtained in a small series of patients with stage T1, T2, and T3 prostate cancer, who received long-term treatment with combined androgen blockade alone. These results were obtained in 26 previously untreated patients diagnosed as having clinically localized prostate cancer but who did not accept randomization to clinical trials including radical prostatectomy[38] or radiation therapy.[37] These patients received combination therapy alone, namely flutamide (250 mg, three times a day) and an LHRH agonist [(D-Trp[6], des-Gly-NH$_2$[10]) LHRH ethylamide] for a median duration of 7.1 years (range 2.8–11.8 years).

As illustrated in Figure 28.6, of the 26 patients, only one showed, during treatment, an increase of serum PSA, the first increase in PSA being observed after 8 years and 4 months of treatment. At 8 years and 4 months, the estimated response rate was thus 90% with a 95% confidence interval of 71–100%.

Since serum PSA remained undetectable up to a treatment duration of 11.8 years (median: 7.1 years) in all other patients, treatment was stopped in 17 patients. These patients have now been followed for a median duration of 2.44 years. As shown in Figure 28.7, four patients have shown progression of serum PSA after the withdrawal of therapy. Combination therapy has been reinstituted in these patients, whereupon serum PSA returned to undetectable levels. Including the median post-treatment follow-up of 2.44 years (up to 4.2 years) in the 17 patients who stopped combination therapy, median overall follow-up is 8.9 years, ranging from 2.8 to 14.1 years. One patient died at 8.4 years from a non-cancer-related cause.

The side effects of combination therapy are well tolerated; they include hot flushes, usually lasting for a few months at start of therapy, impotence, and loss of libido.[11,13,14] Unlike oestrogens, the combination of flutamide and an LHRH agonist leads to an improved lipid profile compared with orchiectomy.[61]

Such data clearly indicate that androgen deprivation is extremely effective for the treatment of clinically localized prostate cancer, its ability to control the disease in 26 patients for up to 8 years being possibly superior to that of radical prostatectomy and radiation therapy alone (Figure 28.8). Although a 15-year follow-up is required to assess the long-term effect of treatment of localized prostate cancer, local recurrence and especially serum PSA can be used as an

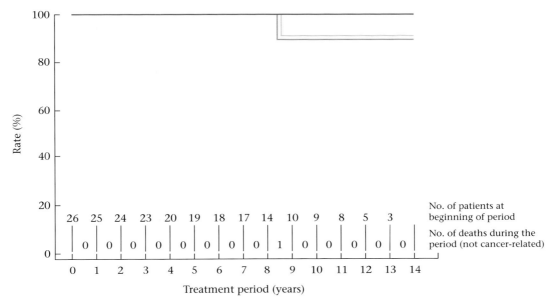

Figure 28.6. Disease-specific survival (———), overall survival (———), and progression-free survival (———) in 26 previously untreated patients with clinically localized prostate cancer who received treatment with combined androgen blockade alone, with the anti-androgen flutamide and the LHRH agonist [D-Trp[6], des-Gly-NH$_2$[10]] LHH ethylamide for the time intervals indicated (median: 7.1 years).

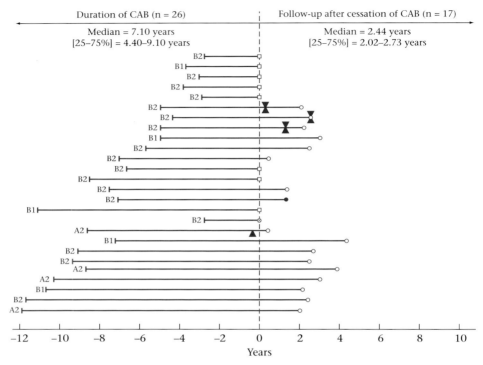

Figure 28.7. Illustration of the duration of endocrine therapy in four stage A2 patients, five stage B1 patients and 17 stage B2 patients with previously untreated prostate cancer, for a median duration of treatment of 7.1 years (up to 11.8 years). The first and only rise in serum PSA while patients were under treatment occurred at 8.3 years. Four patients showed a rising PSA after stopping treatment. No cancer-related death has yet occurred at a median follow-up of 7.1 years (up to 14.1 years). ○, alive evaluation; □, still on CAB at evaluation; ⊗, lost to follow-up; ▲, progression during CAB; ⏳, progression after cessation of CAB; ●, death (from non-cancer related causes).

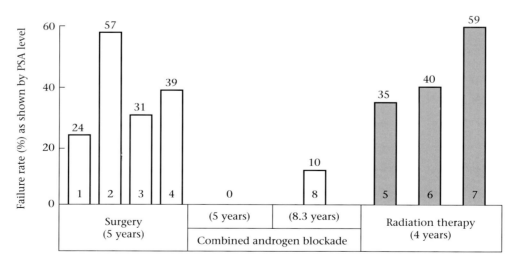

Figure 28.8. Comparison of the failure rate after combined androgen blockade (first failure at 8.3 years in this study versus failure rates of 24%, 57%, 31%, and 39% at 5 years after radical prostatectomy and 35%, 40%, and 59% 4 years after start of radiation therapy: 1-Morton et al., 1991 (ref. 62); 2-Zietman et al., 1994 (ref. 63); 3- Trapassp et al., 1994 (ref. 78); 4-Kupelian et al., 1996 (ref. 79); 5-Zietman et al., 1994 (ref. 64); 6-Kaplan et al., 1993 (ref. 80); 7-Goad et al., 1993 (ref. 81); 8-Labrie et al., 1996 (this study).

interim yardstick to evaluate efficacy.[11,62–64] Moreover, without a randomized study, it is not possible strictly to compare one clinical series with another.

The present data indicate that prostate cancer localized to the prostatic area is (almost) exclusively composed of androgen-sensitive cell clones. In contrast, when prostate cancer becomes metastatic, usually in the bones, it progressively loses its sensitivity to androgens and can grow under the stimulatory influence of other factors, probably local growth factors; thus, the response to androgen ablation progressively wanes.

In addition to survival benefits, combination therapy alone in older men prevents the complications of local recurrence, including urinary obstruction and other signs and symptoms related to enlargement of the tumour in the prostate, thus improving the quality of life. For patients having a longer than 10-year life expectancy and those unwilling to receive continuous combination therapy for such a long period, the present data clearly support the long-term (possibly 5 years) use of neoadjuvant and adjuvant combination therapy in association with radical prostatectomy, radiotherapy or brachytherapy to control extraprostatic micrometastatic disease and thus improve the success of surgery and radiotherapy.

Duration of combination therapy

Inasmuch as there is no doubt that androgen deprivation causes apoptosis or death of prostate cancer cells,[65] it has become equally clear that 3 months of neoadjuvant combination therapy, as used in many studies,[18,38,40] is too short to cause maximal cell death. In fact, after 3 months of combination therapy, 22% of cancers are found not to be organ confined at histopathological examination (Figure 28.5a), thus leaving at least 22% of patients with no cure following radical prostatectomy. Moreover, one should take into account the fact that 15% of organ-confined disease at surgery will ultimately show recurrence of the cancer as indicated by an elevation of serum PSA within 10 years.[66] Since there is a 15% risk of an increase in serum PSA within 10 years after radical prostatectomy in patients with organ-confined disease at surgery, it seems appropriate to reduce by 15% the probability of cure in patients who have organ-confined disease following radical prostatectomy alone (50 – 8 = 42%) as well as following 3 months of combination therapy (78 – 12 = 66%).

Following 3 months of combination therapy, one can thus estimate that only 66% of patients are potentially cured, thus leaving 44% of patients with the risk of recurrence of the disease within 10 years. This is likely to explain the relatively high rate of recurrence of rising PSA in patients who had only 3 months of neoadjuvant endocrine therapy before surgery.[43,50,51] In fact, a difference of potential cure of only 24% (66 vs 42%) can be estimated between the patients who had radical prostatectomy alone and those who had endocrine therapy for 3 months before surgery, thus making it difficult to demonstrate a statistical difference between the two groups in terms of rising PSA at follow-up visits. Moreover, it is likely that rising PSA will be first seen in the more advanced cases in both groups, with potential differences between the groups being expected only on long-term follow-up. A similar situation has been seen in advanced prostate cancer, where the more advanced cases progressed first in both groups and a significant difference between combination therapy and orchiectomy alone was seen clearly at longer follow-up, including a 15.1-month prolongation of cancer-specific survival.[67–69]

Using these numbers, the author has estimated the duration of combination therapy required to cause an optimal or near-100% rate of organ-confined disease.

The calculations illustrated in Figure 28.9 are thus based upon the data obtained regarding organ-confined disease with and without 3 months of neoadjuvant combination therapy (Figure 28.5a). The calculations shown in Figure 28.9 indicate the probability of organ-confined disease during the first 2 years plus 95% confidence interval. For the reasons outlined above, it has been assumed that 15% of organ-confined disease at surgery will ultimately lead to recurrence of the disease as indicated by an elevation of PSA within 10 years.[66] With no neoadjuvant combination therapy, the predicted cure rate is estimated at 42%, increasing to 66 and 79% following 3 and 6 months of combination therapy, respectively. The estimated cure rate then increases to 93% (79–98%) and 99% (91–99.9%) at 12 and 24 months, respectively, of combination therapy.

The previous choice of 3 months of neoadjuvant therapy[36] was motivated by the possibility of growth of prostate cancer while the patients were receiving neoadjuvant combination therapy before proceeding to the removal of the prostate by radical prostatectomy. However, the data now available show that localized prostate cancer does not progress for many years while the patient receives combination therapy alone[70-73] (Figures 28.6, 28.7). As mentioned above, a duration of combination therapy of at least 2 years and possibly 5 years is also supported by the data obtained in an analogous cancer, namely breast cancer, where an 18% increase in survival was observed at 10 years in women who received 5 years compared with 2 years of tamoxifen as adjuvant to surgery.[74]

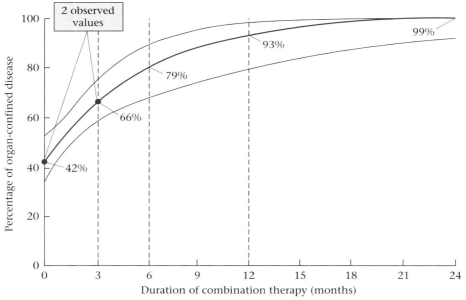

Figure 28.9. Estimate of optimal duration of combination therapy to reach the stage of organ-confined disease in localized prostate cancer. The expected rate of organ-confined disease has been calculated assuming that the benefit of the combination treatment would asymptomatically reach 100% according to a mono-exponential improvement with a non-zero initial value. The equation therefore reads: % organ-confined = 1 – A* exp(–Alpha*Duration), where A is fixed by the initial value that is given by the percentage of organ-confined disease with no treatment (1–A = 49.3% ± 5.9). The time constant is derived from the rate of organ-confined disease at 3 months (77.8% ± 4.4). These data are available from a previous clinical study,[38] and standard deviations are calculated using the normal distribution approximation for rates. Confidence intervals of the model predictions were further obtained by Monte Carlo simulation. The data obtained at time of surgery in the study by Labrie et al.[38] *have been reduced by 15% to take into account the 15% PSA failure following 10 years for organ-confined disease.[66]*

Moreover, women who took tamoxifen for 5 years after surgery for early breast cancer had up to an 18% better chance of surviving without relapse than patients who did not take the drug.[75] This led to the following statement: 'In clinics all over the world, everyone will be using tamoxifen for five years now for sure' (Sandra M. Swaine).

A duration of treatment very much longer than 3 months is also supported by the author's recent data obtained on serum PSA and positive biopsies performed 12 and 24 months following radiation therapy associated with neoadjuvant and adjuvant combination therapy administered for a total of 3 or 10.5 months, respectively. Much better results, although not yet reaching 100% of negative biopsies, were obtained with 10.5 months compared with 3 months of combination therapy, on both the rate of positive biopsies and the PSA level.[37] As main control endpoint, follow-up TRUS-guided needle biopsies were performed 12 and 24 months (when there was sufficient follow-up) after the end of radiation therapy for the three groups of patients. Control biopsies at 12 and 24 months, were performed on 92 and 68 patients, respectively. The biopsy findings are shown in Table 28.2 and are reported as absence of cancer, suspicious, and presence of cancer. Whereas 61.8% of control patients in group 1 were found to have residual cancer, only 30.3 and 4.0% showed residual neoplasm in groups 2 and 3, respectively at 12 months. When looking at 24 months, 65.2, 28.0 and 5.0% of patients in groups 1, 2 and 3, respectively, showed residual cancer (Table 28.2). The differences between all three groups are statistically highly significant at both 12 and 24 months.

Although the choice of 3 months of neoadjuvant combination therapy has enabled the marked induction of apoptosis and downstaging of localized prostate cancer to be demonstrated,[36,38-40,42,44-47,57] it is also clear from the data and calculations outlined above that combination therapy should be given for at least 2 years, and probably 5 years (author's unpublished data) for a reasonable chance of success. This estimate is based upon the best scientific evidence gained from the responses of both prostate and breast cancer to androgen and oestrogen deprivation, respectively.[38,40,74,75] It is equally clear that the best results are obtained with maximal androgen blockade with a pure anti-androgen; monotherapy or a lower degree of androgen blockade cannot achieve a similar level of apoptosis, with the consequent risk of development of androgen-insensitive clones. In agreement with this approach, the greater the reduction in

Table 28.2. Biopsy results 12 and 24 months after external beam radiotherapy associated with neo-adjuvant and adjuvant combination therapy administered for a total of 3 or 10.5 months, respectively

Finding	Group 1		Group 2		Group 3	
	12	24	12	24	12	24
Absence of cancer	10 (29.4)	5 (21.7)	17 (51.5)	18 (72.0)	22 (88.0)	18 (90.0)
Suspicious	3 (8.8)	3 (13.0)	6 (18.2)	0 (0.0)	2 (8.0)	1 (5.0)
Presence of cancer	21 (61.8)	15 (65.2)	10 (30.3)	7 (28.0)	1 (4.0)	1 (5.0)

Values are numbers of patients, with percentage within group in parentheses.
χ^2 statistics: (12 months) $p < 0.001$; group 1 vs 2: $p = 0.033$; group 1 vs 3: $p < 0.001$; group 2 vs 3: $p < 0.006$. (24 months) $p < 0.001$; group 1 vs 2: $p = 0.001$; group 1 vs 3: $p < 0.001$; group 2 vs 3: NS.
Group 1 = radiotherapy alone; group 2 = 3 months of LHRH agonist + flutamide before radiotherapy; group 3 = as for group 2 except that combined androgen blockade was continued for a total of 10.5 months. (From ref. 37 with permission.)

serum PSA following various degrees of androgen deprivation, the longer the time to progression. Moreover, it is well known that suboptimal androgen blockade causes the development of tumours that are unresponsive to combination therapy applied later, at the time of progression.[11]

Conclusions

Androgen blockade is the only treatment of prostate cancer that has been shown to prolong life. Most importantly, the prolongation of life has been achieved at both the localized and advanced stages of the disease. Combined androgen blockade using an optimal dose of a pure anti-androgen in association with medical castration offers a unique opportunity to treat prostate cancer at a clinically localized stage. The duration of treatment should be for a minimum of 2 years (and quite possibly 5 years) and should be associated with radical prostatectomy, radiotherapy or brachytherapy for young and healthy patients, in order to optimize the results. For patients having a life expectancy of less than 10 years, combined androgen blockade alone is a reasonable choice.

References

1. Parker S L, Tong T, Bolden S, Wingo P A. Cancer statistics 1996. CA 1996; 46: 5–27
2. Brown M L, Fintor L, Newman-Horm P A. The economic burden of cancer. J Natl Cancer Inst 1993; 85: 351
3. Huggins C, Hodges C V. Studies of prostatic cancer. I. Effect of castration, estrogen and androgen injections on serum phosphatases in metastatic carcinoma of the prostate. Cancer Res 1941; 1: 293–307
4. Gittes R F. Carcinoma of the prostate. N Engl J Med 1991; 24: 236–245
5. Labrie F, Dupont A, Bélanger A et al. Treatment of prostate cancer with gonadotrophin-releasing hormone agonists. Endocr Rev 1986; 7: 67–74
6. Paulson D, Hodge G B Jr, Hinshaw H et al. Radiation therapy versus delayed androgen deprivation for stage C carcinoma of the prostate. J Urol 1984; 131: 901–902
7. Labrie F, Simard J, Luu-The V et al. Structure, regulation and role of 3β-hydroxysteroid dehydrogenase, 17b-hydroxysteroid dehydrogenase and aromatase enzymes in formation of sex steroids in classical and peripheral intracrine tissues. In: Sheppard MC, Stewart PM (eds) Hormones, enzymes and receptors. Baillière's Clinical Endocrinology and Metabolism. London: Baillière Tindall, 1994: 451–474
8. Labrie F, Simard J, Luu-The V et al. The 3β-hydroxysteroid dehydrogenase/isomerase gene family: lessons from type II 3β-HSD congenital deficiency. In: Hansson V, Levy FO, Taskén K (eds) Signal transduction in testicular cells. Ernst Schering Research Foundation Workshop. Berlin: Springer-Verlag, 1996:185-218 (suppl 2)
9. Labrie F, Luu-The V, Lin S X et al. The key role of 17β-HSDs in sex steroid biology. Steroids 1996: in press (December)
10. Labrie F. Intracrinology. Mol Cell Endocrinol 1991; 78: C113–C118
11. Labrie F, Dupont A, Bélanger A. Complete androgen blockade for the treatment of prostate cancer. In: de Vita VT, Hellman S, Rosenberg SA (eds) Important advances in oncology. Philadelphia: J.B. Lippincott, 1985: 193–217
12. Béland G, Elhilali M, Fradet Y et al. Total androgen blockade versus castration in metastatic cancer of the prostate. In: Motta M, Serio M (eds) Hormonal therapy of prostatic diseases: basic and clinical aspects. Bussum: Medicom, 1988: 302–311
13. Crawford E D, Eisenberger M A, McLeod D G et al. A controlled trial of leuprolide with and without flutamide in prostatic carcinoma. N Engl J Med 1989; 321: 419–424
14. Denis L, Carnelro de Moura J L, Bono A et al. Goserelin acetate and flutamide vs bilateral orchiectomy: a phase III EORTC trial (30853). EORTC GU Group and EORTC Data Center. Urology 1993; 42: 119–129
15. Janknegt R A, Abbou C C, Bartoletti R et al. Orchiectomy and Anandron (Nilutamide) or placebo as treatment of metastatic prostatic cancer in a multinational double-blind randomized trial. J Urol 1993; 149: 77–83

16. Iversen P, Christensen M G, Friis E *et al*. A phase III trial of zoladex and flutamide versus orchiectomy in the treatment of patients with advanced carcinoma of the prostate. Cancer 1990; 66: 1058–1066

17. Lunglmayr G. A multicenter trial comparing the luteinizing hormone releasing hormone analog Zoladex, with Zoladex plus flutamide in the treatment of advanced prostate cancer. The International Prostate Cancer Study Group. Eur Urol 1990; 18 (suppl 3): 28–29

18. Schellhammer P F. Combined androgen blockade for the treatment of metastatic cancer of the prostate. Urology 1996; 47: 622–629

19. Soloway M S, Ishikawa S, van der Zwang R, Todd B. Prognostic factors in patients with advanced prostate cancer. Urology 1989; 33: 53–56

20. Labrie F, Veilleux R, Fournier A. Low androgen levels induce the development of androgen-hypersensitive cell clones in Shionogi mouse mammary carcinoma cells in culture. J Natl Cancer Inst 1988; 80: 1138–1147

21. Osborne C K. Tamoxifen in premenopausal patients. ASCO Education Book, Spring 1996: 166–173

22. Labrie F, Candas B, Cusan L *et al*. Diagnosis of advanced or noncurable prostate cancer can be practically eliminated by prostate-specific antigen. Urology 1996; 47: 212–217

23. Hugosson J, Aus G. Natural evolution of prostate cancer. Endocrine-Related Cancer 1996; 3: 147–155

24. Brawer M K, Lange P H. Adjuvant therapy after radical prostatectomy. Probl Urol 1990; 4: 461–472

25. Gibbons R P, Correa R J Jr, Brannen G E, Weissman R M. Total prostatectomy for clinically localized prostate cancer: long-term results. J Urol 1989; 141: 564–566

26. Lange P H, Narayan P. Understaging and undergrading of prostate cancer. Argument for postoperative radiation as adjuvant therapy. Urology 1983; 21: 113–118

27. Catalona W J, Stein A J. Staging errors in clinically localized prostatic cancer. J Urol 1982; 127: 452–456

28. Veenema R J, Gursel E O, Lattimer J K. Radical retropubic prostatectomy for cancer: a 20-year experience. J Urol 1977; 117: 330–331

29. Elder J S, Jewett H J, Walsh P C. Radical perineal prostatectomy for clinical stage B2 carcinoma of the prostate. J Urol 1982; 127: 704–706

30. Boxer R J, Kaufman J J, Goodwin W E. Radical prostatectomy for carcinoma of the prostate: 1951–1976. A review of 329 patients. J Urol 1977; 117: 208–213

31. Epstein J I, Walsh P C, Carmichael M, Brendler C B. Pathologic and clinical findings to predict tumor extent of nonpalpable (stage T1c) prostate cancer. JAMA 1994; 271: 368–374

32. Stormont T J, Farrow G M, Myers R P *et al*. Clinical stage B0 or T1c prostate cancer: nonpalpable disease identified by elevated serum prostate-specific antigen concentration. Urology 1993; 41: 3–8

33. Labrie F, Dupont A, Bélanger A *et al*. New hormonal therapy in prostatic carcinoma: combined treatment with an LHRH agonist and an antiandrogen. J Clin Invest Med 1982; 5: 267–275

34. Labrie F, Bélanger A, Dupont A *et al*. Science behind total androgen blockade: from gene to combination therapy. Clin Invest Med 1993; 16: 475–492

35. Pilepich M V, Krall J M, Al-Saffaf M *et al*. Androgen deprivation with radiation therapy compared with radiation therapy alone for locally advanced prostatic carcinoma: a randomized comparative trial of the Radiation Therapy Oncology Group. Urology 1995; 45: 616–623

36. Monfette G, Dupont A, Labrie F. Temporary combination therapy with flutamide and Tryptex as adjuvant to radical prostatectomy for the treatment of early stage prostate cancer. In: Labrie F, Lee F, Dupont A (eds) Early stage prostate cancer: diagnosis and choice of therapy. New York: Excerpta Medica, 1989: 41–51

37. Laverdière J, Gomez J L, Cusan L *et al*. Beneficial effect of combination therapy administered prior to, during and following external beam radiation therapy in localized prostate cancer. Int J Radiat Oncol 1996; in press

38. Labrie F, Cusan L, Gomez J L *et al*. Down-staging of early stage prostate cancer before radical prostatectomy: the first randomized trial of neoadjuvant combination therapy with Flutamide and a luteinizing hormone-releasing hormone agonist. Urology 1994; 44: 29–37

39. Labrie F, Dupont A, Cusan L *et al*. Downstaging of localized prostate cancer by neoadjuvant therapy with flutamide and lupron: the first controlled and randomized trial. Clin Invest Med 1993; 16: 499–509

40. Soloway M S, Sharifi R, Wajsman Z *et al.* Randomized prospective study comparing radical prostatectomy alone versus radical prostatectomy preceeded by androgen blockade in clinical stage B2 (T2bNxM0) prostate cancer. J Urol 1995; 154: 424–428

41. Schulman C C, Wildschutz T P. Neoadjuvant hormonal deprivation prior to radical prostatectomy: overview of literature and personal experience on a controversial approach. Endocrine-Related Cancer 1996; 3: 205–209

42. Schulman C C, Sassine A N. Neoadjuvant hormonal deprivation before radical prostatectomy. Clin Invest Med 1993; 16: 523–531

43. Fair W R, Cookson M S, Stroumbakis N *et al.* Update on neoadjuvant androgen deprivation therapy (ADT) and radical prostatectomy in localized prostate cancer. J Urol 1996; 155 (suppl): 677A (abstr 1426)

44. Solomon M H. Radical prostatectomy following androgen blockade. In: Lee F, McLeary RL (eds) Proc 5th Int Symp on Transrectal Ultrasound in the Diagnosis and Management of Prostate Cancer. Chicago: Chicago University Press, 1990: 100

45. Fair W F, Aprikian A G, Cohen D *et al.* Use of neoadjuvant androgen deprivation therapy in clinical localized prostate cancer. Clin Invest Med 1993; 16: 516–522

46. Solomon M H, McHugh T A, Dorr R P *et al.* Hormone ablation therapy as neoadjuvant treatment to radical prostatectomy. Clin Invest Med 1993; 16: 532–538

47. Andros E A, Danesghari F, Crawford E D. Neoadjuvant hormonal therapy in stage C adenocarcinoma of the prostate. Clin Invest Med 1993; 16: 510–515

48. Lee F, Siders D B, Newby J E *et al.* The role of transrectal ultrasound-guided staging biopsy and androgen ablation therapy prior to radical prostatectomy. Clin Invest Med 1993; 16: 458–470

49. Bellavance G, Fradet Y. Influence of neoadjuvant hormonotherapy on PSA response and pathological stage at radical prostatectomy. J Urol 1996; 155 (suppl): 651A (abstr 1360).

50. Klotz L H, Goldenberg Bullock M J, Srigley J R *et al.* Neoadjuvant cyproterone acetate (CPA) therapy prior to radical prostatectomy reduces tumour burden and mar positivity without altering 6 and 12 month posttreatment PSA: results of a randomized trial. J Urol 1996; 155 (suppl): 399A (abstr 356)

51. Soloway M S. Randomized prospective study — radical prostatectomy alone vs radical prostatectomy preceded by androgen blockade in cT2b prostate cancer — initial results. J Urol 1996; 155 (suppl): 555A (abstr 976)

52. Bolla M, Gonzalez D, Warde P *et al.* Immediate hormonal therapy improves locoregional control and survival in patients with locally advanced prostate cancer. Results of a randomized phase III clinical trial of the EORTC radiotherapy and genitourinary tract cancer cooperative groups. J Clin Oncol 1996; 15: 238 (abstr 591)

53. Kolata G. Prostate cancer consensus hampered by lack of data. Science 1987; 236: 1626–1627

54. Labrie F. Endocrine therapy of prostate cancer: optimal form and timing. J Clin Endocrinol Metab 1995; 80: 1066–1071

55. Zietman A L, Prince E A, Nakfoor B M, Shipley W U. Permanent tumor eradication by radiations is enhanced by prior androgen withdrawal in two experimental models. J Urol 1996; 155 (suppl): 509A (abstr 792)

56. Labrie F, Dupont A, Suburu R *et al.* Serum prostatic specific antigen (PSA) as prescreening test for prostate cancer. J Urol 1992; 147: 846–852

57. Labrie F. Endocrine therapy for prostate cancer. Endocrinol Metab Clin North Am 1991; 20: 845–872

58. Labrie F, Bélanger A, Simard J *et al.* Combination therapy for prostate cancer: endocrine and biological basis of its choice as new standard first line therapy. Cancer 1993; 71: 1059–1067

59. Labrie F, Veilleux R. Maintenance of androgen responsiveness by glucocorticoids in Shionogi mammary carcinoma cells in culture. J Natl Cancer Inst 1988; 80: 966–970

60. Noldus J, Ferrari M, Prestigiamoco A, Stamey T A. Effect of Flutamide plus castration on prostate size in patients with previously untreated prostate cancer. Urology 1996; 47: 713–718

61. Moorjani S, Dupont A, Labrie F *et al.* Changes in plasma lipoproteins during various androgen suppression therapies in men with prostatic carcinoma: effects of orchiectomy, estrogen, and combination treatment with LHRH agonist. J Clin Endocrinol Metab 1988; 66: 314–322

62. Morton R A, Steiner M S, Walsh P C. Cancer control following anatomical radical prostatectomy: an interim report. J Urol 1991; 145: 1197–1200
63. Zietman A L, Edelstein R A, Coen J J *et al*. Radical prostatectomy for adenocarcinoma of the prostate: the influence of preoperative and pathologic findings on biochemical disease-free outcome. Urology 1994; 43: 828–833
64. Zietman A L, Shipley W U, Coen J J. Radical prostatectomy and radical radiation therapy for clinical stages T1 to 2 adenocarcinoma of the prostate. New insights into outcome from repeat biopsy and prostate specific antigen follow-up. J Urol 1994; 152: 1806–1812
65. Kerr J F, Wyllie A H, Currie A R. Apoptosis: a basic biological phenomenon with wide-ranging implications in tissue kinetics. Br J Cancer 1972; 26: 239–257
66. Partin A W, Pound C R, Clemens J Q *et al*. PSA after anatomic radical prostatectomy. The Johns Hopkins experience after 10 years. Urol Clin North Am 1993; 20: 713–725
67. Keuppens F, Whelan P, Carneiro de Moura J L *et al*. Orchiectomy versus goserelin plus flutamide in patients with metastatic prostate cancer (EORTC 30853). Cancer 1993; 72: 3863–3869
68. Denis L, Smith P H, De Moura J L *et al*. Orchiectomy vs Zoladex plus flutamide in patients with metastatic prostate cancer. The EORTC GU Group. Eur Urol 1990; 18: 34–40
69. Keuppens F, Denis L, Smith P *et al*. Zoladex vs flutamide versus bilateral orchiectomy: a randomized phase III EORTC trial (30853). Cancer 1990; 66: 1045–1057
70. Têtu B, Labrie F, Dupont A, Monfette G. Histopathologic effect of combination therapy on normal prostate and prostatic adenocarcinoma. In: Labrie F, Dupont A (eds) Early stage prostate cancer: diagnosis and choice of therapy. ICS 841. Amsterdam: Excerpta Medica, 1989: 63–76
71. Têtu B, Srigley J R, Boivin J C *et al*. Effect of combination endocrine therapy (LHRH agonist and Flutamide) on normal prostate and prostatic adenocarcinoma: a histopathologic and immunohistochemical study. Am J Surg Pathol 1991; 15: 111–120
72. Vaillancourt L, Têtu B, Fradet Y *et al*. Effect of neoadjuvant endocrine therapy (combined androgen blockade) on normal prostate and prostatic carcinoma. Am J Surg Pathol 1996; 20: 86–93
73. Gleave M E, Goldenberg S L, Jones E C *et al*. Biochemical and pathological effects of 8 months of neoadjuvant androgen withdrawal therapy before radical prostatectomy in patients with clinically confined prostate cancer. J Urol 1996; 155: 213–219
74. Swedish Breast Cancer Cooperative Group. Randomized trial of two versus five years of adjuvant Tamoxifen for postmenopausal early stage breast cancer. J Natl Cancer Inst 1996; 88: 1543–1549
75. Fisher B, Dignam J, Bryant J *et al*. Five versus more than five years of Tamoxifen therapy for breast cancer patients with negative lymph nodes and estrogen-positive tumors. J Natl Cancer Inst 1996; 88: 1529–1542
76. Labrie F, Cusan L, Gomez J L *et al*. Combination of screening and preoperative endocrine therapy: the potential for an important decrease in prostate cancer mortality. J Clin Endocrinol Metab 1995; 80: 2002–2013
77. Labrie F. Editorial. Endocrine-Related Cancer 1996; 3: 145–146
78. Trapasso JG, deKernion JB, Smith RB, Dorey F. The incidence and significance of detectable levels of serum prostate specific antigen after radical prostatectomy. J Urol 1994; 152: 1821–1825
79. Kupelian P, Katcher J, Levin H, Zippe C. Klein E. Correlation of clinical and pathological factors with rising prostate-specific antigen profiles after radical prostatectomy alone for clinically localized prostate cancer. Urology 1996; 48: 249–260.
80. Kaplan ID, Cox RS, Bagshaw MA: Prostate specific antigen after external beam radiotherapy for prostatic cancer: follow up. J Urol 1993; 149: 519–522
81. Goad JR, Chang SJ, Ohori M, Scardino PT. PSA after definitive radiotherapy for clinically localized prostate cancer. Urol Clin North Am 1993; 20: 727–736

Chapter 29
Evidence-based therapy for prostate cancer: European studies in progress
D. W. W. Newling

Introduction

There is no doubt that the incidence of prostate cancer in all parts of the world is rising.[1] There is also little doubt that more patients are being cured of prostate cancer by radical surgery or radiotherapy. The evidence that has led to the use of these therapeutic manoeuvres remains retrospective and largely anecdotal.[2] In the treatment of patients deemed incurable there are both ongoing and reported prospective randomized studies yielding sound evidence that enables logical choices of therapy to be made. In the investigation of patients with more advanced disease there is a worrying trend to identify activity of compounds at a particular stage of prostate cancer and to translate that into an indication for their use at an entirely different stage. It is hoped that this chapter, by posing certain questions and examining broad areas of therapy, sifts those therapeutic manoeuvres that are truly evidence-based from others that remain largely empirical.

Treatment of curable prostate cancer

With the advent of screening by means of prostate-specific antigen (PSA) and digital rectal examination, more patients are presenting to the urologist with an organ-confined, asymptomatic cancer in the hope of curative therapy. In the United States, six or seven patients present with localized organ-confined disease for every one patient presenting with metastatic disease at the present time.[3] A similar trend is being seen in Europe. Although it is nearly 90 years since the first radical prostatectomy was carried out, it remains one of the greatest indictments of urological practice that, hitherto, no truly prospective, randomized study has been carried out to determine the true place of radical prostatectomy, radical radiotherapy and a watchful waiting policy. The studies of Chodak and Johansson have shown that there is a group of mainly elderly patients, over the age of 70, with well-differentiated tumours, whose cancer appears to impact very little on their anticipated overall survival.[4,5] There remain, however, patients with more aggressive tumours who undoubtedly do require some therapeutic manoeuvre. With the Prostate Intervention or Observation Trial (PIVOT) study in the United States and the Medical Research Council (MRC) study in the United Kingdom, there is an opportunity for truly prospective examination of the role of radical prostatectomy and radiotherapy. Unfortunately, both studies have developed major recruitment problems and are unlikely to be completed. From the large mature studies of radical prostatectomy and radical radiotherapy, certain evidence-based statements can be made. There is little doubt that centres where large number of prostatectomies are carried out have better results than those where fewer than 10 per year are conducted. There is, however, a strong element of selection and, in the larger centres, patients with more advance disease are no longer being offered monotherapy with radical prostatectomy or radiotherapy.[6] A recent study by Schröder of 100 patients with T3, stage C disease, showed that, where radical prostatectomy as monotherapy was used, only 22% remained disease free without evidence of biochemical or clinical progression at a mean time of 44 months. It also stressed the futility of offering radical retropubic prostatectomy to patients with T3 G3 tumours.[7]

Management of locally advanced, non-metastatic disease

Since the VACURG studies of the early 1970s, doubts have existed over the timing of therapy in patients deemed incurable but without symptoms and signs of progressive disease. The data of the Veterans Administration Cooperative Urological Research Group (VACURG) study have been frequently flawed because it has been shown that almost 44% of those patients who were thought not to have received adjuvant therapy had received some form of hormonal therapy, oestrogens or orchiectomy, before the results were eventually examined.[8] Nevertheless, sufficient concern existed to warrant the performance of a number of trials — two major trials that are still ongoing, and one study carried out by the MRC, which has been reported. The European Organization for Research and Treatment of Cancer (EORTC) has two ongoing studies, where patients not deemed suitable for radical cure have been randomized to immediate or delayed hormonal therapy. In the first study, 30891, coordinated by Professor Studer of Berne, patients with locally advanced, possibly metastatic, disease were randomized to orchiectomy or luteinizing hormone-releasing hormone (LHRH) analogue, to be given immediately, or delayed until evidence of progression was seen. The study is not yet completed but over 650 patients of the 750 required have been recruited. That the study continues, after an interim examination, suggests that at this stage there is probably no difference in overall survival. The second study, 30846, coordinated by Professor Schröder of Rotterdam, examines the fate of patients with positive lymph nodes at radical prostatectomy, who were randomized to immediate or delayed hormonal therapy. Again, this study is very nearly complete and a published analysis of a subset of patients[9] has shown that those patients who received immediate hormonal therapy have a longer progression-free survival (of the order of 30 months) than those where therapy was delayed. At present there is no absolute difference in overall survival. In the recently published MRC study, 938 patients (some with metastatic disease but the majority without) were randomized to receive immediate orchiectomy, LHRH agonist plus short-term anti-androgen, or the same therapies delayed until progression occurred. There is a clear trend leading to statistical significance in favour of immediate therapy to improve survival rates in patients with non-metastatic disease. The same cannot be said of patients with metastatic disease, where the timing of therapy appears to have little impact on overall survival. However, the findings that patients who received delayed therapy, with M0 disease, enjoy on average 2 years without the side effects of anti-androgen therapy and that patients with metastatic disease can be saved from some of the more serious effects of their disease by early therapy, are important considerations in terms of the quality of life of patients with this stage of the disease.[10]

Role of neo-adjuvant and adjuvant therapy

In an attempt to improve cure rates for patients with localized prostate cancer, a number of studies of neo-adjuvant and adjuvant hormonal therapy have been carried out. Although Table 29.1 shows that there is considerable evidence for downstaging in many of the studies, overall, surgery has not been found to be any easier and the blood loss during surgery has shown no statistical difference compared with patients not receiving neo-adjuvant therapy. It is difficult to imagine that malignant cells can actually be sucked back into the prostate from neighbouring lymph nodes or from areas outside the prostatic capsule, and so downstaging *per se* seems unlikely to occur in T3 or T4a tumours. That downsizing occurs, possibly giving rise to a suspicion of downstaging, cannot be denied. It is disappointing to reveal that, in the large combined European study, postoperatively, patients in both groups (neo-adjuvant, and prostatectomy alone) appear to be failing biochemically at the same rate. Thus, although neo-adjuvant therapy may have an effect on the primary tumour, the biological behaviour of the tumour, at least in these studies, does not seem to be altered. It has been suggested that one reason may be that neo-adjuvant therapy is not given for long enough, and studies are being undertaken of 3-monthly, 6-monthly and 9-monthly neo-adjuvant therapy, the long-term results of which are awaited. Incidentally, it appears to make little difference what form of hormonal therapy is used in the neo-adjuvant setting.[11,12]

Adjuvant hormonal therapy in patients undergoing radical prostatectomy has been used for a number of years at the Mayo Clinic in the United States and until now in non-randomized studies in Europe. The Mayo figures show an improvement of 20% in symptom-free survival, 5 years after adjuvant orchiectomy for patients with T3 disease.[13] The EORTC has just embarked on an important study in which hormonal therapy will be given to patients with a rising PSA after radical prostatectomy.

The position of neo-adjuvant therapy and of adjuvant hormonal therapy combined with radiotherapy, is at present rather different and more encouraging. In a large randomized study, where patients deemed at risk of early progression following radiotherapy received adjuvant hormonal therapy with an LHRH analogue, an improvement in progression-free survival of 15 months was noted in the patients who received adjuvant therapy. Another study, in which patients with

Table 29.1. Methodological classification of prostate cancer based on hormone sensitivity

Study	Clinical number	Downstaging percentage	Pathological number	Downstaging percentage
Flamm (1991)	0 of 21	0	7 of 31	28
Thompson (1991)	17 of 24	70	3 of 15	20
Morgan (1991)	29 of 36	81	3 of 36	8
Murphy (1991)	NG		5 of 10	50
Van Poppel (1992)	NG		4 of 8	50
McFarlane (1992)	10 of 12	83	3 of 12	25
Rifkin (1992)	NG		15 of 31	48
Vapnek	NG		3 of 28	11
Kennedy	NG		2 of 7	29
Tunn (1992)	NG		0 of 36	0
Schulman (1993)	9 of 15	60	4 of 15	27
Kollerman (1993)	49 of 103	48	40 of 103	39
Hottrie (1993)	45 of 45	100	6 of 45	13
Daheshagari (1993)	NG		13 of 44	30
Labrie (1993)	3 of 10	80	NG	
Fair (1993)	NG		7 of 27	26

NG = not given

capsule penetration and positive lymph nodes, with or without preoperative hormonal therapy, are randomized to receive immediate radiotherapy, or radiotherapy or hormonal therapy delayed until progression, is still in progress.

The latest analysis of the Radiation Therapy Oncology Group (RTOG) study in the United States shows that, in those patients who received neo-adjuvant hormonal therapy prior to radiotherapy, there remains an improvement in progression-free survival at 4 years, although overall survival difference is not yet statistically significant.[3] In 1992, the MRC reported a randomized study in locally advanced disease, comparing radiotherapy with orchiectomy, or the combination of radiotherapy plus orchiectomy. In this study the addition of hormonal therapy to radiotherapy lengthened the time to the onset of metastases and improved disease-specific survival.[15]

Treatment of patients with metastatic disease

Role of orchiectomy

For many years, orchiectomy has been regarded as the gold standard of therapy for metastatic prostate cancer. From the early pioneering work of Hunter, it has seemed the most logical step to prevent proliferation of prostate cancer cells. More recently, however, many workers have examined orchiectomy in the light of its effect on quality of life of patients, accepting that it improves the extent of life of patients with metastatic disease to the order of 2–2.5 years. In a number of EORTC studies, over 500 patients have undergone orchiectomy for metastatic disease and it is clear that a number of important side effects have diminished the quality of the patient's lives.

Orchiectomy gives rise to loss of potency and loss of libido in almost 99% of patients so treated. Hot flushes, although the butt of many comedians' jokes, are regarded as far from amusing by the patients who suffer them. They are distressing and embarrassing, and can be brought about by many day-to-day activities such as eating or moving from one place to another where a different temperature exists. Many patients also object to the loss of muscle mass, increase in adiposity and change in body hair, leading to a female body image over the course of time.

One of the most important features identified by quality-of-life studies is a loss of the ability to concentrate and to carry out a full working day. This is particularly of relevance for younger patients, many of whom find themselves unable to carry on full-time work within 2 years of undergoing orchiectomy.[16]

Finally, orchiectomy is permanent and now that alternative therapies with LHRH analogues, equivalent to orchiectomy, are available it is questionable whether it should remain as the gold standard of therapy.

The advantage of LHRH treatment is that it can be given as first-line therapy and withdrawn if the side effects are particularly troublesome.[17]

Oestrogens

With the demonstration by VACURG, EORTC and other groups, of the serious cardiovascular side effects of oestrogens, this therapy as primary treatment in metastatic prostate cancer fell from favour in the early 1970s. Theoretically, because of their multiplicity of actions, oestrogens are still extremely attractive in the treatment of prostate cancer.[18] Not only do they lower the LH, and therefore testosterone level, block 5α-reductase and the conversion of testosterone to dihydrotestosterone, and increase the concentration of sex hormone-binding globulin, thereby preventing free testosterone from attaching to prostate cancer cells but they have also, very recently, been shown to have a direct cytotoxic effect on prostate cancer cells in culture.[19]

In Scandinavia, oestrogens have continued to be used, given mainly systemically as depot preparations, once or twice a month. In a recent Finnish study, the therapeutic results of which are not yet available, the initial study of toxicity in patients who were randomized to receive orchiectomy or intramuscular Estradurin (estradiol unidecinate) shows no increase in cardiovascular or other serious side effects for those patients receiving the oestrogen compound. A large pan-Scandinavian study, SPCG 5, involving over 400 patients, is also comparing systemic oestrogen with other hormonal therapy, in this case total androgen blockade; and although the study is recruited no results are available as yet (P. Iverson, SPCG Chairman, personal communication). However, it might be construed that, because the study has completed recruitment, it is probable that no clearly disadvantageous side effects have been noted in either arm. It has been clearly demonstrated that the hazard of oestrogen therapy with regard to cardiovascular side effects stems from its first pass through the liver, where it is converted into oestranes and oestrones. If this can be avoided by systemic administration or absorption through the skin, then oestrogens may well, again, become important agents in the therapy of advanced prostate cancer.

Monotherapy with androgen receptor antagonists

Since the seminal work of Huggins and Scott in 1945, the role played by adrenal androgens has been at least partially recognized.[20] In the early 1970s, two classes of androgen receptor antagonists appeared, one being steroidal and the other non-steroidal. These compounds offered the real possibility that, by blocking the androgen receptor on the prostate cancer cell, they could block the influence of both testicular and andrenal androgens.[21] For a variety of reasons, total androgen blockade with such monotherapy does not take place: the steroidal anti-androgen has a tendency to 'fall off' the androgen receptor, thereby allowing adrenal precursors access; the non-steroidal anti-androgen, by blocking the information that returns to the pituitary concerning androgen levels in the blood, causes a secondary rise in luteinizing hormone and testosterone, which may be capable of overriding the receptor mechanism. During the late 1970s and the early 1980s, the EORTC showed that there appeared to be an equivalence in activity between orchiectomy, 1 or 3 mg stilboestrol, and cyproterone acetate (CPA) 250 or 300 mg, in lengthening the time to progression and overall survival of patients with metastatic prostate cancer.[18] As a result of a prognostic factor analysis, it was decided that asymptomatic patients with metastatic disease should take part in another trial of androgen receptor antagonism monotherapy, comparing 300 mg CPA with 750 mg flutamide. This study is fully recruited but the therapeutic results are not yet available. An interesting finding was that those patients who were potent at the beginning of the study, in both arms, retained their potency whether they received a non-steroidal anti-androgen or a steroidal anti-androgen.[22] Elsewhere in Europe, Boccon-Gibod has shown in a small study of 104 patients that monotherapy with flutamide, after 2 years, was just as effective as orchiectomy in preventing progression and lengthening progression-free survival.[23] Only flutamide, of the non-steroidal androgens, and CPA have been approved as monotherapy in Europe, although research on a new anti-androgen, Casodex, in patients at a high risk of recurrence after local therapy, is currently under way.

Maximal androgen blockade

The concept of maximal androgen blockade, although not so named, was introduced in 1977 by Bracchi.[14] The first prospective randomized study of maximal androgen blockade employing orchiectomy plus CPA as the combined therapy arm, was launched by the EORTC in 1980.[18] This study, together with all the other European studies employing a steroidal anti-androgen with LHRH agonist or castration has shown no advantage for this form of total androgen blockade compared with conventional testicular blockade. A number of studies has shown a small advantage for non-steroidal anti-androgens added to castration or LHRH agonists, the most important of which is the EORTC study 30853. The initiative of the EORTC and the American Cancer Society started a meta-analysis of 22 studies, which was reported in 1995. This showed that, in a very heterogeneous group of studies, there was no statistical advantage for maximal androgen blockade in any form compared with conventional testicular ablation either medical or surgical. A common finding in all these studies was that, in those patients with symptomatic metastatic disease, a more rapid response was obtained with maximal androgen blockade than with conventional testicular ablation, without there being a decisive impact on survival.[24] A second meta-analysis is planned for April 1997 but recent information from the second NCI study in the United States, comparing orchiectomy with orchiectomy plus flutamide, suggests that the role of maximal androgen blockade is extremely limited (J.T. Isaacs, 1996, personal communication). It would appear to be of relevance only in patients with painful, widespread metastases, in whom it produces a better subjective response. It should be used over a short period to prevent flare-up, where LHRH agonists are being used alone, and it gives an improvement in survival in patients who have subsequently received definitive radiotherapy for advanced localized disease.[25]

Androgen receptor antagonist withdrawal

This phenomenon, described by Scher and Kelly in 1993,[26] has had a moderate impact on evidence-based treatment of advanced prostate cancer in Europe. The EORTC, in a series of phase II studies, investigated vindesine, mitomycin C (MMC), high- and low-dose epirubicin and methotrexate between 1980 and 1993. A progressively increasing number of patients in that time had been treated in other EORTC studies, using either orchiectomy plus CPA or, latterly, an LHRH agonist plus cyproterone or flutamide, before developing progression and being placed in one of the phase II studies. Although only the studies using high-dose epirubicin and MMC showed a significant number of partial responses, these substances may have to be re-examined in the context of the anti-androgen or endocrine withdrawal syndrome for efficacy. Interestingly, the anti-androgen withdrawal phenomenon has been demonstrated with all anti-androgens, although the mechanism whereby it occurs, in the case of Casodex, may differ from that of other steroidal and non-steroidal anti-androgens. Only one case has been recorded where the endocrine withdrawal symptom has been observed in monotherapy, and that was in a patient who was treated with stilboestrol. Because of the multiplicity of therapeutic effects of stilboestrol it may be considered more a form of total androgen blockade than other monotherapies.[27]

Combination therapies

The combination of an oestrogen plus a nitrogen mustard was first introduced in a single preparation in 1976, by Konyves. The preparation was known as Estracyt and still enjoys wide popularity. Recently, from a number of European studies, it appears that Estracyt must be used in high doses at the start of therapy if it is to have both an oestrogenic and a cytotoxic effect. It has enjoyed widespread popularity, especially in Scandinavia, as primary and secondary therapy in patients with metastatic prostate cancer. At present it appears that, at a dose level of 10⁻ mg/kg, in patients with poorly differentiated prostate cancer, Estracyt is slightly superior to orchiectomy.[28] Eisenberger has shown that, when it is used as second-line therapy, after testicular ablation, objective responses are very few, less than 8% overall; however, subjective responses occur in approximately one-third of the patients so treated.[29] Combination therapy of estramustine with an H3-antagonist and other gut sedatives, considerably reduces the severe gastrointestinal side effects of this compound.

Other combinations of cytotoxic agents with hormonal therapy have been tried. Van Poppel and colleagues and the EORTC have carried out studies of orchiectomy plus MMC in patients with tumours with poor prognostic factors, but have failed to demonstrate any therapeutic advantage from the addition of the cytotoxic agent.[30] Only one European study, carried out by Pummer, has shown an advantage for the addition of chemotherapy to hormonal therapy. In this prospective randomized study of 147 patients he demonstrated a significant increase in progression-free survival for patients receiving a combination of maximal androgen blockade, LHRH plus non-steroidal anti-androgen and the cytotoxic agent epirubicin, when compared with patients receiving maximal androgen blockade alone. Although this is a comparatively small study, the improvement in progression-free survival has already reached statistical significance.[31]

Intermittent therapy

There are anecdotal accounts of patients who, on initial hormonal therapy, reach a steady state without symptoms or signs of progression and continue in that state for some time, without further therapeutic intervention. Bruchovsky, in the androgen-dependent Schonogyi mouse memory tumour line, has shown that intermittent therapy with the same hormonal manipulation can result in secondary and tertiary responses to the same anti-androgen therapy without the development of anti-androgen resistance.[32] The EORTC has just embarked on a phase II feasibility study of intermittent therapy, which will be converted to a phase III study if no problems arise in the monitoring of PSA levels. Similar studies are being carried out in the United States, and South Western Oncology Group (SWOG) has just embarked on a phase III study of intermittent versus continuous therapy. Not only would intermittent therapy prolong the period during which the tumour remains sensitive to a given anti-androgen manipulation but, with patients in the first analysis remaining off therapy for approximately 40% of the time, their quality of life would be greatly improved.[33]

Treatment of patients progressing after hormonal therapy

Patients progressing after initial hormonal therapy present a very heterogeneous group with very variable circulating levels of testosterone; they are, therefore, amenable to an equally heterogeneous group of treatments. Table 29.1 gives a classification of these patients, recently developed at a consensus conference on clinical trials in prostate cancer in Stockholm, Sweden. The possible therapies that are being investigated in Europe at present are summarized in Table 29.2.

In Europe, many of the second-line therapies, particularly cytochrome P-450 inhibitors, other differentiation therapies or pure cytotoxic agents, have been used in patients who have undergone some form of androgen ablation without there being time to allow for the phenomenon of endocrine or anti-androgen withdrawal. The results of these studies may therefore be called into doubt. Two

Table 29.2. Possible therapies for investigations

Second line hormonal therapy
Anti-androgen withdrawal
Differentiation therapies (P54 cytochrome inhibitors e.g. Liarozole)
New cytotoxic combinations incl. Taxol
Combinations of hormone and cytotoxic agents e.g. estramustine
Anti-metastatic agents
Metaloprotease inhibitors (anti-angiogenesis, growth factor inhibitors, e.g. Suramine, Somatostatin, gene therapy

recently completed studies have both been carried out by the EORTC. The first investigated liarozole and showed seven responses in 26 patients who had relapsed after orchiectomy or maximal androgen blockade. This study has not yet been reported and did not allow for the endocrine withdrawal phenomenon.[34] A randomized phase II study of Estracyt versus Estracyt + vinblastine has also just been concluded, prematurely, because of excessive toxicity in the combination arm.[35] This study was the first to be carried out in which time was allowed for anti-androgen withdrawal and stabilization of the PSA with a secondary progression before the second-line therapy was started.

How should we investigate new therapeutic modalities?

Although liarozole has a specific cytostatic effect on rapidly proliferating cells, owing to its effect on retinoic acid metabolism it, along with many of the other preparations (such as anti-angiogenesis agents, antimetastatic agents such as matrix metalloprotease inhibitors) and gene therapy, will probably never be used in patients with advanced hormone-refractory disease but at a much earlier stage to treat hormone-independent cells, present either at the beginning of the disease process or developing during hormonal therapy. It therefore seems inappropriate to look at these agents in patients with very advanced stages of the disease. The agents should probably be investigated by new techniques involving molecular markers of cell proliferation and histological examination of prostate cancers at radical prostatectomy, or by repeated biopsies, after the patient has received one or other of these therapies, as soon as the disease is diagnosed — or even before the disease is diagnosed in patients at high risk of developing it. These techniques must be developed quickly if these new agents are to find their rightful place in the management of prostate cancer.

On the other hand, it is recognized that cytotoxic agents, growth factor inhibitors and some second- and third-line endocrine therapies, need to be tested in patients with advanced disease. There is a growing tendency in Europe as well as in the United States, to use PSA as a surrogate endpoint in patients relapsing after hormonal therapy. As Table 29.3 shows, the PSA is not a genuine surrogate endpoint but merely an indication of activity of agents in advanced disease.[36] Many of the agents mentioned above incidentally have a paradoxical effect on the PSA, and many other agents, such as estramustine mitomycin C (MMC) and growth factor inhibitors, can affect the PSA but not cell proliferation. New agents in patients with advanced progressive disease, after primary hormonal therapy, should probably be screened by PSA monitoring, and a fall in PSA of 50–70%

Table 29.3. Patterns of response to therapeutic agents and hypothetical means of response evaluation in patients with prostate cancer

Criteria	Type of Agent						
	Endocrine	Cytotoxic	Differentiation therapies eg liarozole	Anti-angiogenic	Anti-metastatic	Cyto-static	Radio-therapy
Measurable disease	↓	↓	↔	↔	↔	↔	↓
Bone scan	↓↔(↑)	↔	↔	↔	↔	↔	↓↑
PSA	↓	↓	↑(↔)	any	any	↔	any
Symptoms	↓	↓	↓	↓	↓	↓	↓
Progression-free survival	↑	↑	↑	↑	↑	↑	any

Symbols: ↓ decrease; ↔ no change; (↑) flare; ↑ increase.

would suggest that the compound is active. These agents should then be further investigated in phase II studies where all parameters — biochemical, haematological, quality of life, etc. — should be measured and a parameter identified that correlates with an improvement in survival. This parameter should be investigated further in a phase III study, either against palliative therapy alone or against corticosteroids. The above were the recommendations from the specialists' committee at the recent WHO conference in Stockholm, dealing with hormone-refractory disease.

Conclusions

It is clear that, at many stages of prostate cancer, there are still patients who are being treated empirically, whose therapy is not accompanied by hard evidence of efficacy. With regard to the initial (and, it is hoped, curative) therapy, there is still no evidence as to which patients would benefit from radical prostatectomy or radical radiotherapy rather than a watchful waiting policy. In these patients, molecular markers need to be found that can indicate which patients are particularly at risk of developing progressive disease, before therapy is instituted. In the primary hormonal therapy of incurable prostate cancer, the development of combination therapy is of prime importance, addressing the heterogeneous group of cells present at the onset of local progression leading to metastases.

Finally, all new therapies need to be investigated systematically, particularly their effects at that stage of the disease where they are likely to prove beneficial. Bearing in mind that, in the treatment of advanced disease, all therapies are palliative, quality-of-life issues are often the most important for the patients.

References

1. Prenta K J, Goodson J A, Esper P S. Epidemiology of prostate cancer; molecular and environmental clues. Urology 1996; 48: 676–685
2. Jonler M, Madsen R A, Rhodes P R *et al.* A prospective study and quantifiction of urinary incontinence and quality of life in patients undergoing radical retropubic prostatectomy. Urology 1996; 48: 433–443
3. Porter A F, Zimmerman J, Ruffin M *et al.* Recommendation of the First Michigan Conference on Prostate Cancer. Urology 1996; 48: 519–535

4. Chodak G W, Thisted R, Gerber G. Results of conservative management of clinically localised prostate cancer. N Engl J Med 1994; 330: 242–248

5. Johansson J E. Watchful waiting for early stage prostate cancer. Urology 1994; 43: 138–142

6. Myers R P, Fleming T R. Course of localized prostate cancer treated by radical prostatectomy. Prostate 1983; 4: 461–472

7. Van den Ouden D, Davidson P J T, Hop W C J, Schröder F H. Radical prostatectomy as a monotherapy for locally advanced (stage T3) prostate cancer. J Urol 1994; 151: 646–651

8. Christensen N M, Aagaard J, Madsen P O. Reasons for delay of endocrine treatment in cancer of the prostate (until symptomatic metastases occur). In: Schröder F H (ed) Treatment of prostate cancer — facts and controversies. New York: Wiley-Liss, 1990: 7–14

9. Van den Ouden D, Tribukant B, Blom J H M et al. DNA ploidy of core biopsies and metastatic lymph nodes of prostate cancer patients; impact on time to progression. J Urol 1993; 150: 400–406

10. Kirk D. The MRC Prostate Cancer Working Party and Investigators Group: Hormone therapy in advanced prostate cancer — report of the Medical Research Council; immediate versus deferred treatment — study.

11. Soloway M, Watson R. The role of inductive androgen deprivation prior to radical prostatectomy. Eur Urol 1996; 29(suppl 2); 114–118

12. Wittjes W, Schuurman G, Gerhard F et al. Neo-adjuvant combined androgen deprivation therapy in T2-T3 N0 M0 prostate cancer — early results of an European study. Eur Urol 1996; 30(suppl 2): A775

13. Zincke H. Extended experience with surgical treatment of stage D1 adenocarcinoma of prostate: significant influences of immediate adjuvant hormonal treatment (orchidectomy) on outcome. Urology 1989; 33(suppl): 27–35

14. Bracci U. Present procedures in the treatment of prostatic cancer. In: Bracci U, Di Silverio (eds.). Hormonal Therapy in Prostatic Cancer. Coffese Palermo, 1977: pp 177–192

15. Fellows G J, Clark P B, Beynon L L. Treatment of advanced prostate cancer by orchidectomy, radiotherapy or combined treatment. An MRC study. Br J Urol 1992; 70: 304–309

16. Parmar H, Philips R H, Leitmann S L, Edwards L. How do you like to have an orchiectomy for advanced prostatic cancer? Am J Clin Oncol 1988; 11(suppl 2): 160–168

17. Debruyne F M J. The case for LHRH agonists in Baillières. Clin Oncol 1988; 2: 559–571

18. Robinson M R C, Smith P H, Richards B et al. The Final Analysis of the EORTC Genito-Urinary Tract Cancer Cooperative Group Phase III Clinical Trial (Protocol 30805) comparing orchidectomy, orchidectomy plus cyproterone acetate and low dose stilbestrol in the management of metastatic carcinoma of the prostate. (Pontefact/Leeds/York/Amsterdam/Brussels). Eur Urol 1995; 28: 273–283

19. Robertson C N, Robertson K M, Padilla C M et al. Introduction of apoptosis by diethylstilbestrol in hormone insensitive prostate cancer cells. J Natl Cancer Inst 1996; 88: 908–918

20. Huggins C, Scott W W. Bilateral adrenalectomy in prostatic cancer. Clinical features and urinary excretion of 17-ketosteroids and oestrogens. Ann Surg 1945; 122: 1031–1041

21. Neri R, Kassem N. Biological and clinical properties of antiandrogens. In: Besciani F, King R J B, Lippman M E et al. (eds) Progress in cancer research and therapy. New York: Raven Press, 1984: 507–518

22. Schröder F H. Presentation at the progress and controversies in urological oncology meeting. Rotterdam, 10–12 April, 1996 (unpublished)

23. Boccon-Gibod L et al. Flutamide versus orchidectomy in patients with metastatic prostate carcinoma. Presented at the XIth Congress of the European Association of Urology, July 1994; abstr 25; 13

24. Dalesio O and the Prostate Cancer Trialists' Collaborative Group. Maximum androgen blockade in advanced prostate cancer; an overview of 22 randomised trials with 3283 deaths in 5710 patients. Lancet 1995; 345: 265–269

25. Schröder F H. Letter to all Dutch urologists, Nov 1996 (personal communication)

26. Scher M I, Kelly W K. Flutamide withdrawal syndrome: its impact on clinical trials in prostate cancer. J Clin Oncol 1993; 11: 1566–1572

27. Small E J, Carrol P R. PSA decline after Casodex withdrawal: evidence for an anti-androgen withdrawal syndrome. Urology 1996; 43: 408–410

28. Konyves I. Estramustine phosphate (Estracyt) in the treatment of prostatic carcinoma. Int Urol Nephrol 1989; 21: 393–397

29. Eisenberger M A. Chemotherapy for endocrine resistant cancer of the prostate. In: Schröder F H (ed) Treatment of prostate cancer — facts and controversies. New York: Wiley-Liss, 1990: 155–164

30. Vandenbroucke F, Van Poppel H, Debruyn I *et al*. Interim results of a randomized trial of MMC in combination with orchidectomy for newly diagnosed metastatic prostate cancer. Am J Clin Oncol 1995; 18: 263–266

31. Pummer K. Presentation at the Munich Meeting, 1996. Eur Urol, in press

32. Bruchovsky N, Rennie P S, Coldman A J *et al*. Effects of androgen withdrawal on the stem cell composition of the Schonogyi carcinoma. Cancer Res 1990; 50: 2275–2285

33. Goldenberg S, Bruchovsky N, Gleave M *et al*. Intermittent androgen suppression in the treatment of prostate cancer: a preliminary report. Urology 1995; 45: 639–846

34. Mahler C, Denis L. Treatment of hormone refractory disease. Semin Surg Oncol 1995; 11: 770–783

35. Seidman A D, Scher H I, Petrylak D *et al*. Estramustine and vinblastine: use of prostate specific antigen as a clinical trial end point for hormone refractory prostatic cancer. J Urol 1992; 147: 931–934

36. Wilding G, cited in Eisenberger M A, Nelson W G. How much can we rely on the level of PSA as an endpoint for evaluation of clinical trials? A word of caution! J Natl Cancer Inst 1996; 88: 779–781

Chapter 30

Adjuncts for magnifying the effectiveness of intermittent hormone therapy in early and advanced prostate cancer

R. T. D. Oliver

Introduction

There are reports that treatment with bacillus Calmette–Guérin (BCG) can double 10-year survival in patients with superficial bladder cancer[1,2] and that the chance of achieving this depends on the strength of immune response, as measured by production of interleukin (IL)-2 (ref. 3) and γ-interferon.[4] These data, and the fact that BCG has a negligible effect in metastatic disease, provide the strongest evidence that manipulation of the immune response can influence control of the early stages of cancer development. The fact that reduced or total lack of expression of HLA antigens[5] and other molecules[6,7] that are absolute requisites of successful immunological rejection occurs in the majority of invasive and metastatic tumours provides a possible explanation why there is unlikely to be any gain from use of immunotherapy in such cases. One possible exception to these observations may be tumours arising in individuals who are immunosuppressed, as the little evidence that exists, from a small study of high-grade lymphomas,[8] demonstrates that such tumours have a substantially lower incidence of HLA antigen loss than do spontaneously occurring tumours.

Today, few would consider that there was any likelihood that immune response was relevant to control of hormone-sensitive cancer, whether of the breast or the prostate. There has been little evidence that prostate cancer is increased in patients with HIV disease or on immunosuppressive drugs.[9] However, as the average age of such individuals when first infected is usually only about 30–35 years, a 30-year follow-up would be needed before they reached peak risk of the disease. Equally uninformative, in respect of the role of immune response in prostate cancer, is the lack of information on frequency of spontaneous regression of prostate cancer. There are, however, cases of patients with biopsy-proven tumour who come to surgery and have no evidence of disease in the excised specimen,[10] and who could possibly be examples of spontaneous regression; there are also anecdotal case reports of patients,[11] most notably those receiving cryotherapy to primary tumours,[12] who demonstrate regression of untreated measurable metastatic disease.

The aim of this chapter is to consider the significance of new data on the influence of castration on regeneration of the thymus, and of studies of intermittent hormone therapy, that open up the prospect of a completely new approach to prostate cancer treatment as they suggest that immune response may play a role in determining the duration of response to hormone therapy. Trials to ascertain whether there is any clinical relevance to these observations are considered in the final section.

Castration and regeneration of the human thymus

The association between castration and regeneration of the thymus in experimental animals was first made in the late 19th century by an Italian physiologist studying rabbits,[13] though there has been little research on this issue in humans during the more than 40 years that castration has been routine in both breast and prostate cancer. The first clue that this effect may indeed occur in men was suggested when Sperandio *et al.*,[14] attempting to explain the thymic enlargement seen in testis cancer, observed a correlation between the occurrence of thymic hyperplasia and the level of luteinizing hormone as a measure of Leydig cell damage in the testis of men who had received chemotherapy for testis cancer. In some of these patients the thymic enlargement had been so marked that they had undergone thoracotomy and thymic biopsy.

These observations were then applied to prostate cancer. As it was known, from animal studies, that thymic enlargement was less in older castrated animals,[15] the study initially investigated the effects of castration on circulating levels of lymphocytes (Table 30.1). As judged by the development of lymphopenia in association with the testosterone surge during the first 7 days of LHRH analogue treatment, and lymphocytosis by day 28 when testosterone levels are drastically reduced, it is clear that sex hormones affect circulating lymphocyte levels. However, it would be necessary to investigate T and B lymphocyte subsets in order to confirm that this observation really indicated thymic regeneration. The fact that those who had significant lymphocytosis in this small series of patients had a better prognosis (Table 30.2), although not significant in its own right, does highlight, in the absence of any literature on this issue, how little the work on the role of immune response in prostate cancer has been reported. This ought to be a simple issue that could be explored in databases holding the results of current large-scale clinical trials.

Table 30.1. Influence of prostatic cancer hormone treatment on peripheral blood lymphocytes

Time after starting LHRH analogue (days)	Percentage with post-treatment lymphocytes less than pretreatment	Percentage with post-treatment lymphocytes greater than pretreatment
0 vs 7 (*n* = 12)	58	42
0 vs 28 (*n* = 17)	24	76

Adapted from ref. 15 with permission.

Table 30.2. Impact of hormone-induced lymphocytosis (day 28) on first remission duration

Lymphocytes, day 28	Cases (*n*)	Median remission (months)	Percentage with > 12/12 remission
Increased	13	13	31
Decreased	4	6.5	25

Adapted from ref. 15 with permission.

One group of patients, in whom correlation between clinical outcome and lymphocyte levels could provide important insights into the relevance of lymphocyte immune surveillance and survival in prostate cancer, would be those patients taking part in studies of immediate versus deferred hormone therapy,[16] comparing lymphocyte levels in those who have stable or slowly progressive disease with those who had rapid progression. As the doubling time of prostate-specific antigen (PSA) in selected patients in observation studies may be more than 4 years in 50% of patients,[17] one might expect higher lymphocyte levels in slower growing tumours if there was a component of host response involved.

Intermittent hormone therapy in prostate cancer

Until recently it was held that, because hormone therapy was thought simply to revert the cancer stem cells back to the prepubertal state, any return of hormone inevitably would reignite the cancer; in other words, hormone therapy acted only as a cytostatic therapy. However, if it were possible to consider that hormone therapy refreshed the immune response so that mutated stem cells could be rejected, intermittent therapy could be considered. Two additional observations provide justification for intermittent therapy. First, there is some evidence that hormone-sensitive and insensitive clones, certainly in breast[18] and almost certainly in prostate cancer, behave as separate entities in terms of response to treatment. Chronic use of hormone withdrawal could provide a selection pressure to favour growth of hormone-independent clones, as antibiotics do for antibiotic-insensitive bacteria. Secondly, analysis of prostate tumours in patients relapsing late on continuous hormone therapy has shown a significant increase in androgen receptor overexpression (see Chapter 9).

It is surprising that, in more than 50 years since hormone therapy has been in use, so little has been done to investigate this issue. The author's studies in this area began because of patient pressure after hearing anecdotal stories about celebrities succeeding to do this without apparent harm, and after hearing of the work of Bruchovsky and colleagues.[19–21] Although the author has observed only 20 patients for periods up to 48 months off treatment, 45% remain progression free at 3 years and those relapsing have had a normal response to second treatment.[22] These studies, taken with other reports (see Table 30.3), would suggest that there is a strong case to conduct a randomized trial of intermittent hormone therapy versus continuous therapy, with investigation of host immune response parameters. As there is some evidence, in the author's data supported by the results from Strum *et al.*,[23] that the benefit from intermittent therapy is more pronounced in early cases (Table 30.4), this approach could be an alternative to deferred therapy and might even be an alternative to surgery in operable cases.

Table 30.3. Overview of studies of intermittent hormone therapy

Study (ref. no)	Cases (*n*)	Percentage progression-free at 12 months (mean 30 weeks; range 9–108 weeks)
21	47	N/A
22	20	63
23	21	87

N/A = data not available

Table 30.4. Risk factors and PSA progression-free survival after withdrawal of hormone therapy

Factor	Cases (*n*)	Percentage progression-free off hormones (1 year)
M+	7	29
M0	13	82
No radiation	10	56
Radiation	10	61
Duration on hormones (months)		
< 14	10	80
≥ 14	10	46
Age (years)		
< 66	10	58
≥ 67	10	70

Adapted from ref. 22 with permission.

Preliminary findings, as yet unpublished, on the large UK study of more than 900 asymptomatic patients randomized between immediate and deferred hormone therapy,[24] as well the original retrospective analysis on this issue by Nesbit and Baum,[25] demonstrate that only for early disease patients is there a significant survival advantage for early treatment. These observations, taken with the information (for review see ref. 26) that maximum androgen blockade has a significant impact on survival only in early good-risk patients, provide an added incentive to ascertain whether it might be safe to use hormone therapy intermittently, as there is greater reluctance to use hormones as treatment in such earlier-stage cases.

Prospects for combining hormone therapy with immunotherapy in light of thymic regeneration and intermittent hormone therapy observation

The BCG data in bladder cancer,[1,2] and the observation on loss of HLA antigens and other immune rejection molecules on invasive and metastatic bladder[3-5] and prostate[27] tumours, clearly demonstrate that immune surveillance and immunotherapy are effective only in the setting of early cancer before it has evolved to be completely resistant to immune response. Response to hormone therapy is a marker of a well-differentiated prostate cancer, as androgen sensitivity is the norm for non-malignant prostate cells. There has been no serious attempt in the past to investigate the place of immunotherapy in hormone-sensitive cancer, although one extremely small trial in patients with hormone-sensitive breast cancer using lentinan, a Japanese immunostimulating agent, demonstrates such a marked effect on progression (Table 30.5) that it is surprising that no attempt has been made to repeat this trial.[28] For prostate cancer, with PSA decline providing a particularly accurate and early indication of hormone sensitivity,[29] there should be little difficulty in identifying patients for entry into such a trial. BCG or interferon are the most obvious agents to use in these patients, although the advent of an oral interferon inducer, bropirimine, which has activity in BCG-resistant bladder cancer,[30] offers a particularly interesting alternative.

Table 30.5. *Influence of immunotherapy with lentinan on progression-free survival of breast cancer responders to hormone therapy*

Treatment	Cases (*n*)	Percentage progression-free in primary tumour
Control	16	13
Lentinan polysaccharide	15	47

$\chi^2 = 4.2$, $p < 0.05$
Adapted from ref. 28 with permission.

Significance of these observations to treatment of local disease

Studies of hormones in combination with radiation in advanced disease

With increasing acceptance that, in clinical trials, short-term hormone therapy prior to radiotherapy improves long-term disease control,[31] and animal models suggesting the same (Table 30.6), were BCG or interferon to be shown to improve hormone response, the next stage would be to test the combination in the neo-adjuvant setting prior to radiation, as there is some evidence that immunotherapy might also help to overcome the late consequences of the immunosuppressive effects of radiation on circulating T lymphocytes.[32] There is increasing acceptance that results from use of radiation are best when using small fields with CT scan planning. With increasing recognition of the poor prognosis of persistent cells in the prostate after radiation, there could be a case for increased use of surgery as an additional adjunct of therapy in patients not achieving complete remission, as in bladder cancer,[33] particularly in G3 tumours.

Studies in early cancer detected by PSA screening

With PSA screening detecting cancers in four to five times more people that past mortality studies would have predicted,[34] and evidence from clinical studies[35] that it is the G3 tumours that most benefit from surgery (Table 30.7), the critical issue for the future is to define a way of discrimination that separates the poor-risk from the good-risk cases. Poor-risk patients, as discussed in the previous section, provided that they prove to have localized cancer, would be obvious candidates for radical approaches, combining all three treatment modalities — hormones, radiation and surgery — possibly using the flash radiotherapy technique developed by Whitmore for preoperative treatment of bladder cancer.[36] The fact that the benefits of intermittent therapy and maximum androgen blockade are most clearly demonstrated in the patients with early, well-differentiated cancer

Table 30.6. *Interaction between radiation and endocrine therapy in experimental animal model of prostate cancer*

Treatment	Percentage with progressive tumour
Radiation alone	80
Synchronous orchiectomy and radiation	55
Orchiectomy followed by radiation	35
Radiation followed by orchiectomy	70

Adapted from ref. 60 with permission.

Table 30.7. Literature overview of 10-year survival after radical prostatectomy compared with watchful waiting

Tumours	Watchful waiting		Radical prostatectomy	
	Cases (n)	10-year survival (%)	Cases (n)	10-year survival (%)
T1/2 Grade 1	490	88	519	96*
T1/2 Grade 2	262	87	1597	80†
T1/2 Grade 3	63	35	211	77‡

*p = 0.16; †p = 0.33; ‡p = 0.0004.
Adapted from ref. 35 with permission.

and that these are the patients who have the slowest PSA doubling times when untreated,[17] suggests that short-term therapy (e.g. 2 months hormone therapy combined with immunotherapy) might enable further treatment to be avoided for several years. Given the anxiety raised by fears that tissue trauma, by release of tissue repair cytokines such as epithelial growth factor, even after needle biopsy,[37] could accelerate tumour cell implantation,[38] it might be prudent to avoid the trauma of biopsy for diagnosis, possibly returning to the use of prostatic massage[39] or ejaculates[40] to diagnose such early cases.

Studies in prevention of prostate cancer that are relevant to HIV infection, cervix and penile cancer and prostate cancer

There are two other issues that could magnify the gain from the use of intermittent hormone therapy for treatment of early prostate cancer, which are equally relevant to HIV infection and to cervix and penile cancer. These arise out of increasing understanding from the study of epidemiology of this tumour,[41] which has demonstrated two principal areas of potential preventative intervention, namely modification of diet and sexual habits (Table 30.8). There is clear evidence from a randomized trial in bladder cancer that progression-free survival after BCG immunotherapy of early tumours is enhanced by 'multivitamins',[42] although, probably equally significantly, good nutrition high in

Table 30.8. Overview of dietary and sexual behaviour risk factors for prostate cancer

Risk factor	Relative risk
Obesity	1.25
Meat consumption	1.34
Dairy products consumption	1.30
Total fat consumption	1.31
Animal fat consumption	1.54
Carrot consumption	0.66
Green vegetables consumption	0.93
Early age of 1st intercourse	1.31
Number of sexual partners	1.21
Sexually acquired infection	1.86
Syphilis	0.77
Gonorrhoea	1.22
Vasectomy	1.54

Adapted from ref. 41 with permission.

the appropriate fruits and vegetables but low in animal fats, could be sufficient. Possible mediators of this effect are the fat-soluble vitamins, as vitamin A is known to boost T-lymphocyte function[43] and vitamin D is known to boost macrophage/dendritic cell function.[44] Recently, there has been increased recognition of the importance of dendritic cells in immune resistance to prostate cancer, and reports that it is possible to prime dendritic cells against PSA *in vitro*.[45] Such an approach could be of therapeutic benefit in patients with locally advanced cancer, or in node-positive patients resistant to hormones. An additional aspect of interest relevant to immune response and diet arises from observations demonstrating an inverse correlation between level of sunshine and mortality from prostate cancer in the United States, possibly also mediated via vitamin D production.[46]

The second adjunct to intermittent use of maximum androgen blockade relates to condom use. In 1981 it was demonstrated that condom use can lead to regression of early-stage carcinoma *in situ* of the cervix[47] (Table 30.9). This, taken with reports of increased incidence of prostate cancer after vasectomy,[41] possibly reflecting diminished use of barrier contraception, raises the question whether similar effects may occur in men with prostate premalignant disease. There is no information on such a strategy in early prostate cancer, although one confounding variable that could be a factor in the low incidence of clinically significant, but equal incidence of latent, prostate cancer in the Japanese compared with the European and African Americans (Table 30.10), is that the

Table 30.9. Condom use and spontaneous regression of cervical intraepithelial neoplasia (CIN 1-111)

	Cases* (n)	CR at 2 months (%)	Overall CR[†] (%)	Recurrence[‡] (%)
Cone biopsy and condom	45	NA	100	7.5
Cryosurgery and condom	107	60	100	3.7
Punch biopsy and condom	139	43	100	8.1

CR, complete response; NA, not available.
*CR, 60% CIN III.
[‡]12 of 18 recurrences developed 2nd line CR after further condom use.
[†]Mean time to CR = 4.9 months.
From ref. 47 with permission.

Table 30.10. Comparison of incidence of latent prostate cancer at autopsy with clinical incidence and death rates

Prostate cancer	Year	Race		
		Japanese	American White	American Black
Percentage latent at autopsy	1980*	41	32	34
	1990*	20	33	38
Clinical incidence	1980[†]	3	46	80
	1990[†]	5	55	95
Deaths	1980[†]	1.5	14	25
	1990[†]	2.5	14.5	27

*Age 60–69 years: from ref. 61 with permission.
[†]Adapted from ref. 62 with permission.

Japanese have a very low usage of the contraceptive pill and high usage of barrier contraceptives,[63] in addition to their diet low in animal fat and high in fibre.

There is increasing understanding, from studies of *Helicobacter* in stomach cancer epidemiology, of mechanisms whereby bacteria can act as promoting agents of malignancy.[48] As there is no evidence for any of the well-established genital viral infections being involved in prostate cancer,[49] but some evidence for association of prostatitis with prostate cancer,[50] it is possible that low-grade asymptomatic bacterial infection may be a more significant aetiological factor than previously appreciated. Repeating the study of Breslow *et al.*,[51] looking for latent prostate cancer at post-mortem examination or in live transplant donors from different geographic locations with culture of the prostate, would be one way of investigating this hypothesis.

There is evidence that education in male genital hygiene (Tables 30.11 and 30.12) may be of considerable importance in the prevention of cervical and penile cancer[52,53] and HIV infection.[54,55] In addition, the rates of heterosexual HIV infection and of cervical, penile and prostate cancer are all high in sub-Saharan Africa and South America, but low in the Middle East and Japan. Given that the genital hygiene tradition of the Middle East can be traced back to the time that the Israelites were in Egypt (for review see ref. 56), inclusion of sex-organ-cancer prevention education as part of sex education at the time of puberty ceremonies such as bar mitzvahs could have major benefits in long-term control of all these conditions.

Contribution of progress in genetics to epidemiology

It is now clear (see Chapter 36 and 42) that genetic factors are the most powerful of all the epidemiological risk factors and have a more significant impact in prostate cancer than most other adult cancers, with the possible exception of testis cancer.[57] As in testis cancer,[58,59] for as long as germ line gene therapy is not possible, the prime benefit that will come from knowledge about the genes will be to focus attention on linking genes with functionally relevant mechanisms. Knowledge that immune response is genetically linked could well be relevant to understanding the

Table 30.11. Impact of education on incidence of cancer of the cervix and penis in Madras

Educational level	Cancer (rate/100,000)	
	Cervix	Penis
Illiterate	55	2.3
< 12 years education	19	1.9
> 12 years education	4.7	1.1

Adapted from ref. 52 with permission.

Table 30.12. Impact of religious background on incidence of cancer of the cervix and penis in Madras

Religion	Cancer (rate/100,000)	
	Cervix	Penis
Hindu	35	2.2
Christian	27	0.8
Muslim	14	nil

Adapted from ref. 52 with permission.

mechanism by which persistent infection, such as that postulated in the previous section could be a cofactor. Equally relevant are the group of genes controlling the cytochrome *P*-450 and DNA repair enzymes for explaining the association of prostate cancer with radiation, pesticides and heavy metal exposure.

Conclusions

Arising out of the success of BCG treatment for superficial bladder cancer, it is increasingly accepted that immune surveillance plays a significant role in early cancer. The hypothesis that hormone-sensitive cancer may represent functionally early cancer is leading to the need for new studies to investigate the use of immunotherapy in hormone-sensitive prostate cancer.

The discovery that old observations on regeneration of the thymus after castration in experimental animals also apply in humans, combined with reports that the use of hormone therapy intermittently may be safe, suggest that a complete revision of current approaches to the use of hormone therapy is needed. These observations suggest that there may be greater benefit from short-term intermittent use of hormone therapy in early-stage than there is from its use in advanced prostate cancer. These observations may also apply to oestrogen receptor-positive breast cancer.

The emergence of diet and sexually acquired infections as principal risk factors, from epidemiology studies, has led to the suggestion that the use of diet and barrier contraception, as an adjunct to intermittent hormone therapy in cases of early well-differentiated prostate cancer detected by PSA screening, may well reduce the need for surgery in the four out of five patients in whom disease is potentially not life threatening.

Given increasing evidence that the magnitude of gain from radical surgery is greatest in G3 tumours, and evidence for enhanced radiation response in patients pretreated with hormones, those cases should be considered for new strategies of combined-modality radical therapy at an early stage.

Shared sexual behaviour risk factors between heterosexual HIV infection and cervical, penile and prostate cancer suggest that sex-organ-cancer prevention could be an added gain from the increase use of condoms encouraged by the HIV epidemic. Inclusion of education about these risk factors in sex education at time of puberty ceremonies such as bar mitzvahs is proposed as an approach to reducing the incidence of this disease.

References

1. Herr H W, Schwalb D M, Zhang Z F *et al*. Intravesical bacillus Calmette-Guérin therapy prevents tumour progression and death from superficial bladder cancer: ten-year follow-up of a prospective randomized trial. J Clin Oncol 1995; 13(6): 1404–1408
2. Lamm D L. BCG in perspective — advances in the treatment of superficial bladder cancer. Eur Urol 1995; 27: 2–8
3. Fleishman J D, Kendall M D, Wheeler M J. Urinary interleukins in patients receiving intravesical vacillus Calmette–Guering therapy for superficial bladder cancer. Cancer 1985; 64: 1447–1454
4. Prescot S, James K, Hargreave T B *et al*. Radio-immunoassay detection of interferon gamma in urine after intravesical Evans BCG therapy. J Urol 1990; 144: 1248–1252
5. Nouri A M E, Smith M E F, Crosby D, Oliver R T D. Selective and non-selective immunoregulatory molecules (HLA, B, C antigens and LAFA-3) in transitional cell carcinoma. Br J Cancer 1990; 62: 603–606
6. Oliver R T D, Nouri A M E, Crosby D *et al*. Biological significance of Beta hCG, HLA and other membrane antigen expression on bladder tumours and their relationship to tumour infiltrating lymphocytes (TIL). J Immunogenet 1989; 16: 381–390

7. Nouri A M E, Hussain R F, Dos Santos A V I, Oliver R T D. Defective expression of adhesion molecules on human bladder tumour and human tumour cell lines. Urol Int 1996; 56: 1–5
8. List A F, Spier C M, Miller T P, Grogan T M. Deficient tumour infiltrating T lymphocyte response in malignant lymphoma — relationship to HLA expression and host immunocompetence. Leukemia 1993; 7(3): 398–403
9. Penn I. Cancers complicating organ transplantation. N Engl J Med 1990; 323: 1967–1968
10. Goldstein N S, Begin L R, Grody W W et al. Vanishing cancer phenomenon in radical prostatectomy specimens. Am J Surg Pathol 1995; 19(9): 1002–1009
11. Schurmans J R, Blijenberg B G, Mickisch G J, Schroder F H. Spontaneous remission of a bony metastasis in prostatic adenocarcinoma. Urology 1996; 155: 653
12. Soanes W A, Ablin R J, Gonder M J. Remission of metastatic lesions following cryosurgery in prostatic cancer: immunologic considerations. J Urol 1970; 104: 154–159
13. Grossman C J. Interactions between the gonadal steroids and the immune system. Science 1985; 227: 257–261
14. Sperandio P, Tomio P, Oliver R T D et al. Gonadal atrophy as a cause of thymic hyperplasia after chemotherapy. Br J Cancer 1996; 74: 991–992
15. Oliver R T D, Joseph J V, Gallagher C J. Castration-induced lymphocytosis in prostate cancer: possible evidence for gonad-thymus endocrine interaction in man. Urol Int 1995; 54: 226–229
16. Kirk D. Immediate versus deferred treatment for advanced disease. Cancer Surv 1995; 23: 183
17. Schmid H P. Tumour markers in patients on deferred treatment: prostate specific antigen doubling times. Cancer Surv 1995; 23: 157
18. Bartlett K, Eremin O, Hutcheon A et al. Adjuvant ovarian ablation vs CMF chemotherapy in premenopausal women with pathological stage II breast carcinoma: the Scottish trial. Lancet 1993; 341: 1293–1298
19. Gleave M, Bruchovsky N, Bowden M et al. Intermittent androgen suppression prolongs time to androgen-independent progression in the LNCaP prostate tumour model. J Urol 1994; 151: 457
20. Akakura K, Bruchovsky N, Goldenberg S L et al. Effects of intermittent androgen suppression on androgen dependent tumours. Cancer 1993; 71: 2782–2790
21. Goldenberg S L, Bruchovsky N, Gleave M E et al. Intermittent androgen suppression in the treatment of prostate cancer: a preliminary report. Urology 1995; 45: 839–845
22. Oliver R T D, Grant-Williams G, Paris A M I, Blandy J P. Intermittent androgen deprivation after PSA complete response as a strategy to reduce induction of hormone resistant prostate cancer. Urology 1997; 49: 79–82
23. Strum S B, Scholz M C, Strum M. Prolonged non-detectable PSA in patients treated by androgen deprivation may allow for discontinuation of hormone blockade. Proc Int Symp Recent Adv Diagnosis and Treatment of Prostate Cancer.
24. Kirk D. Hormone therapy in advanced prostate cancer: MRC immediate deferred treatment study. Br J Urol 1996; (suppl 1): abstr 204
25. Nesbit R M, Baum W C. Endocrine control of prostatic carcinoma. Clinical and statistical survey of 1818 cases. JAMA 1950; 143: 1317–1320
26. Denis L. Comment on maximal androgen blockade in prostate cancer — a theory put into practice. Prostate 1995; 27: 233–240
27. Blades R A, Keating P J, McWillian L J et al. Loss of HLA class I expression in prostate cancer: implications for immunotherapy. Urology 1995; 46: 681–686
28. Kosaka A, Hattori Y, Imaizumi A, Yamashita A. Synergistic effect of lentinan and surgical endocrine therapy of the growth of DMBA-induced mammary tumours of rats and of recurrent human breast cancer. Excerpta Medica International Conference 1985; 690: 138–199
29. Matzkin H, Eber P, Todd B, van der Zwaag R, Soloway M S. Prognostic significance of changes in prostate-specific markers after endocrine treatment in stage D2 prostatic cancer. Cancer 1992; 70: 2302
30. Sarosdy M F, Lowe B A, Schellhammer P F et al. Bropiriamine immunotherapy of bladder CIS: positive phase II results of an oral interferon inducer. Proc Annu Meet Am Soc Clin Oncol 1994; 13: A719
31. Pilepich M V, Krall J M, Alsarraf M et al. Androgen deprivation with radiation therapy compared with radiation therapy alone for locally advanced prostatic carcinoma — a randomised comparative trial of the radiation-therapy oncology group. Urology 1995; 45: 616–623

32. DeRuysscher D, Waer M, Vandeputte M et al. Changes of lymphocyte subsets after local irradiation for early stage breast cancer and seminoma testis: long-term increase of activated (HLA-DR+) T cells and decrease of "naive" (CD4-CD45R) T lymphocytes. Eur J Cancer 1992; 28A: 1729–1734

33. Blandy J P, England H R, Evans S J W et al. T3 bladder cancer — the case for salvage cystectomy. Br J Urol 1980; 52: 506–510

34. Parkes C A. An epidemiologist's viewpoint on screening. Cancer Surv 1995; 23: 127

35. Chodak G W, Thisted R A. Comparison of cancer specific survival (CSS) following radical prostatectomy (RP) or watchful waiting (WW) based on two multi-institutional pooled analyses. Proc AUA. J Urol 1996; 155(suppl): abstr 995

36. Whitmore W F, Batata M A, Hilaris B S et al. A comparative study of 2 pre-operative radiation regimens with cystectomy for bladder cancer. Cancer 1977; 40: 1077–1086

37. Fentiman I S, Gregory W M. The hormonal milieu and prognosis in operable breast cancer. Cancer Surv 1993; 18: 149–163

38. Oliver R T D. Does surgery disseminate or accelerate cancer? Lancet 1995; 346: 1506–1507

39. Fergusson J D, Gibson E C. Prostatic smear diagnosis. Br Med J 1956; 1: 822–825

40. Gardiner R A, Smaratunga M L T H, Gwynne R A et al. Abnormal prostatic cells in ejaculates from men with prostatic cancer — a preliminary report. Br J Urol 1996; 78: 414–418

41. Key T. Risk factors for prostate cancer. Cancer Surv 1995; 23: 63–77

42. Lamm D L, Riggs D R, Shriver J S et al. Megadose vitamins in bladder cancer: a double-blind clinical trial. J Urol 1994; 151: 21–26

43. Semba R D, Miotti P C, Chiphangwi J D et al. Maternal vitamin A deficiency and mother to child transmission of HIV-1. Lancet 1994; 343: 1593–1597

44. Rook G A, Steele J, Fraher L, Barker S. Vitamin D3, gamma interferon, and control of proliferation of Mycobacterium tuberculosis by human monocytes. Immunology 1986; 57: 159

45. Tjoa B, Boynton A, Kenny G et al. Presentation of prostate tumor-antigens by dendritic cells stimulates T-cell proliferation and cytotoxicity. Prostate 1996; 28(N1): 65–69

46. Clark L C, Dalkin B L, LaBrec P A et al. An inverse association between incidence of prostate cancer and a clinical index of sun damage. Proc AUA. J Urol 1996; 155(suppl 605a): abstr 1175

47. Richardson A C, Lyon J B. The effect of condom use on squamous cell cervical intra-epithelial neoplasia. Am J Obstet Gynecol 1981; 140: 909–913

48. Forman D. Helicobacter pylori and gastric cancer. Scand J Gastroenterol 1996; 31: 48–51

49. Cuzick J. Human papillomavirus infection of the prostate. Cancer Surv 1995; 23: 91–95

50. Feneley M R, Young M P A, Chinyama C et al. Ki-67 expression in early prostate cancer and associated pathological lesions. J Clin Pathol 1996; 49: 741–748

51. Breslow N, Chan C W, Dhom G, et al. Latent carcinoma of prostate at autopsy in seven areas. Int J Cancer 1977; 20: 680–688

52. Gajalakshmi C K, Shanta V. Association between cervical and penile cancers in Madras, India. Acta Oncol 1993; 32(6): 617–620

53. UK Testicular Cancer Study Group. Social, behavioural and medical factors in the aetiology of testicular cancer: results from the UK study. Br J Cancer 1994; 70: 513–520

54. Cameron D W, Simonsen J N, D'Costa L J. Female to male transmission of human immunodeficiency virus type 1: risk ractors for seroconversion in men. Lancet 1989; 2: 403–407

55. Laga M, Alary M, Azila N et al. Condom promotion, sexually transmitted diseases treatment, and declining incidence of HIV-1 infection in female Zairian sex workers. Lancet 1994; 344: 246–248

56. Blandy J P, Hope-Stone H F, Oliver R T D. Carcinoma of the penis and urethra. In: Oliver R (ed) Urological and genital cancer. Oxford: Blackwell, 1989: 258–271

57. Forman D, Oliver R T D, Brett A R et al. Familial testicular cancer: a report of the UK family register, estimation of risk and an HLA Class 1 sib-pair analysis. Br J Cancer 1992; 65: 255–262

58. Leahy M, Tonks S, Moses J et al. Candidate regions for a testicular cancer susceptibility gene. Hum Mol Genet 1995; 4: 1551–1555

59. Oliver R T D, Oliver J C. Endocrine hypothesis for declining sperm count and rising testis cancer incidence. Lancet 1996; 346: 339–340

60. Zietman A L, Prince E A, Nakfoor B M, Shipley W U. Permanent tumour eradication by radiation is enhanced by prior androgen withdrawal in two experimental models. J Urol 1996; 155: 509 (abstr 792)

61. Oishi K, Yoshida O, Schroeder F H. The geography of prostate cancer and its treatment in Japan. Cancer Surv 1995; 23: 267–280
62. Whittemore A S, Keller J B, Betensky R. Low grade, latent prostate cancer volume: predictor of clinical cancer incidence? J Natl Cancer Inst 1991; 83: 1231–1235
63. Maruyama H, Raphael J H, Djurassi C. Why Japan ought to relegalise the pill. Nature 1996; 379: 579–580

Chapter 31

The Scandinavian Prostate Cancer Group Study #4 (SPCG-4)* and its rationale

J. Adolfsson

Introduction

In January 1989 the Scandinavian Prostate Cancer Group study # 4 (SPCG-4) started to recruit patients. This is a multicentre study randomizing patients with clinically localized low-grade prostate cancer to either radical prostatectomy or deferred endocrine treatment.

Study design

The inclusion criteria are as follows:

- age ≤ 75 years at diagnosis;
- the general health of the patient should permit a radical prostatectomy;
- the patient should have a newly diagnosed adenocarcinoma of the prostate;
- the tumour should be well or moderately differentiated;
- the local tumour stage should be T1d to T2;[1] currently stage T1c is also included;[2]
- the patient should have no detectable distant metastases;
- the prostate-specific antigen value should be less than 50 µg/litre.

The randomization is central. The study is stratified according to the tumour grade because the tumour grade was found to be prognostic in one of the studies forming the basis for the SPCG-4 study.[3] In this setting, it will be possible to investigate not only the prognostic value of tumour grade but also its eventual predictive value for the outcome of the radical prostatectomy.[4] The study hypothesis is that the disease-specific survival rate is improved from 85 to 95% 5 years after the diagnosis in the group treated with radical prostatectomy. To be able to detect this difference with a type I (α) fault of less than 5% with a two-tailed test and a type II (β) fault of 20% or less (power ≥ 80%), with 10% of the patients refusing the assigned treatment, the study needs 233 patients in each arm. It was assumed that another 10% of the patients would be lost to follow-up or erroneously randomized and thus the original study size was agreed as a total of 520 patients.

---

*Steering committee: Hans-Olov Adami, M.D., Fred Helgesen, M.D., Örebro, Lars Holmberg, M.D., Uppsala, Jan-Erik Johannson, M.D. Örebro and Bo-Johan Norlén, M.D., Uppsala, Sweden.

Procedure

The radical prostatectomy is performed via the retropubic approach and all patients randomized to this treatment are subjected to an initial pelvic lymphadenectomy. Frozen sections of the regional lymph nodes are prepared in conjunction with the procedure; if metastases are found, the prostatectomy is discontinued. In the group allocated to deferred treatment, such treatment is given when symptoms arising from the tumour occur.

The patients are followed with clinical and biochemical investigations twice a year and with yearly isotope investigations of the skeleton. The general quality of life of the patients is assessed longitudinally in a subset; the disease-specific quality of life will be analysed in a cross-sectional study when the recruitment of patients is finished. Local progression with obstructive voiding symptoms is treated with transurethral resection of the prostate. Symptomatic local or distant progression after radical prostatectomy is treated with androgen withdrawal. Treatment of progression after deferred endocrine treatment is at the discretion of each investigator.

The primary endpoint of the study is disease-specific survival and the secondary endpoints are metastasis-free survival and quality of life. The first analysis of survival will be performed 5 years after completion of recruitment.This analysis, as well as all subsequent analyses, will be performed according to the intention to treat. The study is funded by the Swedish Cancer Society.

Rationale

The SPCG-4 study was planned and started at the end of the 1980s. At that time there was a clinical impression that early prostate cancer often had a protracted course and that many patients died with their cancer rather than of it. This notion was by that time also documented in studies from Sweden[3,5] and the United Kingdom.[6] Radical prostatectomy was not at that time commonly performed in Scandinavia but acceptance of that procedure was increasing after the changes in surgical technique that were introduced at the start of the 1970s.[7] When the outcome of deferred treatment was compared with that of the (at that time) contemporary series of radical prostatectomies,[8–10] the difference, if any, was minor. There were only two randomized treatment trials up to that time: the Uro-Oncology Research Group compared radical prostatectomy and external radiotherapy, and found a lower rate of progression after radical prostatectomy, although survival was not analysed;[11] and the VACURG study, comparing radical prostatectomy and deferred treatment, had not found any difference in survival at the time of the first follow-up and still have not done so, after more than 20 years of follow-up.[12] Both these studies have flaws in the design and in their procedure, and the results must be regarded with great caution. At the time that the SPCG-4 study was planned, therefore, there was no convincing proof that radical prostatectomy improved the survival of patients with localized prostate cancer.

A survey performed by the Swedish Association of Urology in the mid 1980s showed that a majority of the urologists in Sweden considered deferred treatment to be an acceptable form of management for patients with early prostate cancer beside locally aggressive treatments such as radical prostatectomy and external beam radiation therapy. Thus, it was thought to be feasible to conduct the SPCG-4 study in Sweden.

Progress

Today, almost 7 years after the SPCG-4 study was started, approximately 600 patients have been included. During the time that has elapsed since the study was planned and started, new data from uncontrolled treatment trials and reviews of these trials[13–15] have indicated that the difference in survival outcome between radical prostatectomy and deferred treatment at 5 and 10 years may be less than originally anticipated. If this is true, it will decrease the power of the study. On the other hand, fewer patients than anticipated have refused the allocated treatment and almost no patients have been lost to follow-up, both increasing the power. However, the Steering Committee has decided to enlarge the study size to at least 700 patients to increase the power of the study.

Interim comments

Today, the basic rationale of the study still stands. There is no convincing proof that any treatment for localized prostate cancer is better than any other. No new randomized treatment studies including radical prostatectomy, external radiotherapy or deferred treatment of patients with clinically localized prostate cancer have been reported. There have been several attempts to start such studies: parallel to the SPCG-4 study, a study with a basically similar design but comparing external beam radiation therapy with deferred endocrine treatment has been conducted in Denmark and in Umeå, Sweden; however, this study has had difficulty in recruiting patients and has now been terminated. In the United States, the PIVOT study, randomizing radical prostatectomy versus deferred treatment, has been started but the recruitment rate is not according to plan (M. Brawer, personal communication, December, 1996).

It may well be that the SPCG-4 study will be the only randomized study including deferred treatment with a study size large enough to allow any conclusions regarding survival; however, another 7–10 years must elapse before such data are available, although data on quality of life will be available at an earlier stage.

References

1. UICC. TNM classification of malignant tumors, 3rd edn. Geneva: Union International Contre le Cancer, 1978
2. UICC. TNM classification of malignant tumors, 5th edn. Geneva: Union International Contre le Cancer, 1992
3. Johansson J-E, Andersson S-E, Krusemo U B et al. Natural history of localised prostatic cancer. Lancet 1989; 1(8642): 799–803
4. Steineck G, Adolfsson J, Scher H I, Whitmore W F Jr. Distinguish between prognostic and treatment-predictive information for localized prostate cancer. Urology 1995; 45: 610–615
5. Adolfsson J, Rönström L, Carstensen J et al. The natural course of low-stage, low-grade prostatic carcinoma. Br J Urol 1990; 65: 611–614
6. George N J R. Natural history of localised prostatic cancer managed by conservative therapy alone. Lancet 1988; 5(8584): 494–497
7. Walsh P C, Lepor H, Eggleston J C. Radical prostatectomy with preservation of sexual function: anatomical and pathological considerations. Prostate 1983; 4: 473–485
8. Blute M L, Nativ O, Zincke H et al. Pattern of failure after radical retropubic prostatectomy for clinically and pathologically localized adenocarcinoma of the prostate: influence of tumor deoxyribonucleic acid ploidy. J Urol 1989; 142: 1262–1265
9. Gibbons R P, Correa R J, Brannen G E, Weissman R M. Total prostatectomy for clinically localized prostatic cancer: long-term results. J Urol 1989; 141: 564–566

10. Lepor H, Kimball A W, Walsh P C. Cause-specific actuarial survival analysis: a useful method for reporting survival data in men with clinically localized carcinoma of the prostate. J Urol 1989; 141: 82–84

11. Paulson D F, Lin G H, Hinshaw W, Stephani S. The Uro-Oncology Research Group. Radical surgery versus radiotherapy for adenocarcinoma of the prostate. J Urol 1982; 128: 502–504

12. Iversen P, Madsen P O, Corle D K. Radical prostatectomy versus expectant treatment for early carcinoma of the prostate. Twenty-three year follow-up of a prospective randomized study. Scand J Urol Nephrol 1995; suppl 172: 65–72

13. Adolfsson J, Steineck G, Whitmore W F Jr. Recent results of management of palpable clinically localized prostate cancer. Cancer 1993; 72: 310–322

14. Middleton R G, Thompson I M, Austenfeld M S *et al*. Prostate cancer clinical guidelines panel summary report on the management of clinically localized prostate cancer. J Urol 1995; 154: 2144–2148

15. Wasson J H, Cushman C C, Bruskewitz R C *et al*. A structured literature review of treatment for localized prostate cancer. Arch Fam Med 1993; 2: 487–493

Chapter 32

Immunological targeting for the treatment of prostate cancer

S. F. Slovin, P. O. Livingston, N. Rosen, L. Sepp-Lorenzino, W. K. Kelly, J. Mendelsohn and H. I. Scher

Introduction

Prostate cancers of all stages represent a spectrum of diseases with varied prognoses. For example, within the category of organ-confined disease, some tumours will never affect the quality or quantity of a patient's survival, whereas others are predetermined to metastasize, independent of the local therapy utilized. In each situation, the key to optimal treatment depends on the ability to predict the natural history of the disease for the individual. For patients with more advanced disease, androgen ablation remains a hallmark of treatment. However, despite over five decades of experience, the optimal way(s) to utilize hormonal therapies have not been defined and, used alone, such therapies are unlikely to have any further impact on prostate cancer-specific mortality. Once hormone therapies have failed, the options are limited and, although a number of combination regimens have recently been shown to produce tumour regression,[1] no single agent or combination has been shown to improve survival in a randomized trial. Therefore, novel approaches are needed in an attempt to affect the disease progression.

At the Memorial Sloan-Kettering Cancer Center (MSKCC), the authors have developed a clinical trials programme based on the specific manifestations of the disease and the predicted prognosis based on pretreatment clinical parameters. The trials were derived from laboratory studies investigating the unique features of prostate cancers that might be exploited therapeutically. Thus, for patients with rising PSA values after definitive local therapy, a minimal disease setting, approaches that modulate immune function have been investigated. For those with metastatic 'anaplastic' or 'small cell' tumours of the prostate, which have a distinctly poor prognosis, platinum-based combinations have been investigated.[2] Finally, for patients who have relapsed after androgen ablation, investigation has focused on modulating the signalling pathways that have been shown to contribute to androgen-independent and hormone-independent progression.[3]

Vaccines in minimal residual disease: stimulation of the endogenous immune system

Patients who have progressed after definitive local treatment, with a rising prostate-specific antigen (PSA) as the sole manifestation of disease progression, represent a unique group in whom to evaluate immunological approaches, for several reasons: the disease can be monitored closely through serial measurements of PSA; androgen ablation is tolerated poorly by the 'asymptomatic' patient; furthermore, deferring hormonal therapy does not compromise survival. PSA and acid phosphatase are well-recognized prostate cancer antigens. Less recognized is that prostate cancers express a number of well-defined differentiation antigens on the tumour cell surface that can also be used as therapeutic targets.[4] These include the glycoprotein antigens PSMA (prostate-specific membrane antigen) and MUC-1, and the carbohydrate antigens Globo H, sTn and Le^y. The latter represent biochemically altered 'self' molecules that are also present on other glandular organs. These antigens become overexpressed in the malignant state and often have changes in their carbohydrate residues that allow them to remain immunologically protected from the immune system despite the changes in the amino acid moieties. All have been purified, enabling investigators to generate high-affinity monoclonal antibodies that have been used for tumour targeting and treatment.

Augmentation of the immune response to cancer can be attempted by two basic approaches: these are non-specific immunopotentiation (constituting the bulk of past and current efforts at cancer immunotherapy) and specific immunization, which has not really been evaluated in the treatment of cancer but has contributed much to the control of infectious diseases. It is the knowledge of specific microbial antigens that has permitted the development of successful immunization against infections. Of the many well-defined bacterial antigens studied as targets for vaccine therapy, carbohydrate antigens have proved to be the most clinically relevant and (apart from vaccines against toxins) are the only defined bacterial antigens used in vaccines against bacterial pathogens. More recently, they have proved to be potent targets of immune recognition and for the attack of human cancers.[5] Immunization against carbohydrate antigens results primarily in the generation of an immunoglobulin (Ig)M antibody response. These antibodies can mediate tumour cell lysis, complement-induced inflammation and phagocytosis by the reticulo-endothelial system. To select for potential targets, the authors used antibodies to carbohydrate and glycoprotein antigens to screen human prostate tumour-derived cell lines and human prostate tumour biopsy specimens.[6,7] Once an antigen has been identified and its structure determined, the antigen is synthesized and chemically modified for immunogenicity testing in mice. In these experiments, the chemically modified antigen is conjugated to a carrier molecule and injected with an immune adjuvant.[8] Those constructs that prove to be immunogenic are considered for clinical trial.

The first vaccine in clinical trial targets, MUC-1 (Figure 32.1), is a glycoprotein secreted by glandular organs in the breast, ovary, colon, pancreas, uterus and prostate. In non-transformed cells, mucins are present on the apical surfaces of highly polarized secretory epithelial cells where exposure to the immune system is unlikely. Malignant transformation results in overexpression of an underglycosylated form of mucin over the entire surface of the cell.[9] This abnormal mucin has been isolated and synthesized at MSKCC and consists of a peptide of 32 amino acids that contains the 20-mer tandem repeat unit of the MUC-1 peptide.[10–12] The synthetic peptide was conjugated to keyhole limpet haemocyanin (KLH)[13,14] and the couplet bound to an immune adjuvant, QS-21. QS-21 is a saponin, derived from the bark of a South American tree,[15] that will cause a potentiation of the immune response. Patients with either androgen-dependent disease and rising PSA values, or androgen-independent tumours and low tumour burdens, are considered, with the primary endpoint being the ability to generate high-titre antibodies to the MUC-1 molecule (or the particular carbohydrate of interest) as well as a T-cell response. Secondary endpoints include measurements of antitumour effects such as post-therapy changes in PSA and, if present, measurable disease regression and/or changes in radionuclide bone scan. On an experimental basis, the authors are also monitoring the peripheral blood for the presence or absence of cells expressing the mRNA for PSA both before and after therapy.[16]

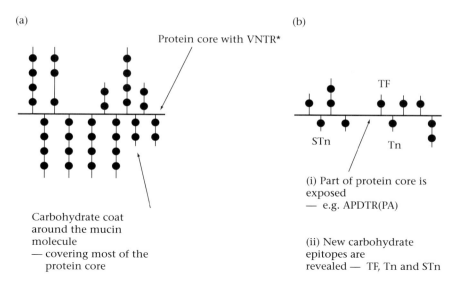

Figure 32.1. The difference between (a) normal mucin molecule and (b) abnormal mucin resulting from malignant transformation. In the abnormal mucin, unmasked immunogenic epitopes occur owing to loss of overlying carbohydrate residues in the malignant state. * = Variable number of terminal repeats. (Modified from ref. 11 with permission.)

The immunization schedule was derived from the authors' studies with carbohydrate vaccines with a similar structure that were previously evaluated in patients with melanoma, colon and breast cancers, and the trial was designed as a dose-escalation study to determine the dose of MUC-1 peptide that generates a maximal response. To date, the first three dose levels have been completed, and immune function assessed for dose levels one and two. Thus far, all 10 patients tested have generated IgM and IgG responses with titres greater than or equal to 1/1280; however, it is too early to report sequential changes in PSA or in other parameters of disease. Additional vaccines are planned. These include clinical trials with the carbohydrate antigens sialylated Tn (sTn),[17–19] a disaccharide antigen expressed O-linked to mucins and Globo H, a hexasaccharide O-linked to -OH groups of serine or threonine to mucins.[20–22]

The authors' ultimate goal is to combine several specific vaccine conjugates into a polyvalent vaccine with the aim of targeting both sides of the immune system (Figure 32.2). The criteria for selecting an optimal vaccine include the percentage of patients making antibody, the antibody titre, antibody class [IgG as opposed to IgM, especially in mediating complement-dependent cytotoxicity and antibody-dependent cellular cytotoxicity (ADCC)] and, most importantly, antibody specificity. It is the authors' hope that a polyvalent vaccine may allow a maximal humoral and/or cytotoxic T-cell response to a number of antigens at the same time, increasing the chances of eliminating the tumour. The primary endpoint will be the ability to generate high-titre antibodies to these antigens. The secondary endpoints will include post-therapy changes in PSA, detection of carcinoma-associated serum antigen (CASA) against circulating serum mucin, cytotoxic T-cell responses against MUC-1 and detection of circulating prostate cancer cells.

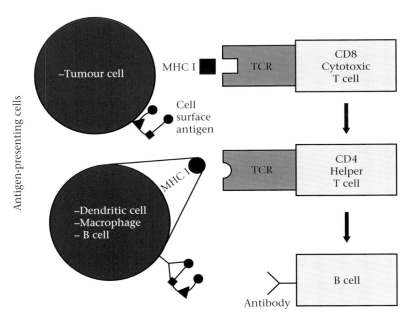

Figure 32.2. Scheme showing the interaction of the humoral and cellular sides of the immune system. Understanding this relationship is an integral part of designing vaccine strategies. TCR = T-cell receptor.

Monoclonal antibodies as targeting agents: radiolabelled antibodies against tumour-associated differentiation antigens in relapsed disease

An alternative to active immunization is passive immunization with monoclonal antibodies that recognize other carbohydrate antigens. For this approach, the authors have been evaluating a radiolabelled antibody, ^{131}I-CC49,[6] which recognizes the carbohydrate antigen s(T)n which is administered to patients after a 1-week pretreatment with interferon-γ (IFN-γ). TAG-72 is a high molecular weight glycoprotein related to the sialylated Tn (sTn) antigen that is expressed by adenocarcinomas of the breast,[23] colon,[24] lung,[25] ovary[26] and prostate.[6,7] It is distinct from carcinoembryonic antigen (CEA) and other tumour-associated differentiation antigens.[27] CC49, a murine IgG$_1$ monoclonal antibody, belongs to a series of monoclonal antibodies developed originally against colon cancer;[24] however, each antibody reacts with a distinct and specific epitope of the TAG-72 antigen.[28,29] The rationale for testing in prostate cancer was based on the localization on paraffin sections of prostate tumours,[30] the observed activity in a phase I trial using ^{131}I-CC49 alone in patients with androgen independent progression,[31] and the observed upregulation of antigen expression by IFN-γ[32,33] Increasing tumour-associated antigen expression has the potential for increasing specific radiation delivery to the tumour. There have been several clinical trials using [131]I- and ^{111}In-labelled CC49 and its related antibodies in patients with metastatic colon and prostate cancer, showing the labelled antibody to be well tolerated with minimal side effects. These studies have demonstrated good tumour localization of the radiolabelled antibody at sites of disease that often correlate with immunohistochemical studies.[29] One approach to improve targeting was by administering IFN-γ. In order to maximize targeting to specific sites the authors, in a phase II trial, made use of the observation of Yan *et al.*[33] that IFN-γ could upregulate the expression of CEA in human colon adenocarcinomas *in vitro*. Not only was the biomarker expression enhanced, based on dose and time dependence, but antiproliferative effects of the tumour cells were noted with maximal CEA expression.[33] In patients with adenocarcinomas, 87% (32 of 37) had positive CEA levels before therapy; of these, 26 (81.3%) showed increased CEA expression after treatment. Similar results were obtained on analysis for TAG-72. Interestingly, 21.9% of tumours that were negative for TAG-72 levels, and 13.3% of patients with negative CEA levels, became positive after treatment with IFN-γ.

On the basis of these observations and those of others,[27,34] the authors sought to assess the following: (1) the ability of CC49 monoclonal antibody to target to sites of metastatic disease in patients with hormone-refractory prostate cancer after daily treatment with IFN-γ; (2) the effect of this therapy on surrogate endpoints that include biochemical parameters such as PSA, as well as stabilization or regression of disease as determined radiographically. In a trial of 14 evaluable patients, myelosuppression was dose-limiting[35] and there was significant targeting to sites of disease in 11 (77%) cases, with palliation of pain in three. It is noteworthy that immunohistochemical staining of bone marrow biopsies containing tumour cells taken before and after interferon treatment revealed an up to sixfold increase in TAG-72 expression in post-treatment biopsies. The estimated radioactivity delivered to each tumour site was of the order of 1000 cGy, indicating a need for repetitive dosing. This could not be accomplished, owing to the development of a HAMA (human anti-mouse antibody) response to the mouse protein.[35] A humanized antibody that can be used repetitively is under development (Dr Jeff Schlom, Bethesda, Maryland, USA, personal communication).

Antibodies against growth factor receptors

When prostate cancers are first diagnosed, it is postulated that they are composed of three distinct cellular phenotypes — androgen dependent, androgen sensitive or androgen independent. Androgen-dependent cancer cells require a threshold level of stimulation by androgens for growth (i.e. without it, these cells undergo apoptosis and die).[36] Androgen-sensitive cells do not succumb, even if no androgen is present; rather, their growth rates decrease, whereas androgen-independent cells grow autonomously, regardless of the level of androgens. It is the latter that are primarily responsible for prostate cancer mortality. In an evolving story, it is now felt that both clonal selection and the adaptation of cells to the low androgen milieu contribute to androgen-independent proliferation. It has also been shown, in experimental models, that chronic androgen deprivation may select for the emergence of a clone of cells with amplified androgen receptors that are more sensitive to low levels of androgen.[37] Specific point mutations have also been found in the hormone-binding domain of the androgen receptor, which change the functional response to different steroid hormones.[38–40] These mutations may change the sensitivity of a cell to different polypeptide growth factors,[41] and are believed to contribute to the paradoxical responses to the withdrawal of anti-androgens, progestational agents and oestrogens in patients with progressive disease and 'castrate' levels of testosterone who are on these medications.[42]

The binding of specific growth factors to their receptors is also believed to contribute to androgen-independent proliferation. These factors include the transmembrane receptor tyrosine kinases such as the epidermal growth factor receptor (EGFr) and its ligand transforming growth factor α (TGFα), the insulin-like growth factors, and members of the fibroblast growth factor families.[43,44] Receptor-mediated signalling through the EGFr and downstream events is illustrated in Figure 32.2. In the clinic, inhibition of receptor function can be achieved through the use of antibodies that prevent the binding of a ligand to its receptor, or by blocking downstream effectors such as the tyrosine kinases (TKs), or *ras*. There are compelling reasons for considering growth factor receptors as targets for immunologic therapy, monoclonal antibodies (MoAbs) in particular. First, these molecules are upregulated in many malignant tumours owing to gene amplification and the overexpression of the receptors.[45,46] Secondly, as is the case in prostate cancer, the overexpression of receptors can cause overproduction of autologous growth factors in an autocrine fashion.[47,48] Third, the upregulation of receptor expression has been associated with a poor prognosis in some malignancies.[49,50]

The authors have targeted the EGFr, which is a protein tyrosine kinase encoded by the C-*erb*-B proto-oncogene and is expressed on many normal and malignant cells.[47] The rationale for evaluating an EGFr-blocking strategy in patients with prostate cancer was based on studies showing that human prostate tumour cells can express EGFr both *in vitro* and *in vivo*,[51–53] that both EGR and TGFα can cause mitogenic effects on cultured cells[49] and that the chimeric monoclonal antibody C225, developed by Dr John Mendelsohn at MSKCC, inhibited the growth of human prostate cancer cell lines despite the fact that these cells express approximately sevenfold fewer receptors than squamous cell carcinoma-derived cell lines. The antibody was also shown to block EGF-induced phosphorylation of the LNCaP cell line, which also has very low levels of receptors. The antibody has also been evaluated against established DU-145 and PC-3 prostate xenografts in nude mice.[47,54] In the case of the DU-145 tumours, five of nine established xenografts were completely eliminated using the antibody alone.[47] For most established tumours (10–20 days) — for example squamous carcinomas, breast carcinomas and colon carcinomas — treatment with anti-EGFR monoclonal antibody produced differing degrees of cytostasis without tumour kill. On the basis of these data, it was suggested that further cytoreductive intervention would be needed concurrently if the anti-EGFR MoAb was to be effective. A report by Baselga and colleagues demonstrated that anti-EGF receptor antibodies were capable of enhancing the effects of the chemotherapeutic agent doxorubicin against well-established A431 squamous cell carcinoma and the MDA 468 breast cancer xenografts which express high levels of the receptor.[49] Other studies have also suggested that cisplatin and taxol, plus the EGFr-blocking antibody had at least additive effects on cell kill.[55,56] Similar results were obtained when doxorubicin was combined with C225 against established PC-3 xenografts.[57]

In human prostate cancers, the authors studied the immunohistochemical staining pattern of EGFr and TGFα in malignant primary and hormone-independent metastatic prostate lesions. Primary malignant prostate epithelial cells in areas with discrete gland formation showed strong EGFr immunostaining, whereas stromal cells were generally non-reactive. In untreated primary tumours, TGFα expression was primarily in the stroma, whereas epithelial cells were weakly positive. In androgen-independent metastatic lesions, EGFr staining was homogeneous, with coexpression of the ligand in 14 of 18 (78%). The data suggested that, unlike the case in primary prostate tumours, where a paracrine relationship predominates, autocrine stimulation may be dominant in relapsed metastatic disease.[52] Taken together, the *in vitro*, *in vivo* and immunohistochemical data provided the background for developing the combination of C225 with doxorubicin in patients with progressive androgen-independent prostate cancer. This followed a phase I trial of the C225 MoAb alone in patients with EGFr-positive tumours.

A single-dose phase I study of C225 MoAb was completed in patients with advanced EGFR-positive tumours, with three evaluable patients enrolled at escalating levels — 5, 20, 50 and 100 mg/m^2. The patients did not experience severe (> grade 3) toxicity. Currently, a phase Ib/IIa dose-escalating study is ongoing at MSKCC, with doses of the MoAb C225 at levels of 20, 50 and 100 mg/m² given in conjunction with either 15 or 20 mg/m² doxorubicin weekly for 6 weeks followed by a 2-week rest period. To date, five dose levels have been completed and dose-limiting toxicities have not been observed. Evidence of an antitumour effect has been observed but, overall, the results are too preliminary to be considered definitive.

The clinical development of compounds that act via 'non-classical' mechanisms is not straightforward. At MSKCC the documentation of progression of disease despite castrate levels of testosterone is required, and, to control for the possibility of a withdrawal response, progression of disease off all agents that act via steroid hormone receptors is also required.[42–58] An attempt is also being made to define the optimal biological dose of the antibody, based on a change in the pharmacokinetics of the antibody that would suggest saturation of the receptor. It is anticipated that the saturating dose will not be the same as the 'maximally tolerated' dose typically defined for traditional chemotherapeutic agents. Alternatively, the direct biological effects of the antibody on the tumour might be assessed; preliminary studies using positron emission tomography, which measures tumour metabolism *in vivo*, are under investigation (H. Scher, D. Golde and S. Larson, 1996). Once a phase II dose for the combination has been defined, and because doxorubicin alone has antitumour activity in relapsed prostate cancer, a randomized comparison of C225 plus doxorubicin vs doxorubicin alone is planned.

Farnesyl transferase inhibitors as a modality for prostate cancer treatment: use of transmembrane tyrosine kinase growth factor receptors (RTKs)

An important role is played by *ras* genes (Figure 32.3) in the development and maintenance of several malignancies. Activating mutations of *ras* are observed in pancreas, colon and other cancers. Although *ras* mutations are rare in prostate

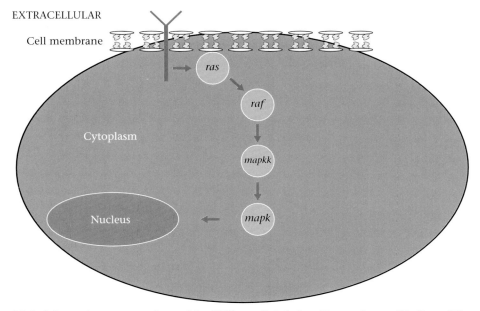

Figure 32.3. Schematic representations of the EGFr-mediated signalling pathway. Binding of the ligand TGFα to the EGFr sets into action a cascade of signal transducing events with the ultimate goal of stimulating and controlling cellular proliferation.

cancer, recent data show that activation of wild-type *ras* is required to maintain the transformed phenotype for a number of cancer cell types, including prostate cancer. Activation of *ras* by an upstream signal results in the accumulation of *ras* in the GTP-bound state. The process proceeds through several enzymatic steps, of which the action of farnesyl transferase is dose limiting (Figure 32.3). As ras requires post-translational modification in order to acquire biological activity, *ras* maturation has become a target for the development of potential inhibitors. The authors are currently studying the target and mechanism of action of farnesyl transferase inhibitors (FTIs) and whether they can be used in combination therapy of human prostate cancer. This is based on the observation that RTK stimulation activates p21 ras protein, which leads to the hypothesis that FTIs would inhibit malignant prostate growth. The authors have shown that FTIs inhibit prostate cancer cell lines *in vitro*, as well as prostate cancer xenografts with no appreciable toxicity to normal tissues. The FTIs inhibited ras processing in four prostate cell lines tested and inhibited the growth and clonogenicity in soft agar of three of the lines.[59] Colleagues at Merck, in parallel experiments, showed that the drug causes regression of ras-dependent tumours in nude mice and prevents the development of tumours in MMTV-*ras* transgenic mice.[60] In both cases, no toxicity to normal tissues was observed.

The mechanism of FTI resistance in cells refractory to the action of this agent is also being investigated. Preliminary data reveal that drug resistance does not result from impaired drug transport or accumulation, nor from amplification or insensitivity of the target enzyme, farnesyl:protein transferase. Furthermore, substrate farnesylation and *ras* function are inhibited by the drug in resistant as well as sensitive cells. It has been noted that EGF activation of MAP (mitogenic activating protein) kinase is inhibited by FTIs only in cells that are sensitive to the drug.[61] The data suggest that resistance may occur in cells that contain a *ras*-independent pathway for activating MAP kinase in response to tyrosine kinases. This also suggests that the key FTI target is upstream of MAP kinase and that inhibitors of upstream tyrosine kinases, such as antireceptor antibodies, might act synergistically with FTIs. Clinical trials in prostate cancer are planned to explore the nature of the drug target(s) and the mechanism through which it inhibits tumour cell growth, and to use this information to design trials in which FTIs are used in combination with anti-androgens, chemotherapeutic drugs or antireceptor antibodies.

Conclusions

The results of clinical trials to date have not shown a survival advantage with any non-hormonal approach. However, the outlook is changing: studies of prostate cancer biology have revealed a number of unique targets that can be exploited therapeutically. These include (but are not limited to) carbohydrate and glycoproteins on the cell surface to which both humoral and cellular responses can be generated. These approaches offer the exciting possibility of treating the disease while maintaining quality of life. As knowledge of the mechanisms responsible for androgen-independent progression increases, the selective targeting of different points on the signal transduction pathway is now possible. The clinical trial with C225 in combination with doxorubicin has shown activity in the phase I trial, and development is continuing. Together with these advances in the understanding of tumour immunobiology, a further consideration is the proper design and execution of clinical trials to determine the role, if any, of these therapies in the treatment of patients with prostate cancers of different stages, thereby defining the target.

The more widespread use of PSA has also allowed the identification of patients at risk of progression, and the ability to intervene at an early stage for patients at risk for disease related morbidity, before these symptoms appear. Equally important will be the design and completion of clinical trials for each stage of the disease, including quality-of-life considerations, so that the impact of a specific intervention can be assessed. For advanced disease, evolving data from phase II studies of non-hormonal approaches using clear-cut endpoints of response show that prostate cancer is not as resistant to treatment as previously believed.[58] Finally, as more is understood of the biology of prostate cancer in different stages, more specific and improved treatments will be developed to improve the outcomes for patients with the disease.

There are several emerging areas regarding the treatment of patients with prostate cancer who have failed first-line therapies such as radiation and prostatectomy. Recent evidence has suggested that growth factors and their receptors represent a promising therapeutic target, both alone and in combination with other standard chemotherapeutic agents. The data regarding the use of antibodies to these, as monotherapy or in a combined-modality approach, have suggested their potential as a possible treatment strategy. Finally, targeting cells at the molecular level using enzyme inhibitors offers an exciting approach in controlling prostate cancer from a cellular level. These all have the potential for improving the therapeutic index for patients with the disease.

Acknowledgements

Supported by CA 05826, Merck Pharmaceuticals, ImClone Systems, CaPCURE and the PepsiCo Foundation.

References

1. Scher H I, Logothetis C J. Management of androgen-independent prostate cancer. In: Raghavan D, Scher H I, Leibel S A et al. (eds) Principles and practice of genitourinary oncology. Philadelphia, Lippincott, 1995; 599–612
2. Frank S J, Amsterdam A, Kelly W K et al. Platinum-based chemotherapy for patients with poorly differentiated hormone-refractory prostate cancers (HRPC): response and pathologic correlations. Proc Annu Meet Am Soc Clin Oncol 1995;14: A601.
3. Scher H I, Steineck G, Kelly W K. Hormone-refractory (D3) prostate cancer: refining the concept. Urology 1995; 46: 142–148
4. Sanda M G, Ayyagari S R, Jaffee E M et al. Demonstration of a rational strategy for human prostate cancer gene therapy. J Urol 1994; 151: 622–628
5. Livingston P O. Augmenting the immunogenicity of carbohydrate tumor antigens. Cancer Biology 1995; 6: 357–366
6. Eklov S, Westlin J, Rikner G et al. Estramustine potentiates the radiation effect in human prostate tumor transplant in nude mice. Prostate 1995; 24: 39–45
7. Brenner P C, Rettig W J, Sanz-Moncasi M P et al. TAG-72 expression in primary, metastatic and hormonally treated prostate cancer as defined by monoclonal antibody CC49. J Urol 1995; 153: 1575–1579
8. Ho S B, Niehans G A, Lyftogt C et al. Heterogeneity of mucin gene expression in normal and neoplastic tissues. Cancer Res 1993; 53: 641–645
9. Yamada O, Oshimi K, Motoji T et al. Telomeric DNA in normal and leukemic blood cells. Am Soc Clin Invest 1995; 95: 1117–1123
10. Gendler S J, Spicer A P, Lalani E-N et al. Structure and biology of a carcinoma-associated mucin, MUC1. Am Rev Respir Dis 1991; 144: S42–S47
11. Apostolopoulos V, McKenzie I F C. Cellular mucins: targets for immunotherapy. CRC Crit Rev Immunol 1995; 14: 293–309
12. Gendler S, Lancaster C, Taylor-Papadimitriou J et al. Molecular cloning and expression of human tumor-associated polymorphic epithelial mucin. J Biol Chem 1990; 265: 15286–15293

13. Mitra A B, Murty V V, Singh V *et al*. Genetic alterations of 5p15: a potential marker for progression of precancerous lesions of the uterine cervix. J Natl Cancer Inst 1995; 17: 742–745

14. Livingston P O, Adluri S, Helling F *et al*. Phase I trial of immunological adjuvant QS-21 with GM2 ganglioside-KLH conjugate vaccines. Immunol Rev 1995; 145: 147–155

15. Livingston P O, Adluri S, Helling F *et al*. Phase I trial of immunological adjuvant QS-21 with a GM2 ganglioside-KLH conjugate vaccine in patients with malignant melanoma. Vaccine 1994; 12: 1275–1280

16. Ghossein R, Scher H, Gerald W *et al*. Detection of circulating tumor cells in patients with localized and metastatic prostatic carcinoma: clinical implications. J Clin Oncol 1995; 13: 1195–1200

17. Zhang S, Walberg L A, Ogata S *et al*. Immune sera and monoclonal antibodies define two configurations for the sialyl Tn tumor antigen. Cancer Res 1995; 55: 3364–3368

18. de Valeriola D. Dose optimization of anthracyclines. Anticancer Res 1995; 14: 2307–2314

19. Livingston P O, Koganty R, Longenecker B M *et al*. Studies on the immunogenicity of synthetic and natural Thomsen–Friedenrich (TF) antigens in mice: augmentation of the response by Quil A and SAF-m adjuvants and analysis of the specificity of the responses. Vaccine Res 1992; 1: 99–109

20. Vlasova E V, Byramova N E, Tuzikov A B *et al*. Monoclonal antibodies directed to the synthetic carbohydrate antigen Ley. Hybridoma 1994; 13: 295–301

21. Martignone S, Menard S, Bedini A *et al*. Study of the expression and function of the tumour-associated antigen CAMBr1 in small cell lung carcinomas. Eur J Cancer 1993; 29A: 2020–2025

22. Perrone F, Menard S, Canevari S *et al*. Prognostic significance of the CaMBr1 antigen on breast carcinoma: relevance of the type of recognised glycoconjugate. Eur J Cancer 1993; 29A: 2113–2117

23. Nuti M, Teramoto Y A, Mariana-Constanti R *et al*. A monoclonal antibody (B72.3) defines patterns of distribution of a novel tumor associated antigen in human mammary carcinoma cell populations. Int J Cancer 1982; 29: 539–545

24. Thor A, Ohuchi N, Szpak C A *et al*. The distribution of oncofetal antigen TAG-72 defined by monoclonal antibody B72.2. Cancer Res 1986; 46: 3118–3124

25. Johnston W W, Szpak C A, Lottich S C *et al*. Use of monoclonal antibody (B72.3) as novel immunohistochemical adjunct for the diagnosis of carcinomas in fine needle aspiration biopsy specimens. Hum Pathol 1986; 17: 501–513

26. Thor A, Gorstein F, Ohuchi N *et al*. Tumor-associated glycoprotein (TAG-72) in ovarian carcinomas defined by monoclonal antibody B72.3. J Natl Cancer Inst 1986; 76: 995–1006

27. Greiner J W, Guadagni F, Goldstein D *et al*. Intraperitoneal administration of interferon-gamma to carcinoma patients enhances expression of tumor-associated glycoprotein-72 and carcinoembryonic antigen on malignant ascites cells. J Clin Oncol 1992; 10: 735–746

28. Stramignoni D, Bowen R, Atkinson B *et al*. Differential reactivity of monoclonal antibodies with human colon adenocarcinomas and adenomas. Int J Cancer 1983; 31: 543–552

29. Divgi C R, Kemeny N, Cordon-Cardo C *et al*. Phase I radioimmunotherapy trial with 131I-labeled monoclonal antibody CC49 in patients with metastatic colorectal carcinoma. Proc Am Soc Clin Oncol 1991; 10: 209 (abstr)

30. Theodoulou M, Reuter V, Drobnjak M *et al*. Epidermal growth factor receptor (EGFr) and TAG-72 expression in hormone-refractory (HR) patients with locally recurrent and metastatic prostate (PR) cancer. J Urol 1995; 153: 450A

31. Meredith R F, Bueschen A J, Khazaeli M B *et al*. Treatment of metastatic prostate carcinoma with radiolabeled antibody CC40. J Nucl Med 1994; 35: 1017–1022

32. Greiner J W, Guadagni F, Noguchi P *et al*. Recombinant interferon enhances antibody-targeting of carcinoma lesions in vivo. Science 1987; 235: 895–898

33. Yan X, Wong J Y C, Esteban J M *et al*. Effects of recombinant human gamma-interferon on carcinoembryonic antigen expression of human colon cancer cells. J Immunotherapy 1991; 11: 77–84

34. Greiner J W, Guadagni F, Goldstein D *et al*. Evidence for the elevation of serum carcinoembryonic antigen and tumor associated glycoprotein-72 in patients administered interferons. Cancer Res 1991; 51: 4155–4163

35. Slovin S F, Larson S, Divgi C *et al*. Monoclonal antibody (MoAb) 131I-CC49 and interferon-gamma (IFN-G): efficacy and therapeutic utility of a phase II trial in hormone insensitive prostate cancer (HIPC). Proc Am Soc Clin Oncol 1996; 15: 444 (abstr)

36. Isaacs J T, Lundmo P I, Berges R *et al.* androgen regulation of programmed cell death of normal and malignant prostatic cells. J Androl 1992; 13: 457–464

37. Visakorpi T, Hyytinen E, Koivisto P *et al.* In vivo amplification of the androgen receptor gene and progression of human prostate cancer. Nature Genet 1995; 9: 401–406

38. Culig Z, Hobisch A, Cronauer M V *et al.* Mutant androgen receptor mutations in an advanced-stage prostatic carcinoma is activated by adrenal androgens and progesterone. Mol Endocrinol 1993; 7: 1541–1550

39. Taplin M E, Bubley G, Frantz M *et al.* Androgen receptor mutations in human hormone-independent prostate cancer. Proc Am Assoc Cancer Res 1994; 34: 1630 (abstr)

40. Tilley W D, Buchanan G, Hickey T E *et al.* Detection of androgen receptor gene mutations in human prostate cancers by immunohistochemistry and PCR-SSP. Proc Am Assoc Cancer Res 1995; 36: 266 (abstr)

41. Culig Z, Hobisch A, Cronauer M V *et al.* Androgen receptor activation in prostatic tumor cell lines by insulin-like growth factor-I, keratinocyte growth factor, and epidermal growth factor. Cancer Res 1994; 54: 5474–5478

42. Scher H I, Zhang Z F, Kelly W K. Hormone and anti-hormone withdrawal therapy: Implications for management of androgen independent prostate cancer. Urology 1996; 47: 61–69

43. Steiner M S. Role of peptide growth factors in the prostate: a review. Urology 1993; 42: 99–110

44. Tanaka A, Miyamoto K, Minamino N *et al.* Cloning and characterization of an androgen-induced growth factor essential for the androgen-dependent growth of mouse mammary carcinoma cells. Proc Natl Acad Sci 1992; 89: 8928–8932

45. Dean C, Modjtahedi H, Eccles S *et al.* Imunotherapy with antibodies to the EGF receptor. Int J Cancer 1994; 8: 103–107

46. Gullick W J. Prevalence of aberrant expression of the epidermal-growth-factor receptor in human cancers. Br Med Bull 1991; 47: 87–98

47. Goldstein N I, Prewett M, Zuklys K *et al.* Biological efficacy of a chimeric antibody to the epidermal growth factor receptor in a human tumor xenograft model. Clin Cancer Res 1995; 1: 1311–1318

48. Sporn M B, Roberts A B. Autocrine growth factors and cancers. Nature 1985; 313: 745–747

49. Baselga J, Norton L, Masui H *et al.* Antitumor effects of doxorubicin in combination with anti-epidermal growth factor receptor monoclonal antibodies. J Natl Cancer Inst 1993; 85: 1327–1333

50. Harris A L, Nicholson S, Sainsbury R *et al.* Epidermal-growth-factor receptor and other oncogenes as prognostic markers. J Natl Cancer Inst Monogr 1992; 11: 181–187

51. Macdonald A, Habib F K. Divergent responses to epidermal growth factor in hormone sensitive and insensitive human prostate cancer cell lines. Br J Cancer 1992; 65: 177–182

52. Scher H I, Sarakis A, Reuter V *et al.* The changing pattern of expression of the epidermal growth factor receptor and transforming growth factor-a in the progression of prostatic neoplasms. Clin Cancer Res 1995; 1: 545–550

53. Ibrahim G K, Kerns B J, MacDonald J A *et al.* Differential immunoreactivity of epidermal growth factor receptor in benign, dysplastic and malignant prostatic tissues. J Urol, 1993; 149: 170–173

54. Prewett M, Rockwell P, O'Connor W O *et al.* A chimeric antibody to the epidermal growth factor receptor inhibits the growth of established human prostatic carcinoma xenografts in nude mice. Clin Cancer Res 1997; in press

55. Aboud-Pirak E, Hurwitz, E, Pirak M E *et al.* Efficacy of antibodies to epidermal growth factor receptor against KB carcinoma in vitro and in nude mice. J Natl Cancer Inst 1988; 80: 1605–1611

56. Hanauske A-R, Osborne C K, Chamness G C *et al.* Alteration of EGF-receptor binding in human breast cancer cells by antineoplastic agents. Eur J Cancer Clin Oncol 1987; 23: 545–551

57. Prewett M, Rockwell P, Rose C *et al.* Altered cell cycle distribution and cyclin-CDK protein expression in A431 epidermoid carcinoma cells treated with doxorubicin and a chimeric monoclonal antibody to the epidermal growth factor receptor. Mol Cell Diff 1996; 4: 167–186

58. Scher H I, Mazumdar M, Kelly W K. Clinical trials in relapsed prostate cancer: defining the target. J Natl Cancer Inst 1996; 88: 1623–1634

59. Scher H, Sepp-Lorenzino L, Bos M *et al.* Farnesylation inhibition reverses the transformd phenotype of malignant prostate epithelial cells. Breast and prostate cancer: basic mechanisms. Keystone Symposium 1996; 46, abstr 426

60. Kohl N E, Scott D, Mosser S *et al.* Selective inhibition of ras-dependent transformation by a farnesyltransferase inhibitor. Science 1993; 260: 1934–1937
61. Sepp-Lorenzino L, Ma Z, Rands E *et al.* A peptidomimetic inhibitor of farnesyl: protein transferase blocks the anchorage-dependent and -independent growth of human tumor cell lines. Cancer Res 1995; 55: 5302–530

Chapter 33
Potential for vaccination therapy in prostate cancer

D. Hrouda and A. G. Dalgleish

Historical background of cancer vaccines

The idea of immunotherapy for cancer is not new. Following the observation that an episode of erysipelas in a patient with a sarcoma coincided with regression of the tumour, William Coley, a surgeon at Cornell University in New York at the end of the last century, began to inject first live bacteria and then the toxins of heat-killed bacteria into patients with tumours and he reported a number of tumour regressions, most of these being sarcomas.[1] Interest in immunotherapy then faded, partly because the results of this treatment were unpredictable but also because of the advent of chemotherapy and radiotherapy.

In 1970, Burnet described the theory of immune surveillance whereby the immune system is responsible for eliminating newly transformed cells and therefore emergence of a tumour is a failure of the immune system.[2] However, the disappointing results of various immunotherapeutic strategies, coupled with the lack of a clear link between immunodeficiency and the major solid tumours, led to disillusionment with the concept. Over the last few years there has been a resurgence of interest in cancer immunotherapy because of a number of advances in our understanding of tumour immunology. These include the increased understanding of tumour-associated antigens (several of which have now been cloned), the identification of cytokines produced by cells in response to infections, the increased understanding of antigen presentation and major histocompatibility complex (MHC) restriction, and the ability to apply new molecular and immunological techniques to well-established tumour models.

Prostate cancer and the immune system

Most studies in the tumour vaccine field have concerned malignant melanoma and renal cell carcinoma, these tumours being relatively immunogenic with reports of occasional spontaneous tumour regression. Initially, prostate cancer may seem an unlikely candidate for vaccine therapy. At one time it was thought that the prostate may be an immunologically privileged site, owing to lack of lymphatics, and therefore not amenable to immunotherapy;[3] however, there is no good evidence to back up this suggestion. Although prostate cancer is poorly immunogenic, compared with melanoma, and spontaneous regressions are unknown, there is now evidence that the immune response may be important.

Vesalainen and colleagues examined a series of 325 prostate adenocarcinomas, with long-term clinical follow-up, for the density of tumour-infiltrating lymphocytes (TILs). TIL density was a prognostic factor independent of tumour grade, patients with absent or weak TIL being at high risk of tumour progression.[4]

There is evidence that prostate cancers may evade immune surveillance by defective antigen presentation. It has been shown that two out of five of the established human metastatic prostate cancer cell lines are defective in cell surface expression of MHC class I,[5] and a study of prostatic tissue from 47 patients with prostate cancer showed that, when individual class I allelic expression was analysed, abnormalities occurred in 85% of primary prostate cancers and 100% of metastases.[6] These findings might explain why prostate cancers that progress fail to stimulate an immune response, but other mechanisms of immune escape described in other tumours may yet prove to be equally or more important. They include secretion of inhibitory substances [e.g. transforming growth factor-β (TGFβ); interleukin (IL)-10],[7,8] abnormal T lymphocyte signal transduction[9] and expression by tumours of Fas ligand which may enable tumour cells to induce apoptosis in Fas-expressing TILs.[10]

Considering past attitudes to the potential of prostate cancer to be immunogenic, it is interesting that non-specific immunotherapy with Bacille Calmette–Guérin (BCG) has been tried previously. BCG given in addition to conventional hormone therapy resulted in a statistically significant increase in survival in one randomized clinical trial in 42 patients with stage D prostate cancer,[11] although a study by another group reported no benefit.[12]

Anti-tumour immune response

Active immunotherapy in the form of a cancer vaccine is aimed at stimulating the patient's immune response to his own established tumour. The concept is based

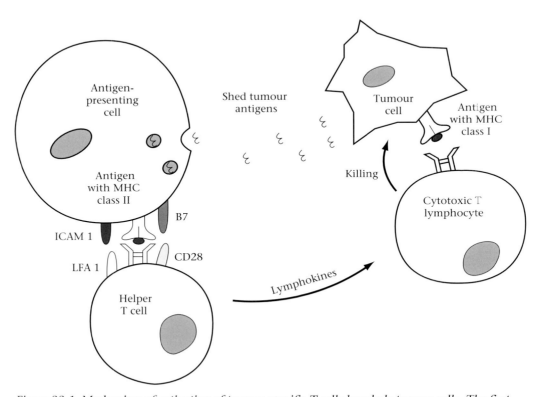

Figure 33.1. Mechanism of activation of tumour-specific T cells by whole tumour cells. The first signal involves presentation of antigen with class I major histocompatibility complex (MHC) on the surface of the tumour cell. Tumour antigens are taken up by antigen-presenting cells (APC) and presented in conjunction with class II MHC to helper T cells. Co-stimulatory molecules on the APC, such as B7 and ICAM I, are important in this interaction. CD28 and LFA 1 are the receptors to these co-stimulatory molecules. The subsequent release of lymphokines stimulates tumour-cell killing by cytotoxic T lymphocytes.

on the theory that tumours possess specific antigens that can be recognized by the immune system. An integral part of antigen presentation is the MHC, which comprises integral membrane glycoproteins of which there are two types, class I and class II. It is now understood that antitumour immunity is largely mediated by cytotoxic T lymphocytes (CD8+).[13] T cells possess specific T-cell receptors on their surface that recognize antigen/MHC complexes. The cytotoxic T lymphocyte (CTL) is activated by two interactions (Figure 33.1). The first, direct pathway, involves the T-cell receptor interacting with the endogenously synthesized antigen, a peptide sequence of 8–11 amino acids, presented on the surface of the cell in the groove of the class I MHC. Activation of the T-cell receptor results in tumour cell killing. However, there is also an indirect pathway whereby tumour antigens are taken up and processed by specialized antigen-presenting cells, e.g. dendritic cells. The antigen is presented with HLA class II MHC to T helper cells (CD4+) and the stimulated T helper cells promote cytotoxic T-cell killing of the tumour cell.[14]

Tumour antigens

The term tumour-associated antigens (TAAs) describes antigens found on human tumours that are also expressed on a small population of normal cells. It has become clear that self proteins aberrantly expressed in tumours can activate CTLs. The majority of TAAs have been identified in melanoma cells but they are beginning to be identified in prostate cancer. One group of self proteins commonly expressed in melanoma cells is the MAGE family.[15] They are normally expressed only in the normal testis and placenta. Two other families, BAGE and GAGE, have a similar distribution of expression. A number of different tumour types have been found to express the *MAGE*, *BAGE* and *GAGE* genes but, until recently, prostate cancer has not been assessed. Recently, *GAGE 7* was found to be expressed in the metastatic prostate cancer cell line LNCaP. A novel gene, designated *PAGE*, which has 45% homology to *GAGE* members, was described by the same authors.[16] Further MAGE, BAGE and GAGE antigens are likely to be described in prostate cancer, but it remains to be seen if expression occurs in a sufficient proportion of tumours for this class of TAAs to be considered good immunotherapeutic targets in prostate cancer.

Another group of TAAs includes tissue-specific proteins such as tyrosinase, Mart-1, gp100 and gp75 in melanoma.[17] Prostate-specific antigen (PSA) and prostate-specific membrane antigen (PSM) could be considered in the same category. It is unclear whether tolerance precludes CTL responses to self proteins that are overexpressed in tumours. If tolerance to such antigens could be broken it would have obvious implications for vaccine therapy in prostate cancer, because PSA and PSM are almost universally expressed by prostate adenocarcinomas. In this regard PSM is a particularly attractive target because it is overexpressed in cancer cells compared with benign cells.[18] The demonstration that within the T-cell repertoire there are populations of T cells that can be activated by certain peptide sequences within PSA (PSA 49–63; PSA 64–78) (ref. 19) and PSM (PSM 4–12) (ref. 20) is an important finding. Fortunately, any autoimmune effects against normal prostate cells expressing these antigens should not have major physiological relevance. In fact, any autoimmune effect would constitute at least a partial 'medical' prostatectomy!

Several other candidate tumour antigens have been described for prostate cancer. TAG-72, an oncofoetal antigen expressed in 80% of prostate adenocarcinomas, is absent from normal adult tissues except secretory endometrium.[21] Prostate carcinoma-associated glycoprotein complex (PAC)[22] and oncogenic antigen 519 (ref. 23) are other antigens commonly expressed in prostate tumours.

Mucins such as MUC1 are being investigated as potential target molecules for cancer immunotherapy in breast carcinoma and a number of other tumours, including prostate cancer. The reason is that not only is MUC1 upregulated in some tumours, but it is also aberrantly glycosylated; therefore tumour-associated mucin is distinct antigenically from the normal mucin.[24] Another advantage is that antigen presentation to T cells is not human leucocyte antigen (HLA) restricted, an observation of relevance to prostate cancer where class I MHC expression is often aberrant or downregulated. Beckett and co-workers have described an antigen that is specific for prostate cancer and prostate intra-epithelial neoplasia (PIN). It has the structure of a mucin and has therefore been called 'prostate mucin antigen', but its potential as an immunotherapeutic target has not been evaluated.[25,26] Another group of antigens that are truly tumour specific and may be considered as potential targets are the products of genes such as mutated *p53* and *ras*, which are different antigenic entities to their wild-type counterparts.

Tumour vaccines

A number of different vaccine strategies are already under clinical investigation. In prostate cancer, autologous whole live irradiated tumour cells transfected to secrete cytokines have received most attention and the strategy is now being assessed in phase I clinical trials. Other antigen specific strategies using peptides, anti-idiotype antibodies, mucins or DNA are all in preclinical or the early stages of clinical evaluation.

Whole tumour cell vaccines: autologous

The aim of transfecting tumour cells with a gene encoding a particular cytokine is to deliver the immunomodulatory cytokine at an effective dose in the vicinity of tumour cells and tumour antigens. Not only can this be an effective way of increasing the immunogenicity of the tumour cells but also it has the advantage of avoiding the side effects associated with the systemic delivery of cytokines. Several different cytokines have been transfected in a number of tumour models. Interleukin-2 (IL-2) and granulocyte macrophage-colony-stimulating factor (GM-CSF) appear to be 'good performers' in several models with GM-CSF found to be superior in the B16-F10 mouse melanoma model.[27] IL-2 is a growth and activation factor for both T cells and NK cells, inducing a CD8+ and NK cell-dependent systemic immune response against murine tumours. GM-CSF is thought to induce differentiation of haematopoietic precursors into dendritic cells and the resulting systemic immune response depends on CD4+ and CD8+ cells.[28]

Investigators have used the immunocompetent Dunning rat model of prostate cancer to assess cytokine-secreting autologous whole-cell vaccines. The R3327 Mat-Ly-Lu tumour, an aggressive androgen-independent tumour, does not induce tumour-specific CTLs and thus does not demonstrate any signs of intrinsic immunogenicity.[29] This model has clear attractions because the low immunogenicity is analogous to human tumours, although there is concern that no other prostate cancers have been found in Copenhagen rats and the original Dunning tumour may not, in fact, be of prostatic origin.[30]

Two groups have reported exciting results when IL-2 or GM-CSF transfected Mat-Ly-Lu cells were used as a therapeutic vaccine in the Dunning rat.[29,31–33] The

Memorial Sloan-Kettering group found that, in the treatment of 3-day-old tumours, an IL-2 secreting vaccine prolonged survival in all rats, with cure rates of up to 100% in some experiments, compared with a cure rate of 40% when a GM-CSF vaccine was used. Rats cured of their tumours were resistant to a second challenge of live tumour cells. The Johns Hopkins group found a 30% cure rate of established tumours and prolonged survival in all animals with a GM-CSF vaccine.[31] Further studies in this model showed that repeated vaccination was required and the ability to delay progression and cure animals was related to total duration of GM-CSF secretion at the subcutaneous site.[33] One concern is that these animal models show excellent results in the treatment of subcutaneously implanted tumours but the response is poor when the tumour is orthotopic.[29,34] This consistent finding remains unexplained but it may be that the ability to cure subcutaneous tumours successfully by vaccination relates to the presence of relatively large numbers of dendritic cells in the dermis.

In the rat prostate cancer model, at least, IL-2 appears to be the superior cytokine to transfect. The drawback of using IL-2 is that the therapeutic range is bell-shaped;[35] therefore, obtaining the correct level of secretion of IL-2 is critical. Recognition that, in human prostate cancer, defective antigen presentation is common, should perhaps guide us to choose a cytokine that allows for antigen presentation that is not class I restricted.

The autologous vaccine approach is being evaluated in a phase I/II study in patients found to have extracapsular disease following radical prostatectomy at Johns Hopkins. Clearly, it will be some time before data from such a study are available. However, the Johns Hopkins group have published the results of their trial of autologous GM-CSF whole-tumour vaccination in advanced renal cell carcinoma. There was one partial response out of 16 patients and they were able to correlate this with the strongest delayed-type hypersensitivity response to the vaccine.[36]

Whole tumour cell vaccines: allogeneic

Although it is often argued that whole tumour cell vaccines must be autologous so that they are both HLA matched and contain the full antigen repertoire of the host, there are major drawbacks to this approach. At present there are still major difficulties in establishing and maintaining human prostate cancer cells *in vitro* or *in vivo*.[37] The ability to obtain reliably, by primary culture, the large quantities of prostate cancer cells required for regular vaccinations remains an elusive objective. There are also doubts as to whether such a labour-intensive, time-consuming customized approach will ever be affordable, even to Western economies. Ideally, one would wish to have a standard vaccine that could be administered to all comers.

If one wishes to pursue the idea of using the whole tumour cell, then allogeneic vaccination using a standard tumour cell line or a mixture of cell lines may be a practical way forward. In order to address whether allogeneic cells can stimulate an immune response against an autologous tumour, the authors conducted a matrix study in murine melanoma models and showed that allogeneic cell vaccination could protect against subsequent lethal dose challenge with autologous tumour cells.[38] This demonstrated that class I MHC restriction could be bypassed by allogeneic vaccination. The expression of highly immunogenic allo-MHC might actually enhance the immunogenicity of tumour-associated antigens, a possible explanation for the good prognosis of bone marrow transplant recipients who develop a severe graft versus host reaction. There have been some reports of regression of concurrent solid tumours in patients with haematological malignancy who received bone marrow transplantation.[39,40] An additional putative advantage would be that a polyvalent vaccine could express an antigenic repertoire more representative of antigens expressed by the patients' metastases than the autologous cells derived from the primary tumour. An NCI phase I/II study being conducted at the Memorial Sloan-Kettering is using MHC class-I matched allogeneic cells transduced to secrete IL-2 and interferon (IFN)γ (NCI-V95-0629).

Peptide-specific vaccines

The identification of tumour-associated antigens has enabled a more antigen-specific vaccine approach to be evaluated. Dendritic cells possess all the necessary antigen-presenting capabilities and are arguably the most efficient antigen-presenting cells known. It has been shown that precursor cells in the peripheral blood of prostate cancer patients can be induced to differentiate *in vitro* into functional dendritic cells by culture in the presence of IL-2.[41] Dendritic cells could be loaded with either autologous tumour cell lysate or an HLA-A2 motif from PSM and this could be used to stimulate proliferation of specific autologous CTLs.[20] This strategy is now to be tested in phase I clinical trials.

The use of peptides offers a much 'cleaner' approach to vaccine therapy. However, the restriction of presentation to a particular HLA allele may limit a particular vaccine to less than 50% of the population even if the peptide is associated with a common HLA type such as HLA-A2. Moreover, peptides are not cheap to produce at the levels required for human administration, especially as responses from multiple epitopes may be required to provide complete protection in humans. Another possible limitation is that because only CTL for one specific antigen will be induced, heterogeneity of antigen expression may allow immune escape. A possible answer to this problem would be to identify multiple peptides that between them bind to most HLA types.

Anti-idiotype antibodies

Anti-idiotype antibodies are directed against determinants expressed on the variable regions of antibodies which themselves recognize a tumour antigen. Therefore the combining site of the anti-idiotype antibody is a mirror image of the epitopes of the TAA. It has been demonstrated that anti-idiotype antibodies can be excellent immunogens for stimulating T-cell mediated immunity against tumours.[42,43] They offer potential advantages over peptides because they are more resistant to proteolytic digestion and have a longer half-life in the circulation, and the Fc region may be preferentially internalized and processed by Fc receptors on antigen-presenting cells. Anti-idiotype antibodies to PSA have been generated and their therapeutic potential is currently under assessment.[44]

DNA vaccines

The injection of cloned DNA to elicit an immune response against the encoded protein was initially demonstrated using DNA encoding flu virus nuclear protein, which was able to protect mice against subsequent challenge with live flu virus.[45] Subsequently, it was shown that this could be applied in cancer, where vaccination with DNA encoding carcinoembryonic antigen was able to protect mice against tumour challenge.[46] It would be interesting to assess this strategy in prostate cancer now that several tumour-associated antigens have been cloned.

In vivo gene therapy and the immune system

In vivo gene therapy includes several different strategies: corrective gene therapy aims to reverse the malignant phenotype by replacing an absent or defective gene, e.g. wild-type *p53*; antisense oligonucleotides complementary to specific DNA or RNA aim to disrupt the expression of target oncogenes; drug-activating suicide genes aim to make the target cells susceptible to a drug, e.g. transfection with the herpes simplex virus thymidine kinase (HSVTK) gene makes the target cells susceptible to the drug ganciclovir.[47]

One of the apparent drawbacks of some *in vivo* gene therapy strategies is the requirement for 100% of the tumour cells to be transfected for eradication of the tumour to occur. The existence of a bystander effect, whereby the percentage of cells killed exceeds the percentage originally transduced, is therefore important.[48] It seems that the bystander effect may be immunologically mediated, at least in one drug-activating suicide gene approach. The HSVTK and ganciclovir combination was more effective in immunocompetent animals than in nude mice challenged with the same melanoma cell line,[49] thus implying that at least part of the tumour cell killing depends on inducing a systemic immune response. Further experiments showed that, whereas *in vitro* tumour cells expressing HSVTK in the presence of ganciclovir die predominantly by necrosis, cells dying *in vivo* induce a pronounced intratumoral infiltrate of lymphocytes and macrophages and their cytokine expression (IL-2, IFN-γ, IL-12 and GM-CSF) is characteristic of the Th1 (cell-mediated) immune response now thought to be important for antitumour effect.[50] In the mouse prostate reconstitution model (an immunocompetent model), HSVTK transfection results in a significant increase in the level of tumour necrosis, marked lymphocytic infiltrate and a doubling of the apoptotic index in treatment animals relative to controls, but with an increase in survival of only 7 days.[51] Phase I studies are beginning in humans, probably using a PSA promoter to allow systemic administration but targeting delivery of the gene to the prostate.

Conclusions

The results of phase I/II trials of autologous IL-2 or GM-CSF whole tumour vaccines are awaited with great interest. It is unlikely that the impressive results in the animal models will immediately translate to human tumours, but those animal models have demonstrated that vaccine therapy for prostate cancer deserves serious further investigation. Advances continue to be made in our understanding of the individual components of anti-tumour responses and how cancer cells may escape immune surveillance. This is already allowing more precise vaccine approaches than the use of whole tumour cells to be investigated, but the best way of dealing with the heterogeneity of antigen expression remains to be established. Experience with cancer immunotherapy to date suggests that vaccines are most likely to show results in low-volume disease, such as patients with extracapsular disease at radical prostatectomy or those suspected to have micrometastatic disease following resection of the primary. Novel therapies often target patients with hormone-escape metastatic prostate cancer; however, the large tumour burden means that the immune system is often considerably impaired and the tumour is likely to be able to outrun the immune response. Vaccines probably need to be evaluated first in early disease if an important therapeutic benefit is not to be missed.

References

1. Coley W B. Treatment of inoperable malignant tumours with the toxins of erysipelas and *Bacillus prodigosus*. Trans Am Surg Assoc 1894; 12: 183
2. Burnet F M. Immunological surveillance. Oxford: Pergamon Press, 1970
3. Gittes R F, McCullough D L. Occult carcinoma of the prostate: an oversight of immune surveillance — a working hypothesis. J Urol 1974; 112: 241–244
4. Vesalainen S, Lipponen P, Talja M *et al*. Histological grade, perineural infiltration, tumour-infiltrating lymphocytes and apoptosis as determinants of long-term prognosis in prostatic adenocarcinoma. Eur J Cancer 1994; 30A(12): 1797–1803
5. Sanda M G, Restifo N P, Walsh J C *et al*. Molecular characterization of defective antigen processing in human prostate cancer [see comments]. J Natl Cancer Inst 1995; 87(4): 280–285
6. Blades R A, Keating P J, McWilliam L J *et al*. Loss of HLA class I expression in prostate cancer: implications for immunotherapy. Urology 1995; 46(5): 681–686; discussion 686–687
7. Mukherji B, Chakraborty N G. Immunobiology and immunotherapy of melanoma [see comments]. Curr Opin Oncol 1995; 7(2): 175–184
8. Huber D, Philipp J, Fontana A. Protease inhibitors interfere with the transforming growth factor-beta-dependent but not the transforming growth factor-beta-independent pathway of tumor cell-mediated immunosuppression. J Immunol 1992; 148(1): 277–284
9. Zier K, Gansbacher B, Salvadori S. Preventing abnormalities in signal transduction of T cells in cancer: the promise of cytokine gene therapy. Immunol Today 1996; 17(1): 39–45
10. Hahne M, Rimoldi D, Schroter M *et al*. Melanoma cell expression of Fas(Apo-1/CD95) ligand: implications for tumor immune escape. Science 1996; 274:1363–1366
11. Guinan P, Toronchi E, Shaw M *et al*. Bacillus calmette-guerin (BCG) adjuvant therapy in stage D prostate cancer. Urology 1982; 20(4): 401–403
12. Brosman S. Nonspecific immunotherapy in GU cancer. In: Crispen R (ed) Neoplasm immunity. Philadelphia: Franklin Institute Press, 1977: 97–107
13. Souberbielle B E, Dalgleish A G. Antitumour immune mechanisms. In: Lewis C E, O'Sullivan C, Barraclough J (eds) The psychoimmunology of cancer. Oxford: Oxford University Press, 1994: 267–290.
14. Huang AY, Golumbek P, Ahmadzadeh M, *et al*. Role of bone marrow-derived cells in presenting MHC class I-restricted tumor antigens. Science 1994; 264(5161): 961-965
15. van der Bruggen P, Traversari C, Chomez P *et al*. A gene encoding an antigen recognized by cytolytic T lymphocytes on a human melanoma. Science 1991; 254(5038): 1643–1647
16. Chen M E, Sikes R A, Troncoso P *et al*. PAGE and GAGE 7 are novel genes expressed in the LNCaP prostatic carcinogenesis model that share homology with melanoma associated antigens. J Urol 1996; 155(5): 624A (abstr 1251)
17. Dalgleish A G, Souberbielle B E. The development of therapeutic vaccines for the management of malignant melanoma. Cancer Surv 1996; 26: 289–319
18. Israeli R S, Powell C T, Corr J G *et al*. Expression of the prostate-specific membrane antigen. Cancer Res 1994; 54(7): 1807–1811
19. Corman J M, Belldegrun A, Sercarz E E *et al*. Prostate specific antigenic peptides induce T cell proliferation in-vitro: a model for the development of prostate specific tumor vaccines. J Urol 1996; 155(5): 528A (abstr 870)
20. Tjoa B, Boynton A, Kenny G *et al*. Presentation of prostate tumor antigens by dendritic cells stimulates T-cell proliferation and cytotoxicity. Prostate 1996; 28(1): 65–69
21. Brenner P C, Rettig W J, Sanz-Moncasi M P *et al*. TAG-72 expression in primary, metastatic and hormonally treated prostate cancer as defined by monoclonal antibody CC49 [see comments]. J Urol 1995; 153(5): 1575–1579
22. Wright G L Jr, Beckett M L, Lipford G B *et al*. A novel prostate carcinoma-associated glycoprotein complex (PAC) recognized by monoclonal antibody TURP-27. Int J Cancer 1991; 47(5): 717–725
23. Shurbaji M S, Kuhajda F P, Pasternack G R *et al*. Expression of oncogenic antigen 519 (OA-519) in prostate cancer is a potential prognostic indicator. Am J Clin Pathol 1992; 97(5): 686–691
24. Burchell J, Graham R, Taylor-Papadimitriou J. Active specific immunotherapy: PEM as a potential target molecule. Cancer Surv 1993; 18: 135–148
25. Beckett M L, Lipford G B, Haley CL *et al*. Monoclonal antibody PD41 recognizes an antigen restricted to prostate adenocarcinomas. Cancer Res 1991; 51(4): 1326–1333

26. Beckett M L, Wright G L Jr. Characterization of a prostate carcinoma mucin-like antigen (PMA). Int J Cancer 1995; 62(6): 703–710

27. Dranoff G, Jaffee E, Lazenby A et al. Vaccination with irradiated tumor cells engineered to secrete murine granulocyte-macrophage colony-stimulating factor stimulates potent, specific, and long-lasting anti-tumor immunity. Proc Natl Acad Sci USA 1993; 90(8): 3539–3543

28. Pardoll D M. Paracrine cytokine adjuvants in cancer immunotherapy. Annu Rev Immunol 1995; 13: 399–415

29. Vieweg J, Rosenthal F M, Bannerji R et al. Immunotherapy of prostate cancer in the Dunning rat model: use of cytokine gene modified tumor vaccines. Cancer Res 1994; 54(7): 1760–1765

30. Pollard M. Commentary on the Dunning tumor. Prostate 1995; 26(6): 287–289

31. Sanda M G, Ayyagari S R, Jaffee E M et al. Demonstration of a rational strategy for human prostate cancer gene therapy. J Urol 1994; 151(3): 622–628

32. Moody D B, Robinson J C, Ewing C M et al. Interleukin-2 transfected prostate cancer cells generate a local antitumor effect in vivo. Prostate 1994; 24(5): 244–251

33. Carducci M A, Ayyagari S R, Sanda M G et al. Gene therapy for human prostate cancer: translational research in the hormone refractory Dunning prostate cancer model. Cancer 1995; 75(suppl 7): 2013–2020

34. Yoshimura I, Weston W D W, Gansbacher B et al. Cytokine mediated immuno-gene therapy in rat prostate cancer model. J Urol 1996; 155(5): 510A (abstr 798)

35. Schmidt W, Schweighoffer T, Herbst E et al. Cancer vaccines: the interleukin 2 dosage effect. Proc Natl Acad Sci USA 1995; 92(10): 4711–4714

36. Marshall F, Jaffee E, Weber C et al. Bioactivity of human GM-CSF gene therapy in metastatic renal carcinoma. J Urol 1996; 155: 582A (abstr 1087)

37. Peehl D M, Stamey T A. Serum-free growth of adult human prostatic epithelial cells. In Vitro Cell Dev Biol 1986; 22(2): 82–90

38. Knight B C, Souberbielle B E, Rizzardi G P et al. Allogeneic murine melanoma cell vaccine: a model for the development of human allogeneic cancer vaccine. Melanoma Res 1996; 6: 299–306

39. Ben-Yosef R, Or R, Nagler A et al. Graft-versus-tumour and graft-versus-leukaemia effect in patient with concurrent breast cancer and acute myelocytic leukaemia. Lancet 1996; 348: 1242–1243

40. Eibl B, Schwaighofer H, Nachbaur D et al. Evidence for a graft-versus-tumor effect in a patient treated with marrow ablative chemotherapy and allogeneic bone marrow transplantation for breast cancer. Blood 1996; 88(4): 1501–1508

41. Tjoa B, Erickson S, Barren R 3rd et al. In vitro propagated dendritic cells from prostate cancer patients as a component of prostate cancer immunotherapy. Prostate 1995; 27(2): 63–69

42. Durrant L G, Doran M, Austin E B et al. Induction of cellular immune responses by a murine monoclonal anti-idiotypic antibody recognizing the 791Tgp72 antigen expressed on colorectal, gastric and ovarian human tumours. Int J Cancer 1995; 61(1): 62–66

43. Buckley D T, Robins A R, Durrant L G. Clinical evidence that the human monoclonal anti-idiotypic antibody 105AD7, delays tumor growth by stimulating anti-tumor T-cell responses. Hum Antibodies Hybridomas 1995; 6(2): 68–72

44. Uemura H, Kitagawa H, Ozono S et al. Generation of anti-idiotype antibodies related to PSA: possible tools for treatment of prostate cancer. J Urol 1995; 153: 380A (abstr 607)

45. Wolff J A, Malone R W, Williams P et al. Direct gene transfer into mouse muscle in vivo. Science 1990; 247(4949 Pt 1): 1465–1468

46. Conry R M, LoBuglio A F, Loechel F et al. A carcinoembryonic antigen polynucleotide vaccine has in vivo antitumor activity. Gene Ther 1995; 2(1): 59–65

47. Hrouda D, Dalgleish A G. Gene therapy for prostate cancer. Gene Ther 1996; 3(10): 845–852

48. Freeman S M, Abboud C N, Whartenby K A et al. The 'bystander effect': tumor regression when a fraction of the tumor mass is genetically modified. Cancer Res 1993; 53(21): 5274–5283

49. Vile R G, Nelson J A, Castleden S et al. Systemic gene therapy of murine melanoma using tissue specific expression of the HSVtk gene involves an immune component. Cancer Res 1994; 54(23): 6228–6234

50. Vile R G, Castleden S, Upton C, Chang H. Generation of an anti-tumour immune response in a non-immunogenic tumour: HSVtk killing in vivo stimulates a lymphocytic

infiltrate and a Th1-like profile of intratumoral cytokine expression. Int J Cancer 1997; 71: 267–274

51. Eastham J A, Chen S-H, Sehgal I *et al.* Prostate cancer gene therapy: herpes simplex virus thymidine kinase gene transduction followed by ganciclovir in mouse and human prostate cancer models. Human Gene Ther 1996; 7: 515–523

Chapter 34
Photodynamic therapy for prostate cancer

S. G. Bown and S. S. C. Chang

Background

Prostate cancer is one of the commonest cancers in men, although its natural history is very variable. Some cancers progress relentlessly and metastasize widely, whereas others lead an indolent course over many years so that the patients die of unrelated causes.[1] At the early stages it is difficult to predict which ones will progress, so there is a major need for an effective, minimally invasive treatment for early disease that carries low morbidity. Unfortunately, the only potentially curative options at present for early disease are radical surgery and radical radiotherapy, both of which carry considerable morbidity.[2,3] Hormone therapy may hold the disease for some time, but is rarely curative. Further, more and more prostate cancers are being detected at the asymptomatic stage, either because the serum prostate-specific antigen (PSA) level is abnormal or because the gland feels abnormal on rectal examination.[4,5] Photodynamic therapy (PDT) is a promising new option that may satisfy some of these needs.

PDT is a technique that combines administration of a photosensitizing drug with subsequent activation of that drug with low-power red light.[6] Neither the drug nor the light has any effect on its own. The drug can be given locally, for example by intravesical administration for treatment of superficial disease in the bladder, or systemically (usually by intravenous injection, but occasionally by mouth). The light used to activate the drug must be of a wavelength that both matches an absorption peak of the drug and penetrates the target tissue well enough to treat all relevant areas. In practice, this usually means using red light, as shorter wavelengths in the blue and green part of the spectrum do not penetrate tissue well enough and the longer wavelengths in the near infrared are not absorbed by currently available photosensitizers. For all applications that require delivery of the light via one or more flexible fibres, lasers are the most convenient source. Laser light is straightforward to control, so it is practical to define the treatment area clearly. Thus, even if the whole patient is sensitized, the PDT effect can be limited to the area exposed to the therapeutic light, although care must be taken to protect skin from bright ambient lights for periods that may vary from a few hours to a month or more, depending on which photosensitizer is used.

The aspect of PDT that attracted most attention initially was the fact that photosensitizers are retained in malignant tissues with some degree of selectivity compared with the adjacent normal tissue in which the tumour arose.[7] When this was combined with the knowledge that photosensitizer and light together led to tissue necrosis, it raised the possibility that cancers could be destroyed without damaging the normal tissue. Unfortunately, under most circumstances, this has proved to be overoptimistic, despite the number of times this possibility has been raised over the last 15 years. Although there is a small degree of selectivity in uptake of photosensitizers, it is rarely feasible to exploit this to achieve selective necrosis.[8] Under the conditions described in most publications on PDT, if tumour and the normal tissue in which the tumour arose are exposed to the same light dose, there is damage to both.[9] However, it is now becoming clear that the real attraction of PDT is the nature of the tissue damage produced, as there is none of the cumulative toxicity associated with radiotherapy or chemotherapy and there is much less damage to connective tissue than with any treatment that produces its effect by heating the tissue, such as diathermy or a high-power laser like the Nd:YAG.[10] This means that there is much less risk of perforating hollow organs.

Despite nearly 20 years of intensive research in the field, it is surprising how few data are available on the nature of PDT effects on normal or neoplastic tissues relevant to clinical practice. Most animal studies have been performed on tumours transplanted to sites convenient for access in small animals (mainly subcutaneously in mice and rats) and the results judged on the disappearance (or otherwise) of the treated tumour and any subsequent regrowth.[11] However, the situation is improving. Once it was clear that normal tissue is not immune to PDT, it became important to understand the biological response of normal and neoplastic tissues and, in particular, to understand what happens in the crucial region where tumour is invading normal tissue. Most interest in PDT to date has been for the treatment of thin or hollow organs such as the urogenital tract, the aerodigestive tract and the skin, but many of the lessons learnt in experimental and clinical studies of these are helpful in understanding the potential for treating prostate cancer.

Urologists were among the first specialists to take an interest in PDT. As the data available on the prostate at present are quite limited, it is useful to review the situation with regard to the application in urology that has received most attention to date, namely its potential for treating carcinoma *in situ* of the bladder — a difficult condition to treat as the disease process can involve the entire urothelium. The first clinical experience was reported in 1976 by Kelly and Snell using the photosensitizer with which most of the early work was done, haematoporphyrin derivative (HpD).[12] They found more fluorescence in papillary tumours and carcinoma *in situ* than in normal areas and could achieve some tumour necrosis with light delivered cystoscopically. However, the procedure was technically difficult and they decided to go back to animal studies to understand the biology better. Other subsequent studies showed that small papillary tumours could be treated successfully. In a series of 19 patients with stage Ta ($n = 17$) and T1 ($n = 22$) disease, Prout *et al.* achieved a 47% complete response rate on assessment 3 months after PDT.[13] Nevertheless, the evidence that PDT was superior to conventional cystoscopic resection was not convincing, particularly as patients were left sensitive to bright lights for several weeks after photosensitization.

Interest next centred more around the possibility of treating widespread disease, such as carcinoma *in situ*, that could not be seen easily macroscopically. The concept was to treat the entire urothelium in the bladder. This was first done by Hisazumi, who used a motor-driven system to achieve a reasonably homogeneous light distribution in the bladder to treat two patients with carcinoma *in situ*.[14] The light dose was much smaller than that used for treating focal disease, but both patients became cytologically and cystoscopically clear of disease. However, both had marked irritative symptoms in the bladder, with frequency of micturition and reduction of bladder capacity that lasted 2–3 months. Other groups have reported very similar results using HpD (or its commercial derivative, Photofrin®), but on occasions the permanent damage to the bladder was severe enough to necessitate a cystectomy, despite the complete ablation of all neoplastic tissue. Harty *et al.* took deep biopsies from treated bladders and showed unequivocally that PDT led to scarring in the muscle layer, so shattering the illusion that, under these treatment conditions, PDT might be able to ablate tumour tissue without damaging adjacent normal areas.[9] These results led to some important experiments designed to understand better the biology of PDT.

The challenge was to see if PDT could produce generalized mucosal ablation in animal bladders without permanent impairment of bladder function. Most studies were conducted with rats. No study has shown any selectivity between the PDT effect on bladder tumours and on the adjacent normal urothelium if both are exposed to the same light dose. However, studies with two newer photosensitizing agents, aluminium sulphonated phthalocyanine (AlSPc) and 5-aminolaevulinic acid (ALA) have shown that, with careful choice of the drug and light doses and of the time interval between drug and light, it is possible to ablate the mucosa without permanently damaging the underlying muscle layer;[15,16] the ablated mucosa healed with regeneration of histologically normal mucosa. Some inflammatory changes were seen in the muscle, but the bladder compliance and capacity returned to normal within 3 months in those treated with the optimum drug and light doses. ALA is just as effective given systemically or intravesically.[16] Groups in Germany have now started clinical trials using intravesical ALA.[17] Others have tried to minimize the damage to muscle in patients by using lower doses of photosensitizer and ingenious systems to ensure uniform distribution of light within the bladder.

The other major result that has come from the experimental work is that connective tissue and, in particular, collagen, in tumour or normal areas, is largely unaffected by PDT. This has been better documented in the GI tract than in the bladder. It has been shown that areas of full-thickness PDT necrosis in the rat colon are mechanically at least as strong as untreated areas at all times after treatment and that, on conventional histology and on electron microscopy, the collagen fibrils remain intact.[10]

The prostate

Most interest in PDT has been for treating superficial disease in hollow organs or the skin, rather than in solid organs. There are two main reasons for this. The red light used has an optical penetration depth of only a few millimetres into most living tissues, so, in general terms, it is difficult to produce a PDT effect more than 5 mm below the surface exposed to the light. This can be overcome by delivering the light interstitially (inserting optical fibres directly into the target tissue through a suitable needle, usually placed percutaneously). Nevertheless, treating a large volume of tissue by this means can require many fibres. The other problem is knowing the precise size and position of a target lesion within a solid organ, which requires sophisticated imaging techniques. However, new photosensitizers and technical developments in light sources and optical fibre light-delivery systems now make it feasible to consider treating lesions in small solid organs such as the prostate.

The biology of PDT on the prostate

The prostate is a glandular organ that has a thick capsule and multiple intralobular septa of connective tissue. From experimental results on the bladder and other organs, one might expect the glandular areas to be destroyed by PDT, but for there to be little effect on the capsule and septa. The only animal with a prostate gland that is even roughly comparable to the human prostate and that can be used for experimental studies is the dog. There is no simple way of producing cancers in the dog prostate, but the most important task is to understand what PDT does to the normal gland. Three groups (the authors' group in the UK and two groups in the USA) have reported recently on PDT experiments on the dog prostate. The authors investigated three different photosensitizers — ALA, AlSPc and meso-tetra-(m-hydroxyphenyl) chlorin (mTHPC),[18,19] Selman and Keck looked at tin (II) etiopurpurin dichloride (SnET2)[20] and Johnson et al. looked at ALA.[21] The authors delivered the light both transurethrally and interstitially via needles inserted through the perineal skin under guidance from transrectal ultrasound; the other groups looked at transurethral light delivery only.

The drug doses used in the authors' experiments were based on experience in other organs. Under general anaesthesia or heavy sedation, percutaneous needle biopsies were taken of the prostate for examination under fluorescence microscopy to measure the distribution and concentration of each photosensitizing agent at a range of times after drug administration, to find the time at which the tissue levels of photosensitizing drug were highest. In general, these times were used for light delivery. In separate experiments, a group of animals was treated with PDT using each of these drugs, together with unsensitized control animals to ensure that the light power and energy used were not causing any thermal effects. The light was delivered either via a single diffuser fibre placed in the urethra, or by up to four fibres positioned in the gland interstitially through needles placed percutaneously under transrectal ultrasound guidance. The time intervals and light doses (for each fibre) used are shown in Table 34.1.

Urinary function after PDT

Some of the animals developed urinary retention 1–2 days after PDT, particularly those that had been treated transurethrally. As dogs will not tolerate prolonged catheterization, these animals were managed by intermittent catheterization, which was satisfactory in all except one animal that had to be killed at 5 days owing to renal failure. The other animals that were scheduled to be kept alive for more than a week were able to pass urine spontaneously again after 5–7 days of intermittent catheterization. No animal became incontinent at any time after PDT. There were no other problems of note attributable to the treatment, although all animals were kept in subdued light to minimize the risk of skin phototoxicity.

Macroscopic findings

The animals were killed at times from 3 days to 3 months after PDT and the prostate and surrounding tissues were examined macroscopically and

Table 34.1. Treatment values used in experiments on normal canine prostates

Drug (dose, mg/kg)	Time (h)	Wavelength (nm)	Light (power, mW)	Light (energy, J)
Controls	–	630 and 650	100 and 300	100–1000
mTHPC (0.3)	72	650	100	100
AlSPc (1.0)	24	675	100	100
ALA (100 and 200)	3 and 8	630	100 and 300	100–1000

microscopically. The capsular structure around the prostate was intact in every case, although sometimes with some hyperaemia and oedema. Two dogs treated transurethrally using mTHPC and killed within a week showed a small rectal ulcer but, in another animal treated similarly and killed at 1 month, there was evidence only of a healed rectal ulcer. There was no suspicion of a fistula at any stage. The problems with urinary retention and rectal ulcers occurred only in animals treated with mTHPC, simply because the lesions produced were so much larger with mTHPC than with the other photosensitizers.

In animals killed within a week of treatment, on sectioning the prostate there were obvious zones of haemorrhagic necrosis around the sites where each fibre tip had been during treatment (Figure 34.1). Using mTHPC and a single diffuser fibre placed transurethrally, the zone of necrosis was up to $30 \times 18 \times 18$ mm in size. Using four fibres placed interstitially, this could be increased to $42 \times 22 \times 20$ mm, which meant that up to 80% of the volume of the prostate had been necrosed. Using AlSPc, the lesions were much smaller (maximum $12 \times 10 \times 10$ mm around a single fibre placed interstitially) but similar in nature. With ALA and a laser power of 100 mW, no lesion larger than 2 mm in diameter could be found. Johnson *et al.*[21] described lesions up to 10 mm in depth using a light dose of 650 mW for 45 min (1755 J) delivered transurethrally with a diffuser fibre 8 hours after 100 mg/kg ALA, with no lesion seen using this light dose in an unsensitized animal. However, in the authors' study when the laser power was increased to 300 mW, as large a lesion resulted in an unsensitized animal as in one that had received ALA, suggesting that the effect was thermal and not photodynamic. These results from different research groups are inconsistent, but it is the authors' impression that there is unlikely to be a useful effect with ALA in the prostate under the conditions tried so far. It is possible that better results would be found by increasing the dose of ALA or fractionating the light.

Histology

In animals killed within a week of PDT, the lesions seen macroscopically corresponded closely to those found microscopically. There was extensive haemorrhagic necrosis in the glandular tissue with a sharp border between normal and necrosed areas (Figure 34.2). In lesions extending across the urethra there was sloughing of the urothelium and infiltration of inflammatory cells in the surrounding tissue (Figure 34.3). These changes evolved slowly. In specimens

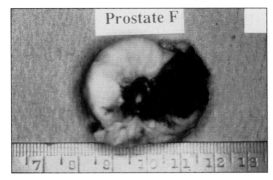

Figure 34.1. Macroscopic section of prostate 7 days after PDT using mTHPC, with two fibres placed interstitially (one just under the capsule and the other close to the urethra). The dark area of haemorrhagic necrosis is sharply defined.

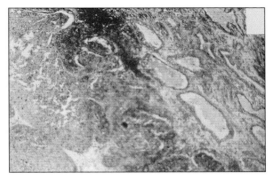

Figure 34.2. Section of prostate 7 days after PDT using mTHPC showing the junction of normal glandular tissue (on the right) and necrosed glandular tissue (on left). H&E stain.

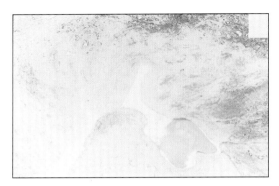

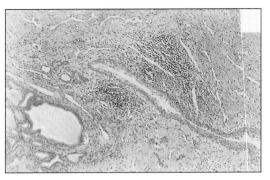

Figure 34.3. Section showing sloughing of the urothelium and necrosis of the surrounding glands 7 days after PDT using mTHPC. H&E stain.

Figure 34.4. Section showing complete regeneration of the urothelium 28 days after PDT with mTHPC. There is very little regeneration of glandular tissue. H&E stain.

Figure 34.5. Section of subcapsular region 28 days after PDT with mTHPC. There is no regeneration of glandular tissue, but the connective tissue in the capsule (pink staining) appears entirely normal. Van Gieson stain.

examined at a month, the urothelium had regenerated without stricture formation (Figure 34.4); however, the glandular elements remained atrophic even at 3 months. The supporting collagenous structure in the capsule and interlobular septa was well preserved at all stages of healing (Figure 34.5). Likewise, the rectal ulcer healed with regeneration of normal mucosa without any breach in the lamina propria at any stage, although some scarring was seen in the muscularis propria.

The results from Selman and Keck using SnET2 were very similar to those of the present authors.[20] Using light delivered transurethrally, they produced lesions up to 20 mm in diameter in the canine prostate, with sloughing of the urothelium that healed without stricturing in 3 weeks. None of their animals developed urinary retention, but they also reported persistent atrophy of the glandular regions of the prostate at the longest time interval studied after PDT, which was 3 weeks.

Significance of experimental results

The experimental work on the canine prostate has shown that in general terms, the effects of PDT seen in the different layers of hollow organs are also seen in a small solid organ like the prostate. There is extensive necrosis of the glandular elements, but little damage to the connective tissue, at least at the interlobular and capsular level. Damage in the region of the urethra causes urothelial sloughing but this heals within a month without stricture formation. Temporary obstruction of urinary flow was seen, most likely owing to periurethral oedema from local inflammation associated with the PDT effect, but this resolved within about a week and the animals were able to resume spontaneous micturition. It was reassuring that no animal became incontinent. Healing was studied only up to 3 months after PDT using mTHPC and only up to 1 month using AlSPc; by this time there was still little evidence of healing of the glandular tissue. This is probably because healing of a roughly spherical zone of necrosis would be expected to be slower than healing of a two-dimensional area in the wall of a hollow organ, where healing can proceed more easily from the edges towards the centre. All treated prostates retained their overall shape, size and texture, but no studies were conducted on the sexual function of treated animals. However, one would not expect effects to be any more severe than after a transurethral resection of the prostate.

A further important factor is the effect of PDT on the neurovascular bundle. There are virtually no published papers on the effects of PDT on peripheral nerves in any part of the body. However, theoretical considerations would suggest that there is unlikely to be much damage. It would be difficult for photosensitizers to diffuse into nerve cells and light would be more likely to be reflected from nerve sheaths than to penetrate into them, although PDT might shut down the microvessels supplying them.

Much more work has been done on the effects of PDT on blood vessels. With many photosensitizers, the main mechanism of PDT necrosis in normal and tumour tissue is shut-down of the microvessels[22] and, even with those like ALA, where the effect is more on individual cells, microvascular shut-down plays a part in the biological effect. Nevertheless, the vessels that are most affected are those without much connective tissue in their wall. Once vessels are large enough to have a defined layer of collagen, elastin or both, then they become much more resistant. Detailed experiments using ALA and AlSPc have shown that arterial endothelium sloughs within a few days of PDT, but regenerates within a week or two without any evidence of an increased risk of thrombus formation at any stage of healing.[23] Further, there is complete necrosis of the smooth muscle cells in the media of the arterial wall. These cells take months to regenerate, but there is no reduction in the mechanical strength of the arterial wall, so no risk of perforation or aneurysm formation.[24] This effect has considerable potential for reducing the proliferation of smooth muscle cells after injury to the wall of arteries, which is one of the main causes of restenosis after balloon angioplasty to coronary or peripheral arteries.

The other urogenital structure that could be at risk from PDT to the prostate is the external sphincter. No animal became incontinent in the authors' experiments, even when almost the entire gland had been necrosed, but the number of animals followed for long enough after PDT for the periurethral oedema to settle and to assess the urinary function subsequently, was very small. Anatomically, the sphincter is far enough from the prostate to avoid exposure to a high light dose, as long as the fibre delivering the laser light is positioned accurately, but there would be a case for deliberately treating the sphincter area in animals using treatment conditions known to produce glandular necrosis to see whether the continence mechanism is damaged.

Outside the urogenital tract, the most important adjacent organ is the rectum. The experiments showed that localized rectal ulceration could be produced, but this healed safely without sequelae. There was some scarring in the muscularis propria of the rectum anteriorly, but as long as the muscle scarring involves only a small percentage of the circumference of the rectum, it is most unlikely to cause any symptoms. The authors' experimental animals showed no sign of bowel problems.

All these experiments were carried out on normal prostates in dogs. Some experiments have been conducted on urological cancers transplanted subcutaneously in small rodents,[11] but none on prostate cancers actually growing in a normal prostate. However, all that is required for these experimental results to be relevant for the treatment of prostate cancers is that the cancer should be at least as sensitive to PDT as the normal tissue from which it arose. Although there is a lack of direct evidence for this at present for the prostate, it is true for every other adenocarcinoma that has been treated with PDT, such as adenocarcinomas of the stomach and colon.[25] There is no need to invoke any selectivity between tumour and normal; even if there is a small degree of selectivity in the uptake of photosensitizer in prostate cancers, there is most unlikely to be any selectivity of necrosis, although if this were seen, it would be a bonus.

The conclusion from the experimental work is that PDT can produce necrosis in the glandular elements of the prostate that heals safely without any unacceptable effects in the surrounding normal tissues. This made it justifiable to start pilot clinical studies in carefully selected patients.

Clinical studies

PDT is a local treatment and so the most suitable patients for initial clinical studies are those with small-volume disease localized to the prostate, in whom other treatment modalities have failed or are considered inappropriate. The patients chosen by the authors' group were those who presented with localized disease and who were treated initially with radical radiotherapy but then subsequently developed recurrent disease that appeared to be confined to the prostate. This programme has only just started and the only data available are preliminary results on two patients; both were considered unsuitable for radical prostatectomy, and the project was approved by the hospital ethics committee.

Case history 1: a 74-year-old man with an incidental finding of an enlarged prostate and elevated PSA, treated with radical radiotherapy (64 Gy in 32 fractions). Recurrent cancer was diagnosed 3 years later from increasing PSA and transrectal ultrasound scan. He was treated with PDT at two sites in each lobe.

Case history 2: a 73-year-old man who presented with increasing prostatic symptoms, a hard prostate and elevated PSA. He was treated with cyproterone acetate and radical radiotherapy (64 Gy in 32 fractions). Local recurrence 3 years later was treated with PDT at three sites.

Both patients were treated in the same way. They were photosensitized with an intravenous injection of mTHPC (0.15 mg/kg) and kept in a room with subdued lighting to minimize the risk of skin photosensitivity. Three days later, under sedation with midazolam and pethidine, the perineal skin was infiltrated with local anaesthetic and needles were inserted percutaneously into the tumour areas in the prostate, with guidance from transrectal ultrasound. With the tip of the needle at the deepest part of the tumour, 0.4 mm optical fibres were passed through each needle and the needles pulled back a few millimetres, leaving the bare tips of the fibres in the tumour. The fibres were then attached to a copper vapour-pumped dye laser giving light at 652 nm in the red part of the visible spectrum (the most suitable wavelength to match an absorption peak of mTHPC and to maximize tissue penetration of the therapeutic light). When one site had been treated, the fibres were pulled back 1 cm and the treatment repeated to cover the tumour area identified on the pretreatment transrectal ultrasound. The light dose down each fibre at each treatment site was 100 mW for 200–250 s (20–25 J). In view of the urinary retention seen in the experimental animals, both patients were catheterized as a precautionary measure, but in each case the catheter was removed without problems within a couple of days and was probably unnecessary, as the treated areas were not very close to the urethra. Both patients felt that the most uncomfortable part of the procedure was the insertion and manipulation of the transrectal ultrasound instrument. As the tissue is not heated during delivery

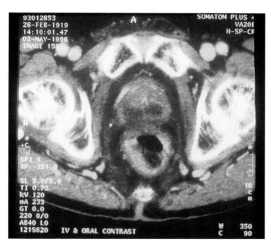

Figure 34.6. Contrast-enhanced CT scan of patient 1, 1 week after interstitial PDT with two fibres placed about 1 cm apart on either side of the urethra. The butterfly-shaped area of reduced enhancement in the centre of the prostate is interpreted as PDT-induced necrosis.

of the low-power laser light used for PDT, this part of the treatment caused no discomfort at all and the only discomfort after treatment was a mild pain in the prostatic area during the first 24 hours. There were no problems with micturition.

The results were assessed by contrast-enhanced CT scans taken 4–7 days after treatment (the CT scan after treatment in patient 1 is shown in Figure 34.6) and by serial measurements of PSA (Table 34.2).

The areas of non-enhancement shown in the post-treatment CT were interpreted as PDT-induced necrosis. The PSA results were slightly disappointing. It was not surprising to see an elevated level immediately after treatment, but no fall below pretreatment levels was seen in the later follow-up specimens. However, as these are the first clinical trials of a new approach to treating this condition, treatments were carried out carefully and conservatively and it is probable that the area of PDT necrosis did not cover the entire tumour. This is effectively a phase I study. More patients will be treated similarly, but what has been shown so far is that PDT can produce necrosis in cancers growing in the prostate, using a procedure that is reasonably comfortable for the patient both during and after treatment and that has shown no complications of note.

Prostate cancer is often a multifocal disease, and cure of early disease localized to the gland would be more likely if all the glandular elements could be necrosed. The authors' experiments suggest that this is feasible using PDT, as necrosis can be produced right up to the prostate capsule without any unacceptable damage to adjacent organs. This will require careful positioning of multiple treatment fibres, perhaps using both the interstitial and transurethral route. Transrectal ultrasound may provide sufficient guidance, but more accurate techniques such as fibre arrays positioned using real-time images from an interventional magnetic resonance (MR) scanner may be needed. Recent studies from Pantelides et al. have shown that red light is scattered extensively within the prostate,[26] and these data combined with the present authors' results and those of Selman et al.[20] suggest that normal-size prostates may be completely ablated with no more than four to six fibre tracks. However, much work must be done, first, to know how to

Table 34.2. PSA measurements (ng/ml) before and after PDT

Case number	Pretreatment	3–4 days after PDT	Later follow-up
1	25.5	43.5	26.5 (5 weeks)
2	5.2	5.1	7.3 (13 weeks)

illuminate every part of the gland sufficiently and, secondly, to interpret the post-treatment scans (CT or MR) to identify the limits of PDT necrosis.

In addition to the relative lack of effect on connective tissue and on organs adjacent to the prostate, one of the greatest attractions of PDT is the lack of cumulative toxicity. If treatment misses an important area, once everything has settled it is possible to re-sensitize the patient and treat the same region again. This is certainly not an option with radical surgery or radical radiotherapy!

The only other published clinical report of PDT for prostate cancer was from Windahl et al. in 1990.[27] They used the photosensitizer Photofrin® and treated two patients with residual cancer in the prostatic bed after two transurethral resections. PSA levels returned to the normal range after treatment and random biopsies taken 3 months after PDT failed to reveal any residual cancer. One patient died of a rapidly progressive lung cancer (undiagnosed at the time of PDT) 6 months later; at post-mortem examination, no cancer could be found in the residual prostatic tissue.

Selman and Keck[20] suggested that PDT might be suitable for treating benign prostatic hypertrophy (BPH); however, the current authors have serious reservations about this, because all their experiments have shown that, as PDT did not affect the prostatic capsule or interlobular septa, the shape and size of the gland was unchanged, even if there was extensive glandular necrosis. Selman et al. did not provide any measurements of gland size or urethral resistance to urine flow before and after PDT, but their photograph of a prostate 3 weeks after PDT suggested that the shape and size of the organ had been preserved, as in the current authors' experiments. The main aim of treatment for BPH is to reduce the bulk of the gland causing obstruction to urinary flow; current data suggest that PDT is most unlikely to achieve this.

In conclusion, PDT is a promising new approach for the treatment of prostate cancer localized to the gland, which has the major advantages of no cumulative toxicity and no unacceptable effects on the prostate capsule or other adjacent tissues. However, much further work is required to establish how best to apply the technique and to demonstrate its effectiveness.

References

1. Chodak G W, Thisted R A, Gerber G S et al. Results of conservative management of clinically localized prostate cancer. N Engl J Med 1994; 330: 242–248
2. Bagshaw M A, Cox R S, Hancock S L. Control of prostate cancer with radiotherapy: Long-term results. J Urol 1994; 152: 1781–1785
3. Murphy G P, Mettlin C, Menck H, Davidson A M. National patterns of prostate cancer treatment by radical prostatectomy: results of a survey by the American College of Surgery Commission on Cancer. J Urol 1994; 152: 1817–1819
4. Parkes C, Wald N J, Murphy P et al. Prospective observational study to assess value of prostate specific antigen as screening test for prostate cancer. Br Med J 1995; 311: 1340–1343
5. Catalona W J, Richie J P, Ahamman F R et al. Comparison of digital rectal examination and serum prostate specific antigen in the early detection of prostate cancer-results of a multicenter clinical trial of 6,630 men. J Urol 1994; 151: 1283–1290
6. Pass H I. Photodynamic therapy in oncology: mechanism and clinical use. J. Natl. Cancer Inst 1993; 85: 443–456
7. Lipson R L, Baldes E J, Olsen A M. The use of a derivative of hematoporphyrin in tumor detection. J Natl Cancer Inst 1961; 26: 1–8
8. Bown S G. Photodynamic therapy to scientists and clinicians — one world or two? J Photochem Photobiol B. Biol 1990; 6: 1–12
9. Harty J I, Amin M, Wieman T J et al. Complications of whole bladder dihematoporphyrin ether photodynamic therapy. J Urol 1989; 141: 1341–1346

10. Barr H, Tralau C J, Boulos P B *et al.* The contrasting mechanisms of colonic damage between photodynamic therapy and thermal injury. Photochem Photobiol 1987; 46: 795–800

11. Morgan A R, Garbo G M, Keck R W, Selman S H. New photosensitisers for photodynamic therapy: combined effect of metallopurpurin derivatives and light on transplantable bladder tumours. Cancer Res 1988; 48: 194–198

12. Kelly J F, Snell M E. Hematoporphyrin derivative: a possible aid in the diagnosis and therapy of carcinoma of the bladder. J Urol 1976; 115: 150–151

13. Prout G R, Lin C-W, Benson R. Photodynamic therapy with hematoporphyrin derivative in the treatment of superficial transitional-cell carcinoma of the bladder. N Engl J Med 1987; 317: 1251–1255

14. Hisazumi H, Miyoshi N, Naito K. Whole bladder wall photoradiation therapy for carcinoma in situ of the bladder: a preliminary report. J Urol 1984; 131: 884–887

15. Pope A J, Bown S G. The morphological and functional changes in rat bladder following photodynamic therapy with phthalocyanine photosensitization. J Urol 1991; 145: 1064–1070

16. Chang S C, MacRobert A J, Bown S G. Photodynamic therapy on rat urinary bladder with intravesical instillation of 5-aminolaevulinic acid: light diffusion and histological changes. J Urol 1996; 155: 1749–1753

17. Kriegmair M, Baumgartner R, Lumper W *et al.* Early clinical experience with 5-amino laevulinic acid for photodynamic therapy of superficial bladder cancer. Br J Urol 1996; 77: 667–671

18. Chang S C, MacRobert A J, Bown S G. Interstitial photodynamic therapy of canine prostate with mesotetra-(m-hydroxyphenyl) chlorin. Int J Cancer 1996; 67: 555–562

19. Chang S, Buonaccorsi G, MacRobert A J, Bown S G. Interstitial photodynamic therapy in the canine prostate with disulphonated aluminium phthalocyanine and ALA induced protoporphyrin IX. Prostate (in press)

20. Selman S H, Keck R W. The effect of transurethral light on the canine prostate after sensitization with the photosensitizer tin(II) etiopurpurin dichloride: a pilot study. J Urol 1994; 152: 2129–2132

21. Johnson S, Motamedi M, Egger N *et al.* Photosensitising the canine prostate with ALA: a new laser prostatectomy? J Urol 1995; 153(suppl): 298A (abstr)

22. Star W M, Marijnissen H P, van den Berg-Blok A E *et al.* Destruction of rat mammary tumor and normal tissue microcirculation by haematoporphyrin derivative photoradiation observed in vitro in sandwich observation chambers. Cancer Res 1986; 4: 2532–2540

23. Nyamekye I, Anglin S, McEwan J *et al.* Photodynamic therapy of normal and balloon injured rat carotid arteries using 5-amino laevulinic acid. Circulation 1995; 91: 417–425

24. Grant W E, Buonaccorsi G, Speight P M *et al.* The effect of photodynamic therapy on the mechanical integrity of normal rabbit carotid arteries. Laryngoscope 1995; 105: 867–871

25. Kato H, Kawaguchi M, Konaka C. Evaluation of photodynamic therapy in gastric cancer. Lasers Med Sci 1986; 1: 67–74

26. Pantelides M L, Whitehurst C, Moore J V *et al.* Photodynamic therapy for localized prostatic cancer: light penetration in the human prostate gland. J Urol 1990; 143: 398–401

27. Windahl T, Andersson S O, Lofgren L. Photodynamic therapy of localised prostate cancer. Lancet 1990; 336: 1139

Chapter 35

The biology of matrix metallo-proteinases and the therapeutic potential of synthetic inhibitors

A. H. Drummond

Introduction

The extracellular matrix is essential for the maintenance of organ integrity and function, acting both as a scaffold for organ growth and cell differentiation and as a barrier that prevents inappropriate cell entry or egress. Its importance is underlined by the complexity of the control mechanisms that have evolved to regulate its content and by the debilitating consequences that result from their failure to operate effectively. Under certain physiological conditions, such as during leucocyte trafficking and trophoblast invasion, motile cells are required to penetrate an intact organ. This can occur, however, only if the invasive cell is able to elaborate, or to stimulate resident cells to elaborate, matrix-degrading enzymes that allow it to move readily into the organ. These enzymes must be subject to strict control if organ homeostasis is not to be imbalanced.

One of the hallmarks of a malignant tumour is the ability of the cancerous cells both to invade locally and to be disseminated throughout the body, seeding in distant organs to set up secondary tumours in the process known as metastasis. The properties of these invasive cells are similar to those of their physiological counterparts mentioned above, with at least two exceptions: proliferative control has been lost and their capacity to regulate matrix-degrading enzymes is impaired.

Members of a number of different enzyme classes, including serine, thiol and metalloproteinases, have the ability to degrade the constituents of extracellular matrix.[1,2] In addition, there is evidence from a range of studies suggesting that, for various human cancers, there is a correlation between the activity or expression of such enzymes and the malignant potential of the tumour.[3,4] In recent years, the matrix-degrading metalloproteinases have been increasingly implicated in this respect and the purpose of this brief review is to summarize our understanding of their role in neoplastic disease and to describe the development of specific matrix metalloproteinase inhibitors. Such agents might be expected to reduce the malignant potential of tumours and, taken chronically, to lead to tumour stabilization.

Matrix metalloproteinases and their natural inhibitors

The matrix metalloproteinases (MMPs) are a growing family of Zn^{2+}-dependent enzymes whose original members were characterized by their ability to degrade extracellular matrix substrates such as the collagens, proteoglycans and laminins. Although the vast majority of the enzymes in the current, enlarged, family would still meet this criterion, direct evidence of matrix-degrading activity is lacking for a few of the more recently identified members (see below) and their identification as MMPs is based on sequence homology rather than on knowledge of their natural substrates. Table 35.1 summarizes the current members of the family. At least 16 proteases or putative proteases have been cloned to date, with three new members having been identified during 1996 alone.

A number of obvious subfamilies exist, based on preferred substrates and/or sequence homology. First, there are the three 'collagenases', which have the rare ability to degrade native, triple-helical, collagen (types I, II, III and X) at neutral pH:[5–7] these are fibroblast collagenase (MMP-1), neutrophil collagenase (MMP-8) and collagenase-3 (MMP-13). Other MMPs are unable to cleave collagens in the triple-helical domain. A second subfamily of MMPs comprising stromelysins 1 and 2 (MMP-3 and -10) and matrilysin (MMP-7) can be identified by their predilection for non-fibrillar collagens, laminin and fibronectin.[8–10] Thirdly, there are the two 'gelatinases', or 'type IV collagenases' (MMP-2 and -9), which avidly hydrolyse denatured interstitial collagens or basement membrane collagens such as types IV and V.[11,12] The remaining family members do not fit readily into any of these categories. Some, such as macrophage metalloelastase (MMP-12),[13] are, like matrilysin, potent elastolytic enzymes. Others, such as stromelysin-3 (MMP-11),[14] which is found expressed at high levels in a variety of human tumours, have, unusually, not been found to hydrolyse any matrix protein efficiently but, like many MMPs, have retained the ability to degrade serine protease inhibitors (serpins) such as α_2-antiplasmin.[15] Lastly, there are at least four enzymes in the MMP family that have the distinguishing characteristic of being cell surface molecules that contain a transmembrane domain, the so-called MT-MMPs.[16–19] One of their roles appears to be in the activation of 72 kDa gelatinase but, shorn of their transmembrane domain, these enzymes retain matrix-degrading

Table 35.1. Matrix metalloproteinases

Enzyme	Number	Metalloproteinase substrates (activation)	Other substrates
Interstitial collagenase	MMP-1		Fibrillar collagens, pro-TNFα
Neutrophil collagenase	MMP-8		Fibrillar collagens
Collagenase-3	MMP-13		Fibrillar collagens
Stromelysin-1	MMP-3	pro MMP-1, pro MMP-13, pro MMP-8	Proteoglycans, laminin, non-fibrillar collagens
Stromelysin-2	MMP-10		Proteoglycans, laminin, non-fibrillar collagens
Stromelysin-3	MMP-11		Serpins
	MMP-18		Undefined
Matrilysin	MMP-7		Elastin, fibronectin, laminins, non-fibrillar collagens, pro-TNFα
Metalloelastase	MMP-12		Elastin, non-fibrillar collagens
72 kDa gelatinase	MMP-2	pro MMP-13	Non-fibrillar collagens, fibronectin
92 kDa gelatinase	MMP-9		Non-fibrillar collagens, elastin
MT1-MMP	MMP-14	pro MMP-13, pro MMP-2	Undefined
MT2-MMP	MMP-15		Undefined
MT3-MMP	MMP-16		Undefined
MT4-MMP	MMP-17		Undefined

potential.[20] It is one of the features of the field that only in a relatively small number of cases are the physiological substrates of the MMPs known with any certainty.

As noted above, overactivity of these enzymes is potentially very damaging and, because of this, a number of regulatory processes have evolved to limit the temporal and geographical scope of their actions.

1. At the genetic level, expression of the MMPs is stimulated by pro-inflammatory cytokines such as tumour necrosis factor α (TNFα) and interleukin (IL)-1β and inhibited by anti-inflammatory agents such as transforming growth factor β (TGFβ), glucocorticoids and inhibitory cytokines such as IL-10. Because of this, expression of the enzymes is rarely constitutive but rather reflects a complex balance between host-derived and, in the case of cancer, tumour-derived factors.

2. The enzymes are first synthesized as latent zymogens that require N-terminal propeptide hydrolysis to become active. It is likely that multiple mechanisms exist for proenzyme activation including MMP-dependent activation of other MMP family members. This is perhaps best exemplified by the case of 72 kDa gelatinase (gelatinase A), which is believed to be activated by cell-surface MT1-MMP,[21] but there is considerable potential for cross-activation (see Table 35.1), a point that needs to be borne in mind when selective MMP inhibitors are being designed.

3. Proteolytically active MMPs can be inhibited by general proteinase inhibitors such as α_2-macroglobulin, found in stoichiometric excess in plasma. In addition, matrix contains, and cells produce, tissue inhibitors of metalloproteinases, TIMPs 1–4.[22–25] These high-affinity inhibitors are believed to play a major role in the pericellular control of MMP activity.

Further detail on the biochemistry and molecular biology of MMPs is to be found in a recent review.[26]

Matrix metalloproteinases: the link to cancer

There is now a very substantial body of evidence citing a role for a range of different matrix metalloproteinases in the local invasion, metastasis and angiogenesis that are associated with tumour progression.[27] These data derive from studies in cancer tissue conducted using a range of techniques that are immunological, biochemical and molecular biological in origin. Because of the complexity of MMP expression and activation and the consequent presence in tissue samples of enzyme–inhibitor complexes in addition to proenzyme and active enzyme, most of the techniques reveal merely that there is increased expression of MMPs in cancer versus normal tissue.

Taking the broad view across a range of human cancers, it is evident that overexpression of MMPs is correlated with a malignant phenotype. In some cases, a correlation has been reported between expression of an MMP and either prognosis or tumour staging,[28,29] but this is not a universal finding, perhaps because our ability to detect reliably the levels of active MMP in a tissue or extract is limited. Indeed, the availability of such a method remains an eagerly sought goal for the future. The ability to select patients that are expressing high levels of active MMPs and who may, as a consequence, have a poor prognosis would simplify and shorten immeasurably the clinical trials required to prove efficacy of an anti-MMP approach in slow-growing cancers such as heart and prostate.

In the case of human prostate cancer, it is evident that both 72 kDa and 92 kDa gelatinases are expressed at high levels in malignant human tissue but are absent in normal prostatic stromal tissue.[30,31] A much higher proportion of patients with skeletal metastasis (64%) showed expression of 92 kDa gelatinase than those with a negative bone scan (17%), emphasizing the potential link with a metastatic phenotype.[30] In patients with benign prostatic hypertrophy, levels of both gelatinases are either undetectable or very low.[30,31] Other MMPs, such as matrilysin, are also known to be expressed in human prostate cancer and, indeed, transfection of the gene for matrilysin into the tumorigenic but non-metastatic human prostatic carcinoma cell line DU-145 leads to the acquisition of invasive behaviour.[32]

In almost all cases in which investigators have probed for the presence of multiple MMPs, this has been confirmed;[27] however, it is unclear whether all contribute to the pathogenesis. In all likelihood, only studies with selective MMP inhibitors will answer this question definitively.

Matrix metalloproteinase inhibitors

From a pharmaceutical perspective, the desire to design specific matrix metalloproteinase inhibitors (MMPIs) predates the body of data linking MMPs and cancer; the initial drive to identify such compounds stemmed from a belief, still unproven in man, that overzealous MMP activity contributes to the joint destruction seen in the arthritides.[33] Nevertheless, as the cancer data on MMPs became ever more compelling, pharmaceutical companies were quick to switch their clinical focus to cancer and it is in this area of therapeutics that the class of inhibitors is now most advanced in clinical evaluation.

The basic design strategy of MMPIs derives from the work that led to the synthesis of specific angiotensin-coverting enzyme (ACE) inhibitors (see Figure 35.1 and for review, ref. 34). This requires a knowledge of the site on MMP substrates that is cleaved by the MMP. The appropriate stereochemistry and amino acid side-chain surrogates in a pseudopeptide containing a strong Zn^{2+}-binding group (often a hydroxamic acid) leads to the identification of specific MMP inhibitors that are inactive against unrelated Zn^{2+} metalloenzymes such as ACE or enkephalinase (illustrated in Figure 35.1 for batimastat).

Batimastat (BB-94) was the first MMPI to be widely profiled for its effectiveness in altering cancer growth in animals.[35] It is a broad-spectrum MMPI which, when administered to rodents by the intraperitoneal (i.p.) route, generates sustained but relatively modest levels in blood (50–100 ng/ml). These levels were, however, adequate to demonstrate not just an antimetastatic effect of batimastat (which might have been predicted from earlier work with the related compound, SC44463[36] but also a strong effect on local tumour growth. It was these latter, striking effects that raised the possibility that an MMPI might be useful not just in blocking metastasis (which would be predicted to have already occurred in the majority of cancer patients at initial presentation) but as cytostatic agents. A good example of the anticancer efficacy of batimastat is provided by the work done on a rat mammary carcinoma line, where the drug was shown to reduce both the haematogenous spread of tumour cells and the growth of secondaries.[37] While lymphatic dissemination was unaffected by the MMPI (there being no matrix barrier between the lymphatic vessel and tissue stroma), subsequent growth in lymphoid tissue was markedly impaired. The work also demonstrated that chronic treatment with batimastat was necessary for a full anticancer effect. Data of a similar, if less striking, nature have been reported with batimastat in a range of human tumours grown in nude mice (data not shown).

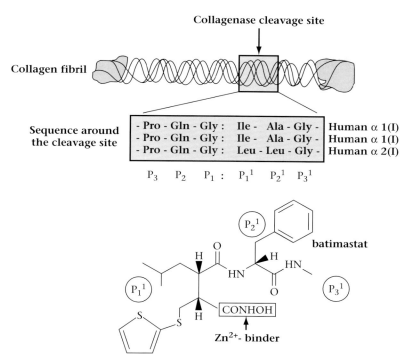

Figure 35.1. Design of matrix metalloproteinase inhibitors.

The mechanism underlying the apparent cytostatic effect of MMPIs such as batimastat remains to be fully resolved. Batimastat is an anti-angiogenic agent when administered directly into tissue undergoing angiogenesis, but is less effective when given systemically.[38] Of some note is the fact that wound healing appears unimpaired in MMPI studies conducted to date. Since angiogenesis is a major component of wound healing, this result would be somewhat surprising if the compound were powerfully anti-angiogenic. It remains possible, however, that tumour angiogenesis is more dependent on MMPs than stromal angiogenesis (where plasmin appears to play a major role). A more likely explanation for the cytostatic effect of batimastat is that it enhances the body's natural fibrotic reaction to a growing tumour. Histological data from a variety of xenograft studies with batimastat indicate a marked build-up of stromal material around growing tumours in the drug-treated animals (data not shown). This is often accompanied by evidence of enhanced necrosis at the centre of the tumour. Further work is necessary to determine if the cytostatic effects of batimastat *in vivo* can be generalized to a single mechanism or whether the mode of action is dependent on the phenotype of the particular tumour.

A number of recent studies indicate that MMP inhibitors may be more effective in combination with established cytotoxic agents. Batimastat and cisplatin were more effective in prolonging survival when administered together in a human ovarian carcinoma model than when given separately (R. Giavazzi, personal communication). Similarly, another synthetic inhibitor, CT1746, enhanced the effect of cyclophosphamide in the murine Lewis lung carcinoma.[39] Other studies using newer agents confirm these general findings, although it remains unclear whether this additivity or synergy between MMPIs and cytotoxic agents in reducing tumour burden can be generalized across all tumour types and across all cytotoxic regimens.

The major outstanding question for pharmaceutical researchers is whether broad-spectrum or selective MMPIs are preferred as anticancer agents. This is currently unresolved but most human tumours *in situ* are associated with the presence of multiple MMP enzymes. Since, in addition, there is considerable substrate overlap between different members of the MMP family, at least *in vitro*, a broad-spectrum MMPI is a sensible starting option. For many years, the major issue has been to obtain orally bioavailable MMPIs of any type, rather than to drive forward the debate regarding selective versus broad-spectrum compounds. The latter consideration is, however, now extremely pertinent since at least one broad-spectrum inhibitor, marimastat (see below), is in phase III clinical trials.

Although both batimastat (BB-94) and a distantly related hydroxamate derivative, GM 6001, reached the clinic (in cancer patients and for corneal damage, respectively), it is marimastat (BB-2516), the first orally active MMPI to enter the clinic,[40] that is now the focus of most attention in this class of agents. Marimastat is rapidly degraded in rodents and, as a consequence, is difficult to study by the oral route in conventional animal cancer models. In human volunteers, however, levels of marimastat in the blood following oral administration are high[40] and it is evident that these are sufficient to test the thesis that an anti-MMP approach will be of value in cancer patients. Further phase II studies in a range of human cancers, including prostate cancer, examined the effect of oral marimastat on the rate of rise of serum cancer antigens (CA-125, CEA, PSA and CA 19-9) over time. Since there was a dose-related fall in the rate of rise of these surrogates of tumour growth over the 28-day period of dosing,[41-43] there was encouragement to proceed to definitive phase III studies in a number of cancer types. Moreover, in gastric cancer, where cancer antigens cannot in general be followed but where biopsies can be readily obtained using a gastroscope, marimastat treatment was associated with fibrotic changes in the tumour that were reminiscent of the animal results referred to above.[44] A number of the patients in this trial appeared to benefit from the drug.

Observation in patients who have received marimastat for lengthy periods are that, in general, the drug is well tolerated. Musculoskeletal pain has been noted after 2–6 months treatment in a proportion of the patients.[44] This appears to be drug related, in that its incidence is dose dependent, but the adverse effects were considered manageable at the dose selected for definitive phase III studies. The musculoskeletal pain resolves rapidly on discontinuation of therapy and treatment can be recommended after a 2–3-week drug-free period. It is currently unclear if this side effect results from the pharmacological mechanism of action of the drug, but this seems likely. As noted above, it will be important to determine whether this is, indeed, the case and whether more selective MMPI compounds can be identified that do not have the propensity to induce the effect. If so, the crucial question will be to determine whether these second-generation oral MMPIs retain the powerful anticancer effects seen with batimastat, marimastat and other broad-spectrum MMPIs.

Conclusions

Novel strategies for anticancer treatment are urgently required, since conventional cytotoxic approaches have proved of limited value in the treatment of the majority of solid tumours. That MMPs are widely overexpressed in human malignant tumours is no longer in question. In addition, the anticancer effects of drugs specifically targeted at matrix metalloproteinases are now well established in animal models. The challenge remaining is to reproduce these effects in the real world of human cancer and, if successful, to determine the best way of combining this novel cytostatic type of therapy with conventional cytoreductive treatments.

References

1. Mignatti P, Tsuboi R, Robbins E, Rifkin D B. In vitro angiogenesis on the human amniotic membrane: requirements for basic fibroblast growth factor-induced proteinases. J Cell Biol 1989; 108: 671–682
2. Mikkelsen T, Yan P S, Ho K L et al. Immunolocalisation of cathepsin B in human glioma—implications for tumour invasion and angiogenesis. J Neurosurg 1995; 83: 285–290
3. Stetler-Stevenson W G, Aznavoorian S, Liotta L A. Tumour cell interactions with the extracellular matrix during invasion and metastasis. Annu Rev Cell Biol 1993; 9: 541–573
4. Sivaparvathi M, Yamamoto M, Nicolson G L et al. Expression and immunohistochemical localisation of cathepsin L during the progression of human gliomas. Clin Exp Metastasis 1996; 14: 27–34
5. Wilhelm S C, Eisen A Z, Teter M et al. Human fibroblast collagenase: glycosylation and tissue-specific levels of enzyme synthesis. Proc Natl Acad Sci USA 1986; 83: 3756–3760
6. Hasty K A, Pourmotabbed T F, Goldberg G I et al. Human neutrophil collagenase: a distinct gene product with homology to other matrix metalloproteinases. J Biol Chem 1990; 265: 11421–11424
7. Freije J M, Biez-Itza I, Balbin M et al. Molecular cloning and expression of collagenase-3, a novel human matrix metalloproteinase produced by breast carcinomas. J Biol Chem 1994; 269: 16766–16773
8. Wilhelm S M, Collier I E, Kronberger A et al. Human skin fibroblast stromelysin: structure, glycosylation, substrate specificity and differential expression in normal and tumorigenic cells. Proc Natl Acad Sci USA 1987; 84: 6725–6729
9. Muller D, Quantin B, Gesnel M C et al. The collagenase gene family consists of at least four members. Biochem J 1988; 253: 187–192
10. Quantin B, Murphy G, Breathnach R. Pump-1 cDNA codes for a protein with characteristics similar to those of classical collagenase family members. Biochemistry 1989; 28: 5325–5334
11. Collier I E, Wilhelm S M, Elzen A Z et al. H-ras oncogene-transformed human bronchial epithelial cells (TBE-1) secrete a single metalloproteinase capable of degrading basement membrane collagen. J Biol Chem 1988; 263: 6579–6587
12. Wilhelm S M, Collier I E, Marmer B L et al. SV-40-transformed human lung fibroblasts secrete a 92-kDa Type IV collagenase which is identical to that secreted by normal human macrophages. J Biol Chem 1989; 264: 17213–17221
13. Shapiro D S, Kobayashi D K, Ley T J. Cloning and characterisation of a unique elastolytic metalloproteinase produced by human alveolar macrophages. J Biol Chem 1993; 268: 23824–23829
14. Basset P, Bellocq J P, Wolf C et al. A novel metalloproteinase gene specifically expressed in stromal cell of breast carcinomas. Nature 1990; 348: 699–704
15. Pei D, Majmudar G, Weiss S J. Hydrolytic inactivation of a breast carcinoma cell-derived serpin by human stromelysin-3. J Biol Chem 1994; 269: 25849–25855
16. Sato H, Takino T, Okada Y et al. A matrix metalloproteinase expressed on the surface of invasive tumour cells. Nature 1994; 370: 61–65
17. Will H, Hinzmann B. cDNA sequence and mRNA tissue distribution of a novel human matrix metalloproteinase with a potential transmembrane segment. Eur J Biochem 1995; 231: 602–608
18. Takino T, Sato H, Shinagawa A, Seiki M. Identification of the second membrane-type matrix metalloproteinase (MT-MMP2) gene from a human placenta cDNA library. MT-MMPs form a unique membrane-type subclass in the MMP family. J Biol Chem 1995; 270: 23013–23020
19. Puente X S, Pendas A M, Llano E et al. Molecular cloning of a novel membrane-type matrix metalloproteinase from a human breast carcinoma. Cancer Res 1996; 56: 944–949
20. Ohuchi E, Imai K, Fujii Y et al. Membrane type 1 matrix metalloproteinase digests interstitial collagens and other extracellular matrix macromolecules. J Biol Chem 1997; 272: 2446–2451
21. Strongin A, Collier I, Bannikov G et al. Mechanism of cell surface activation of 72kDa type IV collagenase. J Biol Chem 1995; 270: 5331–5338

22. Docherty A J P, Lyons A, Smith B J *et al.* Sequence of human tissue inhibitor of metalloproteinases and its identity to erythroid-potentiating activity. Nature 1985; 318: 66–69

23. Stetler-Stevenson W G, Krutzsch H C, Liotta L A. Tissue inhibitor of metalloproteinase (TIMP-2). A new member of the metalloproteinase inhibitor family. J Biol Chem 1989; 264: 17374–17378

24. Apte S S, Mattei M G, Olsen B R. Cloning of the cDNA encoding human tissue inhibitor of metalloproteinases-3 (TIMP-3) and the mapping of the TIMP-3 gene to chromosome 22. Genomics 1994; 19: 86–90

25. Greene J, Wang M S, Lui Y L E *et al.* Molecular cloning and characterisation of human tissue inhibitor of metalloproteinase 4. J Biol Chem 1996; 271: 30375–30380.

26. Kleiner D J, Stetler-Stevenson W G. Structural biochemistry and activation of matrix metalloproteinases. Curr Opin Cell Biol 1993; 5: 891–897

27. Stetler-Stevenson W G, Hewitt R, Corcoran M. Matrix metalloproteinases and tumour invasion: from correlation and casualty to the clinic. Semin Cancer Biol 1996; 7: 147–154

28. Murray G I, Duncan M E, O'Neil P *et al.* Matrix metalloproteinase-1 is associated with poor prognosis in colorectal cancer. Nature Med 2: 461–462

29. Van der Stappen J W J, Hendriks T, Wobbes T. Correlation between collagenolytic activity and grade of histological differentiation in colorectal tumours. Int J Cancer 1990; 45: 1071–1078

30. Hamdy F C, Fadlon E J, Cottam D *et al.* Matrix metalloproteinase-9 expression in primary human prostatic adenocarcinoma and benign prostatic hyperplasia. Br J Cancer 1994; 69: 177–182

31. Stearns M E, Wang M. Type IV collagenase (M(r) 72,000) expression in human prostate: benign and malignant tissue. Cancer Res 1993; 53: 878–883

32. Powell W C, Knox J D, Navre M *et al.* Expression of the metalloproteinase matrilysin in DU-145 cells increases their invasive potential in severe combined immunodeficient mice. Cancer Res 1993; 53: 417–422

33. McCachren S S. Expression of metalloproteinases and metalloproteinase inhibitor in human arthritic synovium. Arthritis Rheum 1991; 34: 1085–1093

34. Beckett R P, Davidson A H, Drummond A H *et al.* Recent advances in matrix metalloproteinase inhibitor research. Drug Dev Today 1996; 1: 16–26

35. Davies B, Brown P D, East N *et al.* A synthetic matrix metalloproteinase inhibitor decreases tumour burden and prolongs survival of mice bearing human ovarian cancer xenografts. Cancer Res 1993; 53: 2087–2091

36. Axelrod J H, Reich R, Miskin R. Expression of human recombinant plasminogen activators enhances invasion and experimental metastasis of H-ras-transformed NIH-3T3 cells. Mol Cell Biol 1989; 9: 2133–2141

37. Eccles S A, Box G M, Court W J *et al.* Control of lymphatic and haematogenous metastasis of a rat mammary carcinoma by the matrix metalloproteinase inhibitor batimastat (BB-94). Cancer Res 1996; 56: 2815–2822

38. Taraboletti G, Garofalo A, Belotti D *et al.* Inhibition of angiogenesis and murine haemangioma growth by batimastat, a synthetic inhibitor of matrix metalloproteinases. J Natl Cancer Inst 1995; 87: 293–298

39. Anderson I C, Shipp M A, Docherty A J P, Teicher B A. Combination therapy including a gelatinase inhibitor and cytotoxic agent reduces local invasion and metastasis of murine Lewis lung carcinoma. Cancer Res 1996; 56: 705–710

40. Drummond A H, Beckett P, Bone E A *et al.* BB-2516: an orally bioavailable matrix metalloproteinase inhibitor with efficacy in animal cancer models. Proc Am Assoc Cancer Res 1995; 36: 100

41. Primrose J, Bleiberg H, Daniel F *et al.* A dose-finding study of marimastat, an oral matrix metalloproteinase inhibitor, in patients with advanced colorectal cancer. Ann Oncol 1996; 7: 35

42. Poole C, Adams M, Barley V *et al.* A dose-finding study of marimastat, an oral matrix metalloproteinase inhibitor, in patients with advanced ovarian cancer. Ann Oncol 1996; 7: 68

43. Millar A, Brown P D. 360 patient meta-analysis of studies of marimastat, a novel matrix metalloproteinase inhibitor. Ann Oncol 1996; 7: 123

44. Parsons S L, Watson S A, Griffin N R, Steele R J C. An open phase I'II study of the oral matrix metalloproteinase inhibitor marimastat in patients with inoperable gastric cancer. Ann Oncol 1996; 7: 47

Chapter 36
Prostate cancer in the Middle East: a perspective from Oman

E. O. Kehinde

Introduction

In the Sultanate of Oman, medical services were very rudimentary until 1970. Before 1970 there was one doctor and one 23-bed hospital serving a population of about 700,000 people scattered over a radius of 1000 km (D. Bosch, personal communication, 1996). However, between 1970 and 1996, the Sultanate was transformed from a near-medieval country to a modern and successful welfare state. The rest of the Middle East has witnessed changes in the past 25 years similar to those in Oman. Two factors combined to set Oman on the road to rapid modernization, namely a high per capita income that resulted from the oil boom of the 1970s and a new purposeful leader from 1970 onwards. However, such rapid modernization and its accompanying urbanization and westernization have also been associated with changes in the pattern of diseases in the Sultanate.

Very little was known about the incidence of various cancers in Oman until about 1990, when a national cancer registry was established. The establishment of the register has revealed that, as with most developing countries, the major causes of morbidity and mortality in the Sultanate remain infectious and parasitic diseases, cardiovascular disorders, diabetes, and natal and perinatal catastrophes[1] (D. Bosch, personal communication, 1996). Furthermore, the true pattern of cancer in 'modern' Oman is now beginning to emerge. Even though the collection of serious data on cancers in Oman is at an early stage (1990–1995), certain trends are noticeable. All data discussed in this chapter relate to Omanis only and exclude cancer occurring in expatriates working in Oman. The total population of Oman according to the 1993 census is about 2.01 million, over 530,000 of whom (26.5%) are expatriates (Table 36.1).

Table 36.1. Composition of the population of Omani males in 1993

Age group (years)	Males (n)	Percentage
0–4	130,207	17.2
5–14	259,222	34.3
15–49	293,821	38.9
50–65	49,495	6.6
Over 65	22,365	3.0
Total	755,110	100

90.4% of Omani males are relatively young, i.e. under 50 years of age.
Total Omani female population in 1993 = 728,116; total Omani male and female population in 1993 = 1,483,226; total population of male and female expatriates in 1993 = 534,848 (i.e. 26.5% of the total national population of 2,018,074).
(From 1993 Census of Population, Ministry of National Planning, Muscat, Oman.)

As with other developing countries, a large proportion of the population of Oman is young (Table 36.1). Since young age groups have a low incidence of malignancies of epithelial origin[2] and a higher incidence of malignancies of non-epithelial origin, such as solid tumours (for example lymphomas and sarcomas), these factors, coupled with improved health care and an ageing population, will lead to an increase in the incidence, as well as a change in the pattern, of malignancies in Oman in the near future. Such a trend has been observed in the neighbouring Arabian Gulf state of Saudi Arabia.[1,3] Consequently, the data in this chapter may need revising in a few years' time.

Descriptive epidemiology of prostate cancer in Oman

Incidence of prostate cancer

The incidence of prostate cancer in Oman was 3.3/100,000 male population/year between 1991 and 1995, compared with 34 and 78/100,000 male population/year for the United Kingdom and the United States of America, respectively, in 1990.[4] This low incidence is in agreement with low figures for other countries in the Middle East (e.g. Kuwait, 5.1/100,000 male population in 1987; Israel, 17.5/100,000 male population in 1982–1986;[5] Saudi Arabia[1]). The low incidence in Oman may be partly due to the fact that 90.4% of the population are below the age of 50 years; thus only 9.6% are above 50 years of age, the group in which one would expect a very high incidence of prostate cancer (Table 36.1).

Increasing longevity (life expectancy was 47 years in 1970 whereas it was 69 years in 1993) may cause the incidence of prostate cancer to rise beyond the current levels in Oman in the near future. Even then, by the year 2025, when 50% of the population of Omani males are expected to be more than 50 years old, the projected incidence of prostate cancer will still be low, at approximately 13.2/100,000 male population/year.

It is interesting to note that, even though prostate cancer is not among the first 10 common cancers in Oman (Figure 36.1), breast cancer, another common 'Western' cancer, is the fourth commonest cancer in Omanis and the commonest

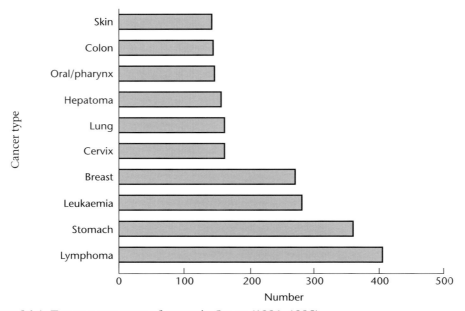

Figure 36.1. Ten common types of cancer in Oman (1991–1995).

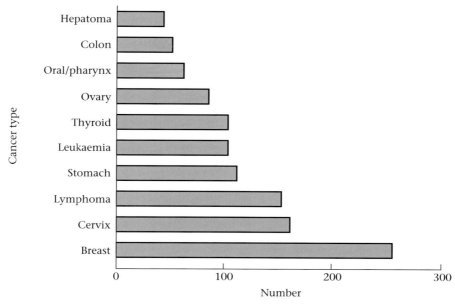

Figure 36.2. Ten common types of cancer in females in Oman (1991–1995).

cancer in Omani females (Figure 36.2). It is intriguing that common aetiological factors in relation to breast cancer, such as nulliparity, low breast-feeding habit, and late age of first pregnancy, are not encountered routinely in the Omani female population.

However, prostate cancer is the fourth commonest cancer in Omani males (Figure 36.3). The prostate is also the fourth commonest site for cancer incidence all over the world after the lung, stomach, colon and rectum.[6] Prostate cancer is the commonest genitourinary tumour in Oman (Table 36.2).

The distribution of prostate cancer by age in Omani men is shown in Figure 36.4. The median age of presentation of prostate cancer is about 66 years, which is

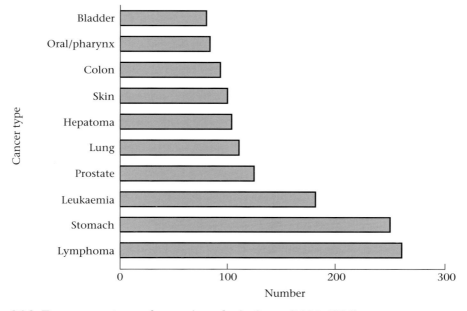

Figure 36.3. Ten common types of cancer in males in Oman (1991–1995).

Table 36.2. Distribution of genitourinary tract tumours in Oman*, 1991–1995

Cancer	No. of cases	Percentage
Prostate	124	41.5
Bladder	106	35.5
Renal[†]	48	16.0
Testicular	19	6.4
Ureteric	1	0.3
Penile[‡]	1	0.3
Total	299	100

*Analysis excludes all expatriates working in Oman.
[†]Consisting of renal cell cancer and transitional cell cancer.
[‡]Circumcision of the male child before 28 days of age is practised in Oman.

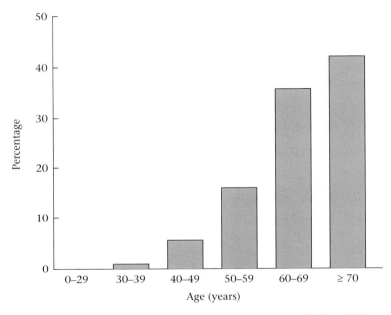

Figure 36.4. Distribution of prostate cancer in Omani men by age (1991–1995).

similar to data from Saudi Arabia[1] and most of Europe and the USA, but a decade earlier in Africans.[7] There has been a 2.5- to three-fold increase in the incidence of prostate cancer in Oman between 1991 and 1995, and this trend, for the reasons stated above, looks set to continue (Figure 36.5).

Late presentation is a feature of prostate cancer in Oman, as about 70% of patients present with stages C and D, only 30% presenting with stages A and B disease. Consequently, commonly employed methods of treatment include orchiectomy, total androgen blockade and other methods of hormone manipulation.

Mortality rate

The rate of mortality from prostate cancer is very difficult to assess in Oman at present as data collection is very rudimentary. Most deaths are not reported at present. It is hoped that the efforts of the national cancer registry will shed light on this important aspect of the descriptive epidemiology of prostate cancer in Oman in the near future.

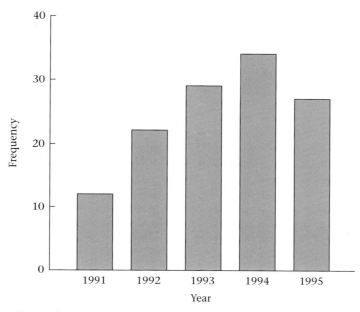

Figure 36.5. Incidence of prostate cancer in Oman (1991–1995).

Prostate cancer screening in Oman

Largely owing to the effect of global communications, a few educated Omanis in their early 50s are requesting prostate cancer screening. Otherwise, prostate cancer screening has not been given any prominence by the Ministry of Health. As in most developed countries, attention has been focused on breast cancer screening in Oman. Considering the statistically significant differences in incidence between the diseases in Oman, unlike the rest of the world, this policy is probably justified.

No geographically discernible differences exist in the incidence of prostate cancer in Oman.

Aetiology of prostate cancer: the Oman experience

It is pertinent at this stage to try to find out why the incidence of prostate cancer is relatively low in Oman. The answer to this question may provide useful clues to preventing the disease in those parts of the world where the disease is assuming epidemic proportions in elderly men. The established risk factors for prostate cancer include, among others, age, family history and ethnic group/country of residence.

The age factor

As stated before, more than 90% of male Omans are under 50 years of age and thus comprise a low-risk age group. The current incidence rate for prostate cancer of 3.3/100,000 male population is probably going to rise exponentially over the next 20–30 years when those currently in the fourth and fifth decades of life enter their seventh and eighth decades, during which prostate cancer is very common. Nevertheless, prostate cancer can occur in younger men; the author currently has in his care a 40-year-old Omani with stage C prostate cancer.

As stated before, by the year 2025 the incidence of prostate cancer in Oman will be about 13.2/100,000 male population. Life expectancy in 2025 is projected to be about 71 years, which does not differ significantly from the current life expectancy of 69 years.

Table 36.3. Incidence of prostate cancer in Oman 1991–1995 compared with other parts of the world (1993)

Country	Incidence/100,000 male population/year	Life expectancy (years)
USA	78.1	76
Switzerland	50.9	78
United Kingdom	34	75
France	29.9	77
Russia	13.9	66
Romania	9.9	70
Japan	7.5	79
Oman	3.3	69
China	1.2	70

Oman has one of the lowest incidence rates for prostate cancer in the world.
Life expectancy in Oman in 1996 is not dissimilar to that in developed countries.

As shown in Table 36.3, even after correcting for differences in life expectancy, Oman has (and probably will continue to have) a low incidence of prostate cancer compared with the very affluent or developed countries such as the USA, Switzerland and the UK. This may indicate an inherent protective factor in Arabs against the development of prostate cancer.

Family history
Personal communications with other urologists in the Sultanate have confirmed four cases of familial prostate cancer. These cases have been in families with well-educated members. A 45-year-old member of one such family has a current prostate-specific antigen (PSA) level of 6.5 ng/ml and he is under investigation to exclude early prostate cancer. Fortunately, the literacy rate in Oman is 60% at present and is set to continue to rise. With better education and increased awareness of prostate cancer it will be interesting to see whether the Western trend of familial prostate cancer will be replicated in Oman.

Ethnic group/country of residence
That Africans living in the USA have a 10- to 20-fold increase in incidence of prostate cancer over that of their counterparts living in West Africa is well known, indicating that environmental factors may play a significant role in the causation of this disease. In the Omani case, the population is actually heterogeneous, made up of indigenous, light-complexioned or coloured Omanis, and Omanis of East African descent who are black. Even though the numbers are small, preliminary data have shown that the incidence of prostate cancer is higher (ratio 3:2) in the African Omanis compared with the Arab Omanis. It is pertinent to note that the two groups have identical patterns of behaviour; they also share a common dietary habit. This again confirms the important role of genetic make-up in the aetiology of the disease[8].

Dietary habit
There is now sufficient evidence to suggest that the 'Western' diet, rich in protein and animal fat but low in fibre, is contributing substantially to the rising incidence of prostate cancer in most developed countries.[8] Similarly, obesity, a by-product of the Western style of living, has been shown to be a relative risk for the development of prostate cancer.[8–10]

Until recently, the Arabian diet consisted of high levels of fibre and low levels of animal fat and protein.[11] The picture has changed, owing to the abrupt rise in purchasing power and is similar to that in the West. Thus the typical Arab in most of the oil-rich Arabian Gulf States now consumes diets rich in animal fat and protein (currently 200–300 g red meat per day in Oman) and low in vegetables[1,11] (K. Dennison and D. Ashfour, 1996, personal communications). This change in dietary habits may contribute in part to the rising incidence of prostate cancer in Oman. It is also pertinent to note that the sight of an obese Arab is a rarity in the older generation of Arabs, that is, the age group with a low incidence of prostate cancer.[12] Unfortunately, today there is evidence of an increased incidence of diseases secondary to obesity, such as hypertension and diabetes mellitus, in very young Arabs.[3,12] It is possible, therefore, that lighter body weight, especially in old age, which has been observed among Arabs for a long time, may have a protective effect against the development of prostate cancer. This has been one of the reasons adduced for the low incidence and rate of mortality of prostate cancer among the Japanese.[13–16]

Sexual behaviour

There is evidence to suggest that increased risk for prostate cancer is associated with high levels of sexual activity and/or a history of sexually transmitted disease (STD) and vasectomy.[8] Unfortunately, because Oman is a strict Islamic country, sexual behavioural patterns are very difficult to determine. However, unlike in the West, where monogamy is the rule, Islam allows men to marry up to four wives. Whether this tenet of Islam helps to reduce sexual promiscuity is difficult to judge. In the more liberal Arab/Islamic countries there is no doubt that STD is more prevalent than in a conservative Islamic country such as Oman. Again from personal observations, this trend is changing, judging by the number of men presenting for treatment of STD in the Urology Outpatients Department. A typical Omani man wants to remain virile for as long as possible; vasectomy (which is erroneously assumed to be associated with decreased libido) is therefore not an accepted method of contraception among Omanis.

Conclusions

Study of the incidence and distribution of cancer in certain populations helps to identify possible causes that might be taken into account in devising preventive tools. All factors considered, the incidence of prostate cancer is very low in Oman, as in the rest of the Middle East. Possible explanations for the low incidence include a predominantly young population, a lower consumption of Western-type diets and possible genetic make-up.

Unfortunately the incidence may be set to rise, owing largely to the adoption of a Western style of living as the result of oil-derived wealth, improved health care and increasing longevity.

Acknowledgements

The author received invaluable help from many colleagues and government bodies in Oman while preparing this paper. He wishes to express his gratitude to all of them and especially to the following: Drs Ali Jafer Mohammed and Matthew M. Koshy of Non-Communicable Disease Section, Directorate General of Health Affairs, Ministry of Health, Oman; Dr Donald Bosch, the first doctor to set up medical practice in Oman as far back as 1954; Drs Salim bin Said Al-Busaidy and

Quassim Al-Busaidy, Senior Consultant Urologists, Ministry of Health, Muscat, Oman; Deena Ashfour, Head of Nutrition Division, Ministry of Health and Kay Dennison, Head of Nutrition Unit, Sultan Qaboos University Hospital. Professor A.S. Daar, Department of Surgery, Sultan Qaboos University, Muscat, Oman, provided valuable guidance and criticism on aspects involving ethical issues in this paper.

References

1. Koriech O M, Al Kuhaymi R. Profile of cancer in Riyadh Armed Forces. Ann of Saudi Med 1994, 14 (3): 187–194
2. La Vecchia C, Negri E, Decarli A, Cislaghi C. Cancer mortality in Italy: an overview of age specific and age standardized trends from 1955 to 1984. Tumori 1990; 76: 87–166
3. Sebai Z A. Cancer in Saudi Arabia. Ann Saudi Med 1989; 9: 55–63
4. Debre B, Gerard M, Flaw T et al. Epidemiology of prostate cancer. J Int Med Res 1990; 18(1): 3–7
5. Brenner H J, Rath P, Tichler T, Nussbaum B. The geography of prostate cancer and its treatment in Israel. In: Oliver R T D, Belldegrun A, Wrigley P F M (eds) Preventing prostate cancer: screening versus chemoprevention. New York: Cold Spring Harbor Laboratory Press 1995: 287–288
6. Parkin D M, Pisani P, Ferlay J. Estimates of the world wide incidence of eighteen major cancers in 1985. Int J Cancer 1993; 54: 594–606
7. Kehinde E O. The geography of prostate cancer and its treatment in Africa. In: Oliver R T D, Belldegrun A, Wrigley P F M (eds) Preventing prostate cancer: screening versus chemoprevention. New York: Cold Spring Harbor Laboratory Press 1995: 281–286
8. Key T. Risk factors for prostate cancer. In: Oliver R T D, Belldegrun A, Wrigley P F M (eds) Preventing prostate cancer: screening versus chemoprevention. New York: Cold Spring Harbor Laboratory Press 1995: 63–77
9. Hayes R B, de Jong F H, Roatgever J et al. Physical characteristics and factors related to sexual development and behaviour and the risk for prostate cancer. Eur J Cancer Prev 1992; 239–245
10. Le Marchand L, Kolonel L N, Wilkens L R et al. Animal fat consumption and prostate cancer: a prospective study in Hawaii. Epidemiology 1994; 5: 276–282
11. Madami K A. Food consumption patterns in Saudi Arabia. In: Musaiger A O, Milach S S (eds) Food consumption patterns and dietary habits in the Arab countries of the Gulf. Cairo: FAO Regional Office for the Near East, 1995: 50–57
12. Al-Shorshan A A. The affluent diet and its consequences: Saudi Arabia — a case in point. World Rev Nutr Diet 1992; 69: 113–165
13. Muir C, Waterhouse J, Mack T et al., (eds). Cancer Incidence in Five Continents. Volume V. IARC Scientific Publication 88, pp 1–20. Lyon: International Agency for Research on Cancer, 1987
14. Pike M C, Krailo M D, Henderson B E et al. Hormonal risk factors, breast tissue age and age incidence of breast cancer. Nature 1983; 303: 767–770
15. Levi F, Lucchini F, La Vecchia C. World wide patterns of cancer mortality. 1985–1989. Eur J Cancer Prev 1994; 3: 109–143
16. La Vecchia C. Epidemiologa del carcinoma della prostata. In: Il Dolore in oncologia: focus sul carcinoma prostatico. Turin: Centro Scientifico Editore, 1994: 87–103

Chapter 37

Health-related quality-of-life in men with prostate cancer: methodological considerations and practical applications

M. S. Litwin and D. F. Penson

Introduction

The traditional goal in the treatment of genitourinary cancer has been to maximize patient survival. However, recent advances in urologic oncology have had a positive impact on prognosis, allowing many patients to live significantly longer with their disease. When critically evaluating interventions in these patients, researchers have typically examined disease-free survival and clinical parameters that focus on disease progression. However, since cancer affects both quantity and quality-of-life, the various components of well-being must also be addressed when treating individual patients with cancer and when conducting cancer clinical trials.[1] Recently, there has been a greater interest in more refined endpoints of treatment than 5- or 10-year survival rates, complete or partial responses, or serum tumour markers. One such endpoint is health-related quality-of-life (HRQOL).

HRQOL is one of several variables commonly studied in the field of medical outcomes research. HRQOL encompasses a wide range of human experience, including the daily necessities of life, individual responses to illness, and activities associated with professional fulfilment and personal happiness.[2] Most importantly, HRQOL involves patients' perceptions of their own health and ability to function in life.

HRQOL is often confused with functional status. Although functional status is one important dimension of HRQOL, it is joined by other aspects of HRQOL such as role function, mental health, vitality, and psychosocial interactions. HRQOL also encompasses the overall sense of satisfaction that an individual experiences in life. Despite the commonly held belief that this type of data cannot be collected in large multicentre trials, patients' compliance with HRQOL questionnaires is usually high.[3]

HRQOL instruments

Whereas quantity of life is relatively easy to assess as survival or progression-free interval, the measurement of quality of life presents more challenges, primarily because it is less familiar to most clinicians.[4] To quantify these qualitative phenomena, the principles of psychometric test theory are applied. This discipline provides the theoretical underpinnings for the science of survey research. Data are collected with HRQOL surveys, called instruments. Instruments typically contain questions, or items, that are organized into scales. Each scale measures a different aspect, or domain, of HRQOL. Some scales comprise dozens of items, whereas others may include only one or two items. Each item contains a stem (which may be a question or a statement) and a response set. A *categorical response set* includes several choices that are mutually exclusive and collectively exhaustive. A *Likert response set* typically includes five levels of agreement or disagreement with the stem. A *visual analogue-response set* is a straight line anchored at each end by words or phrases that represent the range of a given health variable. Patients mark a slash somewhere along the line corresponding to their own perceptions of that variable. Scores are calculated by measuring the distance from one end of the line to the slash. Although visual analogue-response sets are often used in survey research, some patients find this format difficult.

HRQOL instruments may be general or disease specific. General HRQOL domains address the components of overall wellbeing, whereas disease-specific domains focus on the impact of particular organic dysfunctions that affect HRQOL.[5] General HRQOL instruments typically address general health perceptions, sense of overall wellbeing, and function in the physical, emotional and social domains. Disease-specific HRQOL instruments for cancer patients focus on more directly relevant domains, such as anxiety about cancer recurrence, nausea from chemotherapy or urinary incontinence from sphincter damage. Since HRQOL may change over time, longitudinal measurement of these outcomes is critical.[6,7]

Development and evaluation of new HRQOL instruments

The development and validation of new instruments and scales is a long and arduous process that should not be undertaken lightly. It is not adequate simply to write down a list of questions that seem appropriate and give this list to patients; it is always preferable to use established instruments when available. One advantage of using published instruments in the collection of HRQOL data is that they allow researchers to compare the results with those from other previously studied populations with various chronic diseases, including different types of cancer.

When instruments are developed, they are first pilot tested to ensure that the target population can understand and complete them with ease. Pilot testing reveals problems that might otherwise go unrecognized by researchers. For example, many terms that are commonly used by medical professionals are poorly understood by patients. This may result in missing data if patients leave questions blank. Furthermore, since many patients with prostate cancer are older and may have poor eyesight, pilot testing often identifies easily corrected visual barriers such as type size and page layout. Pilot testing is a necessary and valuable phase of instrument development. Instruments are also evaluated for the two fundamental psychometric statistical properties of *reliability* and *validity*.

Reliability

Reliability refers to how reproducible the scale is — that is, what proportion of a patient's test score is true and what proportion is due to individual variation. *Test–retest reliability* is a measure of response stability over time. It is assessed by administering scales to patients at two separate time points, typically a month apart. The correlation coefficients between the two scores reflect the stability of responses. Test–retest reliability is most easily assessed when the domain of interest is unlikely to change over short periods of time. If too long an interval occurs, real change in the variable may artificially deflate test–retest reliability coefficients. Internal consistency reliability is a measure of the similarity of an individual's response across several items, indicating the homogeneity of a scale.[8] The statistic used to quantify the internal consistency, or unidimensionality, of a scale is called Cronbach's coefficient alpha.[9] Generally accepted standards dictate that reliability statistics measured by these two methods should exceed 0.70 (Table 37.1).

Validity

Validity refers to how well the scale or instrument measures the attribute it is intended to measure. Validity provides evidence to support drawing inferences about HRQOL from the scale scores. Three types of validity are usually evaluated in scales and instruments. *Content validity*, sometimes incorrectly referred to as face validity, involves a non-quantitative assessment of the scope and completeness of a proposed scale. It is more superficial than other types of validity and, indeed, is considered by some not to be a true measure of validity at all.[10] Nevertheless, it is almost always included in the early stages of instrument development, even if only as a general review of items by physicians or patients. *Criterion validity* is a more quantitative approach to assessing the performance of scales and instruments. It requires the correlation of scales scores with other measurable health outcomes (predictive validity) and with results from other established tests (concurrent validity). For example, the predictive validity of a new HRQOL scale for physical function might be correlated with the number of

Table 37.1. Types of reliability

Type of reliability	Characteristics	Comments
Test–retest	Measures the stability of responses over time, typically in the same group of respondents	Requires the administration of survey to a sample at two different and appropriate points in time. Time points that are too far apart may produce diminished reliability estimates that reflect actual change over time in the variable interest.
Intra-observer	Measures the stability of responses over time in the same individual respondent	Requires completion of a survey by an individual at two different and appropriate points in time. Time points that are too far apart may produce diminished reliability estimates that reflect actual change over time in the variable of interest.
Alternate-form	Uses differently worded stems or response sets to obtain the same information about a specific topic	Requires two items in which the wording is different but aimed at the same specific variable and at the same vocabulary level
Internal consistency	Measures how well several items in a scale vary together in a sample	Usually requires a computer to carry out calculations
Inter-observer	Measures how well two or more respondents rate the same phenomenon	May be used to demonstrate reliability of a survey or may itself be the variable of interest in a study

Table 37.2. Types of validity

Type of validity	Characteristics	Comments
Face	Casual review of how good an item or group of items appear	Assessed by individuals with no formal training in the subject under study
Content	Formal expert review of how good an item or series of items appear	Usually assessed by individuals with expertise in some aspect of the subject under study
Criterion: concurrent	Measures how well the item or scale correlates with 'gold standard' measures of the same variable	Requires the identification of an established, generally accepted gold standard
Criterion: predictive	Measures how well the item or scale predicts expected future observations	Used to predict outcomes or events of significance that the item or scale might subsequently be used to predict
Construct	Theoretical measure of how meaningful a survey instrument is	Determined usually after years of experience by numerous investigators

subsequent physician visits or hospitalizations. Likewise, the concurrent validity of a new sexual function scale might be correlated with objective performance on infusion cavernosometry or nocturnal penile tumescence testing. A new emotional HRQOL scale might be correlated with an established mental health index. Generally accepted standards dictate that validity statistics should exceed 0.70.

Construct validity is the most valuable, yet most difficult, way of assessing a survey instrument. It is often determined only after years of experience with a survey instrument. It is a measure of how meaningful the scale or survey instrument is when in practical use. Often, it is not calculated as a quantifiable statistic; rather, it is frequently seen as a gestalt of how well a survey instrument performs in a multitude of settings and populations over a number of years. Construct validity is often thought to comprise two other forms of validity — convergent and divergent. *Convergent validity* implies that several different methods for obtaining the same information about a given trait or concept produce similar results. *Divergent validity* means that the scale does not correlate too closely with similar but distinct concepts or traits (Table 37.2).

Collection of HRQOL data

Once an instrument has been thoroughly pilot tested and found to be reliable and valid, it must be administered in a manner that minimizes bias HRQOL data cannot, and should not, be collected from cancer patients directly by the operating surgeon or treating oncologist or radiotherapist. Patients have an unconscious desire to produce responses that their physicians want to hear.[11] This introduces measurement error. No matter how objective the treating physician may claim to be, it is impossible for her or him to collect statistically meaningful outcomes data through direct questioning. Variations in phrasing, inflection, eye contact, rapport, mood, and other factors are difficult or impossible to eliminate. Data must be gathered by disinterested third parties using established psychometric scales and instruments. It is often preferable for instruments to be self-administered by patients, independent of interviewers. Self-assessment of HRQOL frees patient responses from any interviewer bias.

The Southwest Oncology Group (SWOG) has defined the following six principles for HRQOL research in cancer trials: (1) always measure physical functioning, emotional functioning, symptoms, and global quality of life separately; (2) include measures of social functioning and additional protocol-specific measures if resources permit; (3) use patient-based questionnaires; (4) use categorical rather than visual analogue scales; (5) select brief questionnaires, not interviews; (6) select HRQOL measures with published psychometric properties.[12,13]

Using the SWOG guidelines, one can confidently select instruments to assess HRQOL in longitudinal or cross-sectional studies of patients with prostate cancer. The various components of HRQOL should be measured with different scales to assure that each receives adequate attention. Longer instruments yield richer data sets, but they also increase the chance that patients will tire of the survey and provide unreliable or invalid answers. Hence, shorter instruments are generally preferable when obtaining HRQOL data.

It is important to compare results with those from individuals of the same age without known disease. For example, when measuring sexual function after treatment for prostate cancer, it is more helpful to compare outcomes with age-matched control subjects than with a hypothetical state of perfect sexual function. Since sexual function varies with age, it is critical to maintain the appropriate context of the variable under investigation. This principle holds true with other HRQOL domains also.

Established health-related quality-of-life instruments

General HRQOL instruments

General HRQOL instruments have been extensively researched and validated in many types of patients, sick and well. Examples include the RAND Medical Outcomes Study 36-Item Health Survey (also known as the SF-36),[14–19] the Quality of Well-Being scale (QWB),[20–24] the Sickness Impact Profile (SIP)[20,25–27] and the Nottingham Health Profile (NHP).[20,28–32] Each assesses various components of HRQOL, including physical and emotional functioning, social functioning and symptoms. Each has been thoroughly validated and tested.

One of the most commonly used general instruments is the RAND 36-Item Health Survey, which was developed during the Medical Outcomes Study, a large project in which health-related aspects of daily life were examined in many different types of patients.[33] It is a 36-item, self-administered instrument that takes less than 10 minutes to complete and quantifies HRQOL in eight multi-item scales that address different health concepts: these are physical function, social function, bodily pain, emotional well-being, energy/fatigue, general health perceptions, role limitation due to physical problems, and role limitation due to emotional problems. The RAND 36-Item Health Survey is now widely regarded as the 'gold standard' instrument for the measurement of general HRQOL.

The QWB summarizes three aspects of health status (mobility, physical activity and social activity) in terms of quality-adjusted life years, quantifying HRQOL as a single number that may range from death to complete wellbeing. The QWB contains only 18 items, but it requires a trained interviewer.

The SIP measures health status by assessing the impact of sickness on changing daily activities and behaviour. It is self-administered with limited interviewer assistance, but contains 136 items and can take 30 minutes or longer to complete.

The NHP covers six types of experience with illness (pain, physical mobility, sleep, emotional reactions, energy and social isolation) by using a series of weighted yes-or-no items. It contains 38 self-administered items and can be completed fairly quickly.

Cancer-targeted HRQOL instruments

Because of the well-documented association of cancer with psychological stress and emotional anxiety, as well as the deficits in activities of daily living that affect patients living with malignancy, cancer-specific quality of life has also be investigated extensively. Numerous instruments have been developed and tested that measure the special impact of cancer on patients' routine activities. Examples include the Cancer Rehabilitation Evaluation System (CARES),[34–37] the Functional Assessment of Cancer Therapy (FACT)[38–42] and the Functional Living Index for Cancer (FLIC).[43,44] Each has been validated and tested in patients with various types of cancer.

There is consensus on which cancer instrument based measures cancer-specific HRQOL, but they all focus on similar domains that are of particular concern to patients with cancer. For example, the commonly used CARES Short Form (CARES-SF) is a 59-item, self-administered instrument that measures cancer-related HRQOL with five multi-item scales — physical, psychological, medical interaction, marital interaction, and sexual function. A large and valuable database of patients with many different tumours, including urological tumours, has been collected by the authors of the CARES.[45] This information is helpful when comparing the experience of patients with prostate cancer with that of patients with other types of cancer.

The FACT is usually applied as a two-part instrument that includes a general item set pertaining to all cancer patients (FACT-G) and one of several items sets containing special questions for patients with specific tumours. Each item contains a statement with which a patient may agree or disagree across a five-point Likert range. The FACT-G domains include wellbeing in six areas — physical, social–family, relationship with doctor, emotional, functional and miscellaneous. The FACT-G includes 28 items and is self-administered. The authors of the FACT have recently developed two new supplementary disease-targeted HRQOL instruments for patients with bladder or prostate cancer.

The FLIC detects differences in functional states by measuring the physical and emotional quality of cancer patients' daily lives in areas such as coping, fear, depression, pain, nausea, housework and self-perception. Unlike the instruments discussed above, the FLIC uses visual analogue scales.

Other instruments, such as the Sexual Adjustment Questionnaire (SAQ),[46] directly address more specific issues with which cancer patients are concerned. the SAQ is a 108-item self-administered tool that has been shown to be reliable and valid in patients with various cancers and in healthy controls. It measures six domains in patients before, during, and after cancer treatment: these are libido, arousal, activity level, relationships, techniques, and orgasm.

Health-related quality-of-life in men with prostate cancer

Metastatic prostate cancer

Cancer-specific HRQOL has been studied in patients with metastatic prostate cancer by numerous researchers. Cassileth et al.[47,48] used established psychometric instruments (including the FLIC) to show changes in HRQOL after treatment.

Their work suggests that these men are quite interested in considering quality-of-life outcomes when selecting specific hormonal therapy. Herr *et al.*[49] also used established instruments to compare patients receiving hormonal therapy versus observation for metastatic prostate cancer; their research documented better quality-of-life scores among patients who elected to defer treatment over those who underwent early intervention. Tannock *et al.*[50] adapted a series of visual analogue items from an instrument validated in breast cancer patients and applied it, together with the established McGill–Melzack pain questionnaire,[51] to measure qualitative response to prednisone in patients with symptomatic bone metastases from prostate cancer. Although Tannock did not develop his items into scales, he did measure variables such as fatigue, appetite, anxiety, all of which have been shown to contribute to HRQOL in cancer patients. Cleary *et al.*[52] developed a new self-administered patient questionnaire that examined HRQOL in patients with metastatic prostate cancer. He reported on the reliability and validity of this instrument in English and several other languages (Danish, Dutch, German, Norwegian and Swedish). This study suggests that, with certain notable exceptions (domains of sexual interest and function), the scales perform well in various cultural settings. In a recent study of 288 men with prostate cancer, Ganz *et al.*[34] used the CARES to discriminate between various clinical stages of the disease. They also demonstrated that, among patients with prostate, lung, and colorectal cancer, this instrument can be used to document the progressive worsening of quality of life as the cancer advances. These findings were confirmed by Kornblith *et al.*,[53] who used the European Organization for Research and Treatment of Cancer (EORTC) Prostate Cancer Quality of Life Questionnaire to survey patients and spouses, demonstrating that, as disease progresses, steady HRQOL declines among patients are paralleled by increasing psychological distress among their spouses. Fossa *et al.*[52] used an instrument adapted from the EORTC Prostate Quality of Life Questionnaire to compare doctors' and patients' perceptions of patients' HRQOL following chemotherapy for hormone-resistant prostate cancer. The study suggests that physicians tend to underestimate the effects of metastatic prostate cancer on patients' quality of life. daSilva and colleagues[55] summarize the EORTC experience with HRQOL assessment in men with advanced prostate cancer. Fossa[56] also provides a concise summary of this literature.

Localized prostate cancer

In men treated with radical prostatectomy for early-stage disease, Pedersen *et al.*[57] carried out a longitudinal study of HRQOL changes for 18 months following surgery. The initial distress associated with diagnosis of cancer improved over time, although bother from erectile dysfunction persisted. Overall wellbeing was minimally affected.

Assessment of prostate-targeted HRQOL in the sexual, urinary and bowel domains has been documented with a newly established instrument, the UCLA Prostate Cancer Index.[58] It is a 56-item, self-administered, statistically reliable and valid tool that takes about 20 minutes to complete and has been shown to be very robust in men with prostate cancer. The UCLA Prostate Cancer Index was recently used in a large study of men in a managed care population. No differences were seen in general HRQOL when comparing patients who had undergone surgery, radiation, or observation alone for clinically localized prostate cancer or when comparing them with a group of age-matched control subjects without prostate cancer. Among the same patients, significant group differences in HRQOL were identified in the prostate-specific sexual, urinary and bowel domains. Another study,[59] with an early version of the UCLA Prostate Cancer Index, demonstrated that, among men treated with surgery or radiation for localized prostate cancer, urinary dysfunction diminished HRQOL much more than did sexual dysfunction. Although negative functional outcomes were found more commonly than the published literature suggests, the degree of bother experienced by these patients did not necessarily correlate with the level of dysfunction. The UCLA Prostate Cancer Index is now in use in several national and international studies. Rieker and colleagues[60] also used established general HRQOL instruments and newly developed prostate-targeted scales to compare outcomes in men treated with surgery versus radiation for early-stage disease. They have demonstrated that sexual function and bother have a significant impact on quality of life and are distinct from other dimensions. Herr[61] demonstrated that, among men who were incontinent after radical prostatectomy, 26% reported limitations in their usual physical activity and over one-half experienced moderate to severe emotional distress, but 79% of those evaluated less than 5 years after surgery said they would choose surgery again, despite their leakage problems.

Lim and colleagues[62] used the FLIC and the Profile of Mood States (POMS)[63] to look at 136 men who had undergone radical retropubic prostatectomy and 60 men who had received external beam irradiation for clinically localized prostate cancer. They found that the prostatectomy group had worse sexual function and more urinary incontinence, whereas the radiation group had worse bowel function. Radiated patients who were incontinent perceived this as a greater problem than did incontinent patients in the prostatectomy group. When patients were asked if they would have the same treatment again, 92% of prostatectomy patients and 87% of irradiated patients stated that they would.

Using a large national sample of Medicare beneficiaries, Fowler et al.[64,65] and the Prostate Patient Outcomes Research Team (PORT) used reliable and valid psychometric instruments to document that sexual and urinary dysfunctions are much more common after radical prostatectomy than previously reported. These findings have also been documented by Gburek et al.,[66] who reported results from 88 men undergoing surgery, radiation, or both, for early stage disease. They used a series of new disease-targeted questions on sexual, urinary and bowel function, as well as on overall satisfaction with care, to show that the specific complications of prostate cancer treatment are more common than previously reported. There was no difference between the quality-of-life experience of patients undergoing either surgery or radiation, but those receiving both modalities were more likely to suffer more negative HRQOL outcomes. These studies, and others,[67–72] emphasize the significant role for HRQOL research in men with prostate cancer.

Future directions for HRQOL research

Specific research questions begin with the need for basic descriptive analysis of HRQOL in patients treated for prostate cancer. Depiction of the fundamental elements in quality of life for these individuals requires study of their health perceptions and how their daily activities are impacted by both their general health and their cancer. Physical and emotional wellbeing form the cornerstone of this approach, but research must also extend to issues such as eating and sleeping habits, anxiety and fatigue, depression, rapport with physician, interactions with spouse or partner, social interactions, and specific pelvic functions (sexual, urinary and bowel). Characterization of all domains must address not only the actual functions but also the relative importance of these issues to patients and how bothered they are by any dysfunction that is present.

Beyond the descriptive analysis, HRQOL outcomes must be compared in patients undergoing different modes of therapy. General and disease-specific HRQOL must be measured to facilitate comparison with patients treated for diabetes, heart disease, arthritis, and other common chronic conditions. Quality-of-life outcomes must also be risk adjusted for variations in case mix or in sociodemographic variables such as age, race, education, income, insurance status, geographic region and access to health care. In this context, HRQOL may be linked with many factors other than the traditional medical ones. Research initiatives must rely on established HRQOL instruments with proven records of statistical reliability and validity administered by objective third parties. HRQOL can have many different definitions and interpretations, but its measurement must adhere to the strict scientific application of psychometric science.

With better information on quality of life, as well as clinical outcomes, a richer database will be developed that is more useful to patients. Physicians will be better able to evaluate new treatment modalities, educate their patients, and counsel them individually on what to expect when diagnosed and treated for prostate cancer.

References

1. Fayers P M, Jones D R. Measuring and analyzing quality of life in cancer clinical trials: a review. Stat Med 1983; 2: 429–446
2. Osoba D. Measuring the effect of cancer on quality of life. In: Osoba D (ed) Effect of cancer on quality of life. Boca Raton: CRC Press, 1991
3. Sadura A, Pater J, Osoba D et al. Quality of life assessment: patient compliance with questionnaire completion. J Natl Cancer Inst 1992; 84: 1023–1026
4. Litwin M S. Measuring health-related quality of life in men with prostate cancer. J Urol 1994; 152: 1882–1887
5. Patrick D L, Deyo R A. Generic and disease-specific measures in assessing health status and quality of life. Med Care 1989; 27: S217–S232
6. Zwinderman A H. The measurement of change of quality of life in clinical trials. Stat Med 1990; 9: 931–942
7. Olschewski M, Schumacher M. Statistical analysis of quality of life data in cancer clinical trials. Stat Med 1990; 9: 749–763
8. Tulsk D A. An introduction to test theory. Oncology 1990; 4: 43–48
9. Cronback L J. Coefficient alpha and the internal structure of tests. Psychometrika 1951; 16: 297–334
10. Messick S. The one and future issues of validity: assessing the meaning and consequences of measurement. In: Wainer H, Braun H I (eds) Test validity. Hillside, NJ: Lawrence Erlbaum Associates, 1988
11. Tannock I F. Management of breast and prostate cancer: how does quality of life enter the equation? Oncology 1990; 3: 149–156
12. Moinpour C M, Feigl P, Metch B et al. Quality of life endpoints in clinical trials: review and recommendations. J Natl Cancer Inst 1989; 81: 485–495
13. Moinpour C M. Quality of life assessment in Southwest Oncology Group trials. Oncology 1990; 4: 79–89
14. Tarlov A R, Ware J E, Greenfield S et al. Medical outcomes study: an application of methods for evaluating the results of medical care. JAMA 1989; 262: 907–913
15. Ware J E, Sherbourne C D, Davies A R. Developing and testing the MOS 20-item shortform health survey: a general population application. In: Stewart A L, Ware J E (eds) Measuring functioning and well-being: the medical outcomes study approach. Durham, NC: Duke University Press, 1992
16. Stewart A L, Hays R D, Ware J E. The MOS short-form general health survey: Reliability and validity in a patient population. Med Care 1988; 26: 724–735
17. Ware J E, Sherbourne C D. The MOS 36-item short-form health survey (SF-36): I. Conceptual framework and item selection. Med Care 1992; 30: 473–483
18. McHorney C A, Ware J E, Rogers W et al. The validity and relative precision of MOS short- and long-form health status scales and Dartmouth COOP charts in discriminating among

adults with mediacl and psychiatric conditions: results from the medical outcomes study. Med Care 1992; 30(Suppl): MS253–265

19. Hays R D, Hayashi T. Beyond internal consistency reliability: rationale and user's guide for multitrait scaling analysis program on the microcomputer. Behav Res Methods Instr Comput 1990; 22: 167–175

20. McDowell I, Ewell C. Measuring Health: A Guide to Rating Scles and Questionnaires. New York, Oxford University Press, 1987

21. Kaplan R M, Anderson J P. A general health policy model: update and applications. Health Serv Res 1988; 23: 203–235

22. Kaplan R M, Bush J W. Health-related quality of life measurement for evaluation research and policy analysis. Health Psychol 1982; 1: 61–80

23. Hays R M, Shapiro M F. An overview of generic health-related quality of life measures for HIV research. Qual Life Res 1992; 1: 91–98

24. Kaplan R M, Bush J W, Berry C C. Health status: types of validity and the index of wellbeing. Health Serv Res 1976; 11: 478–507

25. Bergner M, Bobbitt R A, Carter W B, Gilson B S. The sickness impact profile: development and final revision of a health status measure. Med Care 1981; 19: 787–805

26. Bergner M, Bobbitt R A, Pollard W E et al. The sickness impact profile: validation of a health status measure. Med Care 1976; 14: 57–67

27. Deyo R A, Inui T S, Leininger J D, Overman S S. Measuring functional outcomes in chronic disease: a comparison of traditional scales and a self-administered health status questionnaire in patients with rheumatoid arthritis. Med Care 1983; 21: 180–192

28. Moinpour C M, Feigle P, Metch B et al. Quality of life end points in cancer clinical trials: review and recommendations. J Natl Cancer Inst 1989; 81: 485–495

29. Martini C J M, McDowell I. Socio-medical measurements of health in primary care. Report submitted to Social Sciences Research Council, London, England, December, 1978

30. Hunt S M, McEwen J, McKenna S P. Measuring health status: a new tool for clinicians and epidemiologists. J R Coll Gen Pract 1985; 35: 185–188

31. McDowell I W, Martini C J M, Waugh W. A method for self-assessment of disability before and after hip replacement operations. Br Med J 1978; 2: 57–58

32. Martini C J, McDowell I. Health status: patient and physician judgements. Health Serv Res 1976; 11: 508–515

33. Stewart A L, Greenfield S, Hays R D. Functional status and well-being of patients with chronic conditions. JAMA 1989; 262: 907–913

34. Ganz P A, Schag C A C, Lee J J, Sim M S. The CARES: a generic measure of health related quality of life for patients with cancer. Qual Life Res 1992; 1: 19–29

35. Schag C A C, Heinrich R L. Development of a comprehensive quality of life measurement tool: CARES. Oncology 1990; 4: 135–138

36. Schag C A C, Heinrich R L. Cancer Rehabilitation Evaluation System (CARES) Manual. Los Angeles: Cares Consultants, 1988

37. Schag C A C, Heinrich R L, Ganz P A. The Cancer Rehabilitation Evaluation System (CARES): the short form (CARES-SF). Proc Am Soc Clin Oncol 1989; 8: 316

38. Cella D F, Tulsky D S. Measuring quality of life today. Oncology 1990; 4: 29–38

39. Tulsky D S, Cella D F, Bonomi A et al. Development and validation of new quality of life measures for patients with cancer. Proc Soc Behav Med 1990; 11: 4546

40. Cella D F, Cherin E A. Quality of life during and after cancer treatment. Compr Ther 1988; 14: 69–75

41. Cella D F, Orofiamma B, Holland J C et al. Relationship of psychological distress, extent of disease, and performance status in patients with lung cancer. Cancer 1987; 60: 239–245

42. Tchekmedyian N S, Cella D F. Quality of Life in Current Oncology Practice and Research. Williston Park, New York: Dominus Publishing, 1991

43. Schipper H, Clinch J, McMurray A, Levitt M. Measuring quality of life in cancer patients: the functional living index-cancer: development and validation. J Clin Oncol 1984; 2: 472–483

44. Finkelstein D M, Cassileth B R, Bonomi P D et al. A pilot study of the functional living index-cancer (FLIC) scale for the assessment of quality of life for metastatic lung cancer patients. Am J Clin Oncol 1988; 11: 630–633

45. Schag C A, Ganz P A, Wing D S et al. Quality of life in adult survivors of lung, colon and prostate cancer. Qual Life Res 1994; 3: 127–141

46. Waterhouse J, Metcalfe M C. Development of the sexual adjustment questionnaire. Oncol Nurs Forum 1986; 13: 53–59

47. Cassileth B R, Soloway M S, Vogelzang N J *et al*. Patients' choice of treatment in stage D prostate cancer. Urology 1989; 33(Suppl): 57–62

48. Cassileth B R, Soloway M S, Vogelzang N J *et al*. Quality of life and psychosocial status in stage D prostate cancer. Qual Life Res 1992; 1: 323–329

49. Herr H W, Kornblith A B, Ofman U. A comparison of the quality of life of patients with metastatic prostate cancer who received or did not receive hormonal therapy. Cancer Suppl 1993; 71: 1143–1150

50. Tannock I F, Gospodarowicz M, Panzarella T *et al*. Treatment of metastatic prostate cancer with low-dose prednisone: evaluation of pain and quality of life as pragmatic indices of response. J Clin Oncol 1989; 7: 1–7

51. Melzack R. The McGill Pain Questionnaire: major properties and scoring methods. Pain 1975; 1: 277–299

52. Cleary P D, Morrissey G, Oster G. Health-related quality of life in patients with advanced prostate cancer: a multinational perspective. Qual Life Res 1995; 4: 207–220

53. Kornblith A B, Herr H W, Ofman U S *et al*. Quality of life of patients with prostate cancer and their spouses. Cancer 1994; 73: 2791–2802

54. Fossa S D, Aaronson N K, Newling D *et al*. Quality of life and treatment of hormone resistant metastatic prostatic cancer. Eur J Cancer 1990; 11: 1133–1136

55. daSilva F C, Fossa S D, Aaronson N K *et al*. The quality of life of ptients with newly diagnosed M1 prostate cancer: experience with EORTC clinical trial 30853. Eur J Cancer 1996; 32A: 72–77

56. Fossa S D. Quality of life in advanced prostate cancer. Semin Oncol 1996; 23(suppl 14): 32–34

57. Pedersen K V, Carlsson P, Rahmquist M, Varenhorst E. Quality of life after radical retropubic prostatectomy for carcinoma of the prostate. Eur Urol 1993; 24: 7–11

58. Litwin M S, Hays R D, Fink A *et al*. Quality of life outcomes in men treated for localized prostate cancer. JAMA 1995; 273: 129–135

59. Litwin M S, Fink A, Hays R D *et al*. Quality of life in men with prostate cancer: a pilot study. J Urol 1993; 149: 494A

60. Rieker P, Clark J, Kalish L *et al*. Health-related quality of life following treatment for early stage prostate cancer. Proc Am Soc Clin Oncol 1993; 12: 452A

61. Herr H A. Quality of life of incontinent men after prostatectomy. J Urol 1994; 151: 652–654

62. Lim A J, Brandon A H, Fiedler J *et al*. Quality of life: radical prostatectomy versus radiation therapy for prostate cancer. J Urol 1995; 154: 1420–1425

63. Jacobson A F, Weiss B L, Steinbook R M *et al*. The measurement of psychological states by use of factors derived from a combination of items from mood and symptom checklists. J Clin Psychol 1978; 34: 677–685

64. Fowler F J, Barry M J, Lu-Yao G *et al*. Patient-reported complications and follow-up treatment after radical prostatectomy. Urology 1993; 42: 622–629

65. Fowler F J, Barry M J, Lu-Yao G *et al*. Effect of radical prostatectomy for prostate cancer on patient quality of life: results from a Medicare survey. Urology 1995; 45: 1007–1015

66. Gburek B, Harmon B, Chodak G W. Quality of life assessment in patients with prostate cancer treated by radical prostatectomy, radiation therapy, or a combination. J Urol 1992; 147: 466A

67. Fossa S, Kaasa S, Calais da Silva F *et al*. Quality of life in prostate cancer patients. Prostate 1992; 4(suppl): 145–148

68. Calais da Silva F, Reis E, Costa T *et al*. Quality of life in patients with prostatic cancer: a feasibility study. Cancer Suppl 1993; 71: 1138–1142

69. Sharp J W. Expanding the definition of quality of life for prostate cancer. Cancer Suppl 1993; 71: 1078–1082

70. Aaronson N K, Calais da Silva F. Prospects for the future: quality of life evaluation in prostatic cancer protocols. Prog Clin Biol Res 1987; 243B: 501–512

71. Friedland J L, Pow-Sang J, Johnson D J, Byrnes J. Quality-of-life issues associated with the treatment of prostate cancer. Cancer Controv 1995; 12: 42–46

72. Chodak G, Sinner M, Rukstalis D B *et al*. Patient-reported outcomes following radical prostatectomy performed at eight academic insitutions. J Urol 1995; 153: 390A

Chapter 38
Diet and prostate cancer

M. Morton

Introduction

Cancer of the prostate is one of a group of diseases that includes breast and colorectal cancer, cardiovascular disease and osteoporosis. These are termed 'Western diseases' because of their more frequent occurrence in the affluent Western countries of Northern Europe, North America and Australasia than in Asian countries and peoples that are less well off. 'Western diseases' have been associated with dietary fat as a causative factor; however, recently it has been recognized that there may be constituents of the more-vegetarian Asian diet that protect against the development of these diseases, and it is the relative lack of such constituents in the Western diet, rather than the high fat content, that is the important factor.

The concept is, therefore, that certain components in the Asian diet — and possibly also in that of the Mediterranean area — are protective against the development of those diseases that are so prevalent in affluent Western countries. This chapter explores the relationship between diet and cancer of the prostate and cites specific components of Asian diets that appear to have a restraining influence on cancer development.

Geographical differences in prostate cancer incidence

Carcinoma of the prostate belongs to the group of hormone-dependent cancers, that also includes cancers of the breast, ovary and endometrium. Prostate cancer is now one of the most commonly diagnosed cancers in the West.[1-3] World-wide, the incidence is rising annually by approximately 2–3%.[4,5] In North American men, prostate cancer is now the second most commonly diagnosed cancer after skin cancer, and the second most common cause of death from cancer after that of the lung. An estimated 200,000 new cases were diagnosed in the United States in 1995 and 40,000 died from the disease that year.[6]

Epidemiological studies have demonstrated considerable geographical variation in the age-adjusted incidence of cancer of the prostate.[7,8] However, autopsy studies reveal that the incidence of latent carcinoma of the prostate, i.e. microscopic foci of cancer cells, is the same in men of all races, from both East and West.[9] The incidence of the clinically malignant disease is highest in the Black North American male,[4,10] some 30-fold greater than in Japanese men,[4] and 120 times greater than that seen in Chinese men in Shanghai.[2,11-13] The incidence rate for cancer of the prostate in Japan is now rising,[2,14] and for Japanese migrants to North America the mortality rate increases to one-half that of the indigenous population within one or two generations.[15,16] The epidemiological phenomena observed in migrating populations appears sufficiently quickly to suggest that dietary and environmental factors, rather than genetic ones, are responsible.

Benign prostatic hyperplasia (BPH) is said to be more common in elderly men from Western countries than in men from the East.[17] However, the prevalence of microscopic BPH, an early clinical event in the development of the disease, is the same in men of all races.[18]

Prostate cancer and BPH clinically present in men over the age of 50. With the prevalence of both diseases later in life, the increasing life expectancy in developed countries suggests that BPH and cancer of the prostate will become serious health-care problems. This further highlights the importance of current research into prevention.

Diet and cancer: general considerations

The 'Western diet' is high in animal fat and protein and refined carbohydrate and low in fibre-rich foodstuffs. In contrast, the low-fat diet of the less prosperous Asian communities is rich in starches, legumes, fruit and vegetables — many of which have a high fibre content.[8,19,20]

Vegetables are a source of fibre, but their protective role[21,22] may also be attributable to other constituents. Evidence[23,24] suggests that certain non-nutrient components of plant products, vegetables and fruits play a preventive role in various carcinogenic processes, particularly relating to endocrine cancers such as those of the breast and prostate, and also colorectal cancer.[21,22,25]

Dietary fat and prostate cancer

Several studies have established a positive correlation between prostatic cancer occurrence and mortality and *per capita* fat consumption.[26] In addition, strong correlations are apparent between prostate cancer mortality rates and those of other cancers suspected as being associated with fat intake, such as those of the breast and ovary.[27]

In the United States Health Professionals Follow-up Study, total fat consumption was directly, though not significantly, related to the risk of advanced cancer. The association was mainly due to animal fat and was not found with vegetable fat; red meat consumption had the strongest association with prostate cancer risk.[28] Positive associations have been reported for animal fat in other studies.[29,30] However, the investigations of Stemmermann and colleagues[31,32] and of Kolonel *et al.*[33] in Hawaii failed to find this association. The recent studies of Whittemore and colleagues[34] claim that differences in saturated fat intake can account for only approximately 10% of the Black–White differences and about 15% of White–Asian–American differences in prostate cancer incidence. This observation suggests that other factors are responsible for interethnic differences in risk for prostate cancer. Dietary fat had no influence on the incidence of prostate cancer in animal models.[35,36]

Vegetables, fruit and cereals and prostate cancer

The long-term studies of 265,118 adults by Hirayama in Japan[37–39] demonstrated that daily consumption of green–yellow vegetables was an important protective factor against cancers of the stomach and prostate, as well as other Western diseases. Green–yellow vegetables were defined as containing more than 600 µg of carotene/100 g, and included pumpkin, carrots, spinach, green lettuce and green asparagus. The standardized mortality rate for cancer of the breast was also reported to be lower when there was an increase in the consumption of soya bean paste soup and soya milk. Hirayama[37] speculated that β-carotene and possibly other components of soya beans and vegetables were implicated in the reduction of mortality.

A case–control study on the effects of diet on breast cancer risk in Singapore[40] indicated that red meat intake was a predisposing factor. However, soya protein, β-carotene and polyunsaturated fatty acids were reported to be protective components of the diet.

The investigations in both Japan[37] and Singapore[40] suggested a protective influence of soya bean products as well as β-carotene on breast cancer risk and drew attention to components of certain vegetables, present in the traditional Asian diet, that may also influence carcinogenesis. A study of Japanese men in Hawaii reported that increased consumption of both rice and tofu were associated with a decreased risk of prostate cancer.[31] Tofu and other soya-based foods are rich sources of isoflavonoid phyto-oestrogens.[41] Several investigators have also demonstrated significant strong negative correlations between mortality from prostate cancer and dietary intake of cereals.[42,43] Cereals contain precursors of the mammalian lignans, another group of dietary phyto-oestrogens.[41] Furthermore, a cohort study of diet, lifestyle and prostate cancer in Seventh-Day Adventist men revealed that increasing consumption of beans, lentils, peas, tomatoes, raisins, dates and other dried foods, were all associated with significantly decreased prostate cancer risk.[29] The Mediterranean-style diet is considered protective against the endocrine cancers[44,45] and features a low animal fat and meat content, with a high intake of fresh fruit, vegetables and pasta. Fresh fruit, citrus fruits and raw vegetables were found to be protective against many cancers, including that of the prostate, in several Italian studies.[46–48] Many fresh fruits and vegetables contain high concentrations of flavonoids, some of which also have oestrogenic properties.[49]

Oestrogenic substances in plants

The presence in plants of non-steroidal substances with oestrogenic activity has been recognized for some time and many hundreds of plants manifest some degree of oestrogenic activity.[50,51] Soya bean and red clover are members of the Leguminosae family and are a major source of isoflavonoids.[51–53] Soya is consumed daily in large amounts in a number of forms in China and Japan, and in Asia generally. Many foods of plant origin contain varying amounts of isoflavonoids, flavonoids and lignans. Some of these polyphenolic phyto-oestrogens possess weak oestrogenic activity and therefore the potential for exerting an influence on hormone-dependent cancers such as those of the breast and prostate.[41]

Soya beans contain the glycoside conjugates of the isoflavonoids genistein and daidzein, which can be metabolized by gut bacteria to the actual aglycones, genistein and daidzein. Genistein can be further metabolized to the non-oestrogenic p-ethylphenol and daidzein is converted to the oestrogenic isoflavan, equol. The aglycones and their metabolites are then absorbed and appear in blood and urine, primarily as glucuronide conjugates, and also as sulphates.[41] Daidzein and genistein were isolated from soya beans more than 60 years ago,[54] and 100 g fat-free soya beans may yield up to 300 mg genistein.[55]

Lignans are another group of polyphenolic plant compounds.[51,56] The plant precursors, matairesinol and secoisolariciresinol, are metabolized by intestinal microflora after ingestion to give rise to the weakly oestrogenic enterolactone and enterodiol, respectively. The lignans are absorbed from the gut to appear in blood and other body fluids.[41] The lignans are very widely distributed in nature and precursors are found in many cereals, grains, fruits and vegetables but the richest source is linseed (flaxseed) and other oilseeds such as sesame.[57]

The flavonoids are closely related in structure to the isoflavonoids, the former having a 2-phenylchroman nucleus and the latter a 3-phenylchroman nucleus.[49] Recently, several commonly occurring plant flavonoids have been shown to possess weak oestrogenic activity.[49] Unlike isoflavonoids, the flavonoids are ubiquitous in nature, and are found in high concentration in many fruits, vegetables and crop species. In particular, apigenin and kaempferol, both of which are oestrogenic, are regarded as major flavonoids because of their common occurrence among plants and their significant concentrations when they are present. Apigenin, for example, is found in the leaves, seeds and fruits of flowering plants, with up to 7% of dry weight in leafy vegetables. Tea-leaves are an excellent source of apigenin.[49]

Isoflavonoids and lignans are normal constituents of body fluids and have been identified in most animal[41] and human body fluids by gas chromatography–mass spectrometry (GC–MS). They are present in urine,[58,59] plasma,[60] saliva[61] and semen.[62] Analysis of expressed prostatic fluid found that enterolactone and equol were constituents,[61] suggesting that dietary oestrogens can accumulate in the prostate.

The levels of isoflavonoids are high in the urine and plasma of the Japanese and Chinese,[63,64] whose traditional foodstuffs contain large amounts of soya in the form of bean curd (tofu), soya bean milk, miso and tempeh. The concentration of lignans is high in the urine of vegetarians,[59] whose diet contains whole-grain cereals, vegetables and fruits. In Western subjects fed 40 g soya daily, the urinary excretion of equol was found to increase 1000-fold from control levels.[53,65] The concentrations of flavonoids in plasma and urine of different populations have yet to be determined; this is an obvious programme for future research. However as tea, fruit and vegetables are the principal sources of flavonoids, it is probable that Asians (with their high consumption of tea) and vegetarians have significant circulating levels of these compounds.

The statistics of the incidence of prostate cancer that have already been quoted show considerable protection afforded to Japanese and Chinese men — and to vegetarians, who also have a lower incidence of prostate cancer than the general Western population. This may be attributable to their intake of phyto-oestrogens.

Biological properties of isoflavonoids, flavonoids and lignans and their relevance to the prevention of prostate cancer

Oestrogenic activity

The mammalian lignans enterolactone and enterodiol, the isoflavonoids daidzein, genistein, coumestrol and equol, and the flavonoids apigenin, kaempferol and phloretin, all possess weak oestrogenic activity.[41,66,67] Some anti-oestrogenic properties have also been described.[68] As weak oestrogens they compete with oestradiol for binding to the nuclear oestrogen receptor[69] and also stimulate the synthesis of sex hormone binding globulin (SHBG) in the liver.[70]

The growth, development and function of the prostate are dependent on the concentration of testosterone (T) in plasma. Although T is the most important plasma androgen, it is the free, non-protein-bound form that is the biologically active moiety.[71–74] For the young adult male, approximately 98% of plasma T is bound to SHBG and other transport proteins;[75–77] the remaining 2% is free and this biologically active fraction passively diffuses into the prostate target cells. An increase in the concentration of SHBG, following ingestion of phyto-oestrogens, for example, decreases the free fraction of testosterone.

Vegetarian[78] and Japanese and Chinese[79] men have higher plasma levels of SHBG and lower concentrations of free T[78] than do Western omnivores.

Inhibition of 5α-reductase

Within the prostate, T is metabolized to 5α-dihydrotestosterone (DHT) by the 5α-reductase enzyme,[80] which is primarily located on the nuclear membrane. DHT has an approximately fivefold greater affinity than T for the intracellular androgen receptor protein (AR) and is the active intracellular androgen in prostate cells.[81-83]

Isoflavonoids and lignans[84] inhibit 5α-reductase and also 17β-hydroxysteroid dehydrogenase. This latter enzyme system catalyses the reversible interconversion of 17β-hydroxy and 17-keto steroids and may have a significant influence on the metabolism of both androgens and oestrogens.

Lower levels of 5α-reductase activity have been observed in young Japanese men in comparison to their Western counterparts.[85] It is likely that daily consumption of phyto-oestrogens results in a small but significant effect on the biological availability and metabolism of androgens such as T and DHT which is relevant to the lower incidence of prostate cancer in Asians. It is also of interest that synthetic 5α-reductase inhibitors, such as finasteride, are currently employed in the treatment of BPH and are being assessed as chemopreventive agents in early prostate cancer.[86]

Inhibition of the aromatase enzyme

Approximately one-third of the plasma oestrogens in the human male are synthesized and secreted by the testes. The remainder is derived from the peripheral conversion of the adrenal C19-steroids dehydroepiandrosterone (DHA) and androstenedione, by the aromatase enzyme system in adipose and muscle tissue. In a similar manner to plasma testosterone, it is the free non-protein-bound oestradiol fraction that diffuses into the prostate cells.

As a man ages, declining testicular activity and increasing aromatization produce a rise in the plasma free oestradiol-17β concentration relative to the level of free testosterone.[77,87,88] This enhanced mid-life 'oestrogenic stimulus' has generally been considered responsible for the increased level of plasma SHBG. This change in the androgen/oestrogen balance may well be a predominant factor in the induction of stromal hyperplasia of the prostate mediated through a synergistic action between oestradiol-17β and DHT.

Adlercreutz et al.[89] have recently shown that enterolactone is an inhibitor of the aromatase enzyme, with an IC_{50} of 14 μM. This lignan was found to bind to, or near to, the active site of the aromatase, thereby competing with the androgen substrate of the enzyme.

A concept might be that naturally ubiquitous weak dietary oestrogens, in Asian and Mediterranean males, influence the pathogenesis of clinical BPH by directly inhibiting the growth-promoting effect of DHT and oestradiol-17β on the stromal tissue of their 'ageing' prostate glands.

Inhibition of tyrosine-specific protein kinases

Tyrosine kinases are necessary for the function of several growth factor receptors, including those for epidermal growth factor, platelet-derived growth factor, insulin and insulin-like growth factors.[90] In addition, several retroviral oncogenes, such as *src*, *abl*, *fps*, *yes*, *fes* and *ros*, code for tyrosine-specific protein kinases.[91] Tyrosine phosphorylation plays an important role in cell proliferation and cell transformation, and tyrosine kinase-specific inhibitors might be used as anticancer agents.[92,93] The isoflavonoid genistein has been shown to be a specific inhibitor of tyrosine kinase activity.[94] In addition, the flavonoids apigenin and kaempferol reverse the transformed phenotypes of v-H-*ras* NIH3T3 cells, an effect mediated via inhibition of tyrosine kinase.[95]

Furthermore, genistein induces apoptosis in human breast tumour cells,[96] inhibits invasion of murine mammary carcinoma cells[97] and enhances adhesion of endothelial cells.[98]

Inhibition of DNA topoisomerases

DNA topoisomerases are enzymes that alter the conformation of DNA and are crucial to cell division.[99] By a process involving strand cleavage, strand passage and religation, these enzymes are able to untangle supercoiled DNA. The soya-derived isoflavonoid genistein is a potent inhibitor of these enzymes and is considered to act by stabilization of a putative 'cleavable complex' between DNA and the topoisomerase enzyme.[100] The flavonoids quercetin fisetin and morin also inhibit DNA topoisomerases I and II, whereas kaempferol inhibits only DNA topoisomerase II.[101] Inhibition of topoisomerases is now the target for the design of new anticancer drugs. In addition, genistein is cytostatic, arresting cell cycle progression in G2-M;[102,103] it also induces apoptosis in immature human thymocytes by inhibiting DNA topoisomerase II.[100] The flavonoid apigenin induces morphological differentiation and G2-M arrest in rat neuronal cells.[104]

Inhibition of angiogenesis

Angiogenesis, or neovascularization, involves the generation of new capillaries, a process invoking the proliferation and migration of endothelial cells. Normally, the process is restricted to wound healing but it is also enhanced in association with cancer growth. Folkman and colleagues[105–107] report that new capillary blood vessels are necessary for a cancer to expand beyond 2 mm in size. Angiogenesis therefore exercises an important role in cancer progression and is essentially seen as the growth towards a focus of cancer of capillary sprouts and columns of endothelial cells from pre-existing capillaries. The process is probably promoted by the production of growth factors by the cancer cells, and fibroblast growth factor (FGF), or members of the FGF family, are recognized as potent angiogenic agents. Genistein inhibits angiogenesis and endothelial cell proliferation.[108] In wound healing, the process is regulated by a balance between angiogenic factors and restraining factors such as transforming growth factor-β. Blocking angiogenesis could inhibit cancer progression, and cortisone and heparin treatment has been reported to suppress the metastatic capacity of experimental tumours by this means;[106] significantly, genistein may have a similar influence. These effects may relate to the inhibition of the tyrosine-kinase associated FGF receptor.[94]

Antioxidant activity

Flavonoids, isoflavonoids and lignans are all polyphenolic compounds and can function as effective antioxidants and radical scavengers. Compounds such as quercetin and cyanidin have antioxidant potentials four times that of trolox, the vitamin E analogue. Removing the ortho-dihydroxy substitution, as in kaempferol for example, or reducing the 2,3 double bond in the C-ring, as in catechin or epicatechin, decreases the antioxidant activity by more than 50%, but these structures are still more effective than α-tocopherol or ascorbate.[109] In addition, flavonoids such as catechin inhibit the oxidation of low-density lipoprotein, an effect consistent with the ability of some flavonoids of similar structure to inhibit lipoxygenases.[110]

Inhibition of tumorigenesis

Soya-bean isoflavones and lignans inhibit experimental carcinogenesis in a wide variety of systems. Of 26 animal studies in which diets containing soy or soybean isoflavones were employed, 17 (65%) reported protective effects.[111] No studies reported that soy intake increased tumour development.

Many *in vitro* tumour model systems, including those for both breast and prostate cancers, are also growth inhibited by isoflavonoids and lignans.[112,113] Genistein and biochanin A, the precursor of genistein, inhibit in culture the growth of androgen-dependent and androgen-independent prostatic cancer cells.[113]

In addition, isoflavonoids and flavonoids inhibit the bioactivation of potent chemical carcinogens. Biochanin A inhibits the metabolic activation of benzo[a]pyrene,[114] and the flavonoid catechins from green and black tea inhibit the activation of the potent tobacco carcinogen 4-(methylnitrosoamino)-1-(3-pyridyl)-1-butanone and subsequent lung tumorigenesis in A/J mice.[115]

Conclusions

This chapter advances dietary factors as responsible for the differences in prostatic cancer incidence and mortality between East and West. The large amounts of isoflavonoids, flavonoids and lignans in the Asian and vegetarian diets and their specific properties may diminish carcinogenesis and suppress cancer of the prostate and other cancers also.

It remains to be determined whether these isoflavonoids, flavonoids and lignans exercise their biological effect as antioxidants, antioestrogens or, indeed, as weak oestrogens. Tamoxifen, as a weak oestrogen, can effectively suppress early breast cancer lesions; concomitantly, as an oestrogen, it can provide a beneficial influence with regard to cardiovascular disease and osteoporosis in women. Hormone replacement therapy, which is essentially low-dose oestrogen therapy, controls menopausal problems, such as hot flushes, and provides longer-term benefits in restraining cardiovascular disease and osteoporosis. It is noteworthy that menopausal Japanese women have a lower frequency of hot flushes than their Western counterparts,[116] presumably because of their soya-based diet and its weak oestrogen content.

Whereas there are these benefits, and others, for the menopausal and post-menopausal woman from such dietary intervention, there might be concern among men regarding the possible occurrence of undesirable side effects, for example feminization phenomena, from these weak oestrogenic influences. Such fears are natural but are reassuringly answerable by the absence of such phenomena in the vast male population of Asia consuming, life long, a traditional soya diet. There is ample evidence that the traditionally eating Asian male lives all aspects of a healthy male life and is abundantly fertile, while at the same time enjoying a significantly reduced risk of prostatic malignancy as well as other benefits, already noted, that may well be linked with his dietary habits.

References

1. Silverberg E, Boring C C, Squires T S. Cancer statistics. CA 1990; 40: 9–26
2. Zaridze D G, Boyle P, Smans M. International trends in prostatic cancer. Int J Cancer 1984; 33: 223–230
3. Sondik E. Incidence. survival and mortality trends in prostate cancer in the United States. In: Coffey D S, Resnick M I, Dorr F A, Karr J P (eds) A multidisciplinary analysis of controversies in the management of prostate cancer. New York: Plenum Press,1988: 9–16
4. Dhom G. Epidemiology of hormone-dependent tumors. In: Voigt K D, Knabbe C (eds) Endocrine dependent tumors. New York: Raven Press, 1991: 1–42

5. Boyle P. Evolution of an epidemic of unknown origin. In: Denis L (ed) Prostate cancer 2000. European School of Oncology Monograph. Heidelberg: Springer Verlag, 1994: 5–11
6. Boring C C, Squires T S, Tong T. Cancer statistics. CA 1994; 44: 7–26
7. Muir C S, Waterhouse J A H, Mack T et al. (eds) Cancer incidence in five continents. In: Volume V, IARC Scientific Publications No. 88. Lyon: IARC, 1987
8. Armstrong B E, Doll R. Environmental factors and cancer incidence and mortality in different countries with special reference to dietary practices. Int J Cancer 1975; 15: 617–631
9. Breslow N, Chan C E, Dhom G et al. Latent carcinoma of the prostate at autopsy in seven areas. Int J Cancer 1977; 20: 680–688
10. Zaridze D G, Boyle P. Cancer of the prostate: epidemiology and aetiology. Br J Urol 1987; 59: 493–503
11. Skeet R G. Epidemiology of urological tumours. In: Williams D I, Chisolm G D (eds) Scientific foundations of urology, Vol.II. London: William Heineman Medical Books, 1976: 199–211
12. Miller G J. Diagnosis of stage A prostatic cancer in the People's Republic of China. In: Coffey D S, Resnick M I, Dorr F A, Karr J P (eds) A multidisciplinary analysis of controversies in the management of prostate cancer. New York: Plenum Press, 1988: 17–24
13. Parkin D M, Muir C S, Whelan S et al. (eds) Cancer incidence in five continents. In: Volume VI, IARC Scientific Publications No. 120. Lyon: IARC, 1992
14. Boyle P, Levi F, Lucchini F, La Vecchia C. Trends in diet-related cancers in Japan: a conundrum. Lancet 1993; 342: 752
15. Haenzel W, Kurihara M. Studies of Japanese migrants. I. Mortality from cancer and other diseases among Japanese in the United States. J Natl Cancer Inst 1968; 40: 43–68
16. Shimizu H, Ropp R K, Bernstein L et al. Cancers of the breast and prostate among Japanese and white immigrants in Los Angeles County. Br J Cancer 1991; 63: 963–966
17. Ekman P. BPH epidemiology and risk factors. Prostate 1989; suppl 2: 23–33
18. Isaacs J T, Coffey D. Etiology and disease process of benign prostatic hyperplasia. Prostate 1989; suppl 2: 33–50
19. Adlercreutz H. Western diet and Western diseases: some hormonal and biochemical mechanisms and associations. Scand J Clin Lab Invest 1990; 50 (suppl 201): 3–23
20. Slavin J L. Epidemiological evidence for the impact of whole grains on health. CRC Crit Rev Food Sci Nutr 1994; 34: 427–434
21. Trock B, Lanza E, Greenwald P. Dietary fibre, vegetables, and colon cancer: critical review and meta-analysis of the epidemiologic evidence. J Natl Cancer Inst 1990; 82: 650–661
22. Macquart-Moulin G, Riboli E, Cornee J et al. Case–control study on colorectal cancer and diet in Marseilles. Int J Cancer 1986; 38: 183–191
23. Steinmetz K, Potter J. Vegetables, fruit and cancer. I. Epidemiology. Cancer Causes Control 1991; 2: 325–357
24. Steinmetz K, Potter J. Vegetables, fruit and cancer. II. Mechanisms. Cancer Causes Control 1991; 2: 427–442
25. Ingram D M, Nottage E, Roberts T. The role of diet in the development of breast cancer: a case–control study of patients with breast cancer, benign epithelial hyperplasia and fibrocystic disease of the breast. Br J Cancer 1991; 641: 187–191
26. Wynder E L, Mabuchi K, Whitmore W F. Epidemiology of cancer of the prostate. Cancer 1971; 28: 344–360
27. Boyle P, Zaridze D G. Risk factors for prostate and testicular cancer. Eur J Cancer 1993; 29A: 1048–1055
28. Giovannucci E, Rimm E B, Colditz G A et al. A prospective study of dietary fat and risk of prostate cancer. J Natl Cancer Inst 1993; 85: 1571–1579
29. Mills P K, Beeson W L, Phillips R L, Frazer G E. Cohort study of diet, lifestyle and prostate cancer in Adventist men. Cancer 1989 ; 64: 598–604
30. Le Marchand L, Kolonel L, Wilkens L R et al. Animal fat consumption and prostate cancer: a prospective study in Hawaii. Epidemiology 1994; 5: 276–282
31. Severson R K, Nomura A M, Grove A S, Stemmerman G N. A prospective study of demographics, diet and prostate cancer among men of Japanese ancestry in Hawaii. Cancer Res 1989 49: 1857–1860
32. Stemmerman G N, Nomura A M, Heilbrun L K. Cancer risk in relation to fat and energy intake among Hawaii Japanese: a prospective study. Int Symp Princess Takamatsu Cancer Res Fund 1985; 16: 265–274
33. Kolonel L N, Hankin J H, Nomura A M, Chu S Y. Dietary fat intake and cancer incidence among five ethnic groups in Hawaii. Cancer Res 1981; 41: 3727–3728

34. Whittemore A S, Wu A H, Kolonel L N *et al.* Family history and prostate cancer risk in black, white and Asian men in the United States and Canada. Am J Epidemiol 1995; 141: 732–740

35. Kroes R, Beems R B, Bosland M C *et al.* Nutritional factors in lung, colon and prostate cancer in animal models. Fed Proc 1986; 45: 136–141

36. Simopoulos A P. Nutritional cancer risks derived from energy and fat. Med Oncol Tumor Pharmacother 1987; 4: 227–239

37. Hirayama T. A large scale cohort study on cancer risks by diet — with special reference to the risk reducing effects of green–yellow vegetable consumption. In: Hayashi Y *et al.* (eds) Diet, nutrition and cancer. Tokyo: Japan Sci. Soc. Press Utrecht: VNU Sci. Press, 1986: 41–53

38. Hirayama T. Epidemiology of prostate cancer with special reference to the role of diet. Natl Cancer Inst Monogr 1979; 3: 149–155

39. Hirayama T. Life-style and cancer: from epidemiological evidence to public behavior change to mortality reduction of target cancers. Natl Cancer Inst Monogr 1992; 12: 65–74

40. Lee H P, Gourley L, Duffy S W *et al.* Dietary effects on breast cancer risk in Singapore. Lancet 1991; 337: 1197–1200

41. Setchell K D R, Adlercreutz H. Mammalian lignans and phytooestrogens. Recent studies on their formation, metabolism and biological role in health and disease. In: Rowland I R (ed) Role of gut flora in toxicity and cancer. London: Academic Press, 1988: 315–345

42. Kodama M, Kodama T. Interrelation between Western type cancers and non-Western type cancers as regards their risk variations in time and space. II Nutrition and cancer risk. Anticancer Res 1990; 10: 1043–1049

43. Rose D P, Boyar A P, Wynder E L. International comparisons of mortality rates for cancer of the breast, ovary, prostate and colon and per capita food consumption. Cancer 1986; 58: 2363–2371

44. Block G, Patterson B, Subar A. Fruit, vegetables and cancer prevention: a review of the epidemiological evidence. Nutr Cancer 1996; 18: 1–29

45. Negri E, La Vecchia C, Franceschi S *et al.* The role of vegetables and fruit in cancer risk. In: Hill M J, Giacosa A, Caygill C P J (eds) Epidemiology of diet and cancer. Chichester: Ellis Horwood, 1994: 327–334

46. Buiatti E, Palli D, De Carli A *et al.* A case–control study of gastric cancer and diet in Italy. Int J Cancer 1989; 44: 611–616

47. Buatti E, Palli D, De Carli A *et al.* A case–control study of gastric cancer and diet in Italy. II. Association with nutrients. Int J Cancer 1990; 45: 896–901

48. La Vecchia C, De Carli A, Negri E, Parazzini F. Epidemiological aspects of diet and cancer: a summary review of case–control studies from Northern Italy. Oncology 1988; 45: 364–370

49. Miksicek R J. Commonly occurring plant flavonoids have estrogenic activity. Mol Pharmacol 1993; 44: 37–43

50. Bradbury R B, White D C. Oestrogens and related substances in plants. Vitam Horm 1954; 12: 207–233

51. Price K R, Fenwick G R. Naturally occurring oestrogens in food — a review. Fd Add Contam 1985; 2: 73–106

52. Verdeal K, Brown R R, Richardson T, Ryan D S. Affinity of phytoestrogens for estradiol-binding proteins and effect of coumestrol on growth of 7,12-dimethylbenz(a)anthracene-induced rat mammary tumors. J Natl Cancer Inst 1980; 64: 285–290

53. Axelson M, Sjovall J, Gustafsson B E, Setchell K D R. A dietary source of the non-steroidal oestrogen equol in man and animals. J Endocrinol 1984; 102: 49–56

54. Walz E. Isoflavon-und Sapogenin-Glucoside in Sojahispida. Justus Liebigs Annln Chem 1931; 489: 118–155

55. Coward L, Barnes N C, Setchell K D R, Barnes S. Genistein, daidzein, and their β-glycoside conjugates: antitumor isoflavones in soybean foods from American and Asian diets. J Agric Food Chem 1993; 41: 1961–1967

56. Rao C B S (ed) The chemistry of lignans. Waltair, India: Andra University Press and Publications, 1978: 1–377

57. Thompson L U, Robb P, Serraino M, Cheung F. Mammalian lignan production from various foods. Nutr Cancer 1991; 16: 43–52

58. Kelly G E, Nelson C, Waring M A *et al.* Metabolites of dietary (soya) isoflavones in human urine. Clin Chim Acta 1993; 223: 9–22

59. Adlercreutz H, Fotsis T, Bannwart C *et al.* Determination of urinary lignans and phytoestrogen metabolites, potential antiestrogens and anticarcinogens, in urine of women on various habitual diets. J Steroid Biochem 1986; 25: 791–797

60. Morton M S, Wilcox G, Wahlquvist M L, Griffiths K. Determination of lignans and isoflavonoids in human female plasma following dietary supplementation. J Endocrinol 1994; 142: 251–259

61. Finlay E M H, Wilson D W, Adlercreutz H, Griffiths K. The identification and measurement of 'phyto-oestrogens' in human saliva, plasma, breast aspirate or cyst fluid, and prostatic fluid using gas chromatography–mass spectrometry. J Endocrinol 1991; 129(suppl): 49

62. Dehennin L, Reiffsteck A, Joudet M, Thibier M. Identification and quantitative estimation of a lignan in human and bovine semen. J Reprod Fertil 1982; 66: 305–309

63. Adlercreutz H, Honjo H, Higashi A et al. Urinary excretion of lignans and isoflavonoid phytoestrogens in Japanese men and women consuming traditional Japanese diet. Am J Clin Nutr 1991; 54: 1093–1100

64. Adlercreutz H, Markkanen H, Watanabe S. Plasma concentrations of phyto-oestrogens in Japanese men. Lancet 1993; 342: 1209–1210

65. Setchell K D R, Borriello S P, Hulme P et al. Nonsteroidal oestrogens of dietary origin: possible roles in hormone-dependent disease. Am J Clin Nutr 1984; 40: 569–578

66. Pope G S, Wright H G. Oestrogenic isoflavones in red clover and subterranean clover. Chem Ind 1954: 1019–1020

67. Bickoff E M. Estrogen-like substances in plants. In: Hissaw F L (ed) Physiology of reproduction. Proc. 22nd Animal Biology Colloquium. Corvallis: Oregon State Univ. Press, 1961: 93–118

68. Waters A P, Knowler J T. Effect of a lignan (HPMF) on RNA synthesis in the rat uterus. J Reprod Fertil 1982; 66: 379–381

69. Martin P M, Horwitz K B, Ryan D S, McGuire W L. Phytoestrogen interaction with estrogen receptors in human breast cancer cells. Endocrinology 1978; 103: 1860–1867

70. Adlercreutz H, Hockerstedt K, Bannwart C et al. Effect of dietary components, including lignans and phytoestrogens on enterohepatic circulation and liver metabolism of estrogens and on sex hormone binding globulin (SHBG). J Steroid Biochem 1987; 27: 1135–1144

71. Cunha G R, Chung L W K, Shannon J M et al. Hormone-induced morphogenesis and growth: role of mesenchymal–epithelial interaction. Recent Prog Horm Res 1983; 39: 559–595

72. Griffiths K, Davies P, Eaton C L et al. Endocrine factors in the initiation, diagnosis and treatment of prostatic cancer. In: Voigt K D, Knabbe C (eds) Endocrine dependent tumors. New York: Raven Press,1991: 83–130

73. Coffey D S. In: Khoury S, Chatelain C, Murphy G, Denis L (eds) The structure and function of the prostate gland and sex accessory tissues in prostate cancer. Paris: FIIS Publ, 1990: 70–103

74. Griffiths K, Davies P, Eaton C L et al. Cancer of the prostate: Endocrine factors. In: Clark J R (ed) Oxford reviews of reproductive biology, Vol. 9. Oxford: Clarendon Press, 1987: 192–259

75. Vermeulen A, Rubens R, Verdonck L. Testosterone secretion and metabolism in male senescence. J Clin Endocrinol Metab 1972; 34: 730–735

76. Rubens R, Dhont M, Vermeulen A. Further studies on Leydig cell function in old age. J Clin Endocrinol Metab 1974; 39: 40–45

77. Vermeulen A, van Camp A, Mattelaer J, De Sy W. Hormonal factors related to abnormal growth of the prostate. In: Coffey D S, Isaacs J T (eds) Prostate cancer. UICC Technical Workshop Series, Vol. 48. Geneva: UICC 1979: 81–92

78. Belanger A, Locong A, Noel C et al. Influence of diet on plasma steroids and sex hormone-binding globulin levels in adult men. J Steroid Biochem 1989; 32: 829–833

79. Vermeulen A. Metabolic effects of obesity in men. Verh K Acad Geneeskd Belg 1993; 55: 393–397

80. Griffiths K, Akaza H, Eaton C L et al. Regulation of prostatic growth. In: Cockett A T K, Khoury S, Aso Y et al. (eds) 2nd International Consultation on Benign Prostatic Hyperplasia (BPH). Paris: S.C.I., 1993: 49–75

81. Bruchovsky N, Wilson J D. The conversion of testosterone to 5-alpha-androstan-17-beta-ol-3-one by rat prostate in vivo and in vitro. J Biol Chem 1968; 243: 2012–2021

82. Bruchovsky N, Wilson J D. The intranuclear binding of testosterone and 5-alpha-androstan-17-beta-ol-3-one by rat prostate. J Biol Chem 1968; 243: 5953–5960

83. Anderson K H, Liao S. Selective retention of dihydrotestosterone by prostatic nuclei. Nature 1968; 219: 277–279

84. Evans B A J, Griffiths K, Morton M. Inhibition of 5α-reductase and 17β-hydroxysteroid dehydrogenase in genital skin fibroblasts by dietary lignans and isoflavonoids. J Endocrinol 1995; 147: 295–302

85. Ross R K, Bernstein L, Lobo R A et al. 5-Alpha-reductase activity and risk of prostate cancer among Japanese and US white and black males. Lancet 1992; 339: 887–889

86. Rittmaster R S. Finasteride. N Engl J Med 1994; 330: 120–125

87. Vermeulen A. Testicular hormone secretion and aging in males. In: Grayshack J T, Wilson J D, Saherbenske M J (eds) Benign prostatic hyperplasia. DHEW Publ. No. (NIH)76–1113. National Institutes of Health, 1976: 177–182

88. Vermeulen A, Deslypere J P, Meirleir K. A new look to the andropause: altered function of the gonadotrophs. J Steroid Biochem 1989; 32: 163–165

89. Adlercreutz H, Bannwart C, Wahala K et al. Inhibition of human aromatase by mammalian lignans and isoflavonoid phytoestrogens. J Steroid Biochem Mol Biol 1993; 44: 147–153

90. Hunter T, Cooper J A. Protein tyrosine kinases. Annu Rev Biochem 1985; 54: 897–930

91. Bishop J M. Cellular oncogenes and retroviruses. Annu Rev Biochem 1985; 52: 301–354

92. Schlessinger J, Schreiber A B, Levi A et al. Regulation of cell proliferation by epidermal growth factor. CRC Crit Rev Biochem 1983; 14: 93–111

93. Kenyon G L, Garcia G A. Design of kinase inhibitors. Med Res Rev 1987; 7: 389–416

94. Akiyama T, Ishida J, Nakagawa S et al. Genistein, a specific inhibitor of tyrosine-specific protein kinases. J Biol Chem 1987; 262: 5592–5595

95. Kuo M L, Lin J K, Huang T S, Yang N C. Reversion of the transformed phenotypes of v-H-ras NIH3T3 cells by flavonoids through attenuating the content of phosphotyrosine. Cancer Lett 1994; 87: 91–97

96. Kiguchi K, Glesne D, Chubb C H et al. Differential induction of apoptosis in human breast cells by okadaic acid and related inhibitors of protein phosphatases 1 and 2A. Cell Growth Differentiation 1994; 5: 995–1004

97. Scholar E M, Toews M L. Inhibition of invasion of murine mammary carcinoma cells by the tyrosine kinase inhibitor genistein. Cancer Lett 1994; 87: 159–162

98. Tiisala S, Majuri M L, Carpen O, Renkonen R. Genistein enhances the ICAM-mediated adhesion by inducing the expression of ICAM-1 and its counter receptors. Biochem Biophys Res Commun 1994; 203: 443–449

99. Cummings J, Smyth J F. DNA topoisomerase I and II as targets for rational design of new anticancer drugs. Ann Oncol 1993; 4: 533–543

100. McCabe M J Jr, Orrenius S. Genistein induces apoptosis in immature human thymocytes by inhibiting topoisomerase-II. Biochem Biophys Res Commun 1993; 194: 944–950

101. Constantinou A, Mehta R, Runyan C et al. Flavonoids as DNA topoisomerase antagonists and poisons: structure–activity relationships. J Nat Prod 1995; 58: 217–225

102. Spinozzi F, Pagliacci M C, Migliorati G et al. The natural tyrosine kinase inhibitor genistein produces cell cycle arrest and apoptosis in Jurkat T-leukemia cells. Leuk Res 1994; 18: 431–439

103. Matsukawa Y, Marui N, Sakai T et al. Genistein arrests cell cycle progression at G2-M. Cancer Res 1993; 53: 1328–1331

104. Sato F, Matsukawa Y, Matsumoto K et al. Apigenin induces morphological differentiation and G-2M arrest in rat neuronal cells. Biochem Biophys Res Commun 1994; 204: 578–584

105. Folkman J, Watson K, Ingber D, Hanahan D. Induction of angiogenesis during the transition from hyperplasia to neoplasia. Nature 1989; 339: 58–61

106. Folkman J. Toward an understanding of angiogenesis: search and discovery. Perspect Biol Med 1985; 29: 10–36

107. Weidner M, Semple JP, Welch WR, Folkman J. Tumour angiogenesis and metaplasia— correlation in invasive breast cancer. N Engl J Med 1991; 324: 1–8

108. Fotsis T, Pepper M, Adlercreutz H et al. Genistein, a dietary-derived inhibitor of in vitro angiogenesis. Proc Natl Acad Sci USA 1993; 90: 2690–2694

109. Rice-Evans C A, Miller N J, Bolwell P G et al. The relative antioxidant activities of plant-derived polyphenolic flavonoids. Free Radic Res Commun 1995; 22: 375–383

110. Mangiapane H, Thomson J, Salter A et al. The inhibition of the oxidation of low density lipoprotein by (+)-catechin, a naturally occurring flavonoid. Biochem Pharmacol 1992; 43: 445–450

111. Messina M J, Persky V, Setchell K D R, Barnes S. Soy intake and cancer risk: a review of the in vitro and in vivo data. Nutr Cancer 1994; 21: 113–130

112. Peterson G, Barnes S. Genistein inhibition of the growth of human breast cancer cells: independence from estrogen receptors and the multi-drug resistant gene. Biochem Biophys Res Commun 1991; 179: 661–667

113. Peterson G, Barnes S. Genistein and biochanin A inhibit the growth of human prostate cancer cells but not epidermal growth factor receptor tyrosine autophosphorylation. Prostate 1993; 22: 335–345

114. Chae Y H, Ho D K, Cassady J M *et al*. Effects of synthetic and naturally occurring flavonoids on metabolic activation of benzo[a]pyrene in hamster cell cultures. Chem Biol Interact 1992; 82: 181–193

115. Shi S T, Wang Z Y, Smith T J *et al*. Effects of green tea and black tea on 4-(methylnitrosoamino)-1-(3-pyridyl)-1-butanone bioactivation, DNA methylation and lung tumorigenesis in A/J mice. Cancer Res 1994; 54: 4641–4647

116. Adlercreutz H, Hamalainen E, Gorbach S, Goldin B. Dietary phyto-oestrogens and the menopause in Japan. Lancet 1992; 339: 1233

Chapter 39
Charity support for prostate cancer

J. Mossman and M. Boudioni

Introduction

Although prostate cancer is the second most common cause of cancer death for men (second to lung cancer), with over 9000 deaths per year in the United Kingdom, very few men (or women) know anything about the prostate, what it does and where it is sited in the body. A diagnosis of prostate cancer suddenly thrusts patients, and those who care for them, into a 'need to know' situation. This is not least because the treatments for prostate cancer can have unwanted effects that many men find absolutely devastating and, added to the anxiety of finding they have cancer, they are faced with difficult decisions about what treatment — if any — to have.

A diagnosis of cancer usually comes as a terrible shock, resulting in the patient feeling isolated and leaving him, his family and friends uncertain about what to expect. Many patients want to know as much as possible about their disease and its treatment and it is well recognized that accurate information helps patients and their families cope better with the disease and plan their lives appropriately.[1,2] Being well informed does not mean having every bit of information, however awful, thrust at the patient as soon as he has been given his diagnosis; rather, it means the provision of information in an appropriate and timely fashion.[3]

BACUP

BACUP (British Association of Cancer United Patients, their relatives and friends) is a voluntary organization that provides information to anyone whose life is affected by cancer. It was set up in 1984 by a young doctor, Vicky Clement-Jones, who had ovarian cancer. At that time there were few sources of information about the realities of living with cancer. Vicky Clement-Jones eloquently described the difficulty of 'trying to lead as normal a life as possible and at the same time contending with going out for a meal and watching one's hair falling out into the minestrone'. She quickly realized that patients and their families could cope with their disease and its treatment when they knew what to expect.[4] Advance knowledge of treatment side effects and how to deal with them allowed people to plan their lives accordingly. There is now some evidence that patients who are well informed about their illness and its treatment fare better, perhaps because they comply better with a treatment for which they understand the need.[5]

Before Vicky Clement-Jones established BACUP, she consulted health professionals, other cancer charities, patients and the Health Departments about the need for such an organization. This widespread consultation ensured that BACUP would have the support of the medical profession and was key to making it an organization to which health professionals would refer their patients. It has also meant that the health professionals are willing to help BACUP by providing accurate and up-to-date information.

Since 1984, the services that BACUP provides have developed considerably. A major element is the provision of information, either written or verbal. There are over 50 booklets on different types of cancer and different treatments, and on aspects of living with cancer. There are also fact-sheets on the less common tumour types and on specific treatments. In the year March 1995 to April 1996, about one-quarter of a million booklets were distributed and the specialist cancer nurses answered over 40,000 enquiries. These enquiries ranged from questions about treatment, to how to get the appropriate social security benefits, to how to find a company that will provide travel insurance. BACUP also provides face-to-face counselling services, currently available in London and in Glasgow.

Clive Bourne, who set up the Prostate Cancer Research Trust as a result of his personal experience of prostate cancer, several years ago wrote: 'Some $3^1/2$ years ago I was diagnosed as suffering from prostate cancer at a stage at which it had already spread to the lymph glands... Being of an enquiring mind, I have of course devoted a considerable portion of my spare time activity to reading and discussions with the medical fraternity.' This attitude — the need to find out about the disease and all the ramifications of being a cancer patient — is a common response of many cancer patients. But, it is not only patients who need to know what is happening: relatives and friends can be equally confused and in need of advice and support. Patients have access to health care professionals; relatives and friends usually do not have such a direct route to help. Because the relatives and friends of a patient play a crucial role in providing support, BACUP's services are available to carers in the widest sense as well as to patients. All BACUP's services are free to patients, their families and friends.

Who uses a support charity?

Data (demographic, tumour site, purpose of call, advice given) are collected from every fifth information enquiry, enabling a profile of the characteristics and needs of patients and their carers to be defined.

Of the 40,000 plus enquiries to BACUP in 1995–96, 2360 (some 6%) were about prostate cancer; in the same period, 28% were concerning breast cancer. (The 1988 incidence in the UK of prostate and breast cancers, respectively, were 13,974 and 30,075.[6] Since the majority of people who contact BACUP are female, it is perhaps not surprising that breast cancer is responsible for proportionately more users; one can speculate that this bias reflects a society in which, traditionally, women are the carers.) The percentage of enquiries relating to prostate cancer is slightly higher than would be expected from the incidence (the observed:expected ratio among BACUP users is 1.16).

For all cancers, the male:female ratio of users is about 1:4; for prostate cancer it is about 1:1, a very different profile. The percentages of patients and of relatives and friends in general are 36 and 46%, whereas for prostate cancer they are 40 and 48%, respectively. This increase in calls from patients may be because they have a greater need for information than do other cancer patients. It is often said that prostate cancer patients are reluctant to talk to families and friends about their illness, but this is not borne out by the high percentage of carers who call BACUP. Another aspect in which prostate cancer callers differ from the profile of callers in general is in the age profile (Table 39.1): it can be seen that the percentage of callers over 60 years is substantially greater for prostate cancer calls than for other cancers.

Table 39.1. Age breakdown for enquiries to BACUP

	Prostate cancer		All cancers	
Age (years)	All enquirers* (%)	Patients (%)	All enquirers* (%)	Patients (%)
< 29	1.9	–	6.4	3.3
30–39	13.8	1.7	21.6	13.6
40–49	14.9	1.7	26.2	25.0
50–59	20.5	17.4	23.1	28.7
60+	49.0	79.2	22.6	29.4

*Excludes calls from health professionals and students, worried, well etc.

The profile of callers in relation to social class shows no difference between all cancer and prostate cancer enquiries. However, for employment status there is a difference: 65% are employed and 14% retired for all cancer enquiries, compared with 50% and 36%, respectively for prostate cancer. Some of this difference may result from the fact that slightly more patients than other categories call about prostate cancer than call in general.

What information do patients want?

People who use BACUP's services confirm that doctors, nurses and other hospital staff often do not have the time to discuss in detail information about the disease and its emotional impact. Even when they do, it is often difficult for patients to take in everything that is said and explained to them. In a recent survey of the impact of a booklet produced by the Royal College of Surgeons on prostate surgery, one patient replied 'Doctors and surgeons talk in a language of their own and they talk quickly and you have to take everything in so fast and at the end you are lost because 80% of what he has been saying to you, you don't understand.'[7]

It is to allow people to access and digest information at their own pace that BACUP produces a range of written information. *Understanding Cancer of the Prostate*[8] is intended to provide the general information that is relevant to any patient diagnosed with prostate cancer and is equally relevant to relatives and friends. There is an explanation of the site, size and function of the prostate and the symptoms of prostate cancer. The diagnostic tests and the types of treatment that may be used are described. After recent consultation with cancer patients (who are becoming more articulate in their search for information), the booklet includes a table describing the unwanted effects that the treatments can produce (Table 39.2). Doctors usually term these 'side effects' but patients who have suffered them consider that this description significantly undervalues the effect they can have on quality-of-life.

The medical aspects of prostate cancer are only part of what patients have to face. There are difficult emotional issues to deal with, such as fear (Am I going to die? Will I be in pain?), blame and guilt (If I hadn't ... this would never have happened) and anger (Why me? And why now?). Some patients find it hard to talk about their illness, and relatives and friends often find it hard to talk to the patient about the illness and their worries. Talking to children can be difficult also. All these aspects are covered in *Understanding Cancer of the Prostate*; in addition, BACUP has separate booklets on these topics that go into greater detail.

Any booklet that is produced for widespread dissemination must, of necessity, be fairly general. Every patient, though, will be different, facing specific problems

Table 39.2. Unwanted effects* of treatment for prostate cancer

Unwanted effects of treatments for prostate cancer — short-term

	TUR	Total prostatectomy	Radiotherapy	Hormone therapy
Urinary incontinence	0	3	1	0
Impotence	0	3	3	3
Diarrhoea/ bowel problems	0	1	2	1
Bladder symptoms	3	3	2	0
Hot flushes	0	0	0	3
Tiredness/ lack of energy	1	1	1	2
Weight gain	0	0	0	0
Sore skin	0	0	3	0

Unwanted effects of treatments for prostate cancer — long-term

	TUR	Total prostatectomy	Radiotherapy	Hormone therapy
Urinary incontinence	0	2	1	0
Impotence	1	3	2	3
Diarrhoea/ bowel problems	0	1	1	1
Bladder symptoms	0	1	1	0
Hot flushes	0	0	0	3
Tiredness/ lack of energy	0	0	0	3
Weight gain	0	0	0	2

*Key:
0 = no effect;
1 = rare effect (less than 10% of people treated);
2 = possible effect (up to 40% of people treated);
3 = common effect (more than 40% of people treated).
(Reproduced from ref. 8 with permission.)

and having individual needs. It is to meet these needs that BACUP has specialist cancer nurses providing an information service. Of the people who used this service, 62% of the people who called about prostate cancer asked about issues relating to treatment and 80% asked about more general aspects or wanted support and reassurance; the corresponding figures for all cancers were 54% and 74%, respectively. (It must be noted that callers can have many queries and up to six can be recorded per caller.)

Looking at these enquiries in relation to prostate cancer in a little more detail (Table 39.3), 24% asked about hormonal therapy and 17% asked about radiotherapy; 19% asked about treatment side effects in general and 12% wanted information on prognosis. Over 42% of callers wanted information about prostate cancer itself and 26% wanted clarification of information they had already been given or had found for themselves; 14% of callers wanted advice on how to communicate with their health professional and 11% on how to communicate with family and friends. Nearly 47% of callers contacted BACUP for emotional support and reassurance. Issues related to sex and sexuality were the subject of 4% of calls; although this may seem low, it is relatively high compared to the less than 1% of calls on the subject from all callers.

Table 39.3. The main enquiries* made by patients and their carers in relation to prostate cancer

Topic of enquiry	Percentage of callers
General treatment	11.7
Surgery	8.3
Radiotherapy	16.9
Chemotherapy	3.2
Hormonal therapy	23.7
Treatment side effects	19.3
Prognosis	11.9
Pain control	9.3
Emotional support/reassurance	46.8
Health professional communications	14.0
Personal/family/friends communications	10.6
Information clarification	26.3
Site-specific information	42.2
Sexuality/sexual problems	4.2

*Up to six items can be coded as subject of enquiry for each person.

Many patients want to be put in touch with other patients who have gone through the same illness, and BACUP can provide contact names and telephone numbers for local self-help and support groups. There are some organizations that deal with prostate cancer only, and BACUP keeps information on these.

What other help can BACUP provide?

In the London and Glasgow offices, face-to-face counselling is available. This is available for those on whom the impact of cancer is such that information is not enough. Counselling can help untangle some of the difficulties and confusion that living with cancer — either for the patient or for a carer — can bring. Patients often find it easier to talk through these difficulties with someone who is independent rather than someone who is close to them. The counselling is short term and is provided by trained counsellors.

BACUP also offers some group counselling and in 1995 ran a prostate counselling group. Since the group completed their counselling with a BACUP counsellor, they have continued to meet as a support group in the BACUP offices. Not unexpectedly, one of the group died and the tribute to him, written by Angus Earnshaw another of the group, is reproduced below.

> Roy Bird was a rare bird,
> bright eyed
> always chirpy
> owl-wise and eagle-eyed
> brooked no condescension from consultants
> nor any prevarication in the group
> mischievous,
> his cheeky chuckle kept us amused
> and ever hopeful
> when he could attend no more we missed him sorely
> always kept an empty chair for our brother in affliction
> we had shared our anger and our grief, bitterness
> determination to be treated with dignity
> and allowed to make or own decisions about our illness
> we shared too our achievements

in accepting the mutilations resulting from our therapies
in fighting back, in comforting one another
now you've left us Roy
may your flight be safe and sure

fare you well

How do people find out about charities such as BACUP?

For most cancer sites, the major source of information about BACUP was from health professionals (24%), whereas for prostate cancer 24% of BACUP users found out about it via the media and 17% from health professionals. Relatives and friends were the source for 19% of all cancer users and 17% of prostate cancer users.

Are charities such as BACUP really needed?

It is often said that if the NHS was doing its job properly, organizations such as BACUP would not be needed. This may be a useful opening gambit for a conversation but it is an invalid assumption.

Many people will have a worry or doubt, at a time that they are at home or at work and do not have an appointment with their doctor for some time. Often, the doubt will be about something that the doctor said and the caller will want to consult someone independent. As one consultant clinical oncologist said, 'I encourage my patients to call BACUP. It's like getting an independent second opinion.' It can be difficult for patients to ask a question that might be thought of as 'challenging' the advice the doctor gave them, and they are reluctant to ask for fear it will alter the way they are treated. BACUP, being independent, can answer their questions openly and honestly without any risk of recrimination.

Health care professionals, however caring and supportive, rarely have the time to sit down and explain everything that might be relevant. They have to make assumptions about what patients want to know and structure their information accordingly. Unfortunately, they are not always correct in their assumptions and do not always use terminology that is readily understood by the lay person.

Further, a patient or carer may need practical information and advice. This might be related to a whole range of issues that crop up between hospital visits, or it may not seem appropriate — or important enough — to ask a doctor or nurse. Sometimes it will be about how to cope with the side effects of treatment and the patient may not have understood what to expect or how to minimize the problems. Although the NHS increasingly recognizes the importance of information, it is not set up to function as an information service.

Conclusions

In the past, the paternalistic attitude of doctors meant that patients often were not told that they had cancer. In 1961, in the United States, a study showed that 90% of surgeons would not routinely discuss a diagnosis of cancer with their patients.[9] Recently, a survey of 250 cancer patients in Glasgow demonstrated that 79% of patients wanted as much information as possible and 96% had a need or an absolute need to know if they had cancer.[7] Most patients wanted to know about the chance of cure and about the side effects of treatment. Although the patients in the survey showed a strong preference for being given the diagnosis by a hospital doctor, the experience at BACUP is that patients need to hear the same information over and over again, and in different ways, for them to really understand it. They also need to hear the information in the type of language they themselves use, and BACUP's nurses are trained to communicate in everyday language.

Although there is an increasing interest among the general public in knowing about the early diagnosis of cancer and where to get the best treatment, there is a real dilemma about widely disseminating information about a serious disease such as cancer to the general public. Each time that there is a media 'splash' about some aspect of cancer, the phone lines at BACUP are overwhelmed by the worried well, often preventing those who are affected by cancer from getting through to a source of help. There needs to be a much more responsible attitude among journalists about the way that information on cancer is presented (avoiding headlines, such as 'The Cancer Lottery', which raise alarm but do little to inform patients about how to get the best treatment).

However — perhaps more importantly — steps need to be taken to ensure that patients have access to the information and support they need. Although the recent changes in the provision of cancer care in England and Wales lay great emphasis on improving the medical aspects of cancer treatment, little, if any, provision is made for information and emotional support. Monies must be made available for information to be distributed to patients and their carers (at the time of diagnosis and at other relevant stages in the progress of the disease) to help them cope with a diagnosis of prostate cancer and the day-to-day aspects of living with cancer.

References

1. Meredith C, Symonds P, Webster L et al. Information needs of cancer patients in west Scotland: cross sectional survey of patients' views. Br Med J 1996; 313: 724–726
2. Audit Commission. What seems to be the matter? Communication between hospitals and patients. NHS report No 12. London: HMSO, 1993
3. BACUP. The Right to Know: a BACUP guide to information and support for people living with cancer. London: November 1995
4. Clement-Jones V. Cancer and beyond: the formation of BACUP. Br Med J 1985; 291: 1021–1023
5. Fallowfield L J, Hall A, Maguire G P. Effects of breast conservation on psychological morbidity associated with diagnosis and treatment of early breast cancer. Br Med J 1986; 293: 1331–1334
6. CRC Factsheet 1: UK Incidence. Cancer Research Campaign, 1994
7. Meredith P, Wood C. Royal College of Surgeons of England Surgical Epidemiology and Audit Unit, November 1996. An investigation into the impact of the booklet: Surgery on the Prostate on a sample of patients undergoing prostatectomy. Personal communication
8. BACUP. Understanding cancer of the prostate. London: BACUP, 1997
9. Oken D. What to tell cancer patients. JAMA 1961: 175: 1120–1128

Index